From the publisher of *Nursing* journal

Nursing™
THE SERIES FOR CLINICAL EXCELLENCE

Interpreting Signs & Symptoms

Wolters Kluwer | Lippincott Williams & Wilkins
Health

Philadelphia · Baltimore · New York · London
Buenos Aires · Hong Kong · Sydney · Tokyo

Staff

Executive Publisher
Judith A. Schilling McCann, RN, MSN

Editorial Director
H. Nancy Holmes

Clinical Director
Joan M. Robinson, RN, MSN

Art Director
Elaine Kasmer

Editorial Project Manager
Jennifer Kowalak

Clinical Manager
Collette Bishop Hendler, RN, BS, CCRN

Clinical Project Manager
Kate Stout, RN, MSN, CCRN

Editor
Naina D. Chohan

Clinical Editors
Mary Perrong, RN, CRNP, MSN, APRN,BC, CPAN;
Marcy Caplin, RN, MSN

Copy Editors
Kimberly Bilotta (supervisor), Scotti Cohn,
Heather Ditch, Jen Fielding, Carolyn Peterson,
Irene Pontarelli, Pamela Wingrod

Designers
Lynn Foulk (project manager and book
design), Joseph John Clark (cover design)

Digital Composition Services
Diane Paluba (manager), Joyce Rossi Biletz,
Donna S. Morris

Manufacturing
Beth J. Welsh

Editorial Assistants
Megan L. Aldinger, Karen J. Kirk,
Linda K. Ruhf

Design Assistant
Georg W. Purvis IV

Indexer
Barbara Hodgson

**Library of Congress
Cataloging-in-Publication Data**

Nursing. Interpreting signs & symptoms.
    p. ; cm. — (Nursing series)
  Includes bibliographical references and index.
    1. Nursing diagnosis—Handbooks, manuals, etc. 2. Nursing assessment—Handbooks, manuals, etc. 3. Symptoms—Handbooks, manuals, etc. 4. Diagnosis—Handbooks, manuals, etc. I. Lippincott Williams & Wilkins. II. Title: Interpreting signs and symptoms. III. Series: Nursing series (Ambler, Pa.)
  [DNLM: 1. Nursing Assessment—Handbooks. 2. Nursing Care--Handbooks. 3. Signs and Symptoms—Handbooks. WY 49 N9757 2007]
  RT48.N866 2007
  616.07'5—dc22
ISBN-13: 978-1-58255-668-0 (alk. paper)
ISBN-10: 1-58255-668-7 (alk. paper)   2006102421

Contents

Contributors and consultants

Helen C. Ballestas, RN, MSN, CRRN, PhD(C)
Nursing Instructor
New York Institute of Technology
Old Westbury

Julie A. Calvery, RN, MSN
Instructor
University of Arkansas
Fort Smith

Kim Cooper, RN, MSN
Nursing Department Program Chair
Ivy Tech Community College
Terre Haute, Ind.

Vivian C. Gamblian, RN, MSN
Professor of Nursing
Collin County Community College
McKinney, Tex.

Dana Reeves, RN, MSN
Assistant Professor
University of Arkansas
Fort Smith

Kendra S. Seiler, RN, MSN
Nursing Instructor
Rio Hondo Community College
Whittier, Calif.

Fernisa Sison, RN, MSN, FNP-BC
Medical/Surgical Instructor
San Joaquin Delta College
Registered Nurse
St. Josephs Medical Center
Stockton, Calif.
Family Nurse Practitioner
Lodi (Calif.) Memorial Hospital

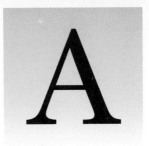

Abdominal distention

Abdominal distention refers to increased abdominal girth—the result of increased intra-abdominal pressure forcing the abdominal wall outward. Distention may be mild or severe, depending on the amount of pressure. It may be localized or diffuse and may occur gradually or suddenly. Acute abdominal distention may signal life-threatening peritonitis or acute bowel obstruction.

Abdominal distention may result from fat, flatus, a fetus, intra-abdominal mass, hemorrhage, stool, or fluid. Fluid and gas are normally present in the GI tract but not in the peritoneal cavity. If fluid and gas can't pass freely through the GI tract, abdominal distention occurs. In the peritoneal cavity, distention may reflect acute bleeding, accumulation of ascitic fluid, or air from perforation of an abdominal organ.

Abdominal distention doesn't always signal pathology. For example, in anxious patients or those with digestive distress, localized distention in the left upper quadrant can result from aerophagia—the unconscious swallowing of air. Generalized distention can result from ingestion of fruits or vegetables with large quantities of unabsorbable carbohydrates, such as legumes, or from abnormal food fermentation by microbes.

ACTION STAT!

 If the patient displays abdominal distention, quickly check for signs of hypovolemia, such as pallor, diaphoresis, hypotension, a rapid thready pulse, rapid shallow breathing, decreased urine output, and altered mentation. Ask the patient if he's experiencing severe abdominal pain or difficulty breathing. Find out about any recent accidents, and observe him for signs of trauma and peritoneal bleeding, such as Cullen's sign or Turner's sign. Then auscultate all abdominal quadrants, noting rapid and high-pitched, diminished, or absent bowel sounds. (If you don't hear bowel sounds immediately, listen for at least 5 minutes in each of the four abdominal quadrants.) Gently palpate the abdomen for rigidity. Remember that deep or extensive palpation may increase pain.

If you detect abdominal distention and rigidity along with abnormal bowel sounds and if the patient complains of pain, begin emergency interventions. Place the patient in the supine position, administer oxygen, and insert an I.V. catheter for fluid replacement. Prepare to insert a nasogastric tube to relieve acute intraluminal distention. Reassure the patient and prepare him for surgery.

History and physical examination

If the patient's abdominal distention isn't acute, ask about its onset and duration and associated signs. A patient with localized distention may report a sensation of pressure, fullness, or tenderness in the affected area. A patient with generalized distention may report a bloated feeling, a pounding heart, and difficulty breathing deeply or when lying flat.

The patient may be unable to bend at the waist. Make sure to ask about abdominal pain, fever, nausea, vomiting, anorexia, altered bowel habits, and weight gain or loss.

Obtain a medical history, noting GI or biliary disorders that may cause peritonitis or ascites, such as cirrhosis, hepatitis, or inflammatory bowel disease. (See *Detecting ascites.*) When did the patient last have a bowel movement? Note chronic constipation. Has the patient recently had abdominal surgery, which can lead to abdominal distention? Ask about recent accidents, even minor ones such as falling off a stepladder.

Perform a complete physical examination. Don't restrict the examination to the abdomen because you could miss important clues to the cause of abdominal distention. Next, stand at the foot of the bed and observe the recumbent patient for abdominal asymmetry to determine if distention is localized or generalized. Then assess abdominal contour by stooping at his side. Inspect for tense, taut skin and bulging flanks, which may indicate ascites. Observe the umbilicus. An everted umbilicus may indicate ascites or umbilical hernia. An inverted umbilicus may indicate distention from gas; it's also common in obesity and pregnancy. Inspect the abdomen for signs of inguinal or femoral hernia and for healed incisions that may point to adhesions. Both may lead to intestinal obstruction. Auscultate for bowel sounds, abdominal friction rubs (indicating peritoneal inflammation), and bruits (indicating an aneurysm). Listen for succussion splash—a splashing sound normally heard in the stomach when the patient moves or when palpation disturbs the viscera. An abnormally loud splash indicates fluid accumulation, suggesting gastric dilation or obstruction.

Next, percuss and palpate the abdomen to determine if distention results from air, fluid, or both. A tympanic note in the left lower quadrant suggests an air-filled descending or sigmoid colon. A tympanic note throughout a generally distended abdomen suggests an air-filled peritoneal cavity. A dull percussion note throughout a generally distended abdomen suggests a fluid-filled peritoneal cavity. Shifting of dullness laterally with the patient in the decubitus position also indicates a fluid-filled abdominal cavity. A pelvic or intra-abdominal mass causes local dullness upon percussion and should be palpable. Obesity causes a large abdomen without shifting dullness, prominent tympany, or palpable bowel or other masses, with generalized rather then localized dullness.

Palpate the abdomen for tenderness, noting whether it's localized or generalized. Watch for peritoneal signs and symptoms, such as rebound tenderness, guarding, rigidity, McBurney's point, obturator sign, and psoas sign. Female patients should undergo a pelvic examination; males, a genital examination. All patients who report abdominal pain should undergo a digital rectal examination with fecal occult blood testing. Finally, measure the patient's abdominal girth for a baseline value. Mark the flanks with a felt-tipped pen as a reference for subsequent measurements.

Detecting ascites

To differentiate ascites from other causes of abdominal distention, check for shifting dullness, fluid wave, and puddle sign, as described here.

Shifting dullness

Step 1. With the patient in a supine position, percuss from the umbilicus outward to the flank, as shown. Draw a line on the patient's skin to mark the change from tympany to dullness.

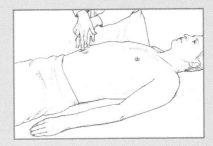

Step 2. Turn the patient onto his side. (Note that this positioning causes ascitic fluid to shift.) Percuss again and mark the change from tympany to dullness. A difference between these lines can indicate ascites.

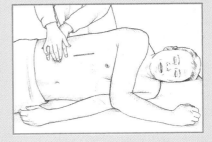

Fluid wave

Have another person press deeply into the patient's midline to prevent vibration from traveling along the abdominal wall. Place one of your palms on one of the patient's flanks. Strike the opposite flank with your other hand. If you feel the blow in the opposite palm, ascitic fluid is present.

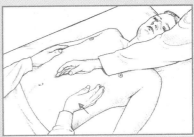

Puddle sign

Position the patient on his elbows and knees, which causes ascitic fluid to pool in the most dependent part of the abdomen. Percuss the abdomen from the flank to the midline. The percussion note becomes louder at the edge of the puddle, or the ascitic pool.

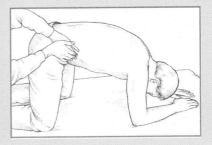

Medical causes

Abdominal cancer. Generalized abdominal distention may occur when the cancer—most commonly ovarian, hepatic, or pancreatic—produces ascites (usually in a patient with a known tumor). It's an indication of advanced disease. Shifting dullness and a fluid wave accompany distention. Associated signs and symptoms may include severe abdominal pain, an abdominal mass, anorexia, jaundice, GI hemorrhage (hematemesis or melena), dyspepsia, and weight loss that progresses to muscle weakness and atrophy.

Abdominal trauma. When brisk internal bleeding accompanies trauma, abdominal distention may be acute and dramatic. Associated signs and symptoms of this life-threatening disorder include abdominal rigidity with guarding, decreased or absent bowel sounds, vomiting, tenderness, and abdominal bruising. Pain may occur over the trauma site, or over the scapula if abdominal bleeding irritates the phrenic nerve. Signs of hypovolemic shock (such as hypotension and rapid, thready pulse) appear with significant blood loss.

Cirrhosis. In cirrhosis, ascites causes generalized distention and is confirmed by a fluid wave, shifting dullness, and a puddle sign. Umbilical eversion and caput medusae (dilated veins around the umbilicus) are common. The patient may report a feeling of fullness or weight gain. Associated findings include vague abdominal pain, fever, anorexia, nausea, vomiting, constipation or diarrhea, bleeding tendencies, severe pruritus, palmar erythema, spider angiomas, leg edema, and possibly splenomegaly. Hematemesis, encephalopathy, gynecomastia, or testicular atrophy may also be seen. Jaundice is usually a late sign. Hepatomegaly occurs initially, but the liver may not be palpable if the patient has advanced disease.

Heart failure. Generalized abdominal distention due to ascites typically accompanies severe cardiovascular impairment and is confirmed by shifting dullness and a fluid wave. Signs and symptoms of heart failure are numerous and depend on the disease stage and degree of cardiovascular impairment. Hallmarks include peripheral edema, jugular vein distention, dyspnea, and tachycardia. Common associated signs and symptoms include hepatomegaly (which may cause right upper quadrant pain), nausea, vomiting, a productive cough, crackles, cool extremities, cyanotic nail beds, nocturia, exercise intolerance, nocturnal wheezing, diastolic hypertension, weight gain, and cardiomegaly.

Irritable bowel syndrome. Irritable bowel syndrome may produce intermittent, localized distention—the result of periodic intestinal spasms. Lower abdominal pain or cramping typically accompanies these spasms. The pain is usually relieved by defecation or by passage of intestinal gas and is aggravated by stress. Other possible signs and symptoms include diarrhea that may alternate with constipation or normal bowel function, nausea, dyspepsia, straining and urgency at defecation, a feeling of incomplete evacuation, and small, mucus-streaked stools.

Large-bowel obstruction. Dramatic abdominal distention is characteristic in this life-threatening disorder; in fact, loops of the large bowel may become visible on the abdomen. Constipation precedes distention and may be the only symptom for days. Associated findings include tympany, high-pitched bowel sounds, and the sudden onset of colicky lower abdominal pain that becomes persistent. Nausea, fecal vomiting, and diminished peristaltic waves and bowel sounds are late signs.

Mesenteric artery occlusion (acute). In this life-threatening disorder, abdominal distention usually occurs several hours after the sudden onset of severe, colicky periumbilical pain accompanied by rapid (even forceful) bowel evacuation. The pain later becomes constant and diffuse. Related signs and symptoms include severe abdominal tenderness with guarding and rigidity, absent bowel sounds and, occasionally, a bruit in the right iliac fossa. The patient may also experience vomiting, anorexia, diarrhea, or constipation. Late signs include fever, tachycardia, tachypnea, hypotension, and cool, clammy skin. Abdominal distention or GI bleeding may be the only clue if pain is absent.

Paralytic ileus. Paralytic ileus, which produces generalized distention with a tympanic percussion note, is accompanied by absent or hypoactive bowel sounds and, occasionally, mild abdominal pain and vomiting. The patient may be severely constipated or may pass flatus and small, liquid stools.

Peritonitis. Peritonitis is a life-threatening disorder in which abdominal distention may be localized or generalized, depending on the extent of the inflammation. Fluid accumulates within the peritoneal cavity and then within the bowel lumen, causing a fluid wave and shifting dullness. Typically, distention is accompanied by sudden and severe abdominal pain that worsens with movement, rebound tenderness, and abdominal rigidity.

The skin over the patient's abdomen may appear taut. Associated signs and symptoms usually include hypoactive or absent bowel sounds, fever, chills, hyperalgesia, nausea, and vomiting. Signs of shock, such as tachycardia and hypotension, appear with significant fluid loss into the abdomen.

Small-bowel obstruction. Abdominal distention is characteristic in small-bowel obstruction, a life-threatening disorder, and is most pronounced during late obstruction, especially in the distal small bowel. Auscultation reveals hypoactive or hyperactive bowel sounds, whereas percussion produces a tympanic note. Accompanying signs and symptoms include colicky periumbilical pain, constipation, nausea, and vomiting; the higher the obstruction, the earlier and more severe the vomiting. Rebound tenderness reflects intestinal strangulation with ischemia. Associated signs and symptoms include drowsiness, malaise, and signs of dehydration. Signs of hypovolemic shock appear with progressive dehydration and plasma loss.

Toxic megacolon (acute). Toxic megacolon is a life-threatening complication of infectious or ulcerative colitis. It produces dramatic abdominal distention that usually develops gradually and is accompanied by a tympanic percussion note, diminished or absent bowel sounds, and mild rebound tenderness. The patient also presents with abdominal pain and tenderness, fever, tachycardia, and dehydration.

Nursing considerations

- Position the patient comfortably, using pillows for support.
- If the patient has flatus, place him on his left side to help flatus escape.
- If the patient has ascites, elevate the head of the bed to ease his breathing.
- Insert a nasogastric tube for bowel compression; monitor amount and type of drainage.
- Administer drugs to relieve pain, and offer emotional support.
- Prepare the patient for diagnostic tests, such as abdominal X-rays, endoscopy, laparoscopy, ultrasonography, computed tomography scan or, possibly, paracentesis.
- Prepare the patient for surgery, if indicated.

Patient teaching

- Teach the patient to use slow deep breathing to help relieve abdominal discomfort.
- If the patient has an obstruction or ascites, tell him which foods and fluids to avoid.
- Emphasize the importance of oral hygiene to prevent dry mouth.
- Explain the underlying disorder and treatment plan.

▐ Abdominal mass

Commonly detected on routine physical examination, an abdominal mass is a localized swelling in one abdominal quadrant. Typically, this sign develops insidiously and may represent an enlarged organ, a neoplasm, an abscess, a vascular defect, or a fecal mass.

Distinguishing an abdominal mass from a normal structure requires skillful palpation. At times, palpation must be repeated with the patient in a different position or performed by a second examiner to verify initial findings. A palpable abdominal mass is an important clinical sign and usually represents a serious—and perhaps life-threatening— disorder.

_{A C T I O N   S T A T !}

 If the patient has a pulsating midabdominal mass and severe abdominal or back pain, suspect an aortic aneurysm. Quickly take his vital signs. Because the patient may require emergency surgery, withhold food or fluids until he's examined. Prepare to administer oxygen and to start an I.V. infusion for fluid and blood replacement. Obtain routine preoperative tests, and prepare the patient for computed tomography scan. Frequently monitor vital signs and urine output.

Be alert for signs of shock, such as altered mental status, tachycardia, hypotension, and cool, clammy skin, which may indicate significant blood loss.

History and physical examination

If the patient's abdominal mass doesn't suggest an aortic aneurysm, continue with a detailed history. Ask the patient if the mass is painful. If so, ask if the pain is constant or if it occurs only on palpation. Is it localized or generalized? Determine if the patient was already aware of the mass. If he was, find out if he noticed any change in the size or location of the mass.

Next, review the patient's medical history, paying special attention to GI disorders. Ask the patient about GI symptoms, such as constipation, diarrhea, rectal bleeding, abnormally colored stools, and vomiting. Has the patient noticed a change in his appetite? If the patient is female, ask whether her menstrual cycles are regular and the first day of her last menses.

A complete physical examination should be performed. Inspect the abdomen for asymmetry, scarring, discoloration, or other skin abnormalities. Also observe for pulsations. Next, auscultate for bowel sounds in each quadrant. Listen for bruits or friction rubs, and check for enlarged veins. Lightly palpate and then deeply palpate the abdomen, assessing any painful or suspicious areas last. Note the patient's position when you locate the mass. Some masses can be detected only with the patient in a supine position; others require a side-lying position.

Estimate the size of the mass in centimeters. Determine its shape. Is it round or sausage shaped? Describe its contour as smooth, rough, sharply defined, nodular, or irregular. Determine the consistency of the mass. Is it doughy, soft, solid, or hard? Percuss the mass. A dull sound indicates a fluid-filled mass; a tympanic sound, an air-filled mass.

Next, determine if the mass moves with your hand or in response to respiration. Is the mass free-floating or attached to intra-abdominal structures? To determine whether the mass is located in the abdominal wall or the abdominal cavity, ask the patient to lift his head and shoulders off the examination table, thereby contracting his abdominal muscles. While these muscles are contracted, try to palpate the mass. If you can, the mass is in the abdominal wall; if you can't, the mass is within the abdominal cavity. (See *Abdominal masses: Locations and common causes,* page 8.)

After the abdominal examination is complete, perform pelvic, genital, and rectal examinations.

Medical causes

Abdominal aortic aneurysm. An abdominal aortic aneurysm may exist for years, producing only a pulsating periumbilical mass with a systolic bruit over the aorta. It may become life-threatening if the aneurysm expands and its walls weaken. In such cases, the patient initially reports constant upper abdominal pain or, less commonly, low back or dull abdominal pain. If the aneurysm ruptures, he'll report severe abdominal and back pain. After rupture, the aneurysm no longer pulsates.

Associated signs and symptoms of rupture include mottled skin below the waist, absent femoral and pedal pulses, lower blood pressure in the legs than in the arms, mild to moderate tenderness with guarding, and abdominal rigidity. Signs of shock—such as altered mental status, tachycardia, and cool, clammy skin—appear with significant blood loss.

Cholecystitis. Deep palpation below the liver border may reveal a smooth,

firm, sausage-shaped mass. With acute inflammation, the gallbladder is usually too tender to be palpated. Cholecystitis can cause severe right upper quadrant pain that may radiate to the right shoulder, chest, or back; abdominal rigidity and tenderness; fever; pallor; diaphoresis; anorexia; nausea; and vomiting. Recurrent attacks usually occur 1 to 6 hours after meals. Murphy's sign (inspiratory arrest elicited when the examiner palpates the right upper quadrant as the patient takes a deep breath) is common.

Colon cancer. A right lower quadrant mass may occur with cancer of the right colon, which may also cause occult bleeding with anemia and abdominal aching, pressure, or dull cramps. Associated findings include weakness, fatigue, exertional dyspnea, vertigo, and signs and symptoms of intestinal obstruction, such as obstipation and vomiting.

Occasionally, cancer of the left colon also causes a palpable mass. It usually produces rectal bleeding, intermittent abdominal fullness or cramping, and rectal pressure. The patient may also report fremitus and pelvic discomfort. Later, he develops obstipation, diarrhea, or pencil-shaped, grossly bloody, or mucus-streaked stools. Typically, defecation relieves pain.

Crohn's disease. With Crohn's disease, tender, sausage-shaped masses are usually palpable in the right lower quadrant and, at times, in the left lower quadrant. Attacks of colicky right lower quadrant pain and diarrhea are common. Associated signs and symptoms include fever, anorexia, weight loss, hyperactive bowel sounds, nausea, abdominal tenderness with guarding, and perirectal, skin, or vaginal fistulas.

Diverticulitis. Most common in the sigmoid colon, diverticulitis may produce a left lower quadrant mass that's usually tender, firm, and fixed. It also

Abdominal masses: Locations and common causes

The location of an abdominal mass provides an important clue to the causative disorder. Here are the disorders most commonly responsible for abdominal masses in each of the four abdominal quadrants.

Right upper quadrant

- Aortic aneurysm (epigastric area)
- Cholecystitis or cholelithiasis
- Gallbladder, gastric, or hepatic carcinoma
- Hepatomegaly
- Hydronephrosis
- Pancreatic abscess or pseudocysts
- Renal cell carcinoma

Left upper quadrant

- Aortic aneurysm (epigastric area)
- Gastric carcinoma (epigastric area)
- Hydronephrosis
- Pancreatic abscess (epigastric area)
- Pancreatic pseudocysts (epigastric area)
- Renal cell carcinoma
- Splenomegaly

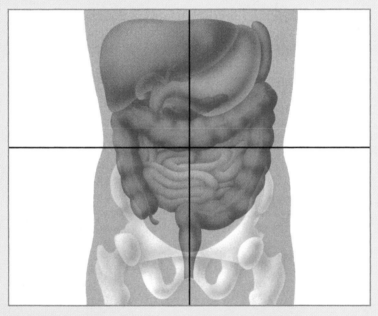

Right lower quadrant

- Bladder distention (suprapubic area)
- Colon cancer
- Crohn's disease
- Ovarian cyst (suprapubic area)
- Uterine leiomyomas (suprapubic area)

Left lower quadrant

- Bladder distention (suprapubic area)
- Colon cancer
- Diverticulitis
- Ovarian cyst (suprapubic area)
- Uterine leiomyomas (suprapubic area)
- Volvulus

produces intermittent abdominal pain that's relieved by defecation or passage of flatus. Other findings may include alternating constipation and diarrhea, nausea, a low-grade fever, and a distended and tympanic abdomen.

Gastric cancer. Advanced gastric cancer may produce an epigastric mass. Early findings include chronic dyspepsia and epigastric discomfort, whereas late findings include weight loss, a feeling of fullness after eating, fatigue and, occasionally, coffee-ground vomitus or melena.

Hepatomegaly. Hepatomegaly produces a firm, blunt, irregular mass in the epigastric region or below the right costal margin. Associated signs and symptoms vary with the causative disorder but commonly include ascites, right upper quadrant pain and tenderness, anorexia, nausea, vomiting, leg edema, jaundice, palmar erythema, spider angiomas, gynecomastia, testicular atrophy and, possibly, splenomegaly.

Hernia. The soft and typically tender bulge is usually an effect of prolonged, increased intra-abdominal pressure on weakened areas of the abdominal wall. An umbilical hernia is typically located around the umbilicus and an inguinal hernia in either the right or left groin. An incisional hernia can occur anywhere along a previous incision. Hernia may be the only sign until strangulation occurs.

Hydronephrosis. Enlarging one or both kidneys, hydronephrosis produces a smooth, boggy mass in one or both flanks. Other findings vary with the degree of hydronephrosis. The patient may have severe colicky renal pain or dull flank pain that radiates to the groin, vulva, or testes. Hematuria, pyuria, dysuria, alternating oliguria and polyuria, nocturia, accelerated hypertension, nausea, and vomiting may also occur.

Ovarian cyst. A large ovarian cyst may produce a smooth, rounded, fluctuant mass, resembling a distended bladder, in the suprapubic region. Large or multiple cysts may also cause mild pelvic discomfort, low back pain, menstrual irregularities, and hirsutism. A twisted or ruptured cyst may cause abdominal tenderness, distention, and rigidity.

Splenomegaly. With splenomegaly, the smooth edge of the enlarged spleen is palpable in the left upper quadrant. Associated signs and symptoms vary with the causative disorder but usually include a feeling of abdominal fullness, left upper quadrant abdominal pain and tenderness, splenic friction rub, splenic bruits, and a low-grade fever.

Uterine leiomyomas (fibroids). If large enough, these common, benign uterine tumors produce a round, multinodular mass in the suprapubic region. The patient's chief complaint is usually menorrhagia; she may also experience a feeling of heaviness in the abdomen, and pressure on surrounding organs may cause back pain, constipation, and urinary frequency or urgency. Edema and varicosities of the lower extremities may develop. Rapid fibroid growth in perimenopausal or postmenopausal women needs further evaluation.

Nursing considerations

- Offer emotional support to the patient and his family as they await the results of diagnostic testing.
- Position the patient comfortably, and administer drugs for pain or anxiety as needed.
- If an abdominal mass causes bowel obstruction, watch for indications of peritonitis—abdominal pain and rebound tenderness—and for signs of shock, such as tachycardia and hypotension.

- Prepare the patient for surgery, if indicated.

Patient teaching
- Explain any diagnostic tests that are needed.
- Teach the patient about the cause of the abdominal mass, once a diagnosis is made. Also explain treatment and potential outcomes.

 # Abdominal pain

Abdominal pain usually results from a GI disorder, but it can be caused by a reproductive, genitourinary (GU), musculoskeletal, or vascular disorder; drug use; or ingestion of toxins. At times, such pain signals life-threatening complications.

Abdominal pain arises from the abdominopelvic viscera, the parietal peritoneum, or the capsules of the liver, kidney, or spleen. It may be acute or chronic, diffuse or localized. Visceral pain develops slowly into a deep, dull, aching pain that's poorly localized in the epigastric, periumbilical, or lower midabdominal (hypogastric) region. In contrast, somatic (parietal, peritoneal) pain produces a sharp, more intense, and well-localized discomfort that rapidly follows the insult. Movement or coughing aggravates this pain. (See *Abdominal pain: Types and locations.*)

Pain may also be referred to the abdomen from another site with the same or similar nerve supply. This sharp, well-localized, referred pain is felt in the skin or deeper tissues and may coexist with skin hyperesthesia and muscle hyperalgesia.

Mechanisms that produce abdominal pain include stretching or tension of the gut wall, traction on the peritoneum or mesentery, vigorous intestinal contraction, inflammation, ischemia, and sensory nerve irritation.

ACTION STAT!

 If the patient is experiencing sudden and severe abdominal pain, quickly take his vital signs and palpate pulses below the waist. Be alert for signs of hypovolemic shock, such as altered mental status, tachycardia, and hypotension. Obtain I.V. access.

Emergency surgery may be required if the patient has mottled skin below the waist and a pulsating epigastric mass or rebound tenderness and rigidity.

History and physical examination

If the patient has no life-threatening signs or symptoms, take his history. Ask him if he has had this type of pain before. Have him describe the pain in his own words. Ask him if the pain is dull, sharp, stabbing, or burning and to rate his pain on a scale, such as the visual analog scale, FACES pain scale, or verbal numeric scale for intensity of pain. Ask if anything relieves the pain or makes it worse. Ask the patient if the pain is constant or intermittent and when the pain began. Constant, steady abdominal pain suggests organ perforation, ischemia, or inflammation or blood in the peritoneal cavity. Intermittent, cramping abdominal pain suggests that the patient may have obstruction of a hollow organ.

If pain is intermittent, find out the duration of a typical episode. In addition, ask the patient to point where the pain is located and if it radiates to other areas.

Find out if movement, coughing, exertion, vomiting, eating, elimination, or walking worsens or relieves the pain. The patient may report abdominal pain as indigestion or gas pain, so have him describe it in detail.

Ask the patient about substance abuse and any history of vascular, GI, GU, or reproductive disorders. Ask the

Abdominal pain: Types and locations

Affected organ	Visceral pain	Parietal pain	Referred pain
Appendix	Periumbilical area	Right lower quadrant	Right lower quadrant
Distal colon	Hypogastrium and left flank for descending colon	Over affected area	Left lower quadrant and back (rare)
Gallbladder	Middle epigastrium	Right upper quadrant	Right subscapular area
Ovaries, fallopian tubes, and uterus	Hypogastrium and groin	Over affected area	Inner thighs
Pancreas	Middle epigastrium and left upper quadrant	Middle epigastrium and left upper quadrant	Back and left shoulder
Proximal colon	Periumbilical area and right flank for ascending colon	Over affected site	Right lower quadrant and back (rare)
Small intestine	Periumbilical area	Over affected site	Midback (rare)
Stomach	Middle epigastrium	Middle epigastrium and left upper quadrant	Shoulders
Ureters	Costovertebral angle	Over affected site	Groin: scrotum in men; labia in women (rare)

female patient about the date of her last menstrual cycle, changes in her menstrual pattern, or dyspareunia.

Ask the patient about appetite changes. Ask about the onset and frequency of nausea or vomiting. Find out about increased flatulence, constipation, diarrhea, and changes in stool consistency. When was the last bowel movement? Ask about urinary frequency, urgency, or pain. Is the urine cloudy or pink?

Perform a physical examination. Take the patient's vital signs, and assess skin turgor and mucous membranes. Inspect his abdomen for distention or visible peristaltic waves and, if indicated, measure his abdominal girth.

Auscultate for bowel sounds and characterize their motility. Percuss all quadrants, noting the percussion sounds. Palpate the entire abdomen for masses, rigidity, and tenderness. Check for costovertebral angle (CVA) tenderness, abdominal tenderness with guarding, and rebound tenderness.

Medical causes

Abdominal aortic aneurysm (dissecting). Initially, this life-threatening disorder may produce dull lower abdominal, lower back, or severe chest pain. Usually, a dissecting abdominal aortic aneurysm produces constant upper abdominal pain, which may worsen when the patient lies down and may abate when he leans forward or sits up. Palpation may reveal an epigastric mass that pulsates before rupture but not after it.

Other findings may include mottled skin below the waist, absent femoral and pedal pulses, lower blood pressure in the legs than in the arms, mild to moderate abdominal tenderness with guarding, and abdominal rigidity. Signs of shock, such as tachycardia and tachypnea, may appear.

Abdominal cancer. Abdominal pain usually occurs late in abdominal cancer. It may be accompanied by anorexia, weight loss, weakness, depression, and abdominal mass and distention.

Abdominal trauma. Generalized or localized abdominal pain occurs with ecchymoses on the abdomen, abdominal tenderness, vomiting and, with hemorrhage into the peritoneal cavity, abdominal rigidity. Bowel sounds are decreased or absent. The patient may have signs of hypovolemic shock, such as hypotension and a rapid, thready pulse.

Adrenal crisis. Severe abdominal pain appears early, along with nausea, vomiting, dehydration, profound weakness, anorexia, and fever. Later signs are progressive loss of consciousness; hypotension; tachycardia; oliguria; cool, clammy skin; and increased motor activity, which may progress to delirium or seizures.

Anthrax, GI. GI anthrax is caused by eating contaminated meat from an infected animal. Initial signs and symptoms include loss of appetite, nausea, vomiting, and fever. Late signs and symptoms include abdominal pain, severe bloody diarrhea, and hematemesis.

Appendicitis. With appendicitis, a life-threatening disorder, pain initially occurs in the epigastric or umbilical region. Anorexia, nausea, or vomiting may occur after the onset of pain. Pain localizes at McBurney's point in the right lower quadrant and is accompanied by abdominal rigidity, increasing tenderness (especially over McBurney's point), rebound tenderness, and retractive respirations. Later signs and symptoms include malaise, constipation (or diarrhea), low-grade fever, and tachycardia.

Cholecystitis. Severe pain in the right upper quadrant may arise suddenly or increase gradually over several hours, usually after meals. It may radiate to the right shoulder, chest, or back. Accompanying the pain are anorexia, nausea, vomiting, fever, abdominal rigidity, tenderness, pallor, and diaphoresis. Murphy's sign (inspiratory arrest elicited when the examiner palpates the right upper quadrant as the patient takes a deep breath) is common.

Cholelithiasis. Patients may suffer sudden, severe, and paroxysmal pain in the right upper quadrant lasting several minutes to several hours. The pain may radiate to the epigastrium, back, or shoulder blades. The pain is accompanied by anorexia, nausea, vomiting (sometimes bilious), diaphoresis, restlessness, and abdominal tenderness with guarding over the gallbladder or biliary duct. The patient may also experience fatty food intolerance and frequent indigestion.

Cirrhosis. Dull abdominal aching occurs early and is usually accompanied by anorexia, indigestion, nausea, vomiting, constipation, or diarrhea. Subsequent right upper quadrant pain worsens when the patient sits up or leans forward. Associated signs include fever, ascites, leg edema, weight gain, hepatomegaly, jaundice, severe pruritus, bleeding tendencies, palmar erythema, and spider angiomas. Gynecomastia and testicular atrophy may also be present.

Crohn's disease. An acute attack in Crohn's disease causes severe cramping pain in the lower abdomen, typically preceded by weeks or months of milder cramping pain. Crohn's disease may also cause diarrhea, hyperactive bowel sounds, dehydration, weight loss, fever, abdominal tenderness with guarding, and possibly a palpable mass in a lower quadrant. Abdominal pain is commonly relieved by defecation. Milder chronic signs and symptoms include right lower quadrant pain with diarrhea, steatorrhea, and weight loss. Complications include perirectal or vaginal fistulas.

Diverticulitis. Mild cases of diverticulitis usually produce intermittent, diffuse left lower quadrant pain, which is sometimes relieved by defecation or passage of flatus and worsened by eating. Other signs and symptoms include nausea, constipation or diarrhea, a low-grade fever and, in many cases, a palpable abdominal mass that's usually tender, firm, and fixed. Rupture causes severe left lower quadrant pain, abdominal rigidity and, possibly, signs and symptoms of sepsis and shock (high fever, chills, and hypotension).

Duodenal ulcer. Localized abdominal pain—described as steady, gnawing, burning, aching, or hunger like—may occur high in the midepigastrium, slightly off center, usually on the right. The pain usually doesn't radiate unless pancreatic penetration occurs. It typically begins 2 to 4 hours after a meal and may cause nocturnal awakening. Ingestion of food or antacids brings relief until the cycle starts again, but it may also produce weight gain. Other symptoms include changes in bowel habits and heartburn or retrosternal burning.

Ectopic pregnancy. Lower abdominal pain may be sharp, dull, or cramping and constant or intermittent in ectopic pregnancy, a potentially life-threatening disorder. Vaginal bleeding, nausea, and vomiting may occur, along with urinary frequency, a tender adnexal mass, and a 1- or 2-month history of amenorrhea. Rupture of the fallopian tube produces sharp lower abdominal pain, which may radiate to the shoulders and neck and become extreme with cervical or adnexal palpation. Signs of shock (such as pallor, tachycardia, and hypotension) may also appear.

Endometriosis. Constant, severe pain in the lower abdomen usually begins 5 to 7 days before the start of menses and may be aggravated by defecation. Depending on the location of the ectopic tissue, the pain may be accompanied by constipation, abdominal tenderness, dysmenorrhea, dyspareunia, and deep sacral pain.

Escherichia coli O157:H7 infection. Signs and symptoms of E. coli O157:H7 infection include watery or bloody diarrhea, nausea, vomiting, fever, and abdominal cramps. In children younger than age 5 and in elderly patients, hemolytic uremic syndrome may develop, and this may ultimately lead to acute renal failure.

Gastric ulcer. Diffuse, gnawing, burning pain in the left upper quadrant or epigastric area commonly occurs 1 or 2 hours after meals and may be relieved by ingestion of food or antacids. Vague bloating and nausea after eating are common. Indigestion, weight change, anorexia, and episodes of GI bleeding also occur.

Gastritis. With acute gastritis, the patient experiences a rapid onset of abdominal pain that can range from mild epigastric discomfort to burning pain in the left upper quadrant. Other typical features include belching, fever, malaise, anorexia, nausea, bloody or coffee-ground vomitus, and melena. Significant bleeding is unusual unless the patient has hemorrhagic gastritis.

Gastroenteritis. Cramping or colicky abdominal pain, which can be diffuse, originates in the left upper quadrant and radiates or migrates to the other quadrants, usually in a peristaltic manner. It's accompanied by diarrhea, hyperactive bowel sounds, headache, myalgia, nausea, and vomiting.

Heart failure. Right upper quadrant pain caused by liver congestion or enlargement commonly accompanies heart failure's hallmarks: jugular vein distention, dyspnea, tachycardia, and peripheral edema. Other findings include nausea, vomiting, ascites, productive cough, crackles, cool extremities, and cyanotic nail beds. Clinical signs are numerous and vary according to the stage of the disease and amount of cardiovascular impairment.

Hepatitis. Liver enlargement from any type of hepatitis causes discomfort or dull pain and tenderness in the right upper quadrant. Associated signs and symptoms may include dark urine, clay-colored stools, nausea, vomiting, anorexia, jaundice, malaise, and pruritus.

Intestinal obstruction. Short episodes of intense, colicky, cramping pain alternate with pain-free intervals with an intestinal obstruction, a life-threatening disorder. Accompanying signs and symptoms may include abdominal distention, tenderness, and guarding; visible peristaltic waves; high-pitched, tinkling, or hyperactive sounds proximal to the obstruction and hypoactive or absent sounds distally; obstipation; and pain-induced agitation. In jejunal and duodenal obstruction, nausea and bilious vomiting occur early. In distal small- or large-bowel obstruction, nausea and vomiting are commonly feculent. Complete obstruction produces absent bowel sounds. Late-stage obstruction produces signs of hypovolemic shock, such as altered mental status, tachycardia, and hypotension.

Irritable bowel syndrome. Lower abdominal cramping or pain is aggravated by ingestion of coarse or raw foods and may be alleviated by defecation or passage of flatus. Related findings include abdominal tenderness, diurnal diarrhea alternating with constipation or normal bowel function, and small stools with visible mucus. Dyspepsia, nausea, and abdominal distention with a feeling of incomplete evacuation may also occur. Stress, anxiety, and emotional lability intensify the symptoms.

Listeriosis. Signs and symptoms of listeriosis include fever, myalgia, abdominal pain, nausea, vomiting, and diarrhea. If the infection spreads to the nervous system, meningitis may develop; signs and symptoms include fever, headache, nuchal rigidity, and change in the level of consciousness.

Mesenteric artery ischemia. Always suspect mesenteric artery ischemia in patients older than age 50 with chronic heart failure, cardiac arrhythmia, cardiovascular infarct, or hypotension who develop sudden, severe abdominal pain after 2 or 3 days of colicky periumbilical pain and diarrhea. Initially, the abdomen is soft and tender with decreased bowel sounds. Associated findings include vomiting, anorexia, alternating periods of diarrhea and constipation and, in late stages, extreme abdominal tenderness with rigidity, tachycardia, tachypnea, absent bowel sounds, and cool, clammy skin.

Norovirus infection. Abdominal pain or cramping is a symptom commonly associated with noroviruses. Transmitted by the fecal-oral route and highly contagious, these viruses that cause gastroenteritis may also produce acute-onset vomiting, nausea, and diarrhea. Less common symptoms include low-grade fever, headache, chills, muscle aches, and generalized fatigue. Individuals who are otherwise healthy usually recover in 24 to 60 hours without suffering lasting effects.

Ovarian cyst. Torsion or hemorrhage causes pain and tenderness in the right or left lower quadrant. Sharp and severe if the patient suddenly stands or stoops, the pain becomes brief and intermittent if the torsion self-corrects or dull and diffuse after several hours if it doesn't. Pain is accompanied by slight fever, mild nausea and vomiting, abdominal tenderness, a palpable abdominal mass and, possibly, amenorrhea. Abdominal distention may occur if the patient has a large cyst. Peritoneal irritation, or rupture and ensuing peritonitis, causes high fever and severe nausea and vomiting.

Pancreatitis. Life-threatening acute pancreatitis produces fulminating, continuous upper abdominal pain that may radiate to both flanks and to the back. To relieve this pain, the patient may bend forward, draw his knees to his chest, or move restlessly about. Early findings include abdominal tenderness, nausea, vomiting, fever, pallor, tachycardia and, in some patients, abdominal rigidity, rebound tenderness, and hypoactive bowel sounds. Turner's sign (ecchymosis of the abdomen or flank) or Cullen's sign (a bluish tinge around the umbilicus) signals hemorrhagic pancreatitis. Jaundice may occur as inflammation subsides.

Chronic pancreatitis produces severe left upper quadrant or epigastric pain that radiates to the back. Abdominal tenderness, a midepigastric mass, jaundice, fever, and splenomegaly may occur. Steatorrhea, weight loss, maldigestion, and hyperglycemia are common.

Pelvic inflammatory disease. Pain in the right or left lower quadrant ranges from vague discomfort worsened by movement to deep, severe, and progres-sive pain. Sometimes, metrorrhagia precedes or accompanies the onset of pain. Extreme pain accompanies cervical or adnexal palpation. Associated findings include abdominal tenderness, a palpable abdominal or pelvic mass, fever, occasional chills, nausea, vomiting, urinary discomfort, and abnormal vaginal bleeding or purulent vaginal discharge.

Perforated ulcer. With perforated ulcer, a life-threatening disorder, sudden, severe, and prostrating epigastric pain may radiate through the abdomen to the back or right shoulder. Other signs and symptoms include boardlike abdominal rigidity, tenderness with guarding, generalized rebound tenderness, absent bowel sounds, grunting and shallow respirations and, in many cases, fever, tachycardia, hypotension, and syncope.

Peritonitis. With peritonitis, a life-threatening disorder, sudden and severe pain can be diffuse or localized in the area of the underlying disorder; movement worsens the pain. The degree of abdominal tenderness usually varies according to the extent of disease. Typical findings include fever; chills; nausea; vomiting; hypoactive or absent bowel sounds; abdominal tenderness, distention, and rigidity; rebound tenderness and guarding; hyperalgesia; tachycardia; hypotension; tachypnea; and positive psoas and obturator signs.

Prostatitis. Vague abdominal pain or discomfort in the lower abdomen, groin, perineum, or rectum may develop with prostatitis. Other findings include dysuria, urinary frequency and urgency, fever, chills, low back pain, myalgia, arthralgia, and nocturia. Scrotal pain, penile pain, and pain on ejaculation may occur in chronic cases.

Pyelonephritis (acute). Progressive lower quadrant pain in one or both sides, flank pain, and CVA tenderness characterize this disorder. Pain may radiate to the lower midabdomen or to the groin. Additional signs and symptoms include abdominal and back tenderness, high fever, shaking chills, nausea, vomiting, and urinary frequency and urgency.

Renal calculi. Depending on the location of calculi, severe abdominal or back pain may occur. The classic symptom is severe, colicky pain that travels from the CVA to the flank, suprapubic region, and external genitalia. The pain may be excruciating or dull and constant. Pain-induced agitation, nausea, vomiting, abdominal distention, fever, chills, hypertension, and urinary urgency with hematuria and dysuria may occur.

Sickle cell crisis. Sudden, severe abdominal pain may accompany chest, back, hand, or foot pain. Associated signs and symptoms include weakness, aching joints, dyspnea, and scleral jaundice.

Smallpox (variola major). Initial signs and symptoms of smallpox include high fever, malaise, prostration, severe headache, backache, and abdominal pain. A maculopapular rash develops on the mucosa of the mouth, pharynx, face, and forearms and then spreads to the trunk and legs. Within 2 days, the rash becomes vesicular and later pustular. The lesions develop at the same time, appear identical, and are more prominent on the face and extremities. The pustules are round, firm, and embedded in the skin. After 8 to 9 days, the pustules form a crust, and later the scab separates from the skin, leaving a pitted scar. In fatal cases, death results from encephalitis, extensive bleeding, or secondary infection.

Splenic infarction. Fulminating pain in the left upper quadrant occurs along with chest pain that may worsen on inspiration. Pain usually radiates to the left shoulder with splinting of the left di-aphragm, abdominal guarding and, occasionally, a splenic friction rub.

Ulcerative colitis. Ulcerative colitis may begin with vague abdominal discomfort that leads to cramping lower abdominal pain. As the disorder progresses, pain may become steady and diffuse, increasing with movement and coughing. The most common symptom—recurrent and possibly severe diarrhea with blood, pus, and mucus—may relieve the pain. The abdomen may feel soft and extremely tender. High-pitched, infrequent bowel sounds may accompany nausea, vomiting, anorexia, weight loss, and mild, intermittent fever.

Other causes

Drugs. Salicylates and nonsteroidal anti-inflammatory drugs commonly cause burning, gnawing pain in the left upper quadrant or epigastric area, along with nausea and vomiting.

Nursing considerations

- Place the patient in a position of comfort.
- Monitor him for tachycardia, hypotension, clammy skin, abdominal rigidity, rebound tenderness, a change in the pain's location or intensity, or sudden relief from the pain since abdominal pain can signal a life-threatening disorder.
- Administer analgesics, as ordered, and evaluate their effect.
- Withhold food and fluids because surgery may be needed.
- Prepare for I.V. infusion and insertion of a nasogastric or other intestinal tube.
- Anticipate the need for peritoneal lavage or abdominal paracentesis.
- Prepare the patient for diagnostic procedures, such as a pelvic and rectal examination; blood, urine, and stool tests; imaging studies; barium studies; ultrasonography; endoscopy; and biopsy.

Patient teaching

- Explain the diagnostic tests the patient will need.
- Explain the underlying disorder and treatment plan.
- Explain which foods and fluids the patient shouldn't have.
- Tell the patient to report any changes in bowel habits.
- Instruct the patient how to position himself to alleviate symptoms.

▌Abdominal rigidity
[Abdominal muscle spasm, involuntary guarding]

Detected by palpation, abdominal rigidity refers to abnormal muscle tension or inflexibility of the abdomen. Rigidity may be voluntary or involuntary. Voluntary rigidity reflects the patient's fear or nervousness upon palpation; involuntary rigidity reflects potentially life-threatening peritoneal irritation or inflammation. (See *Recognizing voluntary rigidity*.)

Involuntary rigidity most commonly results from GI disorders, but may also result from pulmonary and vascular disorders and from the effects of insect toxins. Usually, it's accompanied by fever, nausea, vomiting, and abdominal tenderness, distention, and pain.

ACTION STAT!

 After palpating abdominal rigidity, quickly take the patient's vital signs. Although the patient may not appear gravely ill or have markedly abnormal vital signs, abdominal rigidity calls for emergency evaluation and interventions.

Prepare to administer oxygen and to insert an I.V. catheter for fluid and blood replacement. The patient may require drugs to support blood pressure. Prepare him for urinary catheterization, and monitor intake and output.

A nasogastric tube may need to be inserted to relieve abdominal distention. Because emergency surgery may be necessary, the patient should be prepared for laboratory tests and imaging studies.

History and physical examination

If the patient's condition allows further assessment, take a brief history. Find out when the abdominal rigidity began. Is it associated with abdominal pain? If so, did the pain begin at the same time? Determine whether the abdominal rigidity is localized or generalized. Is it always present? Has its site changed or remained constant? Next, ask about aggra-

Recognizing voluntary rigidity

Distinguishing voluntary from involuntary abdominal rigidity is a must for accurate assessment. Review this comparison so that you can quickly tell the two apart.

Voluntary rigidity
- Usually symmetrical
- More rigid on inspiration (expiration causes muscle relaxation)
- Eased by relaxation techniques, such as positioning the patient comfortably and talking to him in a calm, soothing manner
- Painless when the patient sits up using his abdominal muscles alone

Involuntary rigidity
- Usually asymmetrical
- Equally rigid on inspiration and expiration
- Unaffected by relaxation techniques
- Painful when the patient sits up using his abdominal muscles alone

vating or alleviating factors, such as position changes, coughing, vomiting, elimination, and walking.

Explore other signs and symptoms. Inspect the abdomen for peristaltic waves, which may be visible in very thin patients. Check for a visibly distended bowel loop or pulsations. Next, auscultate bowel sounds. Perform light palpation to locate the rigidity and determine its severity. Avoid deep palpation, which may exacerbate abdominal pain. Finally, check for poor skin turgor and dry mucous membranes, which indicate dehydration.

Medical causes

Abdominal aortic aneurysm (dissecting). Mild to moderate abdominal rigidity occurs with a dissecting abdominal aortic aneurysm, a life-threatening disorder. Typically, it's accompanied by constant upper abdominal pain that may radiate to the lower back. The pain may worsen when the patient lies down and may be relieved when he leans forward or sits up. Before rupture, the aneurysm may produce a pulsating mass in the epigastrium, accompanied by a systolic bruit over the aorta. The mass stops pulsating after rupture. Associated signs and symptoms include mottled skin below the waist, absent femoral and pedal pulses, lower blood pressure in the legs than in the arms, and mild to moderate tenderness with guarding. Significant blood loss causes signs of shock, such as tachycardia, tachypnea, and cool, clammy skin.

Insect toxins. Insect stings and bites, especially black widow spider bites, release toxins that can produce generalized, cramping abdominal pain, usually accompanied by rigidity. These toxins may also cause a low-grade fever, nausea, vomiting, tremors, and burning sensations in the hands and feet. Some patients develop increased salivation, hy-

pertension, paresis, and hyperactive reflexes. Children commonly are restless, have an expiratory grunt, and keep their legs flexed.

Mesenteric artery ischemia. A life-threatening disorder, mesenteric artery ischemia is characterized by 2 or 3 days of persistent, low-grade abdominal pain and diarrhea leading to sudden, severe abdominal pain and rigidity. Rigidity occurs in the central or periumbilical region and is accompanied by severe abdominal tenderness, fever, and signs of shock, such as tachycardia and hypotension. Other findings may include vomiting, anorexia, and diarrhea or constipation. Always suspect this disorder in patients older than age 50 who have a history of heart failure, arrhythmia, cardiovascular infarct, or hypotension.

Peritonitis. Depending on the cause of peritonitis, abdominal rigidity may be localized or generalized. For example, if an inflamed appendix causes local peritonitis, rigidity may be localized in the right lower quadrant. If a perforated ulcer causes widespread peritonitis, rigidity may be generalized and, in severe cases, boardlike.

Peritonitis also causes sudden and severe abdominal pain that can be localized or generalized. In addition, it can produce abdominal tenderness and distention, rebound tenderness, guarding, hyperalgesia, hypoactive or absent bowel sounds, nausea, and vomiting. Usually, the patient also displays fever, chills, tachycardia, tachypnea, and hypotension.

Nursing considerations

▪ Monitor the patient closely for signs of shock.
▪ Place the patient in a position of comfort.
▪ Administer analgesics, as ordered, and evaluate their effect.
▪ Withhold food and fluids.

- Administer an I.V. antibiotic as ordered if emergency surgery is required.
- Prepare the patient for diagnostic tests which may include blood, urine, and stool studies; chest and abdominal X-rays, computed tomography, magnetic resonance imaging, gastroscopy, and colonoscopy.

Patient teaching

- Explain diagnostic tests or surgery the patient will need.
- Tell the patient about any food or fluid restrictions.
- Show him how to position himself for comfort.
- Explain the underlying disorder and treatment plan.

Accessory muscle use

When breathing requires extra effort, the accessory muscles—the sternoclei-domastoid, scalene, pectoralis major, trapezius, internal intercostals, and abdominal muscles—stabilize the thorax during respiration. Some accessory muscle use normally takes place during such activities as singing, talking, coughing, defecating, and exercising. (See *Accessory muscles: Locations and functions,* page 20.)

More pronounced use of these muscles may signal acute respiratory distress, diaphragmatic weakness, or fatigue. It may also result from chronic respiratory disease. Typically, the extent of accessory muscle use reflects the severity of the underlying cause.

ACTION STAT!

 If the patient displays increased accessory muscle use, immediately look for signs of acute respiratory distress. These include a decreased level of consciousness, shortness of breath when speaking, tachypnea, intercostal and sternal retractions, cyanosis, adventitious breath sounds (such as wheezing or stridor), diaphoresis, nasal flaring, and extreme apprehension or agitation. Quickly auscultate for abnormal, diminished, or absent breath sounds. Check for airway obstruction and, if detected, attempt to restore airway patency. Insert an airway or intubate the patient. Then begin suctioning and manual or mechanical ventilation. Assess oxygen saturation using pulse oximetry if available. Administer oxygen; if the patient has chronic obstructive pulmonary disease (COPD), use only a low flow rate for mild COPD exacerbations. You may need to use a high flow rate initially, but be attentive to the patient's respiratory drive. Giving a patient with COPD too much oxygen may decrease his respiratory drive. An I.V. catheter may be required.

History and physical examination

If the patient's condition allows, examine him more closely. Ask him about the onset, duration, and severity of associated signs and symptoms, such as dyspnea, chest pain, cough, sputum production, or fever.

Explore his medical history, focusing on respiratory disorders, such as infection or COPD. Ask about cardiac disorders, such as heart failure, which may lead to pulmonary edema; inquire about neuromuscular disorders, such as amyotrophic lateral sclerosis, which may affect respiratory muscle function. Note a history of allergies or asthma. Because collagen vascular diseases can cause diffuse infiltrative lung disease, ask about such conditions as rheumatoid arthritis and lupus erythematosus.

Ask about recent trauma, especially to the spine or chest. Find out if the patient has recently undergone pulmonary function tests or received respiratory

Accessory muscles: Locations and functions

Physical exertion and pulmonary disease usually increase the work of breathing, taxing the diaphragm and external intercostal muscles. When this happens, accessory muscles provide the extra effort needed to maintain respirations. The upper accessory muscles assist with inspiration, whereas the upper chest, sternum, internal intercostal, and abdominal muscles assist with expiration.

With inspiration, the scalene muscles elevate, fix, and expand the upper chest. The sternocleidomastoid muscles raise the sternum, expanding the chest's anteroposterior and longitudinal dimensions. The pectoralis major elevates the chest, increasing its anteroposterior size, and the trapezius raises the thoracic cage.

With expiration, the internal intercostals depress the ribs, decreasing the chest size. The abdominal muscles pull the lower chest down, depress the lower ribs, and compress the abdominal contents, which exerts pressure on the chest.

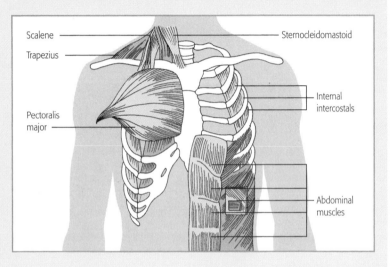

therapy. Ask about smoking and occupational exposure to chemical fumes or mineral dusts such as asbestos. Explore the family history for such disorders as cystic fibrosis and neurofibromatosis, which can cause diffuse infiltrative lung disease.

Perform a detailed chest examination, noting an abnormal respiratory rate, pattern, or depth. Assess the patient's chest for equal expansion during inspiration. Check the trachea for midline position. Assess the color, temperature, and turgor of the patient's skin, and check for clubbing. Auscultate the lungs for adventitious breath sounds.

Medical causes

Acute respiratory distress syndrome (ARDS). In ARDS, a life-threatening disorder, accessory muscle use increases in response to hypoxia. It's accompanied by intercostal, supracostal, and sternal retractions on inspiration and by grunting on expiration. Other characteristics include tachypnea, dyspnea, diaphoresis, diffuse crackles, and a cough with pink, frothy sputum. Worsening hypoxia produces anxiety, tachycardia, and mental sluggishness.

Airway obstruction. Acute upper airway obstruction can be life-threatening—fortunately, most obstructions are subacute or chronic. Typically, obstruction increases accessory muscle use. However, its most telling sign is inspiratory stridor. Associated signs and symptoms include dyspnea, tachypnea, gasping, wheezing, coughing, drooling, intercostal retractions, cyanosis, and tachycardia.

Amyotrophic lateral sclerosis. Typically, this progressive motor neuron disorder affects the diaphragm more than the accessory muscles. As a result, increased accessory muscle use is characteristic. Other signs and symptoms include fasciculations, muscle atrophy and weakness, spasticity, bilateral Babinski's reflex, and hyperactive deep tendon reflexes. Incoordination makes carrying out routine activities difficult for the patient. Associated signs and symptoms include impaired speech, difficulty chewing or swallowing and breathing, urinary frequency and urgency and, occasionally, choking and excessive drooling. (*Note:* Other neuromuscular disorders may produce similar signs and symptoms.) Although the patient's mental status remains intact, his poor prognosis may cause periodic depression.

Asthma. During an acute asthma attack, the patient usually displays increased accessory muscle use. Accompanying it are severe dyspnea, tachypnea, wheezing, a productive cough, nasal flaring, and cyanosis. Auscultation reveals faint or possibly absent breath sounds, musical crackles, and rhonchi. Other signs and symptoms include tachycardia, diaphoresis, and apprehension caused by air hunger. Chronic asthma may also cause barrel chest.

Chronic bronchitis. With chronic bronchitis, a form of COPD, increased accessory muscle use may be chronic and is preceded by a productive cough and exertional dyspnea. Chronic bronchitis is accompanied by wheezing, basal crackles, tachypnea, jugular vein distention, prolonged expiration, barrel chest, and clubbing. Cyanosis and weight gain from edema account for the characteristic label of "blue bloater." A low-grade fever may occur with secondary infection.

Emphysema. Increased accessory muscle use occurs with progressive exertional dyspnea and a minimally productive cough in this form of COPD. Sometimes called a "pink puffer," the patient will display pursed-lip breathing and tachypnea. Associated signs and symptoms include peripheral cyanosis, anorexia, weight loss, malaise, barrel chest, and clubbing. Auscultation reveals distant heart sounds; percussion detects hyperresonance.

Pneumonia. Bacterial pneumonia usually produces increased accessory muscle use. Initially, this infection produces a sudden high fever with chills. Its associated signs and symptoms include chest pain, a productive cough, dyspnea, tachypnea, tachycardia, expiratory grunting, cyanosis, diaphoresis, and fine crackles.

Pulmonary edema. With acute pulmonary edema, increased accessory muscle use is accompanied by dyspnea, tachypnea, orthopnea, crepitant crackles, wheezing, and a cough with pink, frothy sputum. Other findings include restlessness, tachycardia, ventricular gallop, and cool, clammy, cyanotic skin.

Pulmonary embolism. Although signs and symptoms vary with the size, number, and location of the emboli, pulmonary embolism is a life-threatening disorder that may cause increased accessory muscle use. Typically, it produces dyspnea and tachypnea that may be accompanied by pleuritic or substernal chest pain. Other signs and symptoms include restlessness, anxiety, tachycardia, a productive cough, a low-grade fever and, with a large embolus, hemoptysis, cyanosis, syncope, jugular vein distention, scattered crackles, and focal wheezing.

Spinal cord injury. Increased accessory muscle use may occur, depending on the location and severity of the injury. An injury below Ll typically doesn't affect the diaphragm or accessory muscles, whereas an injury between C3 and C5 affects the upper respiratory muscles and diaphragm, causing increased accessory muscle use.
Associated signs and symptoms of spinal cord injury include unilateral or bilateral Babinski's reflex, hyperactive deep tendon reflexes, spasticity, and variable or total loss of pain and temperature sensation, proprioception, and motor function. Horner's syndrome (unilateral ptosis, pupillary constriction, facial anhidrosis) may occur with lower cervical cord injury.

Thoracic injury. Increased accessory muscle use may occur, depending on the type and extent of injury. Associated signs and symptoms of this potentially life-threatening injury include an obvious chest wound or bruising, chest pain, dyspnea, cyanosis, and agitation. Signs of shock, such as tachycardia and hypotension, occur with significant blood loss.

Other causes
Diagnostic tests and treatments. Pulmonary function tests (PFTs), incentive spirometry, and intermittent positive-pressure breathing can increase accessory muscle use.

Nursing considerations
■ If the patient is alert, elevate the head of the bed to make his breathing as easy as possible.

■ Encourage him to get plenty of rest.
■ Reinforce the importance of drinking plenty of fluids to liquefy secretions.
■ Administer oxygen, as ordered.
■ Prepare the patient for such tests as PFTs, chest X-rays, lung scans, arterial blood gas analysis, complete blood count, and sputum culture.

Patient teaching
■ Explain the underlying disorder and treatment plan.
■ Explain how smoking endangers the patient's health, and refer him to an organized program to stop smoking.
■ Teach him the signs and symptoms of infection, when to report them, and about prevention.
■ Explain the purpose of prescribed drugs, such as bronchodilators and mucolytics, and make sure he knows their dosage, schedule, and how to administer them.
■ Teach the patient relaxation techniques to reduce his apprehension and improve breathing.
■ Provide instruction on pursed-lip breathing for patients with chronic lung disorders.
■ Teach the patient coughing and deep-breathing exercises to help keep airways clear.

Agitation

Agitation refers to a state of hyperarousal, increased tension, and irritability that can lead to confusion, hyperactivity, and overt hostility. It can result from a toxic (poisons), metabolic, or infectious cause; brain injury; or a psychiatric disorder. Agitation can also result from pain, fever, anxiety, drug use and withdrawal, hypersensitivity reactions, and various disorders. It can arise gradually or suddenly and last for minutes or months. Whether it's mild or severe, agitation worsens with increased fever, pain, stress, or external stimuli.

Agitation alone merely signals a change in the patient's condition; however, it's a useful indicator of a developing disorder. Obtaining a good history is critical to determining the underlying cause of agitation.

History and physical examination

Determine the severity of the patient's agitation by examining the number and quality of agitation-induced behaviors, such as emotional lability, confusion, memory loss, hyperactivity, and hostility. Obtain a history from the patient or a family member, including diet, known allergies, and all medications, including the use of herbal medicine. Also ask the patient about substance abuse.

Ask if the patient is being treated for any illnesses. Has he had any recent infections, trauma, stress, or changes in sleep patterns? Observe the patient for signs of substance abuse, such as needle tracks, dilated pupils, jaundiced skin, or abdominal ascites. Ask him about alcohol intake. Obtain the patient's baseline vital signs and neurologic status for future comparison.

Medical causes

Alcohol withdrawal syndrome. Mild to severe agitation occurs in alcohol withdrawal syndrome, along with hyperactivity, tremors, and anxiety. With delirium, the potentially life-threatening stage of alcohol withdrawal, severe agitation accompanies hallucinations, insomnia, diaphoresis, and a depressed mood. The patient's pulse rate and temperature rise as withdrawal progresses; status epilepticus, cardiac exhaustion, and shock can occur.

Anxiety. Anxiety produces varying degrees of agitation. The patient may be unaware of his anxiety or may complain of it without knowing its cause. Other findings include nausea, vomiting, diarrhea, cool and clammy skin, frontal headache, back pain, insomnia, and tremors.

Dementia. Mild to severe agitation can result from many common syndromes, such as Alzheimer's and Huntington's diseases. The patient may display a decrease in memory, attention span, problem-solving ability, and alertness. Hypoactivity, wandering behavior, hallucinations, aphasia, and insomnia may also occur.

Drug withdrawal syndrome. Mild to severe agitation occurs in drug withdrawal syndrome. Related findings vary with the drug, but include anxiety, abdominal cramps, diaphoresis, and anorexia. With opioid or barbiturate withdrawal, a decreased level of consciousness (LOC), seizures, and elevated blood pressure, heart rate, and respiratory rate can also occur.

Hepatic encephalopathy. Agitation occurs only with fulminating hepatic encephalopathy. Other findings include drowsiness, stupor, fetor hepaticus, asterixis, and hyperreflexia.

Hypersensitivity reaction. Moderate to severe agitation appears, possibly as the first sign of a reaction. Depending on the severity of the reaction, agitation may be accompanied by urticaria, pruritus, and facial and dependent edema.

With anaphylactic shock, a potentially life-threatening reaction, agitation occurs rapidly along with apprehension, urticaria or diffuse erythema, warm and moist skin, paresthesia, pruritus, edema, dyspnea, wheezing, stridor, hypotension, and tachycardia. Abdominal cramps, vomiting, and diarrhea can also occur.

Hypoxemia. Beginning as restlessness, agitation rapidly worsens. The patient may be confused and have impaired judgment and motor coordination. He may also have tachycardia, tachypnea, dyspnea, and cyanosis.

Increased intracranial pressure (ICP). Agitation usually precedes other early signs and symptoms, such as headache, nausea, and vomiting. Increased ICP produces respiratory changes, such as Cheyne-Stokes, cluster, ataxic, or apneustic breathing; sluggish, nonreactive, or unequal pupils; widening pulse pressure; tachycardia; a decreased LOC; seizures; and motor changes such as decerebrate or decorticate posture.

Post-head trauma syndrome. Shortly after, or even years after a head injury, mild to severe agitation may develop, characterized by disorientation, loss of concentration, angry outbursts, and emotional lability. Other findings include fatigue, wandering behavior, and poor judgment.

Vitamin B$_6$ deficiency. Agitation can range from mild to severe. Other effects include seizures, peripheral paresthesia, and dermatitis. Oculogyric crisis may also occur.

Other causes

Drugs. Mild to moderate agitation, which is commonly dose related, develops as an adverse reaction to central nervous system stimulants—especially appetite suppressants, such as amphetamines and amphetamine-like drugs; sympathomimetics, such as ephedrine; caffeine; and theophylline.

Radiographic contrast media. Reaction to the contrast medium injected during various diagnostic tests produces moderate to severe agitation along with other signs of hypersensitivity.

Nursing considerations

■ Because agitation can be an early sign of many different disorders, monitor the patient's vital signs and neurologic status while the cause is being determined.

■ Eliminate stressors, which can increase agitation.

■ Provide adequate lighting, maintain a calm environment, and allow the patient ample time to sleep.

■ Ensure a balanced diet, and provide vitamin supplements and hydration.

■ Remain calm, nonjudgmental, and nonargumentative.

■ Avoid using restraints, unless absolutely necessary, because they tend to increase agitation.

■ If appropriate, prepare the patient for diagnostic tests, such as a computed tomography scan, skull X-rays, magnetic resonance imaging, and blood studies.

Patient teaching

■ Orient the patient to the unit and its procedures and routines.

■ Explain stress-reduction measures.

■ Offer reassurance and emotional support.

■ Explain all tests and procedures, the underlying cause, and treatment plan.

■ Amenorrhea

The absence of menstrual flow, amenorrhea can be classified as primary or secondary. With primary amenorrhea, menstruation fails to begin before age 16. With secondary amenorrhea, it begins at an appropriate age, but later ceases for 3 or more months in the absence of normal physiologic causes, such as pregnancy, lactation, or menopause.

Pathologic amenorrhea results from anovulation or physical obstruction to menstrual outflow, such as from an imperforate hymen, cervical stenosis, or intrauterine adhesions. Anovulation itself may result from hormonal imbalance, debilitating disease, stress or emotional disturbances, strenuous exercise, malnutrition, obesity, or anatomic abnormalities, such as a congenital absence of the ovaries or uterus. Amenorrhea may also result from drug or hormonal treatments. (See *Understanding disruptions in menstruation,* page 26.)

History and physical examination

Begin by determining whether the amenorrhea is primary or secondary. If it's primary, ask the patient at what age her mother first menstruated because age of menarche is fairly consistent in families. Form an overall impression of the patient's physical, mental, and emotional development because these factors as well as heredity and climate may delay menarche until after age 16.

If menstruation began at an appropriate age but has since ceased, determine the frequency and duration of the patient's previous menses. Ask her about the onset and nature of any changes in her normal menstrual pattern, and determine the date of her last menses. Find out if she has noticed any related signs, such as breast swelling or weight changes.

Determine when the patient last had a physical examination. Review her health history, noting especially any long-term illnesses, such as anemia, or use of hormonal contraceptives. Ask about exercise habits, especially running, and whether she experiences stress on the job or at home. Ask about the patient's eating habits, including the number and size of daily meals and snacks, and ask if she has gained or lost weight recently.

Observe her appearance for secondary sex characteristics or signs of virilization. If you're responsible for performing a pelvic examination, check for anatomic aberrations of the outflow tract, such as cervical adhesions, fibroids, or an imperforate hymen.

Medical causes

Adrenal tumor. Amenorrhea may be accompanied by acne, thinning scalp hair, hirsutism, increased blood pressure, truncal obesity, and psychotic personality changes. Asymmetrical ovarian enlargement in conjunction with the rapid onset of virilizing signs is usually indicative of an adrenal tumor.

Adrenocortical hyperplasia. Amenorrhea precedes characteristic cushingoid signs, such as truncal obesity, moon face, buffalo hump, bruises, purple striae, hypertension, renal calculi, psychiatric disturbances, and widened pulse pressure. Acne, thinning scalp hair, and hirsutism typically appear.

Adrenocortical hypofunction. In addition to amenorrhea, adrenocortical hypofunction may cause fatigue, irritability, weight loss, increased pigmentation (including bluish black discoloration of the areolas and mucous membranes of the lips, mouth, rectum, and vagina), nausea, vomiting, and orthostatic hypotension.

Amenorrhea-lactation disorders. Amenorrhea-lactation disorders, such as Forbes-Albright and Chiari-Frommel syndromes, produce secondary amenorrhea accompanied by lactation in the absence of breast-feeding. Associated features include hot flashes, dyspareunia, vaginal atrophy, and large, engorged breasts.

Anorexia nervosa. Anorexia nervosa can cause either primary or secondary amenorrhea. Related findings include significant weight loss, a thin or emaciated appearance, compulsive behavior patterns, a blotchy or sallow complexion, constipation, reduced libido, decreased pleasure in once-enjoyable activities, dry skin, loss of scalp hair, lanugo on the face and arms, skeletal muscle atrophy, and sleep disturbances.

Congenital absence of the ovaries. Congenital absence of the ovaries results

Understanding disruptions in menstruation

A disruption at any point in the menstrual cycle can produce amenorrhea, as illustrated in this flowchart.

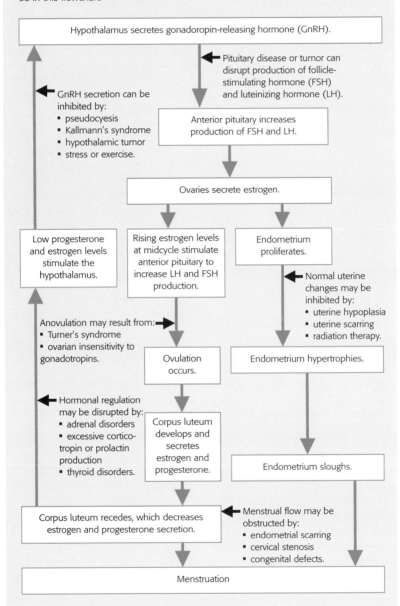

in primary amenorrhea and the absence of secondary sex characteristics.

Congenital absence of the uterus. Primary amenorrhea occurs with congenital absence of the uterus. The patient may develop breasts.

Corpus luteum cysts. Corpus luteum cysts may cause sudden amenorrhea as well as acute abdominal pain and breast swelling. Examination may reveal a tender adnexal mass and vaginal and cervical hyperemia.

Hypothalamic tumor. In addition to amenorrhea, a hypothalamic tumor can cause endocrine and visual field defects, gonadal underdevelopment or dysfunction, and short stature.

Hypothyroidism. Deficient thyroid hormone levels can cause primary or secondary amenorrhea. Typically vague, early findings include fatigue, forgetfulness, cold intolerance, unexplained weight gain, and constipation. Subsequent signs include bradycardia; decreased mental acuity; dry, flaky, inelastic skin; puffy face, hands, and feet; hoarseness; periorbital edema; ptosis; dry, sparse hair; and thick, brittle nails. Other common findings include anorexia, abdominal distention, decreased libido, ataxia, intention tremor, nystagmus, and delayed reflex relaxation time, especially in the Achilles tendon.

Mosaicism. Mosaicism results in primary amenorrhea and the absence of secondary sex characteristics.

Ovarian insensitivity to gonadotropins. A hormonal disturbance, ovarian insensitivity to gonadotropins leads to amenorrhea and an absence of secondary sex characteristics.

Pituitary tumor. Amenorrhea may be the first sign of a pituitary tumor. Associated findings include headache; visual disturbances, such as bitemporal hemianopsia; and acromegaly. Cushingoid signs include moon face, buffalo hump, hirsutism, hypertension, truncal obesity,

bruises, purple striae, widened pulse pressure, and psychiatric disturbances.

Polycystic ovary syndrome. Typically, menarche occurs at a normal age, followed by irregular menstrual cycles, oligomenorrhea, and secondary amenorrhea. Periods of profuse bleeding may alternate with periods of amenorrhea. Obesity, hirsutism, slight deepening of the voice, and enlarged, "oysterlike" ovaries may also accompany this disorder.

Pseudoamenorrhea. An anatomic anomaly, such as imperforate hymen, obstructs menstrual flow, causing primary amenorrhea and, possibly, cyclic episodes of abdominal pain. Examination may reveal a pink or blue bulging hymen.

Pseudocyesis. With pseudocyesis, amenorrhea may be accompanied by lordosis, abdominal distention, nausea, and breast enlargement.

Testicular feminization. Primary amenorrhea may signal this form of male pseudohermaphroditism. The patient, outwardly female but genetically male, shows breast and external genital development but scant or absent pubic hair.

Thyrotoxicosis. Thyroid hormone overproduction may result in amenorrhea. Classic signs and symptoms include an enlarged thyroid (goiter), nervousness, heat intolerance, diaphoresis, tremors, palpitations, tachycardia, dyspnea, weakness, and weight loss despite increased appetite.

Turner's syndrome. Primary amenorrhea and failure to develop secondary sex characteristics may signal this syndrome of genetic ovarian dysgenesis. Typical features include short stature, webbing of the neck, low nuchal hairline, a broad chest with widely spaced nipples and poor breast development, underdeveloped genitalia, and edema of the legs and feet.

Uterine hypoplasia. Primary amenorrhea results from underdevelopment of the uterus, which is detectable on physical examination.

Other causes

Drugs. Busulfan, chlorambucil, injectable or implanted contraceptives, cyclophosphamide, and phenothiazines may cause amenorrhea. Hormonal contraceptives may cause anovulation and amenorrhea after they're discontinued.

Radiation therapy. Irradiation of the abdomen may destroy the endometrium or ovaries, causing amenorrhea.

Surgery. Surgical removal of both ovaries or the uterus produces amenorrhea.

Nursing considerations

■ In patients with secondary amenorrhea, physical and pelvic examinations must rule out pregnancy before diagnostic testing begins.

■ Prepare the patient for tests, such as progestin withdrawal, serum hormone and thyroid function studies, and endometrial biopsy.

Patient teaching

■ Explain to the patient all tests and procedures.

■ Explain the underlying disorder and treatment plan.

■ Encourage the patient to discuss her fears and, if necessary, refer her for psychological counseling.

Amnesia

Amnesia—a disturbance in, or loss of, memory—may be classified as partial or complete and as anterograde or retrograde. Anterograde amnesia denotes memory loss of events that occurred after the onset of the causative trauma or disease; retrograde amnesia, memory loss of events that occurred before the onset. Depending on the cause, amnesia may arise suddenly or slowly and may be temporary or permanent.

Organic (or true) amnesia results from temporal lobe dysfunction, and it characteristically spares patches of memory. A common symptom in patients with seizures or head trauma, organic amnesia can also be an early indicator of Alzheimer's disease. Hysterical amnesia has a psychogenic origin and characteristically causes complete memory loss. Treatment-induced amnesia is usually transient.

History and physical examination

Because the patient typically isn't aware of his amnesia, you'll usually need help in gathering information from his family and friends. Throughout your assessment, notice the patient's general appearance, behavior, mood, and train of thought. Ask when the amnesia first appeared and what the patient is unable to remember. Can he learn new information? How long does he remember it? Does the amnesia encompass a recent or remote period?

Test the patient's recent memory by asking him to identify and repeat three items. Retest after 3 minutes. Test his intermediate memory by asking, "Who was the president before this one?" and "What was the last type of car you bought?" Test remote memory with such questions as "How old are you?" and "Where were you born?"

Take the patient's vital signs and assess his level of consciousness (LOC). Check his pupils: They should be equal in size and should constrict quickly when exposed to direct light. Assess his extraocular movements. Test motor function by having the patient move his arms and legs through their range of motion. Evaluate sensory function with pinpricks on the patient's skin.

Medical causes

Alzheimer's disease. Alzheimer's disease usually begins with retrograde amnesia, which progresses slowly over many months or years to include anterograde amnesia, producing severe and permanent memory loss. Associated findings include agitation, inability to concentrate, disregard for personal hygiene, confusion, irritability, and emotional lability. Later signs include aphasia, dementia, incontinence, and muscle rigidity.

Cerebral hypoxia. After recovery from hypoxia (brought on by such conditions as carbon monoxide poisoning or acute respiratory failure), the patient may experience total amnesia for the event, along with sensory disturbances, such as numbness and tingling.

Head trauma. Depending on the trauma's severity, amnesia may last for minutes, hours, or longer. Usually, the patient experiences brief retrograde and longer anterograde amnesia as well as persistent amnesia about the traumatic event. Severe head trauma can cause permanent amnesia or difficulty retaining recent memories. Related findings may include altered respirations and LOC; headache; dizziness; confusion; visual disturbances, such as blurred or double vision; and motor and sensory disturbances, such as hemiparesis and paresthesia, on the side of the body opposite the injury.

Herpes simplex encephalitis. Recovery from herpes simplex encephalitis commonly leaves the patient with severe and possibly permanent amnesia. Associated findings include signs and symptoms of meningeal irritation, such as headache, fever, and altered LOC, along with seizures and various motor and sensory disturbances (such as paresis, numbness, and tingling).

Hysteria. Hysterical amnesia, a complete and long-lasting memory loss, begins and ends abruptly and is typically accompanied by confusion.

Seizures. In temporal lobe seizures, amnesia occurs suddenly and lasts for several seconds to minutes. The patient may recall an aura or nothing at all. An irritable focus on the left side of the brain primarily causes amnesia for verbal memories, whereas an irritable focus on the right side of the brain causes graphic and nonverbal amnesia. Associated signs and symptoms may include decreased LOC during the seizure, confusion, abnormal mouth movements, and visual, olfactory, and auditory hallucinations.

Wernicke-Korsakoff syndrome. Retrograde and anterograde amnesia can become permanent without treatment in this syndrome. Accompanying signs and symptoms include apathy, an inability to concentrate or to put events into sequence, and confabulation to fill memory gaps. The syndrome may also cause diplopia, decreased LOC, headache, ataxia, and symptoms of peripheral neuropathy, such as numbness and tingling.

Other causes

Drugs. Anterograde amnesia can be precipitated by general anesthetics, especially fentanyl, halothane, and isoflurane; barbiturates, most commonly pentobarbital and thiopental; and certain benzodiazepines, especially triazolam.

Electroconvulsive therapy. The sudden onset of retrograde or anterograde amnesia occurs with electroconvulsive therapy. Typically, the amnesia lasts for several minutes to several hours, but severe, prolonged amnesia occurs with treatments given frequently over a prolonged period.

Temporal lobe surgery. Usually performed on only one lobe, this surgery causes brief, slight amnesia. Removal of both lobes results in permanent amnesia.

Nursing considerations

■ Prepare the patient for diagnostic tests, such as computed tomography scan, magnetic resonance imaging, EEG, or cerebral angiography.
■ Provide reality orientation for the patient with retrograde amnesia, and encourage his family to help by supplying familiar photos, objects, and music.
■ If the patient has severe amnesia, consider basic needs, such as safety, elimination, and nutrition. If necessary, arrange for placement in an extended-care facility.

Patient teaching

■ Adjust your patient-teaching techniques for the patient with anterograde amnesia because he can't acquire new information.
■ Include his family in teaching sessions. In addition, write down all instructions—particularly medication dosages and schedules—so the patient won't have to rely on his memory.

■ Analgesia

Analgesia, the absence of sensitivity to pain, is an important sign of central nervous system disease, commonly indicating a specific type and location of spinal cord lesion. It always occurs with loss of temperature sensation (thermanesthesia) because these sensory nerve impulses travel together in the spinal cord. It can also occur with other sensory deficits—such as paresthesia, loss of proprioception and vibratory sense, and tactile anesthesia—in various disorders involving the peripheral nerves, spinal cord, and brain. When accompanied only by thermanesthesia, analgesia points to an incomplete lesion of the spinal cord.

Analgesia can be classified as partial or total below the level of the lesion and

as unilateral or bilateral, depending on the cause and level of the lesion. Its onset may be slow and progressive with a tumor or abrupt with trauma. Transient in many cases, analgesia may resolve spontaneously.

ACTION STAT!

 Suspect spinal cord injury if the patient complains of unilateral or bilateral analgesia over a large body area, accompanied by paralysis. Immobilize his spine in proper alignment, using a cervical collar and a long backboard, if possible. If a collar or backboard isn't available, position the patient in a supine position on a flat surface and place sandbags around his head, neck, and torso. Use correct technique and extreme caution when moving him to prevent exacerbating spinal injury. Continuously monitor respiratory rate and rhythm, and observe him for accessory muscle use because a complete lesion above the T6 level may cause diaphragmatic and intercostal muscle paralysis. Have an artificial airway and a handheld resuscitation bag on hand, and be prepared to initiate emergency resuscitation measures in case of respiratory failure.

History and physical examination

After you're satisfied that the patient's spine and respiratory status are stabilized—or if the analgesia isn't severe and isn't accompanied by signs of spinal cord injury—perform a physical examination and baseline neurologic evaluation. First, take the patient's vital signs and assess his level of consciousness. Then test pupillary, corneal, cough, and gag reflexes to rule out brain stem and cranial nerve involvement. If the patient is conscious, evaluate his speech, gag reflex, and ability to swallow.

If possible, observe the patient's gait and posture and assess his balance and coordination. Evaluate muscle tone and strength in all extremities. Test for other sensory deficits over all dermatomes (individual skin segments innervated by a specific spinal nerve) by applying light tactile stimulation with a tongue depressor or cotton swab. Perform a more thorough check of pain sensitivity, if necessary, using a pin. (See *Testing for analgesia,* pages 32 and 33.)

Test temperature sensation over all dermatomes, using two test tubes—one filled with hot water, the other with cold water. In each arm and leg, test vibration sense (using a tuning fork), proprioception, and superficial and deep tendon reflexes. Check for increased muscle tone by extending and flexing the patient's elbows and knees as he tries to relax. Focus your history taking on the onset of analgesia (sudden or gradual) and on any recent trauma—a fall, sports injury, or automobile accident. Obtain a complete medical history, noting especially any incidence of cancer in the patient or his family. Obtain a complete drug history.

Medical causes

Anterior cord syndrome. With anterior cord syndrome, analgesia and thermanesthesia occur bilaterally below the level of the lesion, along with flaccid paralysis and hypoactive deep tendon reflexes.

Central cord syndrome. Typically, analgesia and thermanesthesia occur bilaterally in several dermatomes, in many cases extending in a capelike fashion over the arms, back, and shoulders. Early weakness in the hands progresses to weakness and muscle spasms in the arms and shoulder girdle. Hyperactive deep tendon reflexes and spastic weak-

ness of the legs may develop. If the lesion affects the lumbar spine, hypoactive deep tendon reflexes and flaccid weakness may persist in the legs.

With brain stem involvement, additional findings include facial analgesia and thermanesthesia, vertigo, nystagmus, atrophy of the tongue, and dysarthria. The patient may also have dysphagia, urine retention, anhidrosis, decreased intestinal motility, and hyperkeratosis.

Spinal cord hemisection. Contralateral analgesia and thermanesthesia occur below the level of the lesion. In addition, loss of proprioception, spastic paralysis, and hyperactive deep tendon reflexes develop ipsilaterally. The patient may also experience urine retention with overflow incontinence.

Other causes

Drugs. Analgesia may occur with use of a topical or local anesthetic, although numbness and tingling are more common.

Nursing considerations

■ Prepare the patient for spinal X-rays and imaging studies, and maintain spinal alignment and stability during the tests.
■ Focus your care on preventing further injury to the patient because analgesia can mask injury or developing complications.
■ Prevent formation of pressure ulcers through meticulous skin care and frequent repositioning, especially when significant motor deficits impair the patient's mobility.
■ Guard against scalding by testing the patient's bath water temperature before he bathes.

Testing for analgesia

By carefully and systematically testing the patient's sensitivity to pain, you can determine whether his nerve damage has a segmental or peripheral distribution and help locate the causative lesion.

Tell the patient to relax, and explain that you're going to lightly touch areas of his skin with a small pin. Have him close his eyes. Apply the pin firmly enough to produce pain without breaking the skin. (Practice on yourself first to learn how to apply the correct pressure.)

Starting with the patient's head and face, move down his body, pricking his skin on alternating sides. Have the patient report when he feels pain. Use the blunt end of the pin occasionally, and vary your test pattern to gauge the accuracy of his response.

Document your findings thoroughly, clearly marking areas of lost pain sensation either on a dermatome chart (shown below) or on appropriate peripheral nerve diagrams (shown on the next page).

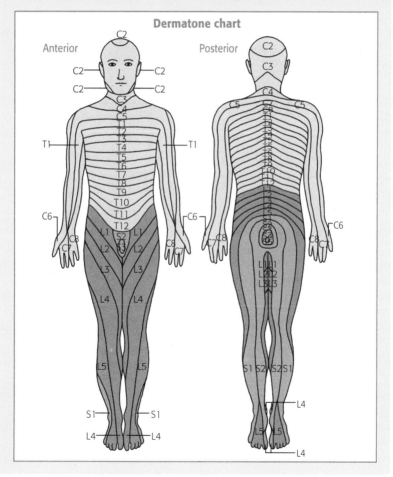

Dermatone chart

Testing for analgesia *(continued)*

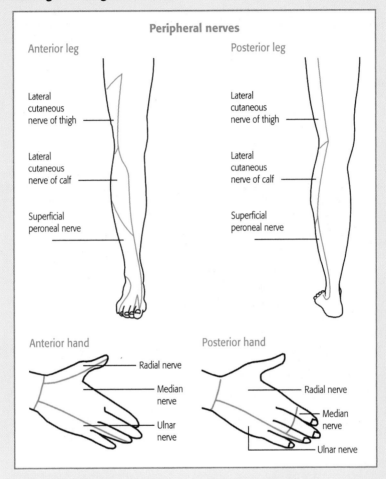

Peripheral nerves

Anterior leg

Lateral cutaneous nerve of thigh

Lateral cutaneous nerve of calf

Superficial peroneal nerve

Posterior leg

Lateral cutaneous nerve of thigh

Lateral cutaneous nerve of calf

Superficial peroneal nerve

Anterior hand

Radial nerve

Median nerve

Ulnar nerve

Posterior hand

Radial nerve

Median nerve

Ulnar nerve

Patient teaching

- Advise the patient to test bath water temperature at home using a thermometer or a body part with intact sensation.
- Explain all tests and procedures.
- Teach the patient about the diagnosis, once established, and the treatment plan.

▊ Anhidrosis

Anhidrosis, an abnormal deficiency of sweat, can be classified as generalized (complete) or localized (partial). Generalized anhidrosis can lead to life-threatening impairment of thermoregulation. Localized anhidrosis rarely interferes with thermoregulation because it affects only a small percentage of the body's eccrine (sweat) glands.

Anhidrosis results from neurologic and skin disorders; congenital, atrophic, or traumatic changes to sweat glands; and the use of certain drugs. Neurologic disorders disturb central or peripheral nervous pathways that normally activate sweating, causing retention of excess body heat and perspiration. The absence, obstruction, atrophy, or degeneration of sweat glands can produce anhidrosis at the skin surface, even if neurologic stimulation is normal.

Anhidrosis may go unrecognized until significant heat or exertion fails to raise sweat. Localized anhidrosis commonly provokes compensatory hyperhidrosis in the remaining functional sweat glands—which, in many cases, is the patient's chief complaint.

ACTION STAT!

 If you detect anhidrosis in a patient whose skin feels hot and flushed, ask him if he's also experiencing nausea, dizziness, palpitations, and substernal tightness. If he is, quickly take his rectal temperature and other vital signs and assess his level of consciousness (LOC). If a rectal temperature higher than 102.2° F (39° C) is accompanied by tachycardia, tachypnea, and altered blood pressure and LOC, suspect life-threatening anhidrotic asthenia (heatstroke). Start rapid cooling measures, such as immersing him in ice or very cold water and giving I.V. fluid replacements. Continue these measures, and check his vital signs and neurologic status frequently, until his temperature drops below 102° F (38.9° C), then place him in an air-conditioned room.

History and physical examination

If anhidrosis is localized or if the patient reports local hyperhidrosis or unexplained fever, take a brief history. Ask the patient to characterize his sweating during heat spells or strenuous activity. Does he usually sweat slightly or profusely? Ask about recent prolonged or extreme exposure to heat and about the onset of anhidrosis or hyperhidrosis. Obtain a complete medical history, focusing on neurologic disorders; skin disorders, such as psoriasis; autoimmune disorders, such as scleroderma; systemic diseases that can cause peripheral neuropathies, such as diabetes mellitus; and drug use.

Inspect skin color, texture, and turgor. If you detect skin lesions, document their location, size, color, texture, and pattern.

Medical causes

Anhidrotic asthenia (heatstroke). A life-threatening disorder, anhidrotic asthenia causes acute, generalized anhidrosis. In early stages, sweating may still occur and the patient may be rational, but his rectal temperature may already exceed 102.2° F (39° C). Associated signs and symptoms include severe headache and muscle cramps, which later disappear; fatigue; nausea and vomiting; dizziness; palpitations; substernal tightness; and elevated blood pressure followed by hypotension. Within minutes, anhidrosis and hot, flushed skin develop, accompanied by tachycardia, tachypnea, and confusion progressing to seizure or loss of consciousness.

Burns. Depending on their severity, burns may cause permanent anhidrosis in affected areas as well as blistering, edema, and increased pain or loss of sensation.

Miliaria crystallina. This usually innocuous form of miliaria causes anhidrosis and tiny, clear, fragile blisters, usually under the arms and breasts.

Miliaria profunda. If severe and extensive, miliaria profunda can progress to life-threatening anhidrotic asthenia.

Typically, it produces localized anhidrosis with compensatory facial hyperhidrosis. Whitish papules appear mostly on the trunk but also on the extremities. Associated signs and symptoms include inguinal and axillary lymphadenopathy, weakness, shortness of breath, palpitations, and fever.

Miliaria rubra (prickly heat). Miliaria rubra typically produces localized anhidrosis, and can also progress to life-threatening anhidrotic asthenia if it becomes severe and extensive; this is a rare occurrence. Small, erythematous papules with centrally placed blisters appear on the trunk and neck and rarely on the face, palms, or soles. Pustules may also appear in extensive and chronic miliaria. Related symptoms include paroxysmal itching and paresthesia.

Peripheral neuropathy. Anhidrosis over the legs usually appears with compensatory hyperhidrosis over the head and neck. Associated findings mainly involve extremities and include glossy red skin; paresthesia, hyperesthesia, or anesthesia in the hands and feet; diminished or absent deep tendon reflexes; flaccid paralysis and muscle wasting; footdrop; and burning pain.

Shy-Drager syndrome. Shy-Drager syndrome causes ascending anhidrosis in the legs. Other signs and symptoms include severe orthostatic hypotension, loss of leg hair, impotence, constipation, urine retention or urgency, decreased salivation and tearing, mydriasis, and impaired visual accommodation. Eventually, focal neurologic signs—such as leg tremors, incoordination, and muscle wasting and fasciculation—may appear.

Spinal cord lesions. Anhidrosis may occur symmetrically below the level of the lesion, with compensatory hyperhidrosis in adjacent areas. Other findings depend on the site and extent of the lesion but may include partial or total loss of motor and sensory function below the lesion as well as impaired cardiovascular and respiratory function.

Other causes

Drugs. Anticholinergics, such as atropine and scopolamine, can cause generalized anhidrosis.

Nursing considerations

- Because even a careful evaluation can be inconclusive, you may need to administer specific tests to evaluate anhidrosis, such as wrapping the patient in an electric blanket or placing him in a heated box to observe the skin for sweat patterns, applying a topical agent to detect sweat on the skin, or administering a systemic cholinergic drug to stimulate sweating.

Patient teaching

- Explain the underlying disorder and treatment plan.
- Advise the patient about ways to stay cool, such as maintaining a cool environment, moving slowly during warm weather, and avoiding strenuous exercise and hot foods.
- Discuss with the patient the anhidrotic effects of drugs he's receiving.
- Explain the signs and symptoms of heatstroke and when to seek medical attention.

■ Anorexia

Anorexia, a lack of appetite in the presence of a physiologic need for food, is a common symptom of GI and endocrine disorders and is characteristic of certain psychological disturbances such as anorexia nervosa. It can also result from such factors as anxiety, chronic pain, poor oral hygiene, increased blood temperature due to hot weather or fever, and changes in taste or smell that normally accompany aging. Anorexia can also result from drug therapy or abuse.

Short-term anorexia rarely jeopardizes health, but chronic anorexia can lead to life-threatening malnutrition and electrolyte disorders.

History and physical examination

Take the patient's vital signs and weight. Find out previous minimum and maximum weights. Ask about involuntary weight loss greater than 10 lb (4.5 kg) in the past month. Explore dietary habits such as when and what the patient eats. Ask what foods he likes and dislikes and why. The patient may identify tastes and smells that nauseate him and cause loss of appetite. Ask about dental problems that interfere with chewing, including poor-fitting dentures. Ask if he has difficulty or pain when swallowing or if he vomits or has diarrhea after meals. Ask the patient how frequently and intensely he exercises.

Check for a history of stomach or bowel disorders, which can interfere with the ability to digest, absorb, or metabolize nutrients. Find out about changes in bowel habits. Ask about alcohol use and drug use and dosage.

If the medical history doesn't reveal an organic basis for anorexia, consider psychological factors. Ask the patient if he knows what's causing his decreased appetite. Situational factors—such as a death in the family or problems at school or at work—can lead to depression and a subsequent loss of appetite. Be alert for signs of malnutrition, consistent refusal of food, and a 7% to 10% loss of body weight in the preceding month. (See *Is your patient malnourished?*)

Medical causes

Acquired immunodeficiency syndrome. An infection or Kaposi's sarcoma affecting the GI or respiratory tract may lead to anorexia. Other findings include fatigue, afternoon fevers, night sweats, diarrhea, cough, lymphadenopathy, bleeding, oral thrush, gingivitis, and skin disorders, including persistent herpes zoster and recurrent herpes simplex, herpes labialis, or herpes genitalis.

Adrenocortical hypofunction. With adrenocortical hypofunction, anorexia may begin slowly and subtly, causing gradual weight loss. Other common signs and symptoms include nausea and vomiting, abdominal pain, diarrhea, weakness, fatigue, malaise, vitiligo, bronze-colored skin, and purple striae on the breasts, abdomen, shoulders, and hips.

Alcoholism. Chronic anorexia commonly accompanies alcoholism, eventually leading to malnutrition. Other findings include signs of liver damage (jaundice, spider angiomas, ascites, edema), paresthesia, tremors, increased blood pressure, bruising, GI bleeding, and abdominal pain.

Anorexia nervosa. Chronic anorexia begins insidiously and eventually leads to life-threatening malnutrition and electrolyte disorders, as evidenced by skeletal muscle atrophy, loss of fatty tissue, constipation, amenorrhea, dry and blotchy or sallow skin, alopecia, sleep disturbances, distorted self-image, anhedonia, decreased libido, and cardiac arrhythmias. Paradoxically, the patient typically exhibits extreme restlessness and vigor and may exercise compulsively. He may have complicated food preparation and eating rituals.

Appendicitis. Anorexia closely follows the abrupt onset of generalized or localized epigastric pain, nausea, and vomiting cause by appendicitis. It can continue as pain localizes in the right lower quadrant (McBurney's point), and other signs and symptoms appear, such as abdominal rigidity, rebound tenderness, constipation (or diarrhea), a slight fever, and tachycardia.

Is your patient malnourished?

When assessing a patient with anorexia, make sure to check for these common signs of malnutrition.

Hair. Dull, dry, thin, fine, straight, and easily plucked; areas of lighter or darker spots and hair loss
Face. Generalized swelling, dark areas on cheeks and under eyes, lumpy or flaky skin around the nose and mouth, enlarged parotid glands
Eyes. Dull appearance; dry and either pale or red membranes; triangular, shiny gray spots on conjunctivae; red and fissured eyelid corners; bloodshot ring around cornea
Lips. Red and swollen, especially at corners
Tongue. Swollen, purple, and raw-looking, with sores or abnormal papillae
Teeth. Missing, or emerging abnormally; visible cavities or dark spots; spongy, bleeding gums
Neck. Swollen thyroid gland

Skin. Dry, flaky, swollen, and dark, with lighter or darker spots, some resembling bruises; tight and drawn, with poor skin turgor
Nails. Spoon-shaped, brittle, and ridged
Musculoskeletal system. Muscle wasting, knock-knee or bowlegs, bumps on ribs, swollen joints, musculoskeletal hemorrhages
Cardiovascular system. Heart rate above 100 beats/minute, arrhythmias, elevated blood pressure
Abdomen. Enlarged liver and spleen
Reproductive system. Decreased libido, amenorrhea
Nervous system. Irritability, confusion, paresthesia in hands and feet, loss of proprioception, decreased ankle and knee reflexes

Cancer. Chronic anorexia occurs along with possible weight loss, weakness, apathy, and cachexia.
Chronic renal failure. With chronic rental failure, chronic anorexia is common and insidious. It's accompanied by changes in all body systems, such as nausea, vomiting, mouth ulcers, ammonia breath odor, metallic taste in the mouth, GI bleeding, constipation or diarrhea, drowsiness, confusion, tremors, pallor, dry and scaly skin, pruritus, alopecia, purpuric lesions, and edema.
Cirrhosis. Anorexia occurs early in cirrhosis and may be accompanied by weakness, nausea, vomiting, constipation or diarrhea, and dull abdominal pain. It continues after these early signs and symptoms subside and is accompanied by lethargy, slurred speech, bleeding tendencies, ascites, severe pruritus,

dry skin, poor skin turgor, hepatomegaly, fetor hepaticus, jaundice, leg edema, gynecomastia, and right upper quadrant pain.
Crohn's disease. With Crohn's disease, chronic anorexia causes marked weight loss. Associated signs vary according to the site and extent of the lesion, but may include diarrhea, abdominal pain, fever, an abdominal mass, weakness, perianal or vaginal fistulas and, rarely, clubbing of the fingers. Acute inflammatory signs and symptoms—right lower quadrant pain, cramping, tenderness, flatulence, fever, nausea, diarrhea (including nocturnal), and bloody stools—mimic those of appendicitis.
Gastritis. With acute gastritis, the onset of anorexia may be sudden. The patient may experience postprandial epi-

gastric distress after a meal, accompanied by nausea, vomiting (commonly with hematemesis), fever, belching, hiccups, and malaise.

Hepatitis. With viral hepatitis (hepatitis A, B, C, or D), anorexia begins in the preicteric phase, accompanied by fatigue, malaise, headache, arthralgia, myalgia, photophobia, nausea and vomiting, a mild fever, hepatomegaly, and lymphadenopathy. It may continue throughout the icteric phase, along with mild weight loss, dark urine, clay-colored stools, jaundice, right upper quadrant pain and, possibly, irritability and severe pruritus.

Signs and symptoms of nonviral hepatitis usually resemble those of viral hepatitis but may vary, depending on the cause and extent of liver damage.

Hypothyroidism. Anorexia is common and usually insidious in patients with a thyroid hormone deficiency. Typically, vague early findings include fatigue, forgetfulness, cold intolerance, unexplained weight gain, and constipation. Subsequent findings include decreased mental stability; dry, flaky, and inelastic skin; edema of the face, hands, and feet; ptosis; hoarseness; thick, brittle nails; coarse, broken hair; and signs of decreased cardiac output such as bradycardia. Other common findings include abdominal distention, menstrual irregularities, decreased libido, ataxia, intention tremor, nystagmus, a dull facial expression, and slow reflex relaxation time.

Ketoacidosis. Anorexia usually arises gradually and is accompanied by dry, flushed skin; a fruity breath odor; polydipsia; polyuria and nocturia; hypotension; a weak, rapid pulse; a dry mouth; abdominal pain; vomiting, and altered level of consciousness.

Pernicious anemia. With pernicious anemia, insidious anorexia may cause considerable weight loss. Related findings include the classic triad of a burning tongue, general weakness, and numbness and tingling in the extremities; alternating constipation and diarrhea; abdominal pain; nausea and vomiting; bleeding gums; ataxia; positive Babinski's and Romberg's signs; diplopia and blurred vision; irritability; headache; malaise; and fatigue.

Other causes

Drugs. Anorexia results from the use of amphetamines, chemotherapeutic agents, sympathomimetics such as ephedrine, and some antibiotics. It also signals digoxin toxicity.

Radiation therapy. Radiation treatments can cause anorexia, possibly as a result of metabolic disturbances.

Total parenteral nutrition (TPN). Maintenance of blood glucose levels by I.V. therapy may cause anorexia.

Nursing considerations

- Because the causes of anorexia are diverse, diagnostic procedures may include thyroid function studies, endoscopy, upper GI series, gallbladder series, barium enema, liver and kidney function tests, hormone assays, computed tomography scans, ultrasonography, blood studies to assess the patient's nutritional status and, possibly, a mental health evaluation.
- Promote protein and calorie intake by providing high-calorie snacks or frequent, small meals.
- Encourage the patient's family to supply his favorite foods to help stimulate his appetite.
- Because the patient may consistently exaggerate his food intake (common in the patient with anorexia nervosa), you'll need to maintain strict calorie and nutrient counts for the patient's meals.
- In severe malnutrition, provide supplemental nutritional support, such as TPN or oral nutritional supplements.

- Because anorexia and poor nutrition increase the patient's susceptibility to infection, monitor his vital signs and white blood cell count and closely observe any wounds.

Patient teaching

- Explain the patient's condition and treatment plan to him and his family.
- Stress the importance of proper nutrition.
- Instruct the patient to perform oral hygiene before meals.
- Teach the patient techniques to help manage the disorder, including establishing a target weight, recording his weight daily, and maintaining a record of his progress by keeping a weight log.
- Encourage the patient to seek psychological and nutritional counseling.

Anuria

Clinically defined as urine output of less than 100 ml in 24 hours, anuria indicates either urinary tract obstruction or acute renal failure due to various mechanisms. (See *Major causes of acute renal failure,* page 40.)

Anuria is rare; even with renal failure, the kidneys usually produce at least 75 ml of urine daily.

Because urine output is easily measured, anuria rarely goes undetected. Without immediate treatment, it can rapidly cause uremia or complications of urine retention.

A C T I O N   S T A T !

 After detecting anuria, your priorities are to determine if urine formation is occurring and to intervene appropriately. Catheterize the patient to relieve any lower urinary tract obstruction and to check for residual urine. You may find that an obstruction hinders catheter insertion or that urine return is cloudy and foul smelling or bloody. If you collect more than 75 ml of urine, suspect lower urinary tract obstruction; if you collect less than 75 ml, suspect renal dysfunction or obstruction higher in the urinary tract.

History and physical examination

Take the patient's vital signs and obtain a complete history. First, ask about changes in his voiding pattern. Determine the amount of fluid he normally ingests each day, the amount of fluid he ingested in the last 24 to 48 hours, and the time and amount of his last urination. Review his medical history, noting previous kidney disease, urinary tract obstruction or infection, prostate enlargement, renal calculi, neurogenic bladder, or congenital abnormalities. Ask about drug use and about abdominal, renal, or urinary tract surgery.

Inspect and palpate the abdomen for asymmetry, distention, or bulging. Inspect the flank area for edema or erythema, and percuss and palpate the bladder. Palpate the kidneys anteriorly and posteriorly, and percuss them at the costovertebral angle. Auscultate over the renal arteries, listening for bruits.

Medical causes

Acute tubular necrosis. Oliguria (occasionally anuria) is a common finding with acute tubular necrosis. It precedes the onset of diuresis, which is heralded by polyuria. Associated findings reflect the underlying cause and may include signs and symptoms of hyperkalemia (muscle weakness, cardiac arrhythmias), uremia (anorexia, nausea, vomiting, confusion, lethargy, twitching, seizures, pruritus, uremic frost, and Kussmaul's respirations), and heart failure (edema, jugular vein distention, crackles, and dyspnea).

Major causes of acute renal failure

Acute renal failure may result from prerenal causes. All conditions that cause prerenal failure impair renal perfusion, resulting in decreased glomerular filtration rate and increased proximal tubular reabsorption of sodium and water. Intrarenal causes damage the kidneys themselves; postrenal causes obstruct urine flow.

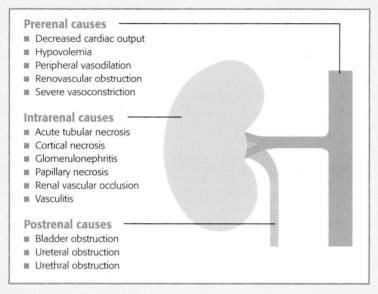

Prerenal causes
- Decreased cardiac output
- Hypovolemia
- Peripheral vasodilation
- Renovascular obstruction
- Severe vasoconstriction

Intrarenal causes
- Acute tubular necrosis
- Cortical necrosis
- Glomerulonephritis
- Papillary necrosis
- Renal vascular occlusion
- Vasculitis

Postrenal causes
- Bladder obstruction
- Ureteral obstruction
- Urethral obstruction

Cortical necrosis (bilateral). Cortical necrosis is characterized by a sudden change from oliguria to anuria, along with gross hematuria, flank pain, and fever.

Glomerulonephritis (acute). Acute glomerulonephritis produces anuria or oliguria. Related effects include a mild fever, malaise, flank pain, gross hematuria, facial and generalized edema, elevated blood pressure, headache, nausea, vomiting, abdominal pain, and signs and symptoms of pulmonary congestion (crackles, dyspnea).

Hemolytic-uremic syndrome. Anuria commonly occurs in the initial stages of hemolytic-uremic syndrome and may last from 1 to 10 days. The patient may experience vomiting, diarrhea, abdominal pain, hematemesis, melena, purpura, fever, elevated blood pressure, hepatomegaly, ecchymoses, edema, hematuria, and pallor. He also may show signs of upper respiratory tract infection.

Renal artery occlusion (bilateral). Renal artery occlusion produces anuria or severe oliguria, commonly accompanied by severe, continuous upper abdominal and flank pain; nausea and vomiting; decreased bowel sounds; a fever up to 102° F (38.9° C); and diastolic hypertension.

Renal vein occlusion (bilateral). Renal vein occlusion occasionally causes anuria; more typical signs and symptoms include acute low back pain, fever, flank tenderness, and hematuria. Development of pulmonary emboli—a common complication—produces sudden dyspnea, pleuritic pain, tachypnea, tachycardia, crackles, pleural friction rub and, possibly, hemoptysis.

Urinary tract obstruction. Severe urinary tract obstruction can produce acute and sometimes total anuria, alternating with or preceded by burning and pain on urination, overflow incontinence or dribbling, increased urinary frequency and nocturia, voiding of small amounts, or an altered urine stream. Associated findings include bladder distention, pain and a sensation of fullness in the lower abdomen and groin, upper abdominal and flank pain, nausea and vomiting, and signs of secondary infection, such as fever, chills, malaise, and cloudy, foul-smelling urine.

Vasculitis. Vasculitis occasionally produces anuria. More typical findings include malaise, myalgia, polyarthralgia, fever, elevated blood pressure, hematuria, proteinuria, arrhythmia, pallor and, possibly, skin lesions, urticaria, and purpura.

Other causes

Diagnostic tests. Contrast media used in radiographic studies can cause nephrotoxicity, producing oliguria and, rarely, anuria.

Drugs. Many classes of drugs can cause anuria or, more commonly, oliguria through their nephrotoxic effects. Antibiotics, especially the aminoglycosides, are the most commonly seen nephrotoxins. Anesthetics, heavy metals, ethyl alcohol, and organic solvents can also be nephrotoxic. Adrenergics and anticholinergics can cause anuria by affecting the nerves and muscles of micturition to produce urine retention.

Nursing considerations

■ If catheterization fails to initiate urine flow, prepare the patient for diagnostic studies—such as ultrasonography, cystoscopy, retrograde pyelography, and renal scan—to detect an obstruction higher in the urinary tract.

■ If diagnostic tests reveal an obstruction, prepare him for immediate surgery to remove the obstruction, or to insert a nephrostomy or ureterostomy tube to drain the urine.

■ If tests fail to reveal an obstruction, prepare the patient for further kidney function studies.

■ Monitor the patient's vital signs and intake and output.

■ Restrict daily fluid allowance to 600 ml more than the previous day's total urine output.

■ Restrict foods and juices high in potassium and sodium, and make sure that the patient maintains a balanced diet with controlled protein levels.

■ Provide low-sodium hard candy to help decrease thirst.

■ Weigh the patient daily.

■ Monitor laboratory studies, especially potassium levels.

■ Monitor cardiac rhythm for arrhythmias.

Patient teaching

■ Teach the patient about maintaining fluid restrictions and about dietary modifications, such as restricting potassium and sodium, as needed.

■ Instruct the patient on nephrostomy tube or ureterostomy tube care if needed.

■ Explain the disorder or cause of anuria and the treatment plan.

Anxiety

Anxiety is the most common psychiatric symptom and can result in significant lifestyle impairment. A subjective reaction to a real or imagined threat, anxiety is a nonspecific feeling of uneasiness or dread. It may be mild, moderate, or severe. Mild anxiety may cause slight physical or psychological discomfort. Severe anxiety may be incapacitating or even life-threatening.

Everyone experiences anxiety from time to time—it's a normal response to actual danger, prompting the body (through stimulation of the sympathetic and parasympathetic nervous systems) to purposeful action. Anxiety is a normal response to physical and emotional stress, which can be produced by virtually any illness. In addition, anxiety can be precipitated or exacerbated by many nonpathologic factors, including lack of sleep, poor diet, and excessive intake of caffeine or other stimulants. Excessive, unwarranted anxiety may indicate an underlying psychological problem or specific type of anxiety disorder.

History and physical examination

If the patient displays acute, severe anxiety, quickly take his vital signs and determine his chief complaint; this will serve as a guide for how to proceed. For example, if the patient's anxiety occurs with chest pain and shortness of breath, you might suspect myocardial infarction and act accordingly. While examining the patient, try to keep him calm. Suggest relaxation techniques, and talk to him in a reassuring, soothing voice. Uncontrolled anxiety can alter vital signs and exacerbate the causative disorder.

If the patient displays mild or moderate anxiety, ask about its duration. Is the anxiety constant or sporadic? Did he notice precipitating factors? Find out if the anxiety is exacerbated by stress, lack of sleep, or caffeine intake or alleviated by rest, tranquilizers, or exercise.

Obtain a complete medical history, especially noting drug use including over-the-counter drugs and herbal supplements. Then perform a physical examination, focusing on any complaints

that may trigger or be aggravated by anxiety.

If the patient's anxiety isn't accompanied by significant physical signs, suspect a psychological basis. Determine the patient's level of consciousness (LOC) and observe his behavior. If appropriate, refer the patient for psychiatric evaluation.

Medical causes

Acute respiratory distress syndrome (ARDS). Acute anxiety occurs with ARDS along with tachycardia, mental sluggishness and, in severe cases, hypotension. Other respiratory signs and symptoms include dyspnea, tachypnea, intercostal and suprasternal retractions, crackles, rhonchi, and decreased pulse oximetry.

Anaphylactic shock. Acute anxiety usually signals the onset of anaphylactic shock. It's accompanied by urticaria, angioedema, pruritus, and shortness of breath. Soon, other signs and symptoms develop: light-headedness, hypotension, tachycardia, nasal congestion, sneezing, wheezing, dyspnea, a barking cough, abdominal cramps, vomiting, diarrhea, and urinary urgency and incontinence.

Angina pectoris. Acute anxiety may either precede or follow an attack of angina pectoris. An attack produces sharp and crushing substernal or anterior chest pain that may radiate to the back, neck, arms, or jaw. The pain may be relieved by nitroglycerin or rest, which eases anxiety.

Asthma. With allergic asthma attacks, acute anxiety occurs with dyspnea, wheezing, a productive cough, accessory muscle use, hyperresonant lung fields, diminished breath sounds, coarse crackles, cyanosis, decreased pulse oximetry, tachycardia, and diaphoresis.

Autonomic hyperreflexia. The earliest signs of autonomic hyperreflexia may be acute anxiety accompanied by severe headache and dramatic hypertension. Pallor and motor and sensory deficits occur below the level of the lesion; flushing occurs above it.

Cardiogenic shock. Acute anxiety in cardiogenic shock is accompanied by cool, pale, clammy skin; tachycardia; a weak, thready pulse; tachypnea; ventricular gallop; crackles; jugular vein distention; decreased urine output; hypotension; narrowing pulse pressure; and peripheral edema.

Chronic obstructive pulmonary disease (COPD). Acute anxiety, exertional dyspnea, cough, wheezing, crackles, hyperresonant lung fields, tachypnea, and accessory muscle use characterize COPD.

Generalized anxiety disorder. Anxiety may be the patient's chief complaint in this type of anxiety disorder. It's characterized by excessive, unrealistic worry lasting 6 months or more. Associated findings include trembling, insomnia, GI disturbances, dizziness, irritability, and muscle aches.

Heart failure. With heart failure, acute anxiety is commonly the first symptom of inadequate oxygenation. Associated findings include restlessness, shortness of breath, tachypnea, decreased LOC, edema, crackles, ventricular gallop, hypotension, diaphoresis, cyanosis, and decreased pulse oximetry.

Hyperthyroidism. Acute anxiety may be an early sign of hyperthyroidism. Classic signs and symptoms include heat intolerance, weight loss despite increased appetite, nervousness, tremor, palpitations, sweating, an enlarged thyroid, and diarrhea. Exophthalmos may occur.

Mitral valve prolapse. Panic may occur in patients with mitral valve prolapse, referred to as the *click-murmur syndrome.* The disorder may also cause paroxysmal palpitations accompanied by sharp, stabbing, or aching precordial pain. Its hallmark is a midsystolic click, followed by an apical systolic murmur.

Myocardial infarction (MI). With MI, a life-threatening disorder, acute anxiety commonly occurs with persistent, crushing substernal pain that may radiate to the left arm, jaw, neck, or shoulder blades. It can be accompanied by shortness of breath, nausea, vomiting, diaphoresis, and cool, pale skin.

Obsessive-compulsive disorder. Chronic anxiety occurs with obsessive-compulsive disorder, along with recurrent, unshakable thoughts or impulses to perform ritualistic acts. The patient recognizes these acts as irrational, but is unable to control them. Anxiety builds if he can't perform these acts and diminishes after he does.

Pheochromocytoma. Acute, severe anxiety accompanies pheochromocytoma's cardinal sign: persistent or paroxysmal hypertension. Common associated signs and symptoms include tachycardia, diaphoresis, orthostatic hypotension, tachypnea, flushing, a severe headache, palpitations, nausea, vomiting, epigastric pain, and paresthesia.

Phobias. With phobias, chronic anxiety occurs along with a persistent fear of an object, activity, or situation that results in a compelling desire to avoid it. The patient recognizes the fear as irrational, but can't suppress it.

Pneumonia. Acute anxiety may occur with pneumonia because of hypoxemia. Other findings include a productive cough, pleuritic chest pain, fever, chills, crackles, diminished breath sounds, and hyperresonant lung fields.

Pneumothorax. Acute anxiety occurs in moderate to severe pneumothorax associated with profound respiratory distress. It's accompanied by sharp pleuritic pain, coughing, shortness of breath, cyanosis, asymmetrical chest expansion, pallor, jugular vein distention, and a weak, rapid pulse.

Postconcussion syndrome. Postconcussion syndrome may produce chronic anxiety or periodic attacks of acute anxiety. Associated signs and symptoms include irritability, insomnia, dizziness, and a mild headache. The anxiety is usually most pronounced in situations demanding attention, judgment, or comprehension.

Posttraumatic stress disorder. Posttraumatic stress disorder produces chronic anxiety of varying severity and is accompanied by intrusive, vivid memories and thoughts of the traumatic event. The patient may relive the event in dreams and nightmares. Insomnia, depression, and feelings of numbness and detachment are common.

Pulmonary edema. With pulmonary edema, acute anxiety occurs with dyspnea, orthopnea, cough with frothy sputum, tachycardia, tachypnea, crackles, decreased pulse oximetry, ventricular gallop, hypotension, and a thready pulse. The patient's skin may be cool, clammy, and cyanotic.

Pulmonary embolism. With pulmonary embolism, acute anxiety is usually accompanied by dyspnea, tachypnea, chest pain, tachycardia, blood-tinged sputum, and a low-grade fever.

Rabies. Anxiety signals the beginning of the acute phase of rabies, a rare disorder, which is commonly accompanied by painful laryngeal spasms associated with difficulty swallowing and, as a result, hydrophobia.

Somatoform disorder. Somatoform disorder is characterized by anxiety and multiple somatic complaints that can't be explained physiologically. The symptoms aren't produced intentionally, but are severe enough to significantly impair functioning. Pain disorder, conversion disorder, and hypochondriasis are examples of somatoform disorder.

Other causes

Drugs. Many drugs cause anxiety, especially sympathomimetics and central nervous system stimulants. In addition, many antidepressants may cause paradoxical anxiety.

Nursing considerations

- Provide supportive care, as indicated by the patient's signs and symptoms.
- Provide a calm, quiet atmosphere.
- Administer medications, as ordered, to reduce anxiety.
- Treat the underlying cause of the patient's anxiety, if known.
- Encourage the patient to express his feelings and concerns.

Patient teaching

- Teach the patient anxiety-reducing measures, such as distraction, relaxation techniques, or biofeedback.
- Teach the patient coping mechanisms to help control his anxiety.
- Explain the underlying causes of his anxiety, if known.

Aphasia
[Dysphasia]

Aphasia, impaired expression or comprehension of written or spoken language, reflects disease or injury of the brain's language centers. (See *Where language originates.*)

Depending on its severity, aphasia may slightly impede communication or may make it impossible. It can be classified as Broca's, Wernicke's, anomic, or global aphasia. Anomic aphasia eventually resolves in more than 50% of patients, but global aphasia is usually irreversible. (See *Identifying types of aphasia,* page 46.)

Quickly look for signs and symptoms of stroke or increased intracranial pressure (ICP), such as pupillary changes, a decreased level of consciousness (LOC), vomiting, seizures, bradycardia, widening pulse pressure, and irregular respirations. If you detect signs of increased ICP, administer mannitol I.V. to decrease cerebral edema. In addition, make sure that emergency resuscitation equipment is readily available to support respiratory and cardiac function if necessary. You may have to prepare the patient for emergency surgery.

History and physical examination

If the patient doesn't display signs of increased ICP or if his aphasia has developed gradually, perform a thorough neurologic examination, starting with his history. You may need to obtain this history from the patient's family or companion because of the patient's impairment. Ask if the patient has a history of headaches, hypertension, seizure disorders, or drug use. Ask about the patient's ability to communicate and to perform routine activities before aphasia began.

Check for obvious signs of neurologic deficit, such as ptosis, fluid leakage from the nose and ears, or motor im-

Where language originates

Aphasia reflects damage to one or more of the brain's primary language centers, which, in most persons, are located in the left hemisphere. *Broca's area* lies next to the region of the motor cortex that controls the muscles necessary for speech. *Wernicke's area* is the center of auditory, visual, and language compre-

hension. It lies between *Heschl's gyrus,* the primary receiver of auditory stimuli, and the *angular gyrus,* a "way station" between the brain's auditory and visual regions. Connecting Wernicke's and Broca's areas is a large nerve bundle, the *arcuate fasciculus,* which enables the repetition of speech.

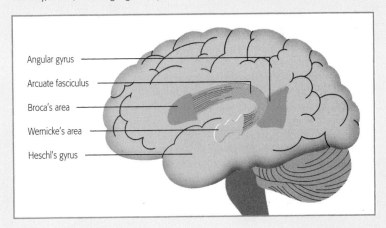

Angular gyrus
Arcuate fasciculus
Broca's area
Wernicke's area
Heschl's gyrus

Identifying types of aphasia

Type	Location of lesion	Signs and symptoms
Anomic aphasia	Temporal-parietal area; may extend to angular gyrus, but sometimes poorly localized	The patient's understanding of written and spoken language is relatively unimpaired. His speech, although fluent, lacks meaningful content. Word-finding difficulty and circumlocution are characteristic. Rarely, the patient also displays paraphasias.
Broca's aphasia (expressive aphasia)	Broca's area; usually in third frontal convolution of the left hemisphere	The patient's understanding of written and spoken language is relatively spared, but speech is nonfluent, evidencing word-finding difficulty, jargon, paraphasias, limited vocabulary, and simple sentence construction. He can't repeat words and phrases. If Wernicke's area is intact, he recognizes speech errors and shows frustration. He's commonly hemiparetic.
Global aphasia	Broca's and Wernicke's areas	The patient has profoundly impaired receptive and expressive ability. He can't repeat words or phrases and can't follow directions. His occasional speech is marked by paraphasias or jargon.
Wernicke's aphasia (receptive aphasia)	Wernicke's area; usually in posterior or superior temporal lobe	The patient has difficulty understanding written and spoken language. He can't repeat words or phrases and can't follow directions. His speech is fluent, but may be rapid and rambling, with paraphasias. He has difficulty naming objects (anomia) and is unaware of speech errors.

pairment. Take the patient's vital signs and assess his LOC. Recognize that dysarthria (impaired articulation due to weakness or paralysis of the muscles necessary for speech) or speech apraxia (inability to voluntarily control the muscles of speech) may accompany aphasia; therefore, speak slowly and distinctly, and allow the patient ample time to respond. Assess the patient's pupillary response, eye movements, and motor function, especially his mouth and tongue movement, swallowing ability, and spontaneous movements and gestures. To best assess motor function, first demonstrate the motions and then have the patient imitate them.

Medical causes

Alzheimer's disease. With Alzheimer's disease, anomic aphasia may begin insidiously and then progress to severe global aphasia. Associated signs and symptoms include behavioral changes, loss of memory, poor judgment, restlessness, myoclonus, and muscle rigidity. Incontinence is usually a late sign.

Brain abscess. Any type of aphasia may occur with brain abscess. Usually, aphasia develops insidiously and may be accompanied by hemiparesis, ataxia, facial weakness, and signs of increased ICP.

Brain tumor. A brain tumor may cause any type of aphasia. As the tumor enlarges, aphasia may occur along with behavioral changes, memory loss, motor weakness, seizures, auditory hallucinations, visual field deficits, and increased ICP.

Creutzfeldt-Jakob disease. Creutzfeldt-Jakob disease is a rapidly progressive dementia accompanied by neurologic signs and symptoms, such as myoclonic jerking, ataxia, aphasia, visual disturbances, and paralysis. It generally affects adults ages 40 to 65.

Encephalitis. Encephalitis usually produces transient aphasia. Its early signs and symptoms include fever, headache, and vomiting. Seizures, confusion, stupor or coma, hemiparesis, asymmetrical deep tendon reflexes, positive Babinski's reflex, ataxia, myoclonus, nystagmus, ocular palsies, and facial weakness may accompany aphasia.

Head trauma. Any type of aphasia may accompany severe head trauma; typically, it occurs suddenly and may be transient or permanent, depending on the extent of brain injury. Associated signs and symptoms include blurred or double vision, headache, pallor, diaphoresis, numbness and paresis, cerebrospinal otorrhea or rhinorrhea, altered respirations, tachycardia, disorientation, behavioral changes, and signs of increased ICP.

Seizures. Seizures and the postictal state may cause transient aphasia if the seizures involve the language centers.

Stroke. The most common cause of aphasia, stroke may produce Wernicke's, Broca's, or global aphasia. Associated findings include decreased LOC, hemiparesis, homonymous hemianopsia, paresthesia, and loss of sensation. Severe hypertension may also be present.

Transient ischemic attack. Transient ischemic attacks can produce any type of aphasia, which occurs suddenly and resolves within 24 hours of the attack. Associated signs and symptoms include transient hemiparesis, hemianopsia, and paresthesia (all usually right-sided), dizziness, and confusion.

Nursing considerations

- If the patient becomes confused or disoriented, help restore a sense of reality by frequently telling him what has happened, where he is and why, and what the date is.
- Expect periods of depression as the patient recognizes his disability.
- Help him to communicate by providing a relaxed, accepting environment with a minimum of distracting stimuli and providing an alternate method of communication, if possible.
- Be alert for sudden outbursts of profanity by the patient reflecting intense frustration with his impairment and deal with such outbursts as gently as possible to ease embarrassment.
- When you speak to the patient, don't assume that he understands you. He may simply be interpreting subtle clues to meaning, such as social context, facial expressions, and gestures.
- To help avoid misunderstanding, use nonverbal techniques, simple phrases, and demonstration to clarify your verbal directions.
- Remember that aphasia is a language disorder, not an emotional or auditory one, so speak to the patient in a normal tone of voice.
- Make sure that he has necessary aids, such as eyeglasses or dentures, to facilitate communication.
- Refer the patient to a speech pathologist to help him cope with and recover, as best as possible, from his aphasia.

Patient teaching

- Carefully explain diagnostic tests, such as skull X-rays, computed tomography scan or magnetic resonance imaging, angiography, and EEG.
- Explain the underlying disorder and treatment plan.
- Teach the patient alternate means of communication, if possible.
- Discuss risk reduction measures for stroke, such as not smoking, eating a healthy diet, exercising regularly, and blood pressure control.

Apnea

Apnea, the cessation of spontaneous respiration, is occasionally temporary and self-limiting, as occurs during Cheyne-Stokes and Biot's respirations. More commonly, it's a life-threatening emergency that requires immediate intervention to prevent death.

Apnea usually results from one or more of six pathophysiologic mechanisms, each of which has numerous causes. Its most common causes include trauma, cardiac arrest, neurologic disease, aspiration of foreign objects, bronchospasm, and drug overdose. (See *Causes of apnea.*)

ACTION STAT!

 If you detect apnea, first establish and maintain a patent airway. Position the patient in a supine position and open his airway using the head-tilt, chin-lift technique. (*Caution:* If the patient has an obvious or suspected head or neck injury, use the jaw-thrust technique to prevent hyperextending the neck.) Next, quickly look, listen, and feel for spontaneous respiration; if it's absent, begin artificial ventilation until it occurs or until mechanical ventilation can be initiated.

Because apnea may result from cardiac arrest (or may cause it), assess the patient's carotid pulse immediately after you've established a patent airway. If the patient is an infant or small child, assess the brachial pulse instead. If you can't palpate a pulse, begin cardiac compression.

History and physical examination

When the patient's respiratory and cardiac status is stable, investigate the underlying cause of apnea. Ask him (or, if he's unable to answer, anyone who witnessed the episode) about the onset of apnea and events immediately preceding it. The cause may be readily apparent, as in trauma.

Take a patient history, noting reports of headache, chest pain, muscle weakness, sore throat, or dyspnea. Ask about a history of respiratory, cardiac, or neurologic disease and about allergies and drug use.

Inspect the head, face, neck, and trunk for soft-tissue injury, hemorrhage, or skeletal deformity. Don't overlook obvious clues, such as oral and nasal secretions reflecting fluid-filled airways and alveoli or facial soot and singed nasal hair suggesting thermal injury to the tracheobronchial tree.

Auscultate all lung fields for adventitious breath sounds, particularly crackles and rhonchi, then percuss for increased dullness or hyperresonance. Next, auscultate the heart for murmurs, pericardial friction rub, and arrhythmias. Check for cyanosis, pallor, jugular vein distention, and edema. If appropriate, perform a neurologic assessment. Evaluate the patient's level of consciousness (LOC), orientation, and mental status; test cranial nerve function and motor function, sensation, and reflexes in all extremities.

Causes of apnea

Apnea may result from a variety of causes, including airway obstruction, brain stem dysfunction, neuromuscular failure, parenchymatous lung disease, pleural pressure gradient disruption, and a decrease in pulmonary capillary perfusion. Each of these causes of apnea can result from a variety of disorders.

Airway obstruction

- Asthma
- Bronchospasm
- Chronic bronchitis
- Chronic obstructive pulmonary disease
- Foreign body aspiration
- Hemothorax or pneumothorax
- Mucus plug
- Obstruction by tongue or tumor
- Obstructive sleep apnea
- Secretion retention
- Tracheal or bronchial rupture

Brain stem dysfunction

- Brain abscess
- Brain stem injury
- Brain tumor
- Central nervous system depressants
- Central sleep apnea
- Cerebral hemorrhage
- Cerebral infarction
- Encephalitis
- Head trauma
- Increased intracranial pressure
- Medullary or pontine hemorrhage or infarction
- Meningitis
- Transtentorial herniation

Neuromuscular failure

- Amyotrophic lateral sclerosis
- Botulism
- Diphtheria
- Guillain-Barré syndrome
- Myasthenia gravis
- Phrenic nerve paralysis
- Rupture of the diaphragm
- Spinal cord injury

Parenchymatous lung disease

- Acute respiratory distress syndrome
- Diffuse pneumonia
- Emphysema
- Near drowning
- Pulmonary edema
- Pulmonary fibrosis
- Secretion retention

Pleural pressure gradient disruption

- Flail chest
- Open chest wounds

Pulmonary capillary perfusion decrease

- Arrhythmias
- Cardiac arrest
- Myocardial infarction
- Pulmonary embolism
- Pulmonary hypertension
- Shock

Medical causes

Airway obstruction. Occlusion or compression of the trachea, central airways, or smaller airways can cause sudden apnea by blocking the patient's airflow and producing acute respiratory failure.

Brain stem dysfunction. Primary or secondary brain stem dysfunction can cause apnea by destroying the brain stem's ability to initiate respirations. Apnea may arise suddenly (as in trauma, hemorrhage, or infarction) or gradually (as in degenerative disease or tumor). Apnea may be preceded by a decreased LOC and by various motor and sensory deficits.

Neuromuscular failure. Trauma or disease can disrupt the mechanics of respiration, causing sudden or gradual apnea. Associated findings include diaphragmatic or intercostal muscle paralysis from injury or respiratory weakness or paralysis from acute or degenerative disease.

Parenchymatous lung disease. An accumulation of fluid within the alveoli produces apnea by interfering with pulmonary gas exchange and producing acute respiratory failure. Apnea may arise suddenly, as in near drowning and acute pulmonary edema, or gradually, as in emphysema. Apnea may be preceded by crackles and labored respirations with accessory muscle use.

Pleural pressure gradient disruption. Conversion of normal negative pleural air pressure to positive pressure by chest wall injuries (such as flail chest) causes lung collapse, producing respiratory distress and, if untreated, apnea. Associated signs include an asymmetrical chest wall and asymmetrical or paradoxical respirations.

Pulmonary capillary perfusion decrease. Apnea can stem from obstructed pulmonary circulation, most commonly due to heart failure or lack of circulatory patency. It occurs suddenly in cardiac arrest, massive pulmonary embolism, and most cases of severe shock. In contrast, it occurs progressively in septic shock and pulmonary hypertension. Related findings include hypotension, tachycardia, and edema.

Other causes

Drugs. Central nervous system (CNS) depressants may cause hypoventilation and apnea. Benzodiazepines may cause respiratory depression and apnea when given I.V. along with other CNS depressants to elderly or acutely ill patients. Drug overdose can lead to respiratory depression and apnea.

Neuromuscular blockers—such as curariform drugs and anticholinesteras-

es—may produce sudden apnea because of respiratory muscle paralysis.

Sleep-related apneas. These repetitive apneas occur during sleep from airflow obstruction or brain stem dysfunction.

Nursing considerations

- Closely monitor the patient's cardiac and respiratory status to prevent further episodes of apnea.
- Provide oxygen and ventilation as necessary, and monitor arterial blood gases and pulse oximetry for effectiveness.

Patient teaching

- Explain the underlying cause and treatment plan.
- Teach safety measures to reduce the risk of aspiration.
- Encourage the patient's family to learn cardiopulmonary resuscitation.
- Teach ways to decrease or avoid episodes of apnea, based on its cause.

Apneustic respirations

Apneustic respirations are characterized by prolonged, gasping inspiration, with a pause at full inspiration. This irregular breathing pattern is an important localizing sign of severe brain stem damage.

Involuntary breathing is primarily regulated by groups of neurons located in respiratory centers in the medulla oblongata and pons. In the medulla, neurons react to impulses from the pons and other areas to regulate respiratory rate and depth. In the pons, two respiratory centers regulate respiratory rhythm by interacting with the medullary respiratory center to smooth the transition from inspiration to expiration and back. The apneustic center in the pons stimulates inspiratory neurons in the medulla to precipitate inspiration. These inspiratory neurons, in turn, stimulate the pneumotaxic center in the pons to precipitate expiration. Destruction of neural pathways by pontine lesions disrupts normal regulation of respiratory rhythm, causing apneustic respirations.

Apneustic respirations must be differentiated from bradypnea and hyperpnea (disturbances in rate and depth, but not in rhythm), Cheyne-Stokes respirations (rhythmic alterations in rate and depth, followed by periods of apnea), and Biot's respirations (irregularly alternating periods of hyperpnea and apnea).

ACTION STAT!

 Your first priority for a patient with apneustic respirations is to ensure adequate ventilation. You'll need to insert an artificial airway and administer oxygen until mechanical ventilation can begin. Next, thoroughly evaluate the patient's neurologic status, using a standardized tool such as the Glasgow Coma Scale. Finally, obtain a brief patient history from a family member if possible.

Medical causes

Pontine lesions. Apneustic respirations usually result from extensive damage to the upper or lower pons due to infarction, hemorrhage, herniation, severe infection, tumor, or trauma. Typically, these respirations are accompanied by profound stupor or coma; pinpoint midline pupils; ocular bobbing (a spontaneous downward jerk, followed by a slow drift up to midline); quadriplegia or, less commonly, hemiplegia with the eyes pointing toward the weak side; a positive Babinski's reflex; negative oculocephalic and oculovestibular reflexes; and, possibly, decorticate posture.

Nursing considerations

- Monitor the patient's neurologic and respiratory status.

- Watch for prolonged periods of apnea or signs of neurologic deterioration.
- Monitor the patient's arterial blood gas levels and pulse oximetry.
- If appropriate, prepare him for neurologic tests, such as EEG and computed tomography scanning or magnetic resonance imaging.

Patient teaching
- Teach the patient and his family about his condition and treatment options.
- Explain all diagnostic tests and procedures.

Arm pain

Arm pain usually results from musculoskeletal disorders, but it can also stem from neurovascular or cardiovascular disorders. (See *Causes of local pain,* page 52.)

In some cases, it may be referred pain from another area, such as the chest, neck, or abdomen. Its location, onset, and character provide clues to its cause. The pain may affect the entire arm or only the upper arm or forearm. It may arise suddenly or gradually and may be constant or intermittent. Arm pain can be described as sharp or dull, burning or numbing, and shooting or penetrating. Diffuse arm pain may be difficult to describe, especially if it isn't associated with injury.

History and physical examination

If the patient reports arm pain after an injury, take a brief history of the injury from the patient. Quickly assess him for severe injuries requiring immediate treatment. If you've ruled out severe injuries, check pulses, capillary refill time, sensation, and movement distal to the affected area because circulatory impairment or nerve injury may require immediate surgery. Inspect the arm for defor-

Causes of local pain

Various disorders cause hand, wrist, elbow, or shoulder pain. In some disorders, pain may radiate from the injury site to other areas.

Hand pain
- Arthritis
- Buerger's disease
- Carpal tunnel syndrome
- Dupuytren's contracture
- Elbow tunnel syndrome
- Fracture
- Ganglion
- Infection
- Occlusive vascular disease
- Radiculopathy
- Raynaud's disease
- Shoulder-hand syndrome (reflex sympathetic dystrophy)
- Sprain or strain
- Thoracic outlet syndrome
- Trigger finger

Wrist pain
- Arthritis
- Carpal tunnel syndrome
- Fracture
- Ganglion
- Sprain or strain
- Tenosynovitis (de Quervain's disease)

Elbow pain
- Arthritis
- Bursitis
- Dislocation
- Fracture
- Lateral epicondylitis (tennis elbow)
- Tendinitis
- Ulnar neuritis

Shoulder pain
- Acromioclavicular separation
- Acute pancreatitis
- Adhesive capsulitis (frozen shoulder)
- Angina pectoris
- Arthritis
- Bursitis
- Cholecystitis or cholelithiasis
- Clavicle fracture
- Diaphragmatic pleurisy
- Dislocation
- Dissecting aortic aneurysm
- Gastritis
- Humeral neck fracture
- Infection
- Pancoast's syndrome
- Perforated ulcer
- Pneumothorax
- Ruptured spleen (left shoulder)
- Shoulder-hand syndrome
- Subphrenic abscess
- Tendinitis

mities, assess the level of pain, and immobilize the arm to prevent further injury.

If the patient reports continuous or intermittent arm pain, ask him to describe it and to relate when it began. Is the pain associated with repetitive or specific movements or positions? Ask him to point out other painful areas because arm pain may be referred. For example, arm pain commonly accompa-

nies the characteristic chest pain of myocardial infarction, and right shoulder pain may be referred from the right upper quadrant abdominal pain of cholecystitis. Ask the patient if the pain worsens in the morning or in the evening, if it prevents him from performing his job, and if it restricts movement. Ask if heat, rest, or drugs relieve it. Finally, ask about preexisting illnesses, a family history of gout or arthritis, and current drug therapy.

Next, perform a focused examination. Observe the way the patient walks, sits, and holds his arm. Inspect the entire arm, comparing it with the opposite arm for symmetry, movement, and muscle atrophy. (It's important to know if the patient is right- or left-handed.) Palpate the entire arm for swelling, nodules, and tender areas. In both arms, compare active range of motion, muscle strength, and reflexes.

If the patient reports numbness or tingling, check his sensation to vibration, temperature, and pinprick. Compare bilateral hand grasps and shoulder strength to detect weakness.

If a patient has a cast, splint, or restrictive dressing, check for circulation, sensation, and mobility distal to the dressing. Ask the patient about edema and if the pain has worsened within the last 24 hours.

Examine the neck for pain on motion, point tenderness, muscle spasms, or arm pain when the neck is extended with the head toward the involved side.

Medical causes

Angina. Angina may cause inner arm pain as well as chest and jaw pain. Typically, the pain follows exertion and persists for a few minutes. Accompanied by dyspnea, diaphoresis, and apprehension, the pain is relieved by rest or vasodilators such as nitroglycerin.

Biceps rupture. Rupture of the biceps after excessive weight lifting or osteoarthritic degeneration of bicipital tendon insertion at the shoulder can cause pain in the upper arm. Forearm flexion and supination aggravate the pain. Other signs and symptoms include muscle weakness, deformity, and edema.

Carpal tunnel syndrome. Median nerve compression in the carpal tendon of the wrist may cause numbness and

tingling in the fingers, along with increasing arm pain. Symptoms usually occur at night, but may increase over time with continued repetitive movement of the hand.

Cellulitis. Typically, cellulitis affects the legs, but it can also affect the arms. It produces pain as well as redness, tenderness, edema and, at times, fever, chills, tachycardia, headache, and hypotension. Cellulitis usually follows an injury or insect bite.

Cervical nerve root compression. Compression of the cervical nerves supplying the upper arm produces chronic arm and neck pain, which may worsen with movement or prolonged sitting. The patient may also experience muscle weakness, paresthesia, and decreased reflex response.

Compartment syndrome. Severe pain with passive muscle stretching is the cardinal symptom of compartment syndrome. It may also impair distal circulation and cause muscle weakness, decreased reflex response, paresthesia, and edema. Ominous signs include paralysis and an absent pulse.

Fractures. In fractures of the cervical vertebrae, humerus, scapula, clavicle, radius, or ulna, pain can occur at the injury site and radiate throughout the entire arm. Pain at a fresh fracture site is intense and worsens with movement. Associated signs and symptoms include crepitus, felt and heard from bone ends rubbing together (don't attempt to elicit this sign); deformity, if bones are misaligned; local ecchymosis and edema; impaired distal circulation; paresthesia; and decreased sensation distal to the injury site. Fractures of the small wrist bones can manifest with pain and swelling several days after the trauma.

Muscle contusion. Muscle contusion may cause generalized pain in the area of injury. It may also cause local swelling and ecchymosis.

Muscle strain. Acute or chronic muscle strain causes mild to severe pain with movement. The resultant reduction in arm movement may cause muscle weakness and atrophy.

Myocardial infarction (MI). MI is a life-threatening disorder in which the patient may complain of left arm pain as well as the characteristic deep and crushing chest pain. He may display weakness, pallor, nausea, vomiting, diaphoresis, altered blood pressure, tachycardia, dyspnea, and feelings of apprehension or impending doom.

Neoplasms of the arm. Neoplasms of the arm produce continuous, deep, and penetrating arm pain that worsens at night. Occasionally, redness and swelling accompany arm pain; later, skin breakdown, impaired circulation, and paresthesia may occur.

Osteomyelitis. Osteomyelitis typically begins with vague and evanescent localized arm pain and fever and is accompanied by local tenderness, painful and restricted movement and, later, swelling. Associated findings include malaise and tachycardia.

Nursing considerations

■ If you suspect a fracture, apply a sling or splint to immobilize the arm, and monitor the patient for worsening pain, numbness, or decreased circulation distal to the injury site.
■ Monitor the patient's vital signs, and be alert for tachycardia, hypotension, and diaphoresis.
■ Withhold food, fluids, and analgesics until potential fractures are evaluated.
■ Promote the patient's comfort by elevating his arm and applying ice.
■ Clean abrasions and lacerations and apply dry, sterile dressings, if necessary.
■ Prepare the patient for X-rays or other diagnostic tests.
■ Administer analgesics, as appropriate, and evaluate their effectiveness.

■ Treat the underlying cause, such as MI, appropriately.

Patient teaching

■ Explain the signs and symptoms of circulatory impairment caused by a tight cast that requires immediate treatment.
■ Discuss the signs and symptoms of an ischemic event.
■ Teach the patient about the cause of arm pain and the treatment plan after the diagnosis is determined.

Asterixis
[Liver flap, flapping tremor]

A bilateral, coarse movement, asterixis is characterized by sudden relaxation of muscle groups holding a sustained posture. This elicited sign is most commonly observed in the wrists and fingers, but may also appear during any sustained voluntary action. Typically, it signals hepatic, renal, or pulmonary disease.

History and physical examination

To elicit asterixis, have the patient extend his arms, dorsiflex his wrists, and spread his fingers (or do this for him if necessary). Briefly observe him for asterixis. Alternatively, if the patient has a decreased level of consciousness (LOC) but can follow verbal commands, ask him to squeeze two of your fingers. Consider rapid clutching and unclutching indications of asterixis, or elevate the patient's leg off the bed and dorsiflex the foot. Briefly check for asterixis in the ankle. If the patient can tightly close his eyes and mouth, watch for irregular tremulous movements of the eyelids and corners of the mouth. If he can stick out his tongue, observe the patient for continuous quivering. (See *Recognizing asterixis.*)

Because asterixis may signal serious metabolic deterioration, quickly evaluate the patient's neurologic status and vital signs. Compare this data with baseline measurements, and watch carefully for acute changes. Continue to closely monitor his neurologic status, vital signs, and urine output.

Watch for signs of respiratory insufficiency, and be prepared to provide endotracheal intubation and ventilatory support. Be alert for complications of end-stage hepatic, renal, or pulmonary disease.

Recognizing asterixis

With asterixis, the patient's wrists and fingers are observed to "flap" because there's a brief, rapid relaxation of dorsiflexion of the wrist.

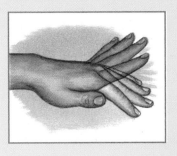

If the patient has hepatic disease, assess him for early indications of hemorrhage, including restlessness, tachypnea, and cool, moist, pale skin. If the patient is jaundiced, check for pallor in the conjunctiva and mucous membranes of the mouth.

It's important to recognize that hypotension, oliguria, hematemesis, and melena are late signs of hemorrhage. Prepare to insert a large-bore I.V. catheter for fluid and blood replacement. Position the patient flat in bed with his legs elevated 20 degrees. Begin or continue to administer oxygen.

If the patient has renal disease, briefly review the therapy he has received. If he's on dialysis, ask about the frequency of treatments to help gauge the severity of disease. Question a family member if the patient's LOC is significantly decreased.

Then assess the patient for hyperkalemia and metabolic acidosis. Look for tachycardia, nausea, diarrhea, abdominal cramps, muscle weakness, hyperreflexia, and Kussmaul's respirations. Prepare to administer sodium bicarbonate, calcium gluconate, dextrose, insulin, or sodium polystyrene sulfonate.

If the patient has pulmonary disease, check for labored respirations, tachypnea, accessory muscle use, and cyanosis, which are critical signs. Prepare to provide oxygen via nasal cannula, mask, or intubation and mechanical ventilation.

Medical causes

Hepatic encephalopathy. A life-threatening disorder, hepatic encephalopathy initially causes mild personality changes and a slight tremor. The tremor progresses into asterixis—a hallmark of hepatic encephalopathy—and is accompanied by lethargy, aberrant behavior, and apraxia. Eventually, the patient becomes stuporous and displays hyperventilation. When he slips into a coma, hyperactive reflexes, a positive Babinski's sign, and fetor hepaticus are characteristic signs. The patient may also experience bradycardia, decreased respirations, and seizures.

Severe respiratory insufficiency. Characterized by life-threatening respiratory acidosis, severe respiratory insufficiency initially produces headache, restlessness, confusion, apprehension, and decreased reflexes. Eventually, the patient becomes somnolent and may demonstrate asterixis before slipping into a coma. Associated signs and symptoms of respiratory insufficiency include difficulty breathing and rapid, shallow respirations. The patient may be hypertensive in early disease but hypotensive later.

Uremic syndrome. A life-threatening disorder, uremic syndrome initially causes lethargy, somnolence, confusion, disorientation, behavior changes, and irritability. Eventually, signs and symptoms appear in diverse body systems. Asterixis is accompanied by stupor, paresthesia, muscle twitching, fasciculations, and footdrop. Other signs and symptoms include polyuria and nocturia followed by oliguria and, then, anuria; elevated blood pressure; signs of heart failure and pericarditis; deep, gasping respirations (Kussmaul's respirations); anorexia; nausea; vomiting; diarrhea; GI bleeding; weight loss; ammonia breath odor; and metallic taste (dysgeusia).

Other causes
Drugs. Certain drugs, such as the anticonvulsant phenytoin, may cause asterixis.

Nursing considerations
■ Provide frequent rest periods to minimize fatigue.
■ Elevate the head of the bed to relieve dyspnea and orthopnea; administer oxygen therapy.
■ Administer oil baths and avoid soap to relieve itching caused by jaundice and uremia.
■ Provide emotional support to the patient and his family.
■ If the patient is intubated or has a decreased LOC, provide enteral or parenteral nutrition.
■ Closely monitor serum and urine glucose levels to evaluate hyperalimentation.

■ Because the patient will probably be on bed rest, reposition him at least once every 2 hours to prevent skin breakdown.
■ Because the patient's debilitated state makes him prone to infection, follow strict hand-washing and aseptic techniques when changing dressings and caring for invasive lines.
■ Discuss end-of-life issues, as appropriate.

Patient teaching
■ Explain the underlying disorder and treatment plan.
■ Teach the patient the importance of planning periods of rest.
■ Explain measures to relieve itching.
■ Discuss measures to reduce the risk of infection with the patient and his family.

Ataxia

Classified as cerebellar or sensory, ataxia refers to incoordination and irregularity of voluntary, purposeful movements. Cerebellar ataxia results from disease of the cerebellum and its pathways to and from the cerebral cortex, brain stem, and spinal cord. It causes gait, trunk, limb, and possibly speech disorders. Sensory ataxia results from impaired position sense (proprioception) due to the interruption of afferent nerve fibers in the peripheral nerves, posterior roots, posterior columns of the spinal cord, or medial lemnisci or, occasionally, caused by a lesion in both parietal lobes. It causes gait disorders. (See *Identifying ataxia.*)

Ataxia occurs in acute and chronic forms. Acute ataxia may result from stroke, hemorrhage, or a large tumor in the posterior fossa. With this life-threatening condition, the cerebellum may herniate downward through the foramen magnum behind the cervical spinal cord or upward through the tentorium

Identifying ataxia

Ataxia may be observed in the patient's speech, in the movements of his trunk and limbs, or in his gait.

Cerebellar ataxia

With cerebellar ataxia, the patient may stagger or lurch in zigzag fashion, turn with extreme difficulty, and lose his balance when his feet are together.

Gait ataxia

With gait ataxia, the patient's gait is wide-based, unsteady, and irregular.

Limb ataxia

With limb ataxia, the patient loses the ability to gauge distance, speed, and power of movement, resulting in poorly controlled, variable, and inaccurate voluntary movements. He may move too quickly or too slowly, or his movements may break down into component parts, giving him the appearance of a puppet or a robot. Other effects include a coarse, irregular tremor in purposeful movement (but not at rest) and reduced muscle tone.

Sensory ataxia

With sensory ataxia, the patient moves abruptly and stomps or taps his feet. This occurs because he throws his feet forward and outward, and then brings them down first on the heels and then on the toes. The patient also fixes his eyes on the ground, watching his steps. However, if he can't watch them, staggering worsens. When he stands with his feet together, he sways or loses his balance.

Speech ataxia

Speech ataxia is a form of dysarthria in which the patient typically speaks slowly and stresses usually unstressed words and syllables. Speech content is unaffected.

Truncal ataxia

Truncal ataxia is a disturbance in equilibrium in which the patient can't sit or stand without falling. Also, his head and trunk may bob and sway (titubation). If he can walk, his gait is reeling.

---

on the cerebral hemispheres. Herniation may also compress the brain stem. Acute ataxia may also result from drug toxicity or poisoning. Chronic ataxia can be progressive and, at times, can result from acute disease. It can also occur in metabolic and chronic degenerative neurologic disease.

If ataxic movements suddenly develop, examine the patient for signs of increased intracranial pressure and impending herniation. Determine his level of consciousness (LOC), and be alert for pupillary changes, motor weakness or paralysis, neck stiffness or pain, and vomiting.

Check his vital signs, especially respirations; abnormal respiratory patterns may quickly lead to respiratory arrest. Elevate the head of the bed. Have emergency resuscitation equipment readily available. Prepare the patient for a computed tomography scan or surgery.

History and physical examination

If the patient isn't in distress, review his history. Ask about multiple sclerosis, diabetes, central nervous system infection, neoplastic disease, previous stroke, and a family history of ataxia. Ask about chronic alcohol abuse or prolonged exposure to industrial toxins such as mercury. Find out if the patient's ataxia developed suddenly or gradually.

If necessary, perform Romberg's test to help distinguish between cerebellar and sensory ataxia. Instruct the patient to stand with his feet together and his arms at his side. Note his posture and balance, first with his eyes open, and then closed. Test results may indicate normal posture and balance (minimal swaying), cerebellar ataxia (swaying and inability to maintain balance with eyes open or closed), or sensory ataxia (increased swaying and inability to maintain balance with eyes closed). Stand close to the patient during this test to prevent his falling.

If you test for gait and limb ataxia, be aware that motor weakness may mimic ataxic movements, so check motor strength as well. Gait ataxia may be severe, even when limb ataxia is minimal. With gait ataxia, ask the patient if he tends to fall to one side, or if falling occurs more frequently at night. With truncal ataxia, remember that the patient's inability to walk or stand, combined with the absence of other signs while he's lying down, may give the impression of hysteria or drug or alcohol intoxication.

Medical causes

Cerebellar abscess. Cerebellar abscess commonly causes limb ataxia on the same side as the lesion as well as gait and truncal ataxia. Typically, the initial symptom is a headache localized behind the ear or in the occipital region, followed by oculomotor palsy, fever, vomiting, an altered LOC, and coma.

Cerebellar hemorrhage. With cerebellar hemorrhage, a life-threatening disorder, ataxia is usually acute but transient. Unilateral or bilateral ataxia affects the trunk, gait, or limbs. The patient initially experiences repeated vomiting, occipital headache, vertigo, oculomotor

palsy, dysphagia, and dysarthria. Later signs, such as a decreased LOC or coma, signal impending herniation.

Creutzfeldt-Jakob disease. Creutzfeldt-Jakob disease is a rapidly progressive dementia accompanied by neurologic signs and symptoms, such as myoclonic jerking, ataxia, aphasia, visual disturbances, and paralysis. It generally affects adults ages 40 to 65.

Diabetic neuropathy. Peripheral nerve damage due to diabetes mellitus may cause sensory ataxia, extremity pain, slight leg weakness, skin changes, and bowel and bladder dysfunction.

Diphtheria. Within 4 to 8 weeks of the onset of symptoms, a life-threatening neuropathy can produce sensory ataxia. Diphtheria can be accompanied by fever, paresthesia, and paralysis of the limbs and, sometimes, the respiratory muscles.

Encephalomyelitis. Encephalomyelitis is a complication of measles, smallpox, chickenpox, or rubella or of rabies or smallpox vaccination that may damage cerebrospinal white matter. Rarely, it's accompanied by cerebellar ataxia. Other signs and symptoms include headache, fever, vomiting, an altered LOC, paralysis, seizures, oculomotor palsy, and pupillary changes.

Friedreich's ataxia. Friedreich's ataxia affects the spinal cord and cerebellum and causes gait ataxia, followed by truncal, limb, and speech ataxia. Other signs and symptoms include pes cavus, kyphoscoliosis, cranial nerve palsy, and motor and sensory deficits. A positive Babinski's reflex may appear.

Guillain-Barré syndrome. Peripheral nerve involvement usually follows a mild viral infection, rarely leading to sensory ataxia. Guillain-Barré syndrome also causes ascending paralysis and possibly respiratory distress.

Hepatocerebral degeneration. Patients who survive hepatic coma are occasionally left with residual neurologic defects, including mild cerebellar ataxia with a wide-based, unsteady gait. Ataxia may be accompanied by an altered LOC, dysarthria, rhythmic arm tremors, and choreoathetosis of the face, neck, and shoulders.

Multiple sclerosis (MS). Nystagmus and cerebellar ataxia commonly occur in MS, but they aren't always accompanied by limb weakness and spasticity. Speech ataxia (especially scanning) may occur as well as sensory ataxia from spinal cord involvement. During remissions, ataxia may subside or may even disappear. During exacerbations, it may reappear, worsen, or even become permanent. MS also causes optic neuritis, optic atrophy, numbness and weakness, diplopia, dizziness, and bladder dysfunction.

Olivopontocerebellar atrophy. Olivopontocerebellar atrophy produces gait ataxia and, later, limb and speech ataxia. Rarely, it produces an intention tremor. It's accompanied by choreiform movements, dysphagia, and loss of sphincter tone.

Poisoning. Chronic arsenic poisoning may cause sensory ataxia, along with headache, seizures, an altered LOC, motor deficits, and muscle aching. Chronic mercury poisoning causes gait and limb ataxia, principally of the arms. It also causes tremors of the extremities, tongue, and lips; mental confusion; mood changes; and dysarthria.

Polyneuropathy. Carcinomatous and myelomatous polyneuropathy may occur before detection of the primary tumor in cancer, multiple myeloma, or Hodgkin's disease. Signs and symptoms include ataxia, severe motor weakness, muscle atrophy, and sensory loss in the limbs. Pain and skin changes may also occur.

Porphyria. Porphyria affects the sensory and, more frequently, the motor nerves, possibly leading to ataxia. It also causes abdominal pain, mental disturbances, vomiting, headache, focal neurologic defects, an altered LOC, generalized seizures, and skin lesions.

Posterior fossa tumor. Gait, truncal, or limb ataxia is an early sign and may worsen as the tumor enlarges. It's accompanied by vomiting, headache, papilledema, vertigo, oculomotor palsy, a decreased LOC, and motor and sensory impairments on the same side as the lesion.

Spinocerebellar ataxia. With spinocerebellar ataxia, the patient may initially experience fatigue, followed by stiff-legged gait ataxia. Eventually, limb ataxia, dysarthria, static tremor, nystagmus, cramps, paresthesia, and sensory deficits occur.

Stroke. In stroke, occlusions in the vertebrobasilar arteries halt blood flow to cause infarction in the medulla, pons, or cerebellum that may lead to ataxia. Ataxia may occur at the onset of stroke and remain as a residual deficit. Worsening ataxia during the acute phase may indicate extension of the stroke or severe swelling. Ataxia may be accompanied by unilateral or bilateral motor weakness, a possible altered LOC, sensory loss, vertigo, nausea, vomiting, oculomotor palsy, and dysphagia.

Wernicke's disease. Wernicke's disease produces gait ataxia and, rarely, intention tremor or speech ataxia. With severe ataxia, the patient may be unable to stand or walk. Ataxia decreases with thiamine therapy. Associated signs and symptoms include nystagmus, diplopia, ocular palsies, confusion, tachycardia, exertional dyspnea, and orthostatic hypotension.

Other causes

Drugs. Toxic levels of anticonvulsants, especially phenytoin, may result in gait ataxia. Toxic levels of anticholinergics and tricyclic antidepressants may also result in ataxia. Aminoglutethimide causes ataxia in about 10% of patients; this effect usually disappears 4 to 6 weeks after drug therapy is discontinued.

Nursing considerations

- Prepare the patient for laboratory studies, such as blood tests for toxic drug levels and radiologic tests.
- If toxic drug levels are the cause, stop the drug.
- Encourage physical therapy to improve function following a stroke.
- If the patient has a brain tumor, prepare him for surgery, chemotherapy, or radiation therapy.

Patient teaching

- Explain the underlying cause and treatment plan.
- Teach the patient and family about ways to promote safety, such as providing a cane or walker for extra support and moving slowly, especially when turning or getting up from a chair.
- Ask the patient's family to check his home for hazards, such as uneven surfaces or the absence of handrails on stairs.
- If appropriate, refer the patient with progressive disease for counseling.

Aura

An aura is a sensory or motor phenomenon, idea, or emotion that marks the initial stage of a seizure or the approach of a classic migraine headache. Auras may be classified as cognitive, affective, psychosensory, or psychomotor. (See *Recognizing types of auras.*)

When associated with a seizure, an aura stems from an irritable focus in the brain that spreads throughout the cortex. Although an aura was once considered a sign of impending seizure, it's now considered the first stage of a

seizure. Typically, it occurs seconds to minutes before the ictal phase. Its intensity, duration, and type depend on the origin of the irritable focus. For example, an aura of bitter taste commonly accompanies a frontal lobe lesion. Unfortunately, an aura is difficult to describe because the postictal phase of a seizure temporarily alters the patient's level of consciousness and may impair his memory of the event.

The aura associated with a classic migraine headache results from cranial blood vessel vasoconstriction. Diagnostically important, it helps distinguish a classic migraine from other types of headaches.

Typically, an aura develops over 10 to 30 minutes and varies in intensity and duration. If the patient recognizes the aura as a warning sign, he may be able to prevent the migraine by taking appropriate drugs.

ACTION STAT!

 When an aura rapidly progresses to the ictal phase of a seizure, quickly evaluate the seizure and be alert for life-threatening complications such as apnea. When an aura heralds a classic migraine, make the patient as comfortable as possible. Place him in a dark, quiet room and administer drugs to prevent the headache if necessary.

History and physical examination

Obtain a thorough history of the patient's headache or seizure history, asking him to describe any sensory or motor phenomena that precede each headache or seizure. Find out how long each headache or seizure typically lasts. Does anything make it worse, such as bright lights, noise, or caffeine? Does anything make it better? Ask the patient about drugs he takes for pain relief.

Recognizing types of auras

Determining whether an aura marks the patient's thought processes, emotions, or sensory or motor function usually requires keen observation. An aura is typically difficult to describe and is only dimly remembered when associated with seizure activity. Here you'll find the types of auras the patient may experience.

Affective auras
- Fear
- Paranoia
- Other emotions

Cognitive auras
- Déjà vu (familiarity with unfamiliar events or environments)
- Flashback of past events
- *Jamais vu* (unfamiliarity with a known event)
- Time standing still

Psychomotor auras
- Automatisms (inappropriate, repetitive movements): lip smacking, chewing, swallowing, grimacing, picking at clothes, climbing stairs

Psychosensory auras
- Auditory: buzzing or ringing in the ears
- Gustatory: acidic, metallic, or bitter tastes
- Olfactory: foul odors
- Tactile: numbness or tingling
- Vertigo
- Visual: flashes of light (scintillations)

Then perform a complete neurologic examination.

Medical causes

Classic migraine headache. A migraine is preceded by a vague premonition and then, usually, a visual aura involving flashes of light. The aura lasts 10 to 30 minutes and may intensify until it completely obscures the patient's vision. A classic migraine may cause numbness or tingling of the lips, face, or hands; slight confusion; and dizziness before the characteristic unilateral, throbbing headache appears. It slowly intensifies; when it peaks, it may cause photophobia, nausea, and vomiting.

Seizure, generalized tonic-clonic. A generalized tonic-clonic seizure may begin with or without an aura. The patient loses consciousness and falls to the ground. His body stiffens (tonic phase), and then he experiences rapid, synchronous muscle jerking and hyperventilation (clonic phase). The seizure usually lasts 2 to 5 minutes.

Nursing considerations

- Advise the patient to keep a diary of factors that precipitate each headache or seizure as well as associated symptoms to help you evaluate the effectiveness of drug therapy and recommend lifestyle changes.

Patient teaching

- Teach the patient stress-reduction measures.
- If the patient recognizes the aura as a warning sign, tell him to prevent the headache by taking appropriate medications.
- Explain diagnostic tests or procedures.
- Explain the underlying disorder and treatment plan.
- If the patient has a seizure disorder, emphasize the importance of taking anticonvulsants as directed.
- Stress the importance of regular follow-up appointments for blood studies.

B

Babinski's reflex
[Extensor plantar reflex]

Babinski's reflex—dorsiflexion of the great toe with extension and fanning of the other toes—is an abnormal reflex elicited by firmly stroking the lateral aspect of the sole with a moderately sharp object. (See *Eliciting Babinski's reflex.*)

In some patients, this reflex can be triggered by noxious stimuli, such as pain, noise, or even bumping the bed. An indicator of corticospinal damage, Babinski's reflex may occur unilaterally or bilaterally and may be temporary or permanent. A temporary Babinski's reflex commonly occurs during the postictal phase of a seizure, whereas a perma-

 Eliciting Babinski's reflex

To elicit Babinski's reflex, stroke the lateral aspect of the sole of the patient's foot with your thumbnail or another moderately sharp object. Normally, this elicits flexion of all toes (a negative Babinski's reflex), as shown below in the left illustration. With a positive Babinski's reflex, the great toe dorsiflexes and the other toes fan out, as shown in the right illustration.

Normal toe flexion

Positive Babinski's reflex

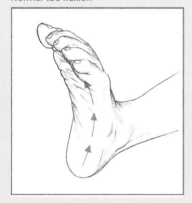 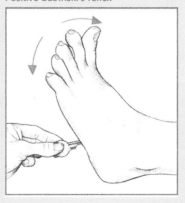

nent Babinski's reflex occurs with corticospinal damage. A positive Babinski's reflex is normal in neonates and in infants up to 24 months old.

History and physical examination

After eliciting a positive Babinski's reflex, evaluate the patient for other neurologic signs. Evaluate muscle strength in each extremity by having the patient push or pull against your resistance. Passively flex and extend the extremity to assess muscle tone. Intermittent resistance to flexion and extension indicates spasticity, and a lack of resistance indicates flaccidity.

Next, check for evidence of incoordination by asking the patient to perform a repetitive activity. Test deep tendon reflexes (DTRs) in the patient's elbow, antecubital area, wrist, knee, and ankle by striking the tendon with a reflex hammer. An exaggerated muscle response indicates hyperactive DTRs; little or no muscle response indicates hypoactivity.

Then evaluate pain sensation and proprioception in the feet. As you move the patient's toes up and down, ask the patient to identify the direction in which the toes have been moved without looking at his feet.

Obtain a complete medical and surgical history as well as a complete drug history.

Medical causes

Amyotrophic lateral sclerosis (ALS). With this progressive motor neuron disorder, bilateral Babinski's reflex may occur with hyperactive DTRs and spasticity. Typically, ALS produces fasciculations accompanied by muscle atrophy and weakness. Incoordination makes carrying out activities of daily living difficult for the patient. Associated signs and symptoms include impaired speech; difficulty chewing, swallowing, and breathing; urinary frequency and urgency; and, occasionally, choking and excessive drooling. Although his mental status remains intact, the patient's poor prognosis may cause periodic depression. Progressive bulbar palsy involves the brain stem and may cause episodes of crying or inappropriate laughter.

Brain tumor. A brain tumor that involves the corticospinal tract may produce Babinski's reflex. The reflex may be accompanied by hyperactive DTRs (unilateral or bilateral), spasticity, seizures, cranial nerve dysfunction, hemiparesis or hemiplegia, decreased pain sensation, an unsteady gait, incoordination, headache, emotional lability, and a decreased level of consciousness (LOC).

Head trauma. Unilateral or bilateral Babinski's reflex may occur as the result of primary corticospinal damage or secondary injury associated with increased intracranial pressure. Hyperactive DTRs and spasticity commonly occur with Babinski's reflex. The patient may also have weakness and incoordination. Other signs and symptoms vary with the type of head trauma and include headache, vomiting, behavior changes, altered vital signs, and decreased LOC with abnormal pupillary size and response to light.

Hepatic encephalopathy. Babinski's reflex occurs late in hepatic encephalopathy when the patient slips into a coma. It's accompanied by hyperactive DTRs and fetor hepaticus.

Meningitis. With meningitis, bilateral Babinski's reflex commonly follows fever, chills, and malaise and is accompanied by nausea and vomiting. As meningitis progresses, it also causes decreased LOC, nuchal rigidity, positive Brudzinski's and Kernig's signs, hyperactive DTRs, and opisthotonos. Associated signs and symptoms include irritability, photophobia, diplopia, delirium, and deep stupor that may progress to coma.

Rabies. Bilateral Babinski's reflex—possibly elicited by nonspecific noxious stimuli alone—appears in the excitation phase of rabies. This phase occurs 2 to 10 days after the onset of prodromal signs and symptoms, such as fever, malaise, and irritability (which occur 30 to 40 days after a bite from an infected animal). Rabies is characterized by marked restlessness and extremely painful pharyngeal muscle spasms. Difficulty swallowing causes excessive drooling and hydrophobia in about 50% of affected patients. Seizures and hyperactive DTRs may also occur.

Spinal cord injury. With acute injury, spinal shock temporarily erases all reflexes. As shock resolves, Babinski's reflex occurs—unilaterally when injury affects only one side of the spinal cord (Brown-Séquard's syndrome), bilaterally when injury affects both sides. Rather than signaling the return of neurologic function, this reflex confirms corticospinal damage. It's accompanied by hyperactive DTRs, spasticity, and variable or total loss of pain and temperature sensation, proprioception, and motor function. Horner's syndrome, marked by unilateral ptosis, pupillary constriction, and facial anhidrosis, may occur with lower cervical cord injury.

Spinal cord tumor. With spinal cord tumor, bilateral Babinski's reflex occurs with variable loss of pain and temperature sensation, proprioception, and motor function. Spasticity, hyperactive DTRs, absent abdominal reflexes, and incontinence are also characteristic. Diffuse pain may occur at the level of the tumor.

Spinal paralytic poliomyelitis. Unilateral or bilateral Babinski's reflex occurs 5 to 7 days after the onset of fever. It's accompanied by progressive weakness, paresthesia, muscle tenderness, spasticity, irritability and, later, atrophy. Resistance to neck flexion is characteris-

tic, as are Hoyne's, Kernig's, and Brudzinski's signs.

Spinal tuberculosis. Spiral tuberculosis may produce bilateral Babinski's reflex accompanied by variable loss of pain and temperature sensation, proprioception, and motor function. It also causes spasticity, hyperactive DTRs, bladder incontinence, and absent abdominal reflexes.

Stroke. Babinski's reflex varies with the site of the stroke. If it involves the cerebrum, it produces unilateral Babinski's reflex accompanied by hemiplegia or hemiparesis, unilateral hyperactive DTRs, hemianopsia, and aphasia. If it involves the brain stem, it produces bilateral Babinski's reflex accompanied by bilateral weakness or paralysis, bilateral hyperactive DTRs, cranial nerve dysfunction, incoordination, and an unsteady gait. Generalized signs and symptoms of stroke include headache, vomiting, fever, disorientation, nuchal rigidity, seizures, and coma.

Syringomyelia. With syringomyelia, bilateral Babinski's reflex occurs with muscle atrophy and weakness that may progress to paralysis. It's accompanied by spasticity, ataxia and, occasionally, deep pain. DTRs may be hypoactive or hyperactive. Cranial nerve dysfunction, such as dysphagia and dysarthria, commonly appears late in the disorder.

Nursing considerations

■ Because Babinski's reflex usually occurs with incoordination, weakness, and spasticity, all of which increase the patient's risk of injury, assist the patient with activity and keep his environment free from obstructions.

■ Prepare the patient for diagnostic tests, such as a computed tomography scan or magnetic resonance imaging of the brain or spine, angiography or myelography and, possibly, a lumbar puncture to clarify or confirm the cause of Babinski's reflex.

Patient teaching

- Caution the patient about the need to call for assistance when getting out of bed.
- Discuss ways to maintain a safe environment.
- Instruct the patient in the use of adaptive devices.
- Explain diagnostic tests and procedures.
- Teach the patient about the disorder and treatment plan after a diagnosis is established.

▌Back pain

Back pain affects an estimated 80% of the population; in fact, it's the second leading reason—after the common cold—for lost time from work. Although this symptom may herald a spondylogenic disorder, it may also result from a genitourinary, GI, cardiovascular, or neoplastic disorder or from trauma or injury. Postural imbalance associated with pregnancy may also cause back pain.

The onset, location, and distribution of pain and its response to activity and rest provide important clues about the cause. Pain may be acute or chronic, constant or intermittent. It may remain localized in the back or radiate along the spine or down one or both legs. Pain may be exacerbated by activity—usually bending, stooping, lifting, or exercising—and alleviated by rest, or it may be unaffected by either.

Intrinsic back pain results from muscle spasm, nerve root irritation, fracture, or a combination of these mechanisms. It usually occurs in the lower back, or lumbosacral area. Back pain may also be referred from the abdomen or flank, possibly signaling a life-threatening per-

forated ulcer, acute pancreatitis, or a dissecting abdominal aortic aneurysm.

 If the patient reports acute, severe back pain, quickly take his vital signs, and then perform a rapid evaluation to rule out life-threatening causes. Ask him when the pain began. Can he relate it to any causes? For example, did the pain occur after eating? After falling on the ice? Have the patient describe the pain. Is it burning, stabbing, throbbing, or aching? Is it constant or intermittent? Does it radiate to the buttocks or legs? Does he have leg weakness? Does the pain seem to originate in the abdomen and radiate to the back? Has he had a pain like this before? What makes it better or worse? Is it affected by activity or rest? Is it worse in the morning or evening? Does it wake him up? Typically, visceral-referred back pain is unaffected by activity and rest. In contrast, spondylogenic-referred back pain worsens with activity and improves with rest. Pain of neoplastic origin is usually relieved by walking and worsens at night.

If the patient describes deep lumbar pain unaffected by activity, palpate for a pulsating epigastric mass. If this sign is present, suspect a dissecting abdominal aortic aneurysm. Withhold food and fluid in anticipation of emergency surgery. Prepare for I.V. fluid replacement and oxygen administration. Monitor the patient's vital signs and peripheral pulses closely.

If the patient describes severe epigastric pain that radiates through the abdomen to the back, assess him for absent bowel sounds and for abdominal rigidity and tenderness. If these occur, suspect a perforated ulcer or acute pancreatitis. Insert an I.V. catheter for fluid and drug replacement, administer oxygen, and insert a nasogastric tube while withholding food.

History and physical examination

If life-threatening causes of back pain are ruled out, continue with a complete history and physical examination. Be aware of the patient's expressions of pain as you do so. Obtain a medical history, including past injuries, surgeries, and illnesses, and a family history. Ask about diet and alcohol intake. Take a drug history, including past and present prescriptions, over-the-counter drugs, and herbal medicines. Ask the patient to rate the pain according to a pain scale and describe the type and location of his pain.

Next, perform a thorough physical examination. Observe skin color, especially in the patient's legs, and palpate skin temperature. Palpate femoral, popliteal, posterior tibial, and pedal pulses. Ask about unusual sensations in the legs, such as numbness and tingling. Observe the patient's posture if pain doesn't prohibit standing. Does he stand erect or tend to lean toward one side? Observe the level of the shoulders and pelvis and the curvature of the back. Ask the patient to bend forward, backward, and from side to side while you palpate for paravertebral muscle spasms. Note rotation of the spine on the trunk. Palpate the dorsolumbar spine for point tenderness. Then ask the patient to walk—first on his heels, then on his toes; protect him from falling as he does so. Weakness may reflect a muscular disorder or spinal nerve root irritation. Place the patient in a sitting position to evaluate and compare patellar tendon (knee), Achilles tendon, and Babinski's reflexes. Evaluate the strength of the extensor hallucis longus by asking the patient to hold up his big toe against re-

sistance. Measure leg length and hamstring and quadriceps muscles bilaterally. Note a difference of more than $3/8''$ (1 cm) in muscle size, especially in the calf.

To reproduce leg and back pain, position the patient in a supine position on the examining table. Grasp his heel and slowly lift his leg. If he feels pain, note its exact location and the angle between the table and his leg when it occurs. Repeat this maneuver with the opposite leg. Pain along the sciatic nerve may indicate disk herniation or sciatica. Note the range of motion of the hip and knee.

Palpate the flanks and percuss with the fingertips or perform fist percussion to elicit costovertebral angle tenderness.

Medical causes
Abdominal aortic aneurysm (dissecting). Life-threatening dissection of this type of aneurysm may initially cause low back pain or dull abdominal pain. More commonly, it produces constant upper abdominal pain. A pulsating abdominal mass may be palpated in the epigastrium; after rupture, however, it no longer pulses. Aneurysmal dissection can also cause mottled skin below the waist, absent femoral and pedal pulses, lower blood pressure in the legs than in the arms, mild to moderate tenderness with guarding, and abdominal rigidity. Signs of shock (such as cool, clammy skin) appear if blood loss is significant.

Ankylosing spondylitis. Ankylosing spondylitis causes sacroiliac pain, which radiates up the spine and is aggravated by lateral pressure on the pelvis. The pain is usually most severe in the morning or after a period of inactivity and isn't relieved by rest. Abnormal rigidity of the lumbar spine with forward flexion is also characteristic. This disorder can cause local tenderness, fatigue, fever, anorexia, weight loss, and occasional iritis.

Appendicitis. Appendicitis is a life-threatening disorder in which a vague and dull discomfort in the epigastric or umbilical region migrates to McBurney's point in the right lower quadrant. With retrocecal appendicitis, pain may also radiate to the back. The shift in pain is preceded by anorexia and nausea and is accompanied by fever, occasional vomiting, abdominal tenderness (especially over McBurney's point), and rebound tenderness. Some patients also have painful, urgent urination.

Cholecystitis. Cholecystitis produces severe pain in the right upper quadrant of the abdomen that may radiate to the right shoulder, chest, or back. The pain may arise suddenly or may increase gradually over several hours, and patients usually have a history of similar pain after a high-fat meal. Accompanying signs and symptoms include anorexia, fever, nausea, vomiting, right upper quadrant tenderness, abdominal rigidity, pallor, and sweating.

Chordoma. A slow-developing malignant tumor, chordoma causes persistent pain in the lower back, sacrum, and coccyx. As the tumor expands, pain may be accompanied by constipation and bowel or bladder incontinence.

Endometriosis. Endometriosis causes deep sacral pain and severe, cramping pain in the lower abdomen. The pain worsens just before or during menstruation and may be aggravated by defecation. It's accompanied by constipation, abdominal tenderness, dysmenorrhea, and dyspareunia.

Intervertebral disk rupture. Intervertebral disk rupture produces gradual or sudden low back pain with or without leg pain (sciatica). It rarely produces leg pain alone. Pain usually begins in the back and radiates to the buttocks and leg. The pain is exacerbated by activity, coughing, and sneezing and is eased by rest. It's accompanied by paresthesia

(most commonly, numbness or tingling in the lower leg and foot), paravertebral muscle spasm, and decreased reflexes on the affected side. This disorder also affects posture and gait. The patient's spine is slightly flexed and he leans toward the painful side. He walks slowly and rises from a sitting to a standing position with extreme difficulty.

Lumbosacral sprain. Lumbosacral sprain causes aching, localized pain and tenderness associated with muscle spasm on lateral motion. The recumbent patient typically flexes his knees and hips to help ease pain. Flexion of the spine intensifies pain, whereas rest helps relieve it. The pain worsens with movement and is relieved by rest.

Metastatic tumors. Metastatic tumors commonly spread to the spine, causing low back pain in at least 25% of patients. Typically, the pain begins abruptly, is accompanied by cramping muscular pain (usually worse at night), and isn't relieved by rest.

Myeloma. Back pain caused by myeloma, a primary malignant tumor, usually begins abruptly and worsens with exercise. It may be accompanied by arthritic signs and symptoms, such as achiness, joint swelling, and tenderness. Other signs and symptoms include fever, malaise, peripheral paresthesia, and weight loss.

Pancreatitis (acute). Pancreatitis is a life-threatening disorder that usually produces fulminating, continuous upper abdominal pain that may radiate to both flanks and to the back. To relieve this pain, the patient may bend forward, draw his knees to his chest, or move restlessly about.

Early associated signs and symptoms include abdominal tenderness, nausea, vomiting, fever, pallor, tachycardia and, in some patients, abdominal guarding, rigidity, rebound tenderness, and hypoactive bowel sounds. A late sign may be jaundice. Occurring as inflammation subsides, Turner's sign (ecchymosis of the abdomen or flank) or Cullen's sign (bluish discoloration of skin around the umbilicus and in both flanks) signals hemorrhagic pancreatitis.

Perforated ulcer. In some patients, perforation of a duodenal or gastric ulcer causes sudden, prostrating epigastric pain that may radiate throughout the abdomen and to the back. This life-threatening disorder also causes board-like abdominal rigidity, tenderness with guarding, generalized rebound tenderness, the absence of bowel sounds, and grunting, shallow respirations. Associated signs include fever, tachycardia, and hypotension.

Prostate cancer. Chronic aching back pain may be the only symptom of prostate cancer. This disorder may also produce hematuria and decrease the urine stream.

Pyelonephritis (acute). Pyelonephritis produces progressive flank and lower abdominal pain accompanied by back pain or tenderness (especially over the costovertebral angle). Other signs and symptoms include high fever and chills, nausea and vomiting, flank and abdominal tenderness, and urinary frequency and urgency.

Renal calculi. The colicky pain of renal calculi usually results from irritation of the ureteral lining, which increases the frequency and force of peristaltic contractions. The pain travels from the costovertebral angle to the flank, suprapubic region, and external genitalia. Its intensity varies but may become excruciating if calculi travel down a ureter. If calculi are in the renal pelvis and calyces, dull and constant flank pain may occur. Renal calculi also cause nausea, vomiting, urinary urgency (if a calculus lodges near the bladder), hematuria, and agitation due to pain. Pain resolves or significantly decreases after calculi move

to the bladder. Encourage the patient to recover the calculi for analysis.

Rift Valley fever. Rift Valley fever may present as several different clinical syndromes. Typical signs and symptoms include fever, myalgia, weakness, dizziness, and back pain. A small percentage of patients may develop encephalitis or may progress·to hemorrhagic fever that can lead to shock and hemorrhage. Inflammation of the retina may result in some permanent vision loss.

Sacroiliac strain. Sacroiliac strain causes sacroiliac pain that may radiate to the buttock, hip, and lateral aspect of the thigh. The pain is aggravated by weight bearing on the affected extremity and by abduction with resistance of the leg. Associated signs and symptoms include tenderness of the symphysis pubis and a limp or gluteus medius or abductor lurch.

Smallpox (variola major). Initial signs and symptoms of smallpox include high fever, malaise, prostration, severe headache, backache, and abdominal pain. A maculopapular rash develops on the mucosa of the mouth, pharynx, face, and forearms and then spreads to the trunk and legs. Within 2 days the rash becomes vesicular and later pustular. The lesions develop at the same time, appear identical, and are more prominent on the face and extremities. The pustules are round, firm, and deeply embedded in the skin. After 8 to 9 days, the pustules form a crust, and later the scab separates from the skin, leaving a pitted scar. In fatal cases, death results from encephalitis, extensive bleeding, or secondary infection.

Spinal neoplasm (benign). Spinal neoplasm typically causes severe, localized back pain and scoliosis.

Spinal stenosis. Resembling a ruptured intervertebral disk, spinal stenosis produces back pain with or without sciatica, which commonly affects both legs.

The pain may radiate to the toes and may progress to numbness or weakness unless the patient rests.

Spondylolisthesis. A major structural disorder characterized by forward slippage of one vertebra onto another, spondylolisthesis may be asymptomatic or may cause low back pain, with or without nerve root involvement. Associated symptoms of nerve root involvement include paresthesia, buttock pain, and pain radiating down the leg. Palpation of the lumbar spine may reveal a "step-off" of the spinous process. Flexion of the spine may be limited.

Transverse process fracture. Transverse process fracture causes severe localized back pain with muscle spasm and hematoma.

Vertebral compression fracture. Initially, vertebral compression fracture may be painless. Several weeks later, it causes back pain aggravated by weight bearing and local tenderness. Fracture of a thoracic vertebra may cause referred pain in the lumbar area.

Vertebral osteomyelitis. Initially, vertebral osteomyelitis causes insidious back pain. As it progresses, the pain may become constant, more pronounced at night, and aggravated by spinal movement. Accompanying signs and symptoms include vertebral and hamstring spasms, tenderness of the spinous processes, fever, and malaise.

Vertebral osteoporosis. Vertebral osteoporosis causes chronic, aching back pain that is aggravated by activity and somewhat relieved by rest. Tenderness may also occur.

Other causes

Neurologic tests. Lumbar puncture and myelography can produce transient back pain.

Nursing considerations

- Monitor the patient closely if the back pain suggests a life-threatening cause.
- Be alert for increasing pain, altered neurovascular status in the legs, loss of bowel or bladder control, altered vital signs, sweating, and cyanosis.
- Withhold food and fluids in case surgery is necessary.
- Administer analgesics, as ordered, and evaluate their effect.
- Make the patient as comfortable as possible by elevating the head of the bed and placing a pillow under his knees.
- Encourage relaxation techniques such as deep breathing.
- Anticipate diagnostic testing, such as routine blood tests, urinalysis, a computed tomography scan, magnetic resonance imaging, appropriate biopsies, and X-rays of the chest, abdomen, and spine.
- Fit the patient for a corset or lumbosacral support.
- Provide heat or cold therapy, a backboard, a convoluted foam mattress, or pelvic traction, as ordered.
- Refer the patient to other professionals, such as a physical therapist, an occupational therapist, or a psychologist, if indicated.

Patient teaching

- Explain pain-relief measures to the patient.
- Teach him about alternatives to analgesic drug therapy, such as biofeedback and transcutaneous electrical nerve stimulation.
- Provide information about use of anti-inflammatory drugs and analgesics.
- Discuss lifestyle changes, such as weight loss or correcting posture.
- Teach relaxation techniques such as deep breathing.
- Instruct the patient on correct use of corset or lumbosacral support.

- Explain diagnostic tests and procedures.
- Teach the patient about the cause of his back pain and the treatment plan.

Barrel chest

In barrel chest, the normal elliptical configuration of the chest is replaced by a rounded one in which the anteroposterior diameter enlarges to approximate the transverse diameter. The diaphragm is depressed and the sternum pushed forward with the ribs attached in a horizontal, not angular, fashion. As a result, the chest appears continuously in the inspiratory position. (See *Recognizing barrel chest.*)

Typically a late sign of chronic obstructive pulmonary disease (COPD), barrel chest results from augmented lung volumes due to chronic airflow obstruction. The patient may not notice it because it develops gradually.

History and physical examination

Begin by asking about a history of pulmonary disease. Note chronic exposure to environmental irritants such as asbestos. Ask about the patient's smoking habits.

Then explore other signs and symptoms of pulmonary disease. Does the patient have a cough? Is it productive or nonproductive? If it's productive, have him describe the sputum's color and consistency. Does the patient experience shortness of breath? Is it related to activity? Although dyspnea is common with COPD, many patients fail to associate it with the disease. Instead, they blame "old age" or "getting out of shape" for causing dyspnea.

Auscultate for abnormal breath sounds, such as crackles and wheezing. Then percuss the chest. Hyperresonant sounds indicate trapped air; dull or flat sounds indicate mucus buildup. Be alert for accessory muscle use, intercostal retractions, and tachypnea, which may signal respiratory distress.

Finally, observe the patient's general appearance. Look for central cyanosis in the cheeks, nose, and mucosa inside the lips. In addition, look for peripheral cyanosis in the nail beds. Also note clubbing of the nail beds, a late sign of COPD.

Medical causes

Asthma. Typically, barrel chest develops only in chronic asthma. An acute asthma attack causes severe dyspnea, wheezing, and a productive cough. It can also cause prolonged expiratory time, accessory muscle use, tachycardia, tachypnea, perspiration, and flushing.

Chronic bronchitis. Barrel chest is a late sign in chronic bronchitis. This form of COPD may also cause productive cough, exertional dyspnea, cyanosis, tachypnea, wheezing, prolonged expiratory time, and accessory muscle use.

Emphysema. Barrel chest is a late sign in this form of COPD. Typically, emphysema begins insidiously, with dyspnea the predominant symptom. Eventually, it may cause chronic cough, anorexia, weight loss, malaise, accessory muscle use, pursed-lip breathing, tachypnea, peripheral cyanosis, and clubbing of the nail beds.

Osteoarthritis. Osteoarthritis of the rib and spine joints may cause rigidity of the chest wall, fixing the rib cage in the inhale position. Other signs and symptoms include joint pain that worsens after exercise, joint swelling, impaired movement, and stiffness in the morning.

Nursing considerations

- To ease breathing, have the patient sit and lean forward, resting his hands on his knees to support the upper torso (tripod position), thus allowing maxi-

Recognizing barrel chest

You can determine whether your patient has a normal chest or a barrel chest by looking at the anteroposterior and transverse chest diameters. In a normal adult chest, the ratio of anteroposterior to transverse (or lateral) diameter is 1:2. In patients with barrel chest, this ratio approaches 1:1 as the anteroposterior diameter enlarges.

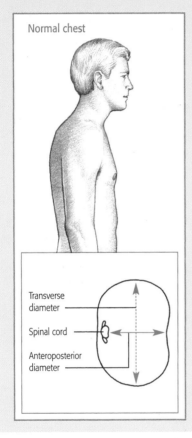

Normal chest

Transverse diameter

Spinal cord

Anteroposterior diameter

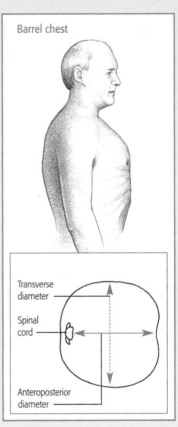

Barrel chest

Transverse diameter

Spinal cord

Anteroposterior diameter

mum diaphragmatic excursion, facilitating chest expansion.

■ Assess pain and provide analgesics as appropriate.

Patient teaching

■ Advise the patient to avoid bronchial irritants, especially smoking, which may exacerbate COPD.

■ Tell him to report purulent sputum production, which may indicate upper respiratory tract infection.

■ Instruct the patient to space his activities to help minimize exertional dyspnea.

■ Explain the underlying disorder and treatment plan.

Battle's sign

Battle's sign—ecchymosis over the mastoid process of the temporal bone—is commonly the only outward sign of a basilar skull fracture. In fact, this type of fracture may go undetected even by skull X-rays. If left untreated, it can be fatal because of associated injury to the nearby cranial nerves and brain stem as well as to blood vessels and the meninges.

Appearing behind one or both ears, Battle's sign is easily overlooked or hidden by the patient's hair. During emergency care of a trauma victim, it may be overshadowed by imminently life-threatening or more apparent injuries. (See *Assessing for Battle's sign.*)

A force that's strong enough to fracture the base of the skull causes Battle's sign by damaging supporting tissues of the mastoid area and causing seepage of blood from the fracture site to the mastoid. Battle's sign usually develops 24 to 36 hours after the fracture and may persist for several days to weeks.

History and physical examination

Perform a complete neurologic examination. Begin with the history. Ask the patient about recent trauma to the head. Did he sustain a severe blow to the head? Was he involved in a motor vehicle accident? Note the patient's level of consciousness as he responds. Does he respond quickly or slowly? Are his answers appropriate, or does he appear confused?

Check the patient's vital signs; be alert for widening pulse pressure and bradycardia, signs of increased intracranial pressure. Assess cranial nerve function in nerves II, III, IV, VI, VII, and VIII. Evaluate pupillary size and response to light as well as motor and verbal responses. Relate these data to the Glasgow Coma Scale. Note cerebrospinal fluid (CSF) leakage from the nose or ears. Ask about postnasal drip, which may reflect CSF drainage down the throat. Look for the halo sign—bloodstain encircled by a yellowish ring—on bed linens or dressings. To confirm that drainage is CSF, test it with a Dextrostix; CSF is positive for glucose, whereas mucus isn't. Follow up the neurologic examination with a complete physical examination to detect other injuries associated with basilar skull fracture.

Medical causes

Basilar skull fracture. Battle's sign may be the only outward sign of basilar skull fracture, or it may be accompanied by periorbital ecchymosis (raccoon eyes), conjunctival hemorrhage, nystagmus, ocular deviation, epistaxis, anosmia, a bulging tympanic membrane (from CSF or blood accumulation), visi-

 ▬▬▬ Assessment tip

Assessing for Battle's sign

When caring for the patient with a traumatic brain injury, be sure to check behind both ears for bruising over the mastoid bone. This sign, known as Battle's sign, is indicative of a basilar skull fracture. Continue to assess for this sign because it may take 24 to 36 hours for the bruising to appear.

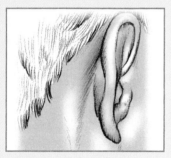

ble fracture lines on the external auditory canal, tinnitus, difficulty hearing, facial paralysis, or vertigo.

Nursing considerations

- Expect a patient with a basilar skull fracture to be on bed rest for several days to weeks. (See *Managing the patient with a basilar skull fracture.*)
- Monitor his neurologic status closely.
- Anticipate that the patient may need skull X-rays and a computed tomography scan to help confirm basilar skull fracture and to evaluate the severity of head injury.
- Although a basilar skull fracture and associated dural tears typically heal spontaneously within several days to weeks, if the patient has a large dural tear, a craniotomy may be necessary to repair the tear with a graft patch.

Patient teaching

- Explain activities the patient should avoid, and emphasize the importance of bed rest.
- Explain to the patient and family the signs and symptoms to look for and report, such as changes in mental status, LOC, or breathing.
- Tell the patient to take acetaminophen for headaches.
- Explain what diagnostic tests the patient may need.
- Discuss surgery with the patient, if indicated, and answer his questions and concerns.

DO'S & DON'TS

 ## Managing the patient with a basilar skull fracture

A basilar skull fracture is a linear fracture that occurs at the base of the skull and involves the anterior or middle fossae. Complications that may result from this type of skull fracture include infection, cranial nerve injury, and dural tear (resulting in leakage of cerebral spinal fluid).

Do's

- Monitor vital signs, oxygen saturation, and neurologic status closely.
- Maintain a patent airway and administer supplemental oxygen as necessary.
- Maintain the patient on bedrest, elevate the head of the bed 30 degrees.
- Administer medications as ordered to decrease intracranial pressure, control pain, and prevent seizures.
- Observe for cerebrospinal fluid (CSF) drainage from the patient's nose or ears (indicates a dural tear), check sheets for a blood-tinged spot surrounded by a lighter ring (halo sign) or test fluid with a reagent strip for glucose.
- Allow CSF to drain naturally or cover lightly the nose or ear with sterile gauze.
- If gastric tube is needed, choose an orogastric tube.
- Assess for signs of infection.

Don'ts

- If the patient has CSF drainage from the nose or ear, don't use packing to stop the drainage; don't allow the patient to blow his nose or cough forcefully.
- To decrease risk of intracranial infection, in cases of suspected or confirmed CSF leak, avoid nasogastric intubation and nasopharyngeal suction.

Biot's respirations
[Ataxic respirations]

A late and ominous sign of neurologic deterioration, Biot's respirations are characterized by an irregular and unpredictable rate, rhythm, and depth. This rare breathing pattern may appear abruptly and may reflect increased pressure on the medulla coinciding with brain stem compression.

ACTION STAT!

 Observe the patient's breathing pattern for several minutes to avoid confusing Biot's respirations with other respiratory patterns. (See *Identifying Biot's respirations*.) Assess the patient's respiratory status and prepare to intubate him and provide mechanical ventilation. Next, take his vital signs, noting especially increased systolic pressure.

History and physical examination

Obtain a brief history from the patient's family. Find out if the patient has experienced a recent head injury or complained of a severe headache. Ask the family when they noticed a change in the patient's neurologic status and how long he has been breathing this way.

Next, perform a physical examination. Evaluate the patient's level of consciousness. Calculate a Glasgow Coma score. Check the patient's skin for pallor or cyanosis. Obtain his vital signs and pulse oximetry level. Note his respiratory rate, rhythm, and depth. Obtain arterial blood gas levels to evaluate oxygenation. Auscultate the patient's lungs for abnormal breath sounds. Place him on a cardiac monitor and interpret his cardiac rhythm.

Medical causes

Brain stem compression. Biot's respirations are characteristic in brain stem compression, a neurologic emergency. Rapidly enlarging lesions may cause ataxic respirations and lead to complete respiratory arrest.

Nursing considerations

- Monitor the patient's vital signs frequently, including oxygen saturation.
- Administer oxygen and support ventilation as necessary.
- Elevate the head of the patient's bed 30 degrees to help reduce intracranial pressure.
- Prepare the patient for emergency surgery to relieve pressure on the brain stem.
- Anticipate diagnostic testing, such as computed tomography scans or magnet-

Identifying Biot's respirations

Biot's respirations, also known as *ataxic respirations,* have a completely irregular pattern. Shallow and deep breaths occur randomly, with haphazard, irregular pauses. The respiratory rate tends to be slow and may progressively decelerate to apnea.

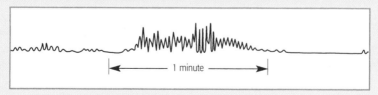

1 minute

ic resonance imaging, to confirm the cause of brain stem compression.

■ Discuss end-of-life issues with the patient's family.

Patient teaching

■ Because Biot's respirations typically reflect a grave prognosis, give the patient's family information and emotional support.

Bladder distention

Bladder distention—abnormal enlargement of the bladder—results from an inability to excrete urine, which results in its accumulation. Distention can be caused by a mechanical or anatomic obstruction, neuromuscular disorder, or the use of certain drugs. Relatively common in all ages and both sexes, it's most common in older men with prostate disorders that cause urine retention.

Distention usually develops gradually, but it occasionally has a sudden onset. Gradual distention usually remains asymptomatic until stretching of the bladder produces discomfort. Acute distention produces suprapubic fullness, pressure, and pain. If severe distention isn't corrected promptly by catheterization or massage, the bladder rises within the abdomen, its walls become thin, and renal function can be impaired.

Bladder distention is aggravated by the intake of caffeine, alcohol, large quantities of fluid, and diuretics.

ACTION STAT!

 If the patient has severe distention, insert an indwelling urinary catheter to help relieve discomfort and prevent bladder rupture. If more than 700 ml is emptied from the bladder, compressed blood vessels dilate and may make the patient feel faint. Typically, the indwelling urinary catheter is clamped for 30 to 60 minutes to permit vessel compensation.

History and physical examination

If distention isn't severe, begin by reviewing the patient's voiding patterns. Find out the time and amount of the patient's last voiding and the amount of fluid consumed since then. Ask if he has difficulty urinating. Does he use Valsalva's maneuver or Credé's method to initiate urination? Does he urinate with urgency or without warning? Is urination painful or irritating? Ask about the force and continuity of his urine stream and whether he feels that his bladder is empty after voiding.

Explore the patient's history of urinary tract obstruction or infections; venereal disease; neurologic, intestinal, or pelvic surgery; lower abdominal or urinary tract trauma; and systemic or neurologic disorders. Note his drug history, including his use of over-the-counter drugs and herbal medicines.

Take the patient's vital signs, and percuss and palpate the bladder. (Remember that if the bladder is empty, it can't be palpated through the abdominal wall.) Inspect the urethral meatus, and measure its diameter. Describe the appearance and amount of any discharge. Finally, test for perineal sensation and anal sphincter tone; in male patients, digitally examine the prostate gland.

Medical causes

Benign prostatic hyperplasia (BPH). With BPH, bladder distention gradually develops as the prostate enlarges. Occasionally, its onset is acute. Initially, the patient experiences urinary hesitancy, straining, and frequency; reduced force of and the inability to stop the urine stream; nocturia; and postvoiding dribbling. As the disorder progresses, it produces prostate enlargement, sensations of suprapubic fullness and incomplete bladder emptying, perineal pain, constipation, and hematuria.

Bladder calculi. Bladder calculi may produce bladder distention, but more commonly pain is the only symptom. The pain is usually referred to the tip of the penis, the vulvar area, the lower back, or the heel. It worsens during walking or exercise and abates when the patient lies down. It can be accompanied by urinary frequency and urgency, terminal hematuria, and dysuria. Pain is usually most severe when micturition ceases.

Bladder cancer. By blocking the urethral orifice, neoplasms can cause bladder distention. Associated signs and symptoms include hematuria (most common sign); urinary frequency and urgency; nocturia; dysuria; pyuria; pain in the bladder, rectum, pelvis, flank, back, or legs; vomiting; diarrhea; and sleeplessness. A mass may be palpable on bimanual examination.

Multiple sclerosis. With multiple sclerosis, a neuromuscular disorder, urine retention and bladder distention result from the interruption of upper motor neuron control of the bladder. Associated signs and symptoms include optic neuritis, paresthesia, impaired position and vibratory senses, diplopia, nystagmus, dizziness, abnormal reflexes, dysarthria, muscle weakness, emotional lability, Lhermitte's sign (transient, electric-like shocks that spread down the body when the head is flexed), Babinski's sign, and ataxia.

Prostate cancer. Prostate cancer eventually causes bladder distention in about 25% of patients. Usual signs and symptoms include dysuria, urinary frequency and urgency, nocturia, weight loss, fatigue, perineal pain, constipation, and induration of the prostate or a rigid, irregular prostate on digital rectal examination. For some patients, urine retention and bladder distention are the only signs.

Prostatitis. With acute prostatitis, bladder distention occurs rapidly along with perineal discomfort and suprapubic fullness. Other signs and symptoms include perineal pain; a tense, boggy, tender, and warm enlarged prostate; decreased libido; impotence; decreased force of the urine stream; dysuria; hematuria; and urinary frequency and urgency. Additional signs and symptoms include fatigue, malaise, myalgia, fever, chills, nausea, and vomiting.

With chronic prostatitis, bladder distention is rare; however, it may be accompanied by sensations of perineal discomfort and suprapubic fullness, prostatic tenderness, decreased libido, urinary frequency and urgency, dysuria, pyuria, hematuria, persistent urethral discharge, ejaculatory pain, and a dull pain radiating to the lower back, buttocks, penis, or perineum.

Spinal neoplasms. Disrupting upper neuron control of the bladder, spinal neoplasms cause neurogenic bladder and resultant distention. Associated signs and symptoms include a sense of pelvic fullness, continuous overflow dribbling, back pain that typically mimics sciatica pain, constipation, tender vertebral processes, sensory deficits, and muscle weakness, flaccidity, and atrophy. Signs and symptoms of urinary tract infection (dysuria, urinary frequency and urgency, nocturia, tenesmus, hematuria, and weakness) may also occur.

Urethral calculi. With urethral calculi, urethral obstruction leads to bladder distention. The patient experiences interrupted urine flow. The obstruction causes pain radiating to the penis or vulva and referred to the perineum or rectum. It may also produce a palpable stone and urethral discharge.

Urethral stricture. Urethral stricture results in urine retention and bladder distention with chronic urethral discharge (most common sign), urinary frequency (also common), dysuria, urgency, decreased force and diameter of the urine stream, and pyuria. Urinoma and urosepsis may also develop.

Other causes

Catheterization. Using an indwelling urinary catheter can result in urine retention and bladder distention. While the catheter is in place, inadequate drainage due to kinked tubing or an occluded lumen may lead to urine retention. In addition, a misplaced urinary catheter or irritation with catheter removal may cause edema, thereby blocking urine outflow.

Drugs. Parasympatholytics, anticholinergics, ganglionic blockers, sedatives, anesthetics, and opiates can produce urine retention and bladder distention.

Nursing considerations
- Insert a urinary catheter to relieve distention. If a catheter is already in place, irrigate or replace it to improve function.
- Monitor the patient's vital signs, intake and output, and the extent of bladder distention.
- Encourage the patient to change positions to alleviate discomfort.
- Administer an analgesic, as appropriate.
- Prepare the patient for diagnostic tests (such as cystoscopy and radiologic studies) to determine the cause of bladder distention.
- Prepare the patient for surgery if interventions fail to relieve bladder distention and obstruction prevents catheterization.
- Provide privacy for voiding and encourage a normal voiding position.

Patient teaching
- Explain the underlying cause and treatment plan.
- Teach the patient to use Valsalva's maneuver or Credé's method to empty the bladder.
- Explain how to stimulate voiding or perform self-catheterization as appropriate.

Blood pressure, decreased
[Hypotension]

Low blood pressure refers to inadequate intravascular pressure to maintain the oxygen requirements of the body's tissues. Although commonly linked to shock, this sign may also result from a cardiovascular, respiratory, neurologic, or metabolic disorder. Hypoperfusion states especially affect the kidneys, brain, and heart, and may lead to renal failure, a change in the patient's level of consciousness (LOC), or myocardial ischemia. Low blood pressure may be drug-induced or may accompany diagnostic tests—most commonly those using contrast media. It may stem from stress or change of position—specifically, rising abruptly from a supine or sitting position to a standing position (orthostatic hypotension).

Normal blood pressure varies considerably; what qualifies as low blood pressure for one person may be normal for another. Consequently, every blood pressure reading must be compared against the patient's baseline. Typically, a reading below 90/60 mm Hg, or a drop of 30 mm Hg from the baseline, is considered low blood pressure.

Low blood pressure can reflect an expanded intravascular space (as in severe infections, allergic reactions, or adrenal insufficiency), reduced intravascular volume (as in dehydration and hemorrhage), or decreased cardiac output (as in impaired cardiac muscle contractility). Because the body's pressure-regulating mechanisms are complex and interrelated, a combination of these factors usually contributes to low blood pressure.

ACTION STAT!

 If the patient's systolic pressure is less than 80 mm Hg, or 30 mm Hg below his baseline, suspect shock. Quickly evaluate the patient for a decreased LOC. Check his apical pulse for tachycardia and his respirations for tachypnea. Inspect the patient for cool, clammy skin. Elevate the patient's legs above the level of his heart, or place him in Trendelenburg's position if the bed can be adjusted. Then insert a large-bore I.V. catheter to replace fluids and blood or to administer drugs. Prepare to administer oxygen with mechanical ventilation if necessary. Monitor the patient's intake and output and insert an indwelling urinary catheter to accurately measure urine output. The patient may need a central venous catheter or a pulmonary artery catheter to facilitate monitoring of his fluid status. Prepare for cardiac monitoring to evaluate cardiac rhythm. Be ready to insert a nasogastric tube to prevent aspiration in the comatose patient. Throughout emergency interventions, keep the patient's spinal column immobile until spinal cord trauma is ruled out.

History and physical examination

If the patient is conscious, ask him about associated symptoms. For example, does he feel unusually weak or fatigued? Has he had nausea, vomiting, or dark or bloody stools? Is his vision blurred? Is his gait unsteady? Does he have palpitations? Does he have chest or abdominal pain or difficulty breathing?

Has he had episodes of dizziness or fainting? Do these episodes occur when he stands up suddenly? If so, take the patient's blood pressure while he's lying down, sitting, and then standing; compare readings. (See *Ensuring accurate blood pressure measurement.*)

A drop in systolic or diastolic pressure of 10 to 20 mm Hg or more and an increase in heart rate of more than 15 beats/minute between position changes suggest orthostatic hypotension.

Next, continue with a physical examination. Inspect the skin for pallor, sweating, and clamminess. Palpate peripheral pulses. Note paradoxical pulse—an accentuated fall in systolic pressure during inspiration—which suggests pericardial tamponade. Then auscultate for abnormal heart sounds (gallops, murmurs), rate (bradycardia, tachycardia), or rhythm. Auscultate the lungs for abnormal breath sounds (diminished sounds, crackles, wheezing), rate (bradypnea, tachypnea), or rhythm (agonal or Cheyne-Stokes respirations). Look for signs of hemorrhage, including visible bleeding and palpable masses, bruising, and tenderness. Assess the patient for abdominal rigidity and rebound tenderness; auscultate for abnormal bowel sounds. Carefully assess the patient for possible sources of infection such as open wounds.

Medical causes

Acute adrenal insufficiency. Orthostatic hypotension is characteristic with acute adrenal insufficiency, accompanied by fatigue, weakness, nausea, vomiting, abdominal discomfort, weight loss, fever, and tachycardia. The patient may also have hyperpigmentation of fingers, nails, nipples, scars, and body folds; pale, cool, clammy skin; restlessness; decreased urine output; tachypnea; and coma.

Ensuring accurate blood pressure measurement

When taking the patient's blood pressure, begin by applying the cuff properly, as shown here.

■ For accuracy and consistency, position your patient with his upper arm at heart level and his palm turned up.

■ Apply the cuff snugly, 1″ (2.5 cm) above the brachial pulse, as shown in the top photo.

■ Position the manometer in line with your eye level.

■ Palpate the brachial or radial pulse with your fingertips while inflating the cuff.

■ Inflate the cuff to 30 mm Hg above the point where the pulse disappears.

■ Place the bell of your stethoscope over the point where you felt the pulse, as shown in the bottom photo. Using the bell helps you hear Korotkoff sounds, which indicate pulse.

■ Release the valve slowly and note the point at which Korotkoff sounds reappear. The start of the pulse sound indicates the systolic pressure.

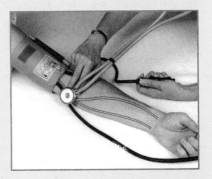

■ The sounds will become muffled and then disappear. The last Korotkoff sound you hear is the diastolic pressure.

Anaphylactic shock. Following exposure to an allergen, such as penicillin or insect venom, a dramatic fall in blood pressure and narrowed pulse pressure signal anaphylactic reaction. Initially, anaphylactic shock causes anxiety, restlessness, a feeling of doom, intense itching (especially of the hands and feet), and pounding headache. Later, it may also produce weakness, sweating, nasal congestion, coughing, difficulty breathing, nausea, abdominal cramps, involuntary defecation, seizures, flushing, change or loss of voice due to laryngeal edema, urinary incontinence, and tachycardia.

Anthrax (inhalation). Inhalation anthrax is caused by inhalation of aerosolized spores. Initial signs and symptoms are flulike and include fever, chills, weakness, cough, and chest pain. The disease generally occurs in two stages with a period of recovery after the initial signs and symptoms. The second stage develops abruptly with rapid deterioration marked by fever, dyspnea, stridor, and hypotension, generally leading to death within 24 hours. Radiologic findings include mediastinitis and symmetric mediastinal widening.

Cardiac arrhythmias. With an arrhythmia, blood pressure may fluctuate between normal and low readings. Dizziness, chest pain, difficulty breathing, light-headedness, weakness, fatigue, and palpitations may also occur. Auscultation typically reveals an irregular rhythm and a pulse rate greater than 100 beats/minute or less than 60 beats/minute. A life-threatening arrhythmia may cause absence of a pulse and no palpable blood pressure and requires emergency resuscitation measures.

Cardiac contusion. With cardiac contusion, low blood pressure occurs along with tachycardia and, at times, anginal pain and dyspnea.

Cardiac tamponade. An accentuated fall in systolic pressure (more than 10 mm Hg) during inspiration, known as *paradoxical pulse,* is characteristic in patients with cardiac tamponade. This disorder also causes restlessness, cyanosis, tachycardia, jugular vein distention, muffled heart sounds, dyspnea, and Kussmaul's sign (increased venous distention with inspiration).

Cardiogenic shock. A fall in systolic pressure to less than 80 mm Hg or to 30 mm Hg less than the patient's baseline because of decreased cardiac contractility is characteristic in patients with cardiogenic shock. Accompanying low blood pressure are tachycardia, narrowed pulse pressure, diminished Korotkoff sounds, peripheral cyanosis, and pale, cool, clammy skin. Cardiogenic shock also causes restlessness and anxiety, which may progress to disorientation and confusion. Associated signs and symptoms include angina, dyspnea, jugular vein distention, oliguria, ventricular gallop, tachypnea, and a weak, rapid pulse.

Cholera. Cholera may be mild and with uncomplicated diarrhea or severe and life-threatening. Signs include abrupt watery diarrhea and vomiting. Severe fluid and electrolyte loss leads to thirst, weakness, muscle cramps, decreased skin turgor, oliguria, tachycardia, and hypotension. Without treatment, death can occur within hours.

Diabetic ketoacidosis. Hypovolemia triggered by osmotic diuresis in hyperglycemia is responsible for the low blood pressure associated with diabetic ketoacidosis, which is usually present in patients with type 1 diabetes mellitus. It commonly produces polydipsia, polyuria, polyphagia, dehydration, weight loss, abdominal pain, nausea, vomiting, breath with fruity odor, Kussmaul's respirations, tachycardia, seizures, confusion, and stupor that may progress to coma.

Heart failure. With heart failure, blood pressure may fluctuate between normal and low readings. A precipitous drop in blood pressure may signal cardiogenic shock. Other signs and symptoms of heart failure include exertional dyspnea, dyspnea of abrupt or gradual onset, paroxysmal nocturnal dyspnea or difficulty breathing in the supine position (orthopnea), fatigue, weight gain, pallor or cyanosis, sweating, and anxiety. Auscultation reveals ventricular gallop, tachycardia, bilateral crackles, and tachypnea. Dependent edema, jugular vein distention, increased capillary refill time, and hepatomegaly may also occur.

Hyperosmolar hyperglycemic nonketotic syndrome (HHNS). HHNS, which is common in the patient with type 2 diabetes mellitus, decreases blood pressure—at times dramatically—if he loses significant fluid from diuresis due to severe hyperglycemia and hyperosmolarity. It also produces dry mouth, poor skin turgor, tachycardia, confusion progressing to coma and, occasionally, generalized tonic-clonic seizure.

Hypovolemic shock. A fall in systolic pressure to less than 80 mm Hg or 30 mm Hg less than the patient's baseline, secondary to acute blood loss or dehydration, is characteristic in hypovolemic shock. Accompanying it are diminished Korotkoff sounds, a narrowed pulse pressure, and a rapid, weak, and irregular pulse. Peripheral vasoconstriction causes cyanosis of the extremities and pale, cool, clammy skin. Other signs and symptoms include oliguria, confusion, disorientation, restlessness, and anxiety.

Hypoxemia. Initially, blood pressure may be normal or slightly elevated, but as hypoxemia becomes more pronounced, blood pressure drops. The patient may display tachycardia, tachypnea, dyspnea, and confusion and may progress from stupor to coma.

Myocardial infarction (MI). With MI, a life-threatening disorder, blood pressure may be low or high. A precipitous drop in blood pressure may signal cardiogenic shock. Associated signs and symptoms include chest pain that may radiate to the jaw, shoulder, arm, or epigastrium; dyspnea; anxiety; nausea or vomiting; sweating; and cool, pale, or cyanotic skin. Auscultation may reveal an atrial gallop, a murmur and, occasionally, an irregular pulse.

Neurogenic shock. The result of sympathetic denervation due to cervical injury or anesthesia, neurogenic shock produces low blood pressure and bradycardia. The patient's skin remains warm and dry because of cutaneous vasodilation and sweat gland denervation. Depending on the cause of shock, there may also be motor weakness of the limbs or diaphragm.

Pulmonary embolism. Pulmonary embolism causes sudden, sharp chest pain and dyspnea accompanied by a cough and, occasionally, a low-grade fever. Low blood pressure occurs with a narrowed pulse pressure and diminished Korotkoff sounds. Associated signs include tachycardia, tachypnea, a paradoxical pulse, jugular vein distention, and hemoptysis.

Septic shock. Initially, septic shock produces fever and chills. Low blood pressure, tachycardia, and tachypnea may also develop early, but the patient's skin remains warm. Low blood pressure becomes increasingly severe—less than 80 mm Hg or 30 mm Hg less than the patient's baseline—and is accompanied by narrowed pulse pressure. Other late signs and symptoms include pale skin, cyanotic extremities, apprehension, thirst, oliguria, and coma.

Vasovagal syncope. Vasovagal syncope is the transient loss or near-loss of consciousness that's characterized by low blood pressure, pallor, cold sweats, nausea, palpitations or slowed heart rate, and weakness following stressful, painful, or claustrophobic experiences.

Other causes

Diagnostic tests. Diagnostic tests include the gastric acid stimulation test using histamine and X-ray studies using contrast media. The latter may trigger an allergic reaction, which causes low blood pressure.

Drugs. Calcium channel blockers, diuretics, vasodilators, alpha- and beta-adrenergic blockers, general anesthetics, opioid analgesics, monoamine oxidase inhibitors, anxiolytics (such as benzodiazepines), tranquilizers, and most I.V. antiarrhythmics (especially bretylium tosylate) can cause low blood pressure.

Nursing considerations

- Check the patient's vital signs frequently to determine if low blood pressure is constant or intermittent.
- If blood pressure is extremely low, assist in the insertion of an arterial catheter to allow close monitoring of pressures; alternatively, a Doppler flowmeter may be used.
- Prepare the patient for laboratory tests, which may include urinalysis, routine blood studies, an electrocardiogram, and

chest, cervical, and abdominal X-rays or computed tomography scans.

■ Administer fluid, blood products, and medication as ordered to improve blood pressure.

Patient teaching

■ Advise the patient with orthostatic hypotension to stand up slowly from a sitting or lying position.

■ For the patient with vasovagal syncope, discuss how to avoid triggers.

■ Emphasize the importance of dangling the feet and rising slowly when getting out of bed.

■ Explain diagnostic tests and procedures.

■ Explain the underlying disorder and treatment plan.

▮ Blood pressure, increased
[Hypertension]

Elevated blood pressure or hypertension (an intermittent or sustained increase in blood pressure of 140/90 mm Hg) strikes more men than women and twice as many Blacks as Whites. By itself, this common sign is easily ignored by the patient; after all, he can't see or feel it; however, its causes can be life-threatening.

Elevated blood pressure may develop suddenly or gradually. A sudden, severe rise in pressure (exceeding 180/110 mm Hg) may indicate life-threatening hypertensive crisis; however, even a less dramatic rise may be equally significant if it heralds a dissecting aortic aneurysm, increased intracranial pressure, myocardial infarction, eclampsia, or thyrotoxicosis.

Usually associated with essential hypertension, elevated blood pressure may also result from a renal or endocrine disorder; a treatment that affects fluid status, such as dialysis; or a drug's adverse effect. Ingestion of large amounts of certain foods, such as black licorice and cheddar cheese, may temporarily elevate blood pressure. (See *Pathophysiology of elevated blood pressure*.)

Sometimes, elevated blood pressure may simply reflect inaccurate blood pressure measurement. Careful measurement alone doesn't ensure a clinically useful reading. To be useful, each blood pressure reading must be compared with the patient's baseline. Serial readings may be necessary to establish elevated blood pressure.

History and physical examination

If you detect sharply elevated blood pressure, quickly rule out possible life-threatening causes. (See *Managing elevated blood pressure*, page 84.)

After ruling out life-threatening causes, complete a history and physical examination. Determine if the patient has a history of cardiovascular or cerebrovascular disease, diabetes, or renal disease. Ask about a family history of high blood pressure—a likely finding with essential hypertension, pheochromocytoma, or polycystic kidney disease. Then ask about its onset. Did high blood pressure appear abruptly? Ask the patient's age. The sudden onset of high blood pressure in middle-aged or elderly patients suggests renovascular stenosis. Although essential hypertension may begin in childhood, it typically isn't diagnosed until near age 35. Pheochromocytoma and primary aldosteronism usually occur between ages 40 and 60. If you suspect either, check for orthostatic hypotension. Take the patient's blood pressure with him lying down, sitting, and then standing. Normally, systolic pressure falls and diastolic pressure rises on standing. With orthostatic hypotension, both pressures fall.

Note headache, palpitations, blurred vision, and sweating. Ask about wine-

Pathophysiology of elevated blood pressure

Blood pressure—the force blood exerts on vessels as it flows through them—depends on cardiac output, peripheral resistance, and blood volume. A brief review of its regulating mechanisms—nervous system control, capillary fluid shifts, kidney excretion, and hormonal changes—will help you understand how elevated blood pressure develops.

■ *Nervous system control* involves the sympathetic system, chiefly baroreceptors and chemoreceptors, which promotes moderate vasoconstriction to maintain normal blood pressure. When this system responds inappropriately, increased vasoconstriction enhances peripheral resistance, resulting in elevated blood pressure.

■ *Capillary fluid shifts* regulate blood volume by responding to arterial pressure. Increased pressure forces fluid into the interstitial space; decreased pressure allows it to be drawn back into the arteries by osmosis. However, this fluid shift may take several hours to adjust blood pressure.

■ *Kidney excretion* also helps regulate blood volume by increasing or decreasing urine formation. Normally, an arterial pressure of about 60 mm Hg maintains urine output. When pressure drops below this reading, urine formation ceases, thereby increasing blood volume. Conversely, when arterial pressure exceeds this reading, urine formation increases, thereby reducing blood volume. Like capillary fluid shifts, this mechanism may take several hours to adjust blood pressure.

■ *Hormonal changes* reflect stimulation of the kidney's renin-angiotensin-aldosterone system in response to low arterial pressure. This system affects vasoconstriction, which increases arterial pressure, and stimulates aldosterone release, which regulates sodium retention—a key determinant of blood volume.

Elevated blood pressure signals the breakdown or inappropriate response of these pressure-regulating mechanisms. Its associated signs and symptoms concentrate in the target organs and tissues illustrated below.

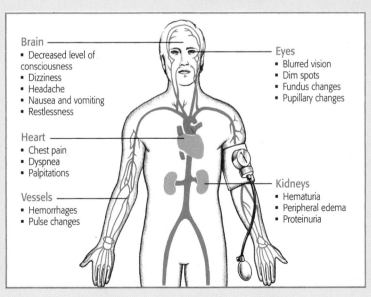

Brain
• Decreased level of consciousness
• Dizziness
• Headache
• Nausea and vomiting
• Restlessness

Heart
• Chest pain
• Dyspnea
• Palpitations

Vessels
• Hemorrhages
• Pulse changes

Eyes
• Blurred vision
• Dim spots
• Fundus changes
• Pupillary changes

Kidneys
• Hematuria
• Peripheral edema
• Proteinuria

ACTION STAT!

Managing elevated blood pressure

Elevated blood pressure can signal various life-threatening disorders. If pressure exceeds 180/110 mm Hg, the patient may be experiencing hypertensive crisis and may require prompt treatment. Maintain a patent airway in case the patient vomits, and institute seizure precautions. Prepare to administer an I.V. antihypertensive and diuretic. You'll need to insert an indwelling urinary catheter to accurately monitor urine output.

In preeclampsia or eclampsia

If blood pressure is less severely elevated, continue to rule out other life-threatening causes. If the patient is pregnant, suspect preeclampsia or eclampsia. Place her on bed rest and insert an I.V. catheter. Administer magnesium sulfate (to decrease neuromuscular irritability) and an antihypertensive. Monitor her vital signs closely for the next 24 hours. If diastolic blood pressure continues to exceed 100 mm Hg despite drug therapy, you may need to prepare the patient for induced labor and delivery or for cesarean birth. Offer emotional support if she must face delivery of a premature neonate.

In hyperthyroidism

If the patient isn't pregnant, quickly observe for equally obvious clues. Assess the patient for exophthalmos and an enlarged thyroid gland. If these signs are present, ask about a history of hyperthyroidism. Then look for other associated signs and symptoms, including tachycardia, widened pulse pressure, palpitations, severe weakness, diarrhea, fever exceeding 100° F (37.8° C), and nervousness. Prepare to administer an antithyroid drug orally or by nasogastric tube, if necessary. Evaluate fluid status; look for signs of dehydration such as poor skin turgor. Prepare the patient for I.V. fluid replacement and temperature control using a cooling blanket, if necessary.

In increased ICP

If the patient shows signs of increased intracranial pressure (ICP) (such as a decreased level of consciousness and fixed or dilated pupils), ask him or a family member if he has recently experienced head trauma. Then check for an increased respiratory rate and bradycardia. You'll need to maintain a patent airway in case the patient vomits. In addition, institute seizure precautions, and prepare to give an I.V. diuretic. Insert an indwelling urinary catheter, and monitor intake and output. Check his vital signs every 15 minutes until he's stable.

In dissecting aortic aneurysm

If the patient has absent or weak peripheral pulses, ask about chest pressure or pain, which suggests a dissecting aortic aneurysm. Enforce bed rest until a diagnosis has been established. As appropriate, give the patient an I.V. antihypertensive or prepare him for surgery.

colored urine and decreased urine output; these signs suggest glomerulonephritis, which can cause elevated blood pressure.

Obtain a drug history, including past and present prescriptions, herbal medicines, and over-the-counter drugs (especially decongestants). If the patient is already taking an antihypertensive, determine how well he complies with the regimen. Ask about his perception of elevated blood pressure. How serious does he believe it is? Does he expect drug therapy to help? Explore psychosocial or environmental factors that may impact blood pressure control.

Follow up the history with a thorough physical examination. Using a funduscope, check for intraocular hemorrhage, exudate, and papilledema, which characterize severe hypertension. Perform a thorough cardiovascular assessment. Check for carotid bruits and jugular vein distention. Assess skin color, temperature, and turgor. Palpate peripheral pulses. Auscultate for abnormal heart sounds (such as gallops, louder second sound, or murmurs), rate (for example, bradycardia or tachycardia), or rhythm. Then auscultate for abnormal breath sounds (such as crackles or wheezing), rate (for example, bradypnea or tachypnea), or rhythm.

Palpate the abdomen for tenderness, masses, or liver enlargement. Auscultate for abdominal bruits. Renal artery stenosis produces bruits over the upper abdomen or in the costovertebral angles. Easily palpable, enlarged kidneys and a large, tender liver suggest polycystic kidney disease. Obtain a urine sample to check for microscopic hematuria.

Medical causes

Anemia. Accompanying elevated systolic pressure in anemia are pulsations in the capillary beds, bounding pulse, tachycardia, systolic ejection murmur, pale mucous membranes and, in patients with sickle cell anemia, ventricular gallop and crackles.

Aortic aneurysm (dissecting). Initially, this life-threatening disorder causes a sudden rise in systolic pressure (which may be the precipitating event), but no change in diastolic pressure; however, this increase is brief. The body's ability to compensate fails, resulting in hypotension.

Other signs and symptoms vary, depending on the type of aortic aneurysm. An abdominal aneurysm may cause persistent abdominal and back pain, weakness, sweating, tachycardia, dyspnea, a pulsating abdominal mass, restlessness, confusion, and cool, clammy skin. A thoracic aneurysm may cause a ripping or tearing sensation in the chest, which may radiate to the neck, shoulders, lower back, or abdomen; pallor; syncope; blindness; loss of consciousness; sweating; dyspnea; tachycardia; cyanosis; leg weakness; murmur; and absent radial and femoral pulses.

Atherosclerosis. With atherosclerosis, systolic pressure rises while diastolic pressure commonly remains normal or slightly elevated. The patient may show no other signs, or he may have a weak pulse, flushed skin, tachycardia, angina, and claudication.

Cushing's syndrome. Cushing's syndrome causes elevated blood pressure and widened pulse pressure as well as truncal obesity, moon face, and other cushingoid signs. It's usually caused by corticosteroid use.

Hypertension. Essential hypertension develops insidiously and is characterized by a gradual increase in blood pressure from decade to decade. Except for this high blood pressure, the patient may be asymptomatic or (rarely) may complain of suboccipital headache, light-headedness, tinnitus, and fatigue.

With malignant hypertension, diastolic pressure abruptly rises above 120 mm Hg, and systolic pressure may exceed 200 mm Hg. Typically, the patient has pulmonary edema marked by jugular vein distention, dyspnea, tachypnea, tachycardia, and coughing of pink, frothy sputum. Other characteristic signs and symptoms include severe headache, confusion, blurred vision, tinnitus, epistaxis, muscle twitching, chest pain, nausea, and vomiting.

Increased intracranial pressure (ICP). Increased ICP causes an increased respiratory rate initially, followed by increased systolic pressure and widened pulse pressure. Increased ICP affects the heart rate last, causing bradycardia (Cushing's reflex). Associated signs and symptoms include headache, projectile vomiting, a decreased level of consciousness, and fixed or dilated pupils.

Metabolic syndrome. Blood pressure that exceeds 135/85 mm Hg is one of the conditions associated with metabolic syndrome (previously called *syndrome X*). Other conditions that define this syndrome are obesity, abnormal cholesterol level, and high blood insulin level. Individuals with this combination of risk factors are at a significantly greater risk for developing heart disease, stroke, peripheral vascular disease, and type 2 diabetes. Factors contributing to these conditions include physical inactivity, excessive weight gain, and genetic predisposition.

Myocardial infarction (MI). MI is a life-threatening disorder that may cause high or low blood pressure. Common findings include crushing chest pain that may radiate to the jaw, shoulder, arm, or epigastrium. Other findings include dyspnea, anxiety, nausea, vomiting, weakness, diaphoresis, atrial gallop, and murmurs.

Pheochromocytoma. Paroxysmal or sustained elevated blood pressure characterizes pheochromocytoma and may be accompanied by orthostatic hypotension. Associated signs and symptoms include anxiety, diaphoresis, palpitations, tremors, pallor, nausea, weight loss, and headache.

Polycystic kidney disease. With polycystic kidney disease, elevated blood pressure is typically preceded by flank pain. Other signs and symptoms include enlarged kidneys; an enlarged, tender liver; and intermittent gross hematuria.

Preeclampsia and eclampsia. Potentially life-threatening to the mother and fetus, preeclampsia and eclampsia characteristically increase blood pressure. They're defined as a reading of 140/90 mm Hg or more in the first trimester, a reading of 130/80 mm Hg or more in the second or third trimester, an increase of 30 mm Hg above the patient's baseline systolic pressure, or an increase of 15 mm Hg above the patient's baseline diastolic pressure. Accompanying elevated blood pressure are generalized edema, sudden weight gain of 3 lb (1.4 kg) or more per week during the second or third trimester, severe frontal headache, blurred or double vision, decreased urine output, proteinuria, midabdominal pain, neuromuscular irritability, nausea and, possibly, seizures.

Renovascular stenosis. Renovascular stenosis produces abruptly elevated systolic and diastolic pressures. Other characteristic signs and symptoms include bruits over the upper abdomen or in the costovertebral angles, hematuria, and acute flank pain.

Thyrotoxicosis. Accompanying the elevated systolic pressure associated with thyrotoxicosis, a potentially life-threatening disorder, are widened pulse pressure, tachycardia, bounding pulse, pulsations in the capillary nail beds, palpitations, weight loss, exophthalmos, an enlarged thyroid gland, weakness, diarrhea, a fever over 100° F (37.8° C), and warm, moist skin. The patient may appear nervous and emotionally unstable, displaying occasional outbursts or even psychotic behavior. Heat intolerance, exertional dyspnea and, in females, decreased or absent menses may also occur.

Other causes

Drugs. Central nervous system stimulants (such as amphetamines), sympathomimetics, corticosteroids, nonsteroidal anti-inflammatory drugs, hormonal contraceptives, monoamine oxidase inhibitors, and over-the-counter cold remedies can increase blood pressure, as can cocaine abuse.

Treatments. Kidney dialysis and transplantation cause transient elevated blood pressure.

Nursing considerations

- If routine screening detects elevated blood pressure, prepare the patient for routine blood tests, urinalysis, and depending on the suspected cause of the increased blood pressure, radiographic studies, especially of the kidneys.
- Administer antihypertensives, as ordered, and evaluate their effect.

Patient teaching

- Explain the importance of regular blood pressure monitoring and keeping follow-up appointments.
- Explain how to take prescribed antihypertensives correctly and adverse effects that should be reported.
- Instruct the patient not to discontinue medications without contacting the practitioner.
- Emphasize the importance of weight loss and regular exercise.
- Explain the need for sodium restriction.
- Discuss stress management.
- Discuss ways of reducing other risk factors for coronary artery disease, such as smoking cessation and lowering elevated cholesterol levels.

Bowel sounds, absent
[Silent abdomen]

Absent bowel sounds refers to an inability to hear any bowel sounds with a stethoscope in any quadrant after listening for at least 5 minutes in each quadrant. Bowel sounds cease when mechanical or vascular obstruction or neurogenic inhibition halts peristalsis. When peristalsis stops, gas from bowel contents and fluid secreted from the intes-

tinal walls accumulate and distend the lumen, leading to life-threatening complications (such as perforation, peritonitis, and sepsis) or hypovolemic shock.

Simple mechanical obstruction, resulting from adhesions, hernia, or tumor, causes loss of fluids and electrolytes and induces dehydration. Vascular obstruction cuts off circulation to the intestinal walls, leading to ischemia, necrosis, and shock. Neurogenic inhibition, affecting innervation of the intestinal wall, may result from infection, bowel distention, or trauma. It may also follow mechanical or vascular obstruction or metabolic derangement such as hypokalemia.

Abrupt cessation of bowel sounds, when accompanied by abdominal pain, rigidity, and distention, signals a life-threatening crisis requiring immediate intervention. Absent bowel sounds following a period of hyperactive sounds are equally ominous and may indicate strangulation of a mechanically obstructed bowel.

ACTION STAT!

 If you fail to detect bowel sounds and the patient reports sudden, severe abdominal pain and cramping or exhibits severe abdominal distention, prepare to insert a nasogastric (NG) or intestinal tube to suction lumen contents and decompress the bowel. (See *Are bowel sounds really absent?* page 88.) Administer I.V. fluids and electrolytes to offset dehydration and imbalances caused by the dysfunctioning bowel.

Because the patient may require surgery to relieve an obstruction, withhold food and fluids. Take the patient's vital signs, and be alert for signs of shock, such as hypotension, tachycardia, and cool, clammy skin. Measure abdominal girth as a baseline for gauging subse-

Are bowel sounds really absent?

Before concluding that the patient has absent bowel sounds, ask yourself these questions.

Did you use the diaphragm of your stethoscope to ausculate for the bowel sounds?
The diaphragm detects high-frequency sounds, such as bowel sounds, whereas the bell detects low-frequency sounds, such as a vascular bruit or venous hum.

Did you listen for at least 5 minutes in each quadrant for the presence of bowel sounds?
Normally, bowel sounds occur every 5 to 15 seconds, but the duration of a single sound may be less than 1 second.

Did you listen for bowel sounds in all quadrants?
Bowel sounds may be absent in one quadrant but present in another.

---

quent changes. If the patient vomits, be sure to check it for occult blood.

History and physical examination

If the patient's condition permits, proceed with a brief history. Start with abdominal pain: When did it begin? Has it gotten worse? Where does he feel it? Ask about a sensation of bloating and about flatulence. Find out if the patient has had diarrhea or has passed pencil-thin stools—possible signs of a developing luminal obstruction. The patient may have had no bowel movements at all—a possible sign of complete obstruction or paralytic ileus.

Ask about conditions that commonly lead to mechanical obstruction, such as abdominal tumors, hernias, and adhesions from past surgery. Determine if the patient was involved in an accident— even a seemingly minor one, such as falling off a stepladder—that may have caused vascular clots. Check for a history of acute pancreatitis, diverticulitis, or gynecologic infection, which may have led to intra-abdominal infection and bowel dysfunction. Be sure to ask about previous toxic conditions, such as uremia, and about spinal cord injury, which can lead to paralytic ileus.

If the patient's pain isn't severe or accompanied by other life-threatening signs or symptoms, obtain a detailed medical and surgical history and perform a complete physical examination followed by an abdominal assessment and pelvic examination.

Start your assessment by inspecting the abdominal contour. Stoop at the recumbent patient's side and then at the foot of his bed to detect localized or generalized distention. Auscultate for bowel sounds in all quadrants, listening for 5 minutes in each quadrant. Percuss and palpate the abdomen gently. Listen for dullness over fluid-filled areas and tympany over pockets of gas. Palpate for abdominal rigidity and guarding, which suggest peritoneal irritation that can lead to paralytic ileus.

Medical causes
Complete mechanical intestinal obstruction. Absent bowel sounds follow a period of hyperactive bowel sounds in this potentially life-threatening disorder. This silence accompanies

acute, colicky abdominal pain that arises in the quadrant of obstruction and may radiate to the flank or lumbar regions. Associated signs and symptoms include abdominal distention, and bloating, constipation, and nausea and vomiting (the higher the blockage, the earlier and more severe the vomiting). In late stages, signs of shock may occur with fever, rebound tenderness, and abdominal rigidity.

Mesenteric artery occlusion. With mesenteric artery occlusion, a life-threatening disorder, bowel sounds disappear after a brief period of hyperactive sounds. Sudden, severe midepigastric or periumbilical pain occurs next, followed by abdominal distention, bruits, vomiting, constipation, and signs of shock. Fever is common. Abdominal rigidity may appear later.

Paralytic (adynamic) ileus. The cardinal sign of paralytic (adynamic) ileus is absent bowel sounds. In addition to abdominal distention, associated signs and symptoms include generalized discomfort and constipation or the passage of small, liquid stools. If paralytic ileus follows acute abdominal infection, the patient may also experience fever and abdominal pain.

Other causes

Abdominal surgery. Bowel sounds are normally absent after abdominal surgery—the result of anesthetic use and surgical manipulation.

Nursing considerations

- After NG or intestinal tube insertion, elevate the head of the bed at least 30 degrees.
- Ensure tube patency by checking for drainage and properly functioning suction devices, and irrigate accordingly.
- Administer I.V. fluids and electrolytes and monitor laboratory values, as indicated.

- Prepare the patient for X-ray and imaging studies and blood work to determine the cause of absent bowel sounds.
- Administer analgesics, as ordered.
- Withhold food and fluids, as indicated.

Patient teaching

- Explain diagnostic tests and therapeutic procedures.
- Discuss any food or fluid restrictions.
- Explain the need for postoperative ambulation.
- Teach the patient about the cause of absent bowel sounds and the treatment plan after the diagnosis is established.

Bowel sounds, hyperactive

Sometimes audible without a stethoscope, hyperactive bowel sounds reflect increased intestinal motility (peristalsis). They're commonly characterized as rapid, rushing, gurgling waves of sounds. (See *Characteristics of bowel sounds,* page 90.)

They may stem from life-threatening bowel obstruction or GI hemorrhage or from GI infection, inflammatory bowel disease (which usually follows a chronic course), food allergies, or stress.

ACTION STAT!

 After detecting hyperactive bowel sounds, quickly check the patient's vital signs and ask him about associated symptoms, such as abdominal pain, vomiting, and diarrhea. If he reports cramping abdominal pain or vomiting, continue to auscultate for bowel sounds. If bowel sounds stop abruptly, suspect complete bowel obstruction. Prepare to assist with GI suction and decompression, to give I.V. fluids and electrolytes and, possibly, prepare the patient for surgery.

Characteristics of bowel sounds

The sounds of swallowed air and fluid moving through the GI tract are known as *bowel sounds*. These sounds usually occur every 5 to 15 seconds, but their frequency may be irregular. For example, bowel sounds are normally more active just before and after a meal. Bowel sounds may last less than 1 second or up to several seconds.

Normal bowel sounds can be characterized as murmuring, gurgling, or tinkling. *Hyperactive bowel sounds* can be characterized as loud, gurgling, splashing, and rushing; they're higher pitched and occur more frequently than normal sounds. *Hypoactive bowel sounds* can be characterized as softer or lower in tone and less frequent than normal sounds.

If he has diarrhea, record its frequency, amount, color, and consistency. If you detect excessive watery diarrhea or bleeding, prepare to administer an antidiarrheal, I.V. fluids and electrolytes and, possibly, blood transfusions.

History and physical examination

If you've ruled out life-threatening conditions, obtain a detailed medical and surgical history. Ask the patient if he has had a hernia or abdominal surgery because these may cause mechanical intestinal obstruction. Does he have a history of inflammatory bowel disease? Ask about recent eruptions of gastroenteritis among family members, friends, or coworkers. If the patient has traveled recently, even within the United States, was he aware of any endemic illnesses?

In addition, determine whether stress may have contributed to the patient's problem. Ask about food allergies and recent ingestion of unusual foods or fluids. Check for fever, which suggests infection. Having already auscultated, now gently inspect, percuss, and palpate the abdomen.

Medical causes

Crohn's disease. Hyperactive bowel sounds usually arise insidiously. Associated signs and symptoms include diarrhea, cramping abdominal pain that may be relieved by defecation, anorexia, a low-grade fever, abdominal distention and tenderness and, in many cases, a fixed mass in the right lower quadrant. Perianal and vaginal lesions are common. Muscle wasting, weight loss, and signs of dehydration may occur as Crohn's disease progresses.

Food hypersensitivity. Malabsorption—typically lactose intolerance—may cause hyperactive bowel sounds. Associated signs and symptoms include diarrhea and, possibly, nausea and vomiting, angioedema, and urticaria.

Gastroenteritis. Hyperactive bowel sounds follow sudden nausea and vomiting and accompany "explosive" diarrhea. Abdominal cramping or pain is common, usually after a peristaltic wave. Fever may occur, depending on the causative organism.

GI hemorrhage. Hyperactive bowel sounds provide the most immediate indication of persistent upper GI bleeding. Other findings include hematemesis, coffee-ground vomitus, abdominal distention, bloody diarrhea, rectal passage of bright red clots and jellylike material or melena, and pain during bleeding. Decreased urine output, tachycardia, and hypotension accompany significant blood loss.

Mechanical intestinal obstruction. Hyperactive bowel sounds occur simultaneously with cramping abdominal pain every few minutes in patients with mechanical intestinal obstruction, a potentially life-threatening disorder; bowel sounds may later become hypoactive and then disappear. With small-bowel obstruction, nausea and vomiting occur earlier and with greater severity than in large-bowel obstruction. With complete bowel obstruction, hyperactive sounds are also accompanied by abdominal distention and constipation, although the part of the bowel distal to the obstruction may continue to empty for up to 3 days.

Ulcerative colitis (acute). Hyperactive bowel sounds arise abruptly in patients with acute ulcerative colitis and are accompanied by bloody diarrhea, anorexia, abdominal pain, nausea and vomiting, fever, and tenesmus. Weight loss, arthralgias, and arthritis may occur.

Nursing considerations

■ Prepare the patient for diagnostic tests, such as laboratory studies, imaging studies, endoscopy, barium X-rays, or stool analysis.
■ If the patient has diarrhea, administer I.V. fluids and electrolytes to replace losses.
■ Restrict food and fluids to rest the GI tract, as indicated.
■ If the patient has GI bleeding, restrict food and fluids and administer I.V. fluids, blood, and vasopressors.

Patient teaching

■ Explain dietary changes, such as food and fluid restrictions, clear liquid diet, or bland diet.
■ Teach stress reduction and relaxation techniques.
■ Discuss any activity restrictions.
■ Explain diagnostic tests and procedures.
■ Teach the patient about the cause of hyperactive bowel sounds and the treatment plan after a diagnosis is established.

■ Bowel sounds, hypoactive

Hypoactive bowel sounds, detected by auscultation, are diminished in regularity, tone, and loudness from normal bowel sounds. They don't herald an emergency; in fact, they're considered normal during sleep. Hypoactive bowel sounds may portend absent bowel sounds, which can indicate a life-threatening disorder.

Hypoactive bowel sounds result from decreased peristalsis, which, in turn, can result from a developing bowel obstruction. The obstruction may be mechanical (as from a hernia, tumor, or twisting), vascular (as from an embolism or thrombosis), or neurogenic (as from mechanical, ischemic, or toxic impairment of bowel innervation). Hypoactive bowel sounds can also result from the use of certain drugs, abdominal surgery, and radiation therapy.

History and physical examination

After detecting hypoactive bowel sounds, look for related symptoms. Ask the patient about the location, onset, duration, frequency, and severity of any pain. Cramping or colicky abdominal pain usually indicates a mechanical bowel obstruction, whereas diffuse abdominal pain usually indicates intestinal distention related to paralytic ileus.

Ask the patient about any recent vomiting. When did it begin? How often does it occur? Does the vomitus look bloody? Ask about changes in bowel habits. Does he have a history of constipation? When was the last time he had a bowel movement or expelled gas?

Obtain a detailed medical and surgical history of conditions that may cause mechanical bowel obstruction, such as an abdominal tumor or hernia. Does the patient have a history of severe pain; trauma; conditions that can cause paralytic ileus, such as pancreatitis; bowel inflammation or gynecologic infection, which may produce peritonitis; or toxic conditions such as uremia? Has he recently had radiation therapy or abdominal surgery or ingested a drug, such as an opiate, which can decrease peristalsis and cause hypoactive bowel sounds?

After the history is complete, perform a physical examination. Inspect the abdomen for distention, noting surgical incisions and obvious masses. Gently percuss and palpate the abdomen for masses, gas, fluid, tenderness, and rigidity. Measure abdominal girth to detect any subsequent increase in distention. Check for poor skin turgor, hypotension, narrowed pulse pressure, and other signs of dehydration and electrolyte imbalance, which may result from paralytic ileus.

Medical causes

Mechanical intestinal obstruction. Bowel sounds may become hypoactive after a period of hyperactivity. The patient may also have acute colicky abdominal pain in the quadrant of obstruction, possibly radiating to the flank or lumbar region; nausea and vomiting (the higher the obstruction, the earlier and more severe the vomiting); constipation; and abdominal distention and bloating. If the obstruction becomes complete, signs of shock may occur.

Mesenteric artery occlusion. After a brief period of hyperactivity, bowel sounds become hypoactive and then quickly disappear, signifying a life-threatening crisis. Associated signs and symptoms include fever; a history of colicky abdominal pain leading to sudden and severe midepigastric or periumbilical pain, followed by abdominal distention and possible bruits; vomiting; constipation; and signs of shock. Abdominal rigidity may appear late.

Paralytic (adynamic) ileus. Bowel sounds are hypoactive and may become absent. Associated signs and symptoms include abdominal distention, generalized discomfort, and constipation or passage of small, liquid stools and flatus. If the disorder follows acute abdominal infection, fever and abdominal pain may occur.

Other causes

Drugs. Certain classes of drugs reduce intestinal motility and thus produce hypoactive bowel sounds. These include opiates, such as codeine; anticholinergics, such as propantheline bromide; phenothiazines, such as chlorpromazine; and vinca alkaloids such as vincristine. General or spinal anesthetics produce transient hypoactive sounds.

Radiation therapy. Hypoactive bowel sounds and abdominal tenderness may occur after irradiation of the abdomen.

Surgery. Hypoactive bowel sounds may occur after manipulation of the bowel. Motility and bowel sounds in the small intestine usually resume within 24 hours; colonic bowel sounds, in 3 to 5 days.

Nursing considerations

- Frequently assess for indications of shock, such as thirst; anxiety; restlessness; tachycardia; cool, clammy skin; and weak, thready pulse.
- Monitor vital signs and auscultate for bowel sounds every 2 to 4 hours.
- If severe pain, abdominal rigidity, guarding, and fever accompany hypoactive bowel sounds, perform emergency interventions to treat paralytic ileus from peritonitis.
- If GI suction and decompression are needed using a nasogastric or intestinal

tube, restrict oral intake, maintain tube patency, monitor drainage, provide oral and nasal hygiene, keep the head of the bed elevated, and turn the patient to facilitate passage of the tube through the GI tract.

- Prepare the patient for diagnostic studies, such as X-ray studies and endoscopic procedures.
- Provide comfort measures as needed, such as placing the patient with paralytic ileus in semi-Fowler's position.

Patient teaching

- Encourage the patient to ambulate to stimulate peristalsis or, if he can't tolerate ambulation, range-of-motion exercises or turning from side to side may stimulate peristalsis.
- Explain all diagnostic procedures and the need to withhold food and fluids.
- Teach the patient about the cause of hypoactive bowel sounds and the treatment plan after a diagnosis is established.

Bradycardia

Bradycardia refers to a heart rate of less than 60 beats/minute. It occurs normally in young adults, trained athletes, and elderly people as well as during sleep. It's a normal response to vagal stimulation caused by coughing, vomiting, or straining during defecation. When bradycardia results from these causes, the heart rate rarely drops below 40 beats/minute. When it results from pathologic causes (such as cardiovascular disorders), the heart rate may be slower.

By itself, bradycardia is a nonspecific sign. In conjunction with such symptoms as chest pain, dizziness, syncope, and shortness of breath, it can signal a life-threatening disorder.

History and physical examination

After detecting bradycardia, check for related signs of life-threatening disorders. (See *Managing severe bradycardia,* page 94.)

If the patient's bradycardia isn't accompanied by untoward signs, ask the patient if he or a family member has a history of a slow pulse rate because this may be inherited. Find out if he has an underlying metabolic disorder, such as hypothyroidism, which can precipitate bradycardia. Ask which medications he's taking and if he's complying with the prescribed schedule and dosage. Monitor his vital signs, temperature, pulse, respirations, blood pressure, and oxygen saturation.

Medical causes

Cardiac arrhythmia. Depending on the type of arrhythmia and the patient's tolerance of it, bradycardia may be transient or sustained, benign or life-threatening. Related findings may include hypotension, palpitations, dizziness, weakness, syncope, and fatigue.

Cardiomyopathy. Cardiomyopathy is a potentially life-threatening disorder that may cause transient or sustained bradycardia. Other findings include dizziness, syncope, edema, fatigue, jugular vein distention, orthopnea, dyspnea, and peripheral cyanosis.

Hypothermia. Bradycardia usually appears when the core temperature drops below 89.6° F (32° C). It's accompanied by shivering, peripheral cyanosis, muscle rigidity, bradypnea, and confusion leading to stupor.

Hypothyroidism. Hypothyroidism causes severe bradycardia in addition to fatigue, constipation, unexplained weight gain, and sensitivity to cold. Related signs include cool, dry, thick skin; sparse, dry hair; facial swelling; perior-

Managing severe bradycardia

Bradycardia can signal a life-threatening disorder when accompanied by pain, shortness of breath, dizziness, syncope, or other symptoms; prolonged exposure to cold; or head or neck trauma. Take the patient's vital signs. Connect him to a cardiac monitor and insert an I.V. catheter. Depending on the cause of bradycardia, you'll need to initiate transcutaneous pacing, administer fluids, atropine, or thyroid medication. If indicated, insert an indwelling urinary catheter. Intubation or mechanical ventilation may be needed if the patient's respiratory rate falls.

Fnding the cause

If appropriate, perform a focused evaluation to help locate the cause of bradycardia. For example, ask about pain. Viselike pressure or crushing or burning chest pain that radiates to the arms, back, or jaw may indicate an acute

myocardial infarction (MI); a severe headache, increased intracranial pressure. Ask about nausea, vomiting, or shortness of breath—signs and symptoms associated with an acute MI and cardiomyopathy. Observe the patient for peripheral cyanosis, edema, or jugular vein distention, which may indicate cardiomyopathy. Look for a thyroidectomy scar because severe bradycardia may result from hypothyroidism caused by failure to take thyroid hormone replacements.

Providing supportive care

If the cause of bradycardia is evident, provide supportive care. For example, keep the hypothermic patient warm by applying blankets, and monitor his core temperature until it reaches 99° F (37.2° C); stabilize the head and neck of a trauma patient until cervical spinal injury is ruled out.

bital edema; thick, brittle nails; and confusion leading to stupor.

Myocardial infarction (MI). Sinus bradycardia is the most common arrhythmia associated with an acute MI. Accompanying signs and symptoms of an MI include an aching, burning, or viselike pressure in the chest that may radiate to the jaw, shoulder, arm, back, or epigastric area; nausea and vomiting; cool, clammy, and pale or cyanotic skin; anxiety; and dyspnea. Blood pressure may be elevated or decreased. Auscultation may reveal abnormal heart sounds.

Other causes

Diagnostic tests. Cardiac catheterization and electrophysiologic studies can induce temporary bradycardia.

Drugs. Beta-adrenergic blockers and some calcium channel blockers, cardiac glycosides, topical miotics (such as pilo-

carpine), protamine, quinidine and other antiarrhythmics, and sympatholytics may cause transient bradycardia. Failure to take thyroid replacements may cause bradycardia.

Invasive treatments. Suctioning can induce hypoxia and vagal stimulation, causing bradycardia. Cardiac surgery can cause edema or damage to conduction tissues, causing bradycardia.

Nursing considerations

- Monitor the patient's vital signs, cardiac rhythm, and level of consciousness frequently.
- Prepare the patient for laboratory tests, such as complete blood count; cardiac markers, serum electrolyte, blood glucose, blood urea nitrogen, arterial blood gas, and blood drug levels; and thyroid function tests.

- Prepare the patient for a 12-lead electrocardiogram and possibly 24-hour Holter monitoring.

Patient teaching

- Inform the patient about signs and symptoms he should report.
- Teach him to take his pulse as well as the parameters for calling the practitioner or seeking emergency care.
- Provide instructions for care of a permanent pacemaker, if appropriate.
- Teach the patient about the cause of his bradycardia and the treatment plan after a diagnosis is established.

Bradypnea

Commonly preceding life-threatening apnea or respiratory arrest, bradypnea is a pattern of regular respirations with a rate of fewer than 10 breaths/minute. This sign results from neurologic and metabolic disorders and drug overdose, which depress the brain's respiratory control centers. (See *How the nervous system controls breathing,* page 96.)

ACTION STAT!

 Depending on the degree of central nervous system (CNS) depression, the patient with severe bradypnea may require constant stimulation to breathe. If the patient seems excessively sleepy, try to arouse him by shaking and instructing him to breathe. Quickly take the patient's vital signs. Assess his neurologic status by checking pupil size and reactions and by evaluating his level of consciousness (LOC) and his ability to move his extremities.

Place the patient on an apnea monitor and pulse oximeter, keep emergency airway equipment available, and be prepared to assist with endotracheal intubation and mechanical ventilation if spontaneous respirations cease. To prevent aspiration, position the patient on his side or keep his head elevated 30 degrees higher than the rest of his body, and clear his airway with suctioning if needed. Administer opioid antagonists, as ordered.

History and physical examination

Obtain a brief history from the patient if possible. Alternatively, obtain this information from whoever accompanied him to the facility. Ask if he's experiencing a drug overdose and, if so, try to determine what drugs he took, how much, when, and by what route. Check his arms for needle marks, indicating possible drug abuse. You may need to administer I.V. naloxone, an opioid antagonist.

If you rule out a drug overdose, ask about chronic illnesses, such as diabetes and renal failure. Check for a medical identification bracelet or an I.D. card that identifies an underlying condition. Ask whether the patient has a history of head trauma, brain tumor, neurologic infection, or stroke.

Perform a complete physical examination, especially noting abnormalities of the respiratory system.

Medical causes

Diabetic ketoacidosis. Bradypnea occurs late in patients with severe, uncontrolled diabetes. Patients with severe ketoacidosis may experience Kussmaul's respirations. Associated signs and symptoms include a decreased LOC, fatigue, weakness, a fruity breath odor, and oliguria.

Hepatic failure. Occurring with end-stage hepatic failure, bradypnea may be accompanied by coma, hyperactive reflexes, asterixis, a positive Babinski's sign, fetor hepaticus, and other signs.

Increased intracranial pressure (ICP). A late sign of increased ICP, a life-

How the nervous system controls breathing

Stimulation from external sources and from higher brain centers acts on respiratory centers in the pons and medulla. These centers, in turn, send impulses to the various parts of the respiratory system to alter respiration patterns.

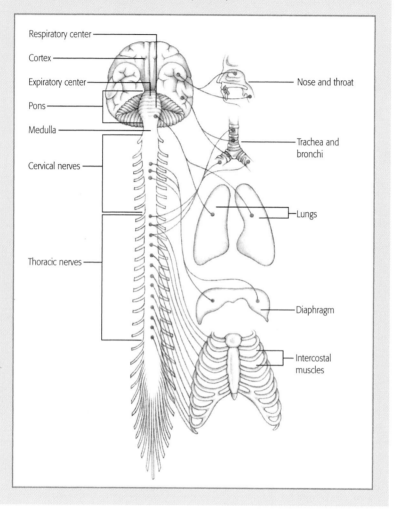

threatening condition, bradypnea is preceded by a decreased LOC, deteriorating motor function, and fixed, dilated pupils. The triad of bradypnea, bradycardia, and hypertension is a classic sign of late medullary strangulation.

Renal failure. Occurring with end-stage renal failure, bradypnea may be accompanied by convulsions, a decreased LOC, GI bleeding, hypotension or hypertension, uremic frost, and diverse other signs.

Respiratory failure. Bradypnea occurs with end-stage respiratory failure along with cyanosis, diminished breath sounds, tachycardia, mildly increased blood pressure, and a decreased LOC.

Other causes
Drugs. Overdose with an opioid analgesic or, less commonly, a sedative, barbiturate, phenothiazine, or other CNS depressant can cause bradypnea. The use of any of these drugs with alcohol can also cause bradypnea.

Nursing considerations
▪ Check the patient's respiratory status frequently and be prepared to give ventilatory support if necessary.
▪ Don't leave the patient unattended, especially if his LOC is decreased.
▪ Obtain blood for arterial blood gas analysis, electrolyte studies, and a possible drug screen.
▪ Ready the patient for chest X-rays and, possibly, a computed tomography scan of the head.
▪ Administer prescribed drugs and evaluate their effect.
▪ Avoid giving a CNS depressant because it can exacerbate bradypnea.
▪ Administer oxygen, being judicious in the patient with chronic carbon dioxide retention (such as chronic obstructive pulmonary disease) because excess oxygen therapy can decrease respiratory drive.
▪ Review all drugs and dosages given during the last 24 hours.

Patient teaching
▪ Explain the complications of opioid therapy such as bradypnea.
▪ Discuss the signs and symptoms of opioid toxicity.
▪ Teach the patient about the cause of bradypnea and the treatment plan after a diagnosis is established.

■ Breast dimpling

Breast dimpling—the puckering or retraction of skin on the breast—results from abnormal attachment of the skin to underlying tissue. It suggests an inflammatory or malignant mass beneath the skin surface and usually represents a late sign of breast cancer; benign lesions usually don't produce this effect. Dimpling usually affects women older than age 40, but also occasionally affects men.

Because breast dimpling occurs over a mass or induration, the patient usually discovers other signs before becoming aware of the dimpling. A thorough breast examination may reveal dimpling and alert the patient and nurse to a problem.

History and physical examination
Obtain a medical, reproductive, and family history, noting factors that place the patient at a high risk for breast cancer. Ask about pregnancy history because women who haven't had a full-term pregnancy before age 30 are at higher risk for developing breast cancer. Has her mother or a sister had breast cancer? Has she herself had a previous malignancy, especially cancer in the other breast?

Ask the patient if she has noticed changes in the shape of her breast. Is any area painful or tender, and is the pain cyclic? If she's breast-feeding, has she recently experienced high fever, chills, malaise, muscle aches, fatigue, or other flulike signs or symptoms? Can she remember sustaining trauma to the breast?

Carefully inspect the dimpled area. Is it swollen, red, or warm to the touch? Do you see bruises or contusions? Ask the patient to tense her pectoral muscles by pressing her hips with both hands or by raising her hands over her head. Does the puckering increase? Gently pull the skin upward toward the clavicle. Is the dimpling exaggerated?

Observe the breast for nipple retraction. Do both nipples point in the same direction? Are the nipples flattened or inverted? Does the patient report nipple discharge? If so, ask her to describe the color and character of the discharge. Observe the contour of both breasts. Are they symmetrical?

Examine both breasts with the patient lying down, sitting, and then leaning forward. Does the skin move freely over both breasts? If you can palpate a lump, note its size, location, consistency, mobility, and delineation. What relation does the lump have to the breast dimpling? Gently mold the breast skin around the lump. Is the dimpling exaggerated? Examine breast and axillary lymph nodes, noting any enlargement.

Medical causes

Breast abscess. Breast dimpling sometimes accompanies a chronic breast abscess. Associated findings include a firm, irregular, nontender lump and signs of nipple retraction, such as deviation, inversion, or flattening. Axillary lymph nodes may be enlarged.

Breast cancer. Breast dimpling is an important but somewhat late sign of breast cancer. A neoplasm that causes dimpling is usually close to the skin and at least 1 cm in diameter. It feels irregularly shaped and fixed to underlying tissue, and it's usually painless. Other signs of breast cancer include peau d'orange, changes in breast symmetry or size, nipple retraction, and a unilateral, spontaneous, nonmilky nipple discharge that's serous or bloody. (A bloody nipple discharge in the presence of a lump is a classic sign of breast cancer.) Axillary lymph nodes may be enlarged. Pain may be present, but isn't a reliable symptom

of breast cancer. A breast ulcer may appear as a late sign.

Fat necrosis. Breast dimpling from fat necrosis follows inflammation and trauma to the fatty tissue of the breast (although the patient usually can't remember such trauma). Tenderness, erythema, bruising, and contusions may occur. Other findings include a hard, indurated, poorly delineated lump, which is fibrotic and fixed to underlying tissue or overlying skin as well as signs of nipple retraction. Fat necrosis is difficult to differentiate from breast cancer.

Mastitis. Breast dimpling may signal bacterial mastitis, which usually results from duct obstruction and milk stasis during breast-feeding. Heat, erythema, swelling, induration, pain, and tenderness usually accompany mastitis. Dimpling is more likely to occur with diffuse induration than with a single hard mass. The skin on the breast may feel fixed to underlying tissue. Other possible findings include nipple retraction, nipple cracks, a purulent discharge, and enlarged axillary lymph nodes. Flulike signs and symptoms (such as fever, malaise, fatigue, and aching) commonly occur.

Nursing considerations

- Because any breast problem can arouse fears of altered body image, mutilation, loss of sexuality, and death, allow the patient to express her feelings and provide emotional support.
- Prepare the patient for diagnostic testing, such as mammography, thermography, biopsy, ultrasonography, and cytology of nipple discharge.

Patient teaching

- Explain what to expect during diagnostic testing.
- Explain the importance of clinical breast examination and mammography

following the American Cancer Society guidelines.

■ Teach the patient how to perform breast self-examination.

■ If the patient breast-feeds and has mastitis, advise her to pump her breasts to prevent milk stasis, to discard the milk, and to substitute formula until the breast infection resolves.

■ Teach the patient about the cause of breast dimpling and the treatment plan after a diagnosis is established.

▋ Breast nodule
[Breast lump]

A commonly reported gynecologic sign, a breast nodule has two chief causes: benign breast disease and cancer. Benign breast disease, the leading cause of nodules, can stem from cyst formation in obstructed and dilated lactiferous ducts, hypertrophy or tumor formation in the ductal system, inflammation, or infection.

Although fewer than 20% of breast nodules are malignant, the signs and symptoms of breast cancer aren't easily distinguished from those of benign breast disease. Breast cancer is a leading cause of death among women, but can occur occasionally in men, with signs and symptoms mimicking those found in women. Thus, breast nodules in both sexes should always be evaluated.

A woman who's familiar with the feel of her breasts and performs monthly breast self-examination can detect a nodule 6.4 mm or less in size, considerably smaller than the 1-cm nodule that's readily detectable by an experienced examiner. However, a woman may fail to report a nodule because of the fear of breast cancer.

History and physical examination

If the patient reports a lump, ask her how and when she discovered it. Does the size and tenderness of the lump vary with her menstrual cycle? Has the lump changed since she first noticed it? Has she noticed other breast signs, such as a change in breast shape, size, or contour; a discharge; or nipple changes?

Is she breast-feeding? Does she have fever, chills, fatigue, or other flulike signs or symptoms? Ask her to describe any pain or tenderness associated with the lump. Is the pain in one breast only? Has she sustained recent trauma to the breast?

Explore the patient's medical and family history for factors that increase her risk of breast cancer. These include having a mother or sister with breast cancer or having a history of cancer, especially cancer in the other breast. Other risk factors include nulliparity and a first pregnancy after age 30.

Next, perform a thorough breast examination. Pay special attention to the upper outer quadrant of each breast, where one-half of the ductal tissue is located. This is the most common site of malignant breast tumors.

Carefully palpate a suspected breast nodule, noting its location, shape, size, consistency, mobility, and delineation. Does the nodule feel soft, rubbery, and elastic or hard? Is it mobile, slipping away from your fingers as you palpate it, or firmly fixed to adjacent tissue? Does the nodule seem to limit the mobility of the entire breast? Note the nodule's delineation. Are the borders clearly defined or indefinite? Does the area feel more like a hardness or diffuse induration than a nodule with definite borders?

Do you feel one nodule or several small ones? Is the shape round, oval, lobular, or irregular? Inspect and palpate the skin over the nodule for warmth, redness, and edema. Palpate the lymph nodes of the breast and axilla for enlargement.

Observe the contour of the breasts, looking for asymmetry and irregularities. Be alert for signs of retraction, such as skin dimpling and nipple deviation, retraction, or flattening. (To exaggerate dimpling, have your patient raise her arms over her head or press her hands against her hips.) Gently pull the breast skin toward the clavicle. Is dimpling evident? Mold the breast skin and again observe the area for dimpling.

Be alert for a nipple discharge that's spontaneous, unilateral, and nonmilky (for example, serous, bloody, or purulent). Be careful not to confuse it with the grayish discharge that can be elicited from the nipples of a woman who has been pregnant.

Medical causes

Adenofibroma. The extremely mobile or "slippery" feel of this benign neoplasm helps distinguish it from other breast nodules. The nodule usually occurs singly and characteristically feels firm, elastic, and round or lobular, with well-defined margins. It doesn't cause pain or tenderness, can vary from pinhead size to very large, commonly grows rapidly, and usually lies around the nipple or on the lateral side of the upper outer quadrant.

Areolar gland abscess. Areolar gland abscess is a tender, palpable mass on the periphery of the areola following an inflammation of the sebaceous glands of Montgomery. Fever may also be present.

Breast abscess. A localized, hot, tender, fluctuant mass with erythema and peau d'orange typifies an acute abscess. Associated signs and symptoms include fever, chills, malaise, and generalized discomfort. With a chronic abscess, the nodule is nontender, irregular, and firm and may feel like a thick wall of fibrous tissue. It's commonly accompanied by skin dimpling, peau d'orange, nipple retraction and, sometimes, axillary lymphadenopathy.

Breast cancer. A hard, poorly delineated nodule that's fixed to the skin or underlying tissue suggests breast cancer. Malignant nodules typically cause breast dimpling, nipple deviation or retraction, or flattening of the nipple or breast contour. Between 40% and 50% of malignant nodules occur in the upper outer quadrant.

Nodules usually occur singly, although satellite nodules may surround the main one. They're usually nontender. Nipple discharge may be serous or bloody. (A bloody nipple discharge in the presence of a nodule is a classic sign of breast cancer.) Additional findings include edema (peau d'orange) of the skin overlying the mass, erythema, tenderness, and axillary lymphadenopathy. A breast ulcer may occur as a late sign. Breast pain, an unreliable symptom, may be present.

Fibrocystic breast disease. The most common cause of breast nodules, this fibrocystic condition produces smooth, round, slightly elastic nodules, which increase in size and tenderness just before menstruation. The nodules may occur in fine, granular clusters in both breasts or as widespread, well-defined lumps of varying sizes. A thickening of adjacent tissue may be palpable. Cystic nodules are mobile, which helps differentiate them from malignant ones. Because cystic nodules aren't fixed to underlying breast tissue, they don't produce retraction signs, such as nipple deviation or dimpling. Signs and symptoms of premenstrual syndrome—including headache, irritability, bloating, nausea, vomiting, and abdominal cramping—may also be present.

Mammary duct ectasia. The rubbery breast nodule in mammary duct ectasia, a menopausal or postmenopausal disorder, usually lies under the areola. It's commonly accompanied by transient pain, itching, tenderness, and erythema of the areola; thick, sticky, multicolored nipple discharge from multiple ducts; and nipple retraction. The skin overlying the mass may be bluish green or exhibit peau d'orange. Axillary lymphadenopathy is possible.

Mastitis. With mastitis, breast nodules feel firm and indurated or tender, flocculent, and discrete. Gentle palpation defines the area of maximum purulent accumulation. Skin dimpling and nipple deviation, retraction, or flattening may be present, and the nipple may show a crack or abrasion. Accompanying signs and symptoms include breast warmth, erythema, tenderness, and peau d'orange as well as a high fever, chills, malaise, and fatigue.

Paget's disease. Paget's disease is a slow-growing intraductal carcinoma that begins as a scaling, eczematoid unilateral nipple lesion. The nipple later becomes reddened and excoriated and may eventually be completely destroyed. The process extends along the skin as well as in the ducts, usually progressing to a deep-seated mass.

Nursing considerations

- Provide a simple explanation of your examination, and encourage the patient to express her feelings.
- Prepare the patient for diagnostic tests, which may include transillumination, mammography, thermography, needle aspiration or open biopsy, and cytologic examination of nipple discharge.
- Postpone teaching the patient how to perform breast self-examination until she overcomes her initial anxiety at discovering a nodule.

- Although most nodules occurring in the breast-feeding patient result from mastitis, the possibility of cancer demands careful evaluation.

Patient teaching

- Advise the patient with mastitis to pump her breasts to prevent further milk stasis, to discard the milk, and to substitute formula until the infection responds to antibiotics.
- Explain the importance of clinical breast examination and mammography following the American Cancer Society guidelines.
- Teach the patient how to perform breast self-examination.
- Explain how to treat mastitis.
- Teach the patient about the cause of the breast nodule and the treatment plan after a diagnosis is established.

Breast pain
[Mastalgia]

An unreliable indicator of cancer, breast pain commonly results from benign breast disease. It may occur during rest or movement and may be aggravated by manipulation or palpation. (Breast tenderness refers to pain elicited by physical contact.) Breast pain may be unilateral or bilateral; cyclic, intermittent, or constant; and dull or sharp. It may result from surface cuts, furuncles, contusions, or similar lesions (superficial pain); nipple fissures or inflammation in the papillary ducts or areolae (severe localized pain); stromal distention in the breast parenchyma; a tumor that affects nerve endings (severe, constant pain); or inflammatory lesions that distend the stroma and irritate sensory nerve endings (severe, constant pain). Breast pain may radiate to the back, the arms and, sometimes, the neck.

Breast tenderness in women may occur before menstruation and during pregnancy. Before menstruation, breast pain or tenderness stems from increased mammary blood flow due to hormonal changes. During pregnancy, breast tenderness and throbbing, tingling, or pricking sensations may occur, also from hormonal changes. In men, breast pain may stem from gynecomastia (especially during puberty and senescence), reproductive tract anomalies, or organic disease of the liver or pituitary, adrenal cortex, or thyroid glands.

History and physical examination

Begin by asking the patient if breast pain is constant or intermittent. For either type, ask about onset and character. If it's intermittent, determine the relationship of pain to the phase of the menstrual cycle. Is the patient breast-feeding? If not, ask about any nipple discharge and have her describe it. Is she pregnant? Has she reached menopause? Has she recently experienced flulike symptoms or sustained injury to the breast? Has she noticed a change in breast shape or contour?

Ask the patient to describe the pain. She may describe it as sticking, stinging, shooting, stabbing, throbbing, or burning. Determine if the pain affects one breast or both, and ask the patient to point to the painful area.

Instruct the patient to place her arms at her sides, and inspect the breasts. Note their size, symmetry, and contour and the appearance of the skin. Remember that breast shape and size vary and that breasts normally change during menses, pregnancy, and lactation and with aging. Are the breasts red or edematous? Are the veins prominent?

Note the size, shape, and symmetry of the nipples and areolae. Do you detect ecchymosis, a rash, ulceration, or a discharge? Do the nipples point in the same direction? Do you see signs of re-traction, such as skin dimpling or nipple inversion or flattening? Repeat your inspection, first with the patient's arms raised above her head and then with her hands pressed against her hips.

Palpate the breasts, first with the patient seated and then with her lying down and a pillow placed under her shoulder on the side being examined. Use the pads of your fingers to compress breast tissue against the chest wall. Proceed systematically from the sternum to the midline and from the axilla to the midline, noting any warmth, tenderness, nodules, masses, or irregularities. Palpate the nipple, noting tenderness and nodules, and check for discharge. Palpate axillary lymph nodes, noting any enlargement.

Medical causes

Areolar gland abscess. Areolar gland abscess is a tender, palpable mass on the periphery of the areola following an inflammation of the sebaceous glands of Montgomery. Fever may also occur.

Breast abscess (acute). In the affected breast, local pain, tenderness, erythema, peau d'orange, and warmth are associated with a nodule. Malaise, fever, and chills may also occur.

Breast cyst. A breast cyst that enlarges rapidly may cause acute, localized, and usually unilateral pain. A palpable breast nodule may be present.

Fat necrosis. Local pain and tenderness may develop in fat necrosis, a benign disorder. A history of trauma usually is present. Associated findings include ecchymosis; erythema of the overriding skin; a firm, irregular, fixed mass; and skin retraction signs, such as skin dimpling and nipple retraction. Fat necrosis may be hard to differentiate from cancer.

Fibrocystic breast disease. Fibrocystic breast disease is a common cause of breast pain that's associated with the development of cysts that may cause pain before menstruation and are asymptomatic afterward. Later in the course of the disorder, pain and tenderness may persist throughout the cycle. The cysts feel firm, mobile, and well defined. Many are bilateral and found in the upper outer quadrant of the breast, but others are unilateral and generalized. Signs and symptoms of premenstrual syndrome—including headache, irritability, bloating, nausea, vomiting, and abdominal cramping—may also be present.

Mammary duct ectasia. Burning pain and itching around the areola may occur, although ectasia is commonly asymptomatic at first. The history may include one or more episodes of inflammation with pain, tenderness, erythema, and acute fever, or with pain and tenderness alone, which develop and then subside spontaneously within 7 to 10 days. Other findings include a rubbery, subareolar breast nodule; swelling and erythema around the nipple; nipple retraction; a bluish green discoloration or peau d'orange of the skin overlying the nodule; a thick, sticky, multicolored nipple discharge from multiple ducts; and axillary lymphadenopathy. A breast ulcer may occur in late stages.

Mastitis. Unilateral pain may be severe, particularly when the inflammation occurs near the skin surface. Breast skin is typically red and warm at the inflammation site; peau d'orange may be present. Palpation reveals a firm area of induration. Skin retraction signs—such as breast dimpling and nipple deviation, inversion, or flattening—may be present. Systemic signs and symptoms—such as high fever, chills, malaise, and fatigue—may also occur.

Sebaceous cyst (infected). Breast pain may be reported with sebaceous cyst, a cutaneous cyst. Associated symptoms include a small, well-delineated

nodule, localized erythema, and induration.

Nursing considerations
- Provide emotional support for the patient.
- Prepare the patient for diagnostic tests, such as mammography, ultrasonography, thermography, cytology of nipple discharge, biopsy, or culture of any aspirate.

Patient teaching
- Explain the importance of clinical breast examination and mammography following the American Cancer Society guidelines.
- Teach the patient how to perform breast self-examination.
- Explain the use of warm or cold compresses.
- Instruct the patient on the correct type of brassiere.
- Teach the patient about the cause of her breast pain and the treatment plan after a diagnosis is established.

Breast ulcer

Appearing on the nipple, areola, or the breast itself, an ulcer indicates destruction of the skin and subcutaneous tissue. A breast ulcer is usually a late sign of cancer, appearing well after the confirming diagnosis. Breast ulcers can also result from trauma, infection, or radiation.

History and physical examination
Begin the history by asking when the patient first noticed the ulcer and if it was preceded by other breast changes, such as nodules, edema, or nipple discharge, deviation, or retraction. Does the ulcer seem to be getting better or worse? Does it cause pain or produce drainage? Has she noticed any change in breast

shape? Has she had a skin rash? If she has been treating the ulcer at home, find out how.

Review the patient's personal and family history for factors that increase the risk of breast cancer. Ask, for example, about previous cancer, especially of the breast, and mastectomy. Determine whether the patient's mother or sister has had breast cancer. Ask the patient's age at menarche and menopause because more than 30 years of menstrual activity increases the risk of breast cancer. Ask about pregnancy because nulliparity or birth of a first child after age 30 also increases the risk of breast cancer.

If the patient recently gave birth, ask if she breast-feeds her infant or has recently weaned him. Ask if she's currently taking an oral antibiotic and if she's diabetic. All these factors predispose the patient to *Candida* infections.

Inspect the patient's breast, noting any asymmetry or flattening. Look for a rash, scaling, cracking, or red excoriation on the nipples, areola, and inframammary fold. Check especially for skin changes, such as warmth, erythema, or peau d'orange. Palpate the breast for masses, noting any induration beneath the ulcer. Then carefully palpate for tenderness or nodules around the areola and the axillary lymph nodes.

Medical causes

Breast cancer. A breast ulcer that doesn't heal within a month usually indicates breast cancer. Ulceration along a mastectomy scar may indicate metastatic cancer; a nodule beneath the ulcer may be a late sign of a fulminating tumor. Other signs include a palpable breast nodule, skin dimpling, nipple retraction, bloody or serous nipple discharge, erythema, peau d'orange, and enlarged axillary lymph nodes.

Breast trauma. Tissue destruction from breast trauma with inadequate healing may produce breast ulcers. Associated signs depend on the type of trauma, but may include ecchymosis, lacerations, abrasions, swelling, and hematoma.

Candida albicans *infection.* Severe *Candida* infection can cause maceration of breast tissue followed by ulceration. Well-defined, bright-red papular patches—usually with scaly borders—characterize the infection, which can develop in the breast folds. In breast-feeding women, cracked nipples predispose them to infection. Women describe the pain, felt when the infant sucks, as a burning pain that penetrates into the chest wall.

Paget's disease. Bright-red nipple excoriation can extend to the areola and ulcerate. Serous or bloody nipple discharge and extreme nipple itching may accompany ulceration. Symptoms are usually unilateral.

Other causes

Radiation therapy. After treatment, the breasts appear "sunburned." Subsequently, the skin ulcerates and the surrounding area becomes red and tender.

Nursing considerations

- If breast cancer is suspected, provide emotional support and encourage the patient to express her feelings.
- Prepare her for diagnostic tests, such as ultrasonography, thermography, mammography, nipple discharge cytology, and breast biopsy.
- If a *Candida* infection is suspected, prepare her for skin or blood cultures.

Patient teaching

- Teach the patient how to apply a topical antifungal or antibacterial ointment or cream.

- Instruct her to keep the ulcer dry to reduce chafing and to wear loose-fitting undergarments.
- Explain the importance of clinical breast examination and mammography following the American Cancer Society guidelines.
- Teach the patient about the cause of the breast ulcer and the treatment plan after a diagnosis is established.

Breath with ammonia odor
[Uremic fetor]

The odor of ammonia on the breath—described as urinous or "fishy" breath—typically occurs in end-stage chronic renal failure. This sign improves slightly after hemodialysis and persists throughout the course of the disorder, but isn't of great concern.

Ammonia breath odor reflects the long-term metabolic disturbances and biochemical abnormalities associated with uremia and end-stage chronic renal failure. It's produced by metabolic end products blown off by the lungs and the breakdown of urea (to ammonia) in the saliva. A specific uremic toxin hasn't been identified. In animals, breath odor analysis has revealed toxic metabolites, such as dimethylamine and trimethylamine, which contribute to the "fishy" odor. The source of these amines, although still unclear, may be intestinal bacteria acting on dietary chlorine.

History and physical examination

When you detect ammonia breath odor, the diagnosis of chronic renal failure will probably be well established. Look for associated GI symptoms so that palliative care and support can be individualized.

Inspect the patient's oral cavity for bleeding, swollen gums or tongue, and ulceration with drainage. Ask the patient if he has experienced a metallic taste, loss of smell, increased thirst, heartburn, difficulty swallowing, loss of appetite at the sight of food, or early morning vomiting. Because GI bleeding is common in patients with chronic renal failure, ask about bowel habits, noting especially melanous stools or constipation.

Take the patient's vital signs. Watch for indications of hypertension (the patient with end-stage chronic renal failure is usually somewhat hypertensive) or hypotension. Be alert for other signs of shock (such as tachycardia, tachypnea, and cool, clammy skin) and altered mental status. Significant changes can indicate complications, such as massive GI bleeding or pericarditis with tamponade.

Medical causes

End-stage renal disease. Ammonia breath odor is a late finding symptom in end-stage renal disease. Accompanying signs and symptoms include anuria, skin pigmentation changes and excoriation, brown arcs under the nail margins, tissue wasting, Kussmaul's respirations, neuropathy, lethargy, somnolence, confusion, disorientation, behavior changes with irritability, and mood lability. Later neurologic signs that signal impending uremic coma include muscle twitching and fasciculation, asterixis, paresthesia, and footdrop. Cardiovascular findings include hypertension, myocardial infarction, signs of heart failure, pericarditis, and even sudden death and stroke. GI findings include anorexia, nausea, heartburn, vomiting, constipation, hiccups, and a metallic taste, with oral signs and symptoms, such as stomatitis, gum ulceration and bleeding, and a coated tongue. The patient has an increased risk of peptic ulceration and acute pancreatitis. Weight loss is common; uremic frost, pruritus, and signs of hormonal changes, such as impotence or amenorrhea, also appear.

Nursing considerations
▪ Maximize dietary intake by offering the patient frequent small meals of his favorite foods, within dietary limitations.
▪ Provide mouth care if the patient is unable to do it himself.

Patient teaching
▪ Instruct the patient to perform frequent mouth care, particularly before meals because reducing foul mouth taste and odor may stimulate his appetite.
▪ Tell him to use a half-strength hydrogen peroxide mixture or lemon juice gargle to help neutralize the ammonia.
▪ Recommend the use of commercial lozenges or breath sprays or to suck on hard candy to freshen his breath.
▪ Advise him to use a soft toothbrush or sponge to prevent trauma. If he's unable to perform mouth care, do it for him and teach his family members how to assist him.
▪ Teach the patient about the cause of the ammonia breath odor after a diagnosis is established.

Breath with fecal odor

Fecal breath odor typically accompanies fecal vomiting associated with a long-standing intestinal obstruction or gastro-jejunocolic fistula. It represents an important late diagnostic clue to a potentially life-threatening GI disorder because complete obstruction of any part of the bowel, if untreated, can cause death within hours from vascular collapse and shock.

When the obstructed or adynamic intestine attempts self-decompression by regurgitating its contents, vigorous peristaltic waves propel bowel contents backward into the stomach. When the stomach fills with intestinal fluid, further reverse peristalsis results in vomiting. The odor of feculent vomitus lingers in the mouth.

Fecal breath odor may also occur in patients with a nasogastric (NG) or intestinal tube. The odor is detected only while the underlying disorder persists and abates soon after its resolution.

ACTION STAT!

 Because fecal breath odor signals a potentially life-threatening intestinal obstruction, you'll need to quickly evaluate the patient's condition. Monitor his vital signs, and be alert for signs of shock, such as hypotension, tachycardia, narrowed pulse pressure, and cool, clammy skin. Ask the patient if he's experiencing nausea or has vomited. Find out the frequency of vomiting as well as the color, odor, amount, and consistency of the vomitus. Have an emesis basin nearby to collect and accurately measure the vomitus.

Anticipate possible surgery to relieve an obstruction or repair a fistula, and withhold all food and fluids. Be prepared to insert an NG or intestinal tube for GI tract decompression. Insert a peripheral I.V. catheter for vascular access, or assist with central line insertion for large-bore access and central venous pressure monitoring. Obtain a blood sample and send it to the laboratory for complete blood count and electrolyte analysis because large fluid losses and shifts can produce electrolyte imbalances. Maintain adequate hydration and support circulatory status with additional fluids. Give a physiologic solution—such as lactated Ringer's or normal saline solution or Plasmanate—to prevent metabolic acidosis from gastric losses and metabolic alkalosis from intestinal fluid losses.

History and physical examination

If the patient's condition permits, ask about previous abdominal surgery because adhesions can cause an obstruction. Ask about loss of appetite. Is the patient experiencing abdominal pain? If so, have him describe its onset, duration, intensity, and location. Ask if the pain is intense, persistent, or spasmodic. Have the patient describe his normal bowel habits, especially noting constipation, diarrhea, or leakage of stool. Ask when the patient's last bowel movement occurred, and have him describe the stool's color and consistency.

Auscultate for bowel sounds—hyperactive, high-pitched sounds may indicate impending bowel obstruction, whereas hypoactive or absent sounds occur late in obstruction and paralytic ileus. Inspect the abdomen, noting its contour and any surgical scars. Measure abdominal girth to provide baseline data for subsequent assessment of distention. Palpate for tenderness, distention, and rigidity. Percuss for tympany, indicating a gas-filled bowel, and dullness, indicating fluid.

Rectal and pelvic examinations should be performed. All patients with a suspected bowel obstruction should have a flat and upright abdominal X-ray; some will also need a chest X-ray, sigmoidoscopy, and barium enema.

Medical causes

Distal small-bowel obstruction.

With late small-bowel obstruction, nausea is present although vomiting may be delayed. Vomitus initially consists of gastric contents, then changes to bilious contents, followed by fecal contents with resultant fecal breath odor. Accompanying symptoms include achiness, malaise, drowsiness, and polydipsia. Bowel changes (ranging from diarrhea to constipation) are accompanied by abdominal distention, persistent epigastric or periumbilical colicky pain, and hyperactive bowel sounds and borborygmi. As the obstruction becomes complete, bowel sounds become hypoactive or absent. Fever, hypotension, tachycardia, and rebound tenderness may indicate strangulation or perforation.

Gastrojejunocolic fistula. With gastrojejunocolic fistula, symptoms may be variable and intermittent because of temporary plugging of the fistula. Fecal vomiting with resulting fecal breath odor may occur, but the most common chief complaint is diarrhea, accompanied by abdominal pain. Related GI findings include anorexia, weight loss, abdominal distention and, possibly, marked malabsorption.

Large-bowel obstruction. Vomiting is usually absent initially with a large-bowel obstruction, but fecal vomiting with resultant fecal breath odor occurs as a late sign. Typically, symptoms develop more slowly than in small-bowel obstruction. Colicky abdominal pain appears suddenly, followed by continuous hypogastric pain. Marked abdominal distention and tenderness occur, and loops of large bowel may be visible through the abdominal wall. Although constipation develops, defecation may continue for up to 3 days after complete obstruction because of stool remaining in the bowel below the obstruction. Leakage of stool is common with partial obstruction.

Nursing considerations

■ After an NG or intestinal tube has been inserted, keep the head of the bed elevated at least 30 degrees and turn the patient to facilitate passage of the intestinal tube through the GI tract.

- Ensure tube patency by monitoring drainage and watching that suction devices function properly. Irrigate as required.
- Monitor GI drainage, and send serum specimens to the laboratory for electrolyte analysis.
- Prepare the patient for diagnostic tests, such as abdominal X-rays, barium enema, and proctoscopy.

Patient teaching

- Explain all procedure and treatments to the patient.
- Teach the techniques of good oral hygiene.
- Explain food and fluid restrictions.
- Assure the patient that the fecal odor is temporary and will abate after treatment of the underlying condition.
- Teach the patient about the cause of fecal breath odor and the treatment plan after a diagnosis is established.

▌ Breath with fruity odor

Fruity breath odor results from respiratory elimination of excess acetone. This sign characteristically occurs with ketoacidosis—a potentially life-threatening condition that requires immediate treatment to prevent severe dehydration, irreversible coma, and death.

Ketoacidosis results from the excessive catabolism of fats for cellular energy in the absence of usable carbohydrates. This process begins when insulin levels are insufficient to transport glucose into the cells, as in diabetes mellitus, or when glucose is unavailable and hepatic glycogen stores are depleted, as in low-carbohydrate diets and malnutrition. Lacking glucose, the cells burn fat faster than enzymes can handle the ketones, the acidic end products. As a result, the ketones (acetone, beta-hydroxybutyric acid, and acetoacetic acid) accumulate

in the blood and urine. To compensate for increased acidity, Kussmaul's respirations expel carbon dioxide with enough acetone to flavor the breath. Eventually, this compensatory mechanism fails, producing ketoacidosis.

ACTION STAT!

 When you detect fruity breath odor, check for Kussmaul's respirations and examine the patient's level of consciousness (LOC). Take his vital signs and check skin turgor. Be alert for fruity breath odor that accompanies rapid, deep respirations; stupor; and poor skin turgor. Try to obtain a brief history, noting especially diabetes mellitus, nutritional problems such as anorexia nervosa, and fad diets with little or no carbohydrates. Obtain venous blood samples for glucose, complete blood count, and electrolyte, acetone, and arterial blood gas (ABG) levels. Administer I.V. fluids and electrolytes to maintain hydration and electrolyte balance and, in the patient with diabetic ketoacidosis, give regular insulin to reduce blood glucose levels.

If the patient is obtunded, you'll need to insert endotracheal and nasogastric (NG) tubes. Suction as needed. Insert an indwelling urinary catheter, and monitor intake and output. Insert central venous pressure and arterial lines to monitor the patient's fluid status and blood pressure. Place the patient on a cardiac monitor, monitor his vital signs and neurologic status, and draw blood as ordered to check glucose, electrolyte, acetone, and ABG levels.

History and physical examination

If the patient isn't in severe distress, obtain a thorough history. Ask about the onset and duration of fruity breath odor. Find out about changes in breathing pattern. Ask about increased thirst, frequent urination, weight loss, fatigue, and abdominal pain. Ask the female patient if she has had candidal vaginitis or vaginal secretions with itching. If the patient has a history of diabetes mellitus, ask about stress, infections, and noncompliance with therapy—the most common causes of ketoacidosis in known diabetics. If the patient is suspected of having anorexia nervosa, obtain a dietary and weight history.

Medical causes

Anorexia nervosa. Severe weight loss associated with anorexia nervosa may produce fruity breath, usually with nausea, constipation, and cold intolerance as well as dental enamel erosion and scars or calluses in the dorsum of the hand, both related to induced vomiting.

Ketoacidosis. Fruity breath odor accompanies alcoholic ketoacidosis, which is usually seen in poorly nourished alcoholics with vomiting, abdominal pain, and only minimal food intake over several days. Kussmaul's respirations begin abruptly and accompany dehydration, abdominal pain and distention, and absent bowel sounds. Blood glucose levels are normal or slightly decreased.

With diabetic ketoacidosis, fruity breath odor commonly occurs as ketoacidosis develops over 1 or 2 days. Other findings include polydipsia, polyuria, nocturia, a weak and rapid pulse, hunger, weight loss, weakness, fatigue, nausea, vomiting, and abdominal pain. Eventually, Kussmaul's respirations, orthostatic hypotension, dehydration, tachycardia, confusion, and stupor occur. Signs and symptoms may lead to coma.

Starvation ketoacidosis is a potentially life-threatening disorder that has a gradual onset. Besides fruity breath odor, typical findings include signs of cachexia and dehydration, a decreased

LOC, bradycardia, and a history of severely limited food intake.

Other causes

Drugs. Any drug known to cause metabolic acidosis, such as nitroprusside and salicylates, can result in fruity breath odor.

Low-carbohydrate diets. These diets, which encourage little or no carbohydrate intake, may cause ketoacidosis and the resulting fruity breath odor.

Nursing considerations

- Provide emotional support for the patient and his family.
- When the patient is more alert and his condition stabilizes, remove the NG tube and start him on an appropriate diet.
- Switch his insulin from the I.V. to the subcutaneous route.

Patient teaching

- Explain tests and treatments to the patient.
- Discuss the signs and symptoms of hyperglycemia and actions to take.
- Emphasize the importance of wearing medical identification.
- Refer the patient with starvation ketoacidosis to a psychologist or support group.
- Teach the patient about the cause of fruity breath odor after a diagnosis is established.

Brudzinski's sign

A positive Brudzinski's sign (flexion of the hips and knees in response to passive flexion of the neck) signals meningeal irritation. Passive flexion of the neck stretches the nerve roots, causing pain and involuntary flexion of the knees and hips.

Brudzinski's sign is a common and important early indicator of life-threatening meningitis and subarachnoid hemorrhage. It can be elicited in children as well as adults, although more reliable indicators of meningeal irritation exist for infants.

Testing for Brudzinski's sign isn't part of the routine examination, unless meningeal irritation is suspected. (See *Testing for Brudzinski's sign.*)

ACTION STAT!

 If the patient is alert, ask him about headache, neck pain, nausea, and vision disturbances (such as blurred or double vision and photophobia)—all indications of increased intracranial pressure (ICP). Next, observe the patient for signs and symptoms of increased ICP, such as an altered level of consciousness (LOC) (for example, restlessness, irritability, confusion, lethargy, personality changes, and coma), pupillary changes, bradycardia, widened pulse pressure, irregular respiratory patterns (such as Cheyne-Stokes or Kussmaul's respirations), vomiting, and moderate fever.

Keep artificial airways, intubation equipment, a handheld resuscitation bag, and suction equipment on hand because the patient's condition may suddenly deteriorate. Elevate the head of his bed 30 to 60 degrees to promote venous drainage. Administer an osmotic diuretic, such as mannitol, to reduce cerebral edema.

Monitor ICP and be alert for ICP that continues to rise. You may have to provide mechanical ventilation and administer a barbiturate and additional doses of a diuretic. Cerebrospinal fluid (CSF) may have to be drained.

History and physical examination

Continue your neurologic examination by evaluating the patient's cranial nerve function, noting motor or sensory deficits. Be sure to look for Kernig's sign (resistance to knee extension after flexion of the hip), which is a further indication of meningeal irritation. Look for signs of central nervous system infection, such as fever and nuchal rigidity.

Ask the patient or his family, if necessary, about a history of hypertension, spinal arthritis, or recent head trauma. Ask about dental work and abscessed teeth (a possible cause of meningitis), open-head injury, endocarditis, and I.V. drug abuse. Ask about sudden onset of headaches, which may be associated with subarachnoid hemorrhage.

Medical causes

Arthritis. With severe spinal arthritis, a positive Brudzinski's sign can occasionally be elicited. The patient may also report back pain (especially after weight bearing) and limited mobility.

Meningitis. A positive Brudzinski's sign can usually be elicited 24 hours after the onset of meningitis, a life-threatening disorder. Accompanying findings may include headache, a positive Kernig's sign, nuchal rigidity, irritability or restlessness, deep stupor or coma, vertigo, fever (high or low, depending on the severity of the infection), chills, malaise, hyperalgesia, muscular hypotonia, opisthotonos, symmetrical deep tendon reflexes, papilledema, ocular and facial palsies, nausea and vomiting, photophobia, diplopia, and unequal, sluggish pupils. As ICP rises, arterial hypertension, bradycardia, widened pulse pressure, Cheyne-Stokes or Kussmaul's respirations, and coma may develop.

Subarachnoid hemorrhage. Brudzinski's sign may be elicited within minutes after initial bleeding in subarachnoid hemorrhage, a life-threatening disorder. Accompanying signs and symptoms include the sudden onset of severe headache, nuchal rigidity, altered

ASSESSMENT TIP

 Testing for Brudzinski's sign

Here's how to test for Brudzinski's sign when you suspect meningeal irritation:

With the patient
in a supine posi-
tion, place your
hands behind her
neck and lift her
head toward her
chest (as shown
at right).

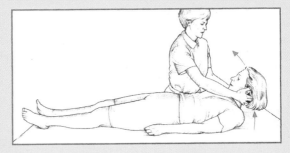

If your patient has
meningeal irrita-
tion, she'll flex
her hips and
knees in re-
sponse to the
passive neck flex-
ion (as shown at
right).

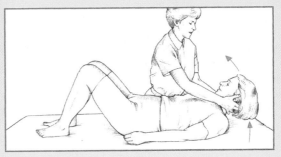

LOC, dizziness, photophobia, cranial nerve palsies (as evidenced by ptosis, pupil dilation, and limited extraocular muscle movement), nausea and vomiting, fever, and a positive Kernig's sign. Focal signs—such as hemiparesis, vision disturbances, or aphasia—may also occur. As ICP rises, arterial hypertension, bradycardia, widened pulse pressure, Cheyne-Stokes or Kussmaul's respirations, and coma may develop.

Nursing considerations
- Provide constant ICP monitoring and perform frequent neurologic checks.
- Monitor vital signs, intake and output, and cardiorespiratory status.
- To promote patient comfort, maintain low lights and minimal noise and elevate the head of the bed.

- Prepare the patient for diagnostic tests, such as blood, urine, and sputum cultures to identify bacteria; lumbar puncture to assess CSF and relieve pressure; and computed tomography scan, magnetic resonance imaging, cerebral angiography, and spinal X-rays to locate a hemorrhage.

Patient teaching
- Discuss the signs and symptoms of meningitis and subdural hematoma, if these are the cause of Brudzinski's sign.
- Advise the patient and his family to seek immediate medical attention if these signs and symptoms occur.

Bruits

Commonly an indicator of life- or limb-threatening vascular disease, bruits are swishing sounds caused by turbulent blood flow. They're characterized by location, duration, intensity, pitch, and the time of onset in the cardiac cycle. Loud bruits produce intense vibration and a palpable thrill. A thrill doesn't provide a further clue to the causative disorder or to its severity.

Bruits are most significant when heard over the abdominal aorta; the renal, carotid, femoral, popliteal, or subclavian artery; or the thyroid gland. (See *Preventing false bruits.*)

They're also significant when heard consistently despite changes in patient position and when heard during diastole.

History and physical examination

If you detect bruits over the abdominal aorta, check for a pulsating mass or a bluish discoloration around the umbilicus (Cullen's sign). Either of these signs—or severe, tearing pain in the abdomen, flank, or lower back—may signal life-threatening dissection of an aortic aneurysm. Check peripheral pulses, comparing intensity in the upper versus lower extremities.

If you suspect dissection, monitor the patient's vital signs constantly, and withhold food and fluids until a definitive diagnosis is made. Watch for signs and symptoms of hypovolemic shock, such as thirst; hypotension; tachycardia; a weak, thready pulse; tachypnea; an altered level of consciousness (LOC); mottled knees and elbows; and cool, clammy skin.

If you detect bruits over the thyroid gland, ask the patient if he has a history of hyperthyroidism or signs and symptoms of it, such as nervousness, tremors, weight loss, palpitations, heat intolerance, and (in females) amenorrhea. Watch for signs and symptoms of life-threatening thyroid storm, such as tremor, restlessness, diarrhea, abdominal pain, and hepatomegaly.

If you detect carotid artery bruits, be alert for signs and symptoms of a transient ischemic attack (TIA), including dizziness, diplopia, slurred speech, flashing lights, and syncope. These findings may indicate an impending stroke. Be sure to evaluate the patient frequently for changes in LOC and muscle function.

If you detect bruits over the femoral, popliteal, or subclavian artery, watch for signs and symptoms of decreased or absent peripheral circulation, such as edema, weakness, and paresthesia. Ask the patient if he has a history of intermittent claudication. Frequently check distal pulses and skin color and temperature. Watch for the sudden absence of pulse, pallor, or coolness, which may indicate a threat to the affected limb.

If you detect a bruit, make sure to check for further vascular damage and perform a thorough cardiac assessment.

Medical causes

Abdominal aortic aneurysm. A pulsating periumbilical mass accompanied by a systolic bruit over the aorta characterizes abdominal aortic aneurysm. Associated signs and symptoms include a rigid, tender abdomen; mottled skin; diminished peripheral pulses; and claudication. Sharp, tearing pain in the abdomen, flank, or lower back signals imminent dissection.

Abdominal aortic atherosclerosis. Loud systolic bruits in the epigastric and midabdominal areas are common with abdominal aortic atherosclerosis. They may be accompanied by leg weakness, numbness, paresthesia, or paralysis; leg pain; or decreased or absent femoral,

Preventing false bruits

Auscultating bruits accurately requires practice and skill. These sounds typically stem from arterial luminal narrowing or arterial dilation, but they can also result from excessive pressure applied to the stethoscope's bell during auscultation. This pressure compresses the artery, creating turbulent blood flow and a false bruit.

To prevent false bruits, place the bell lightly on the patient's skin. If you're auscultating for a popliteal bruit, help the patient to a supine position, place your hand behind his ankle, and lift his leg slightly before placing the bell behind the knee.

Normal blood flow, no bruit

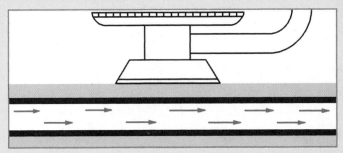

Turbulent blood flow and resultant bruit caused by aneurysm

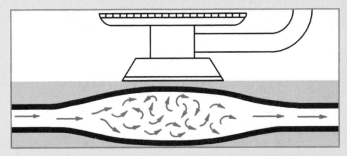

Turbulent blood flow and false bruit caused by compression of artery

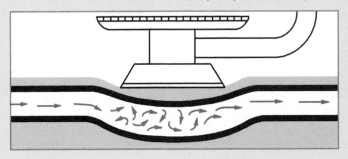

popliteal, or pedal pulses. Abdominal pain is rarely present.

Anemia. In patients with severe anemia, short systolic bruits may be heard over both carotid arteries and may be accompanied by headache, fatigue, dizziness, pallor, jaundice, palpitations, mild tachycardia, dyspnea, nausea, anorexia, and glossitis.

Carotid artery stenosis. Systolic bruits can be heard over one or both carotid arteries with carotid artery stenosis. Other signs and symptoms may be absent. Dizziness, vertigo, headache, syncope, aphasia, dysarthria, sudden vision loss, hemiparesis, or hemiparalysis signals a TIA and may herald a stroke.

Carotid cavernous fistula. A carotid cavernous fistula causes characteristic continuous bruits heard over the eyeballs and temples. Vision disturbances and protruding, pulsating eyeballs are also common.

Peripheral arteriovenous fistula. A rough, continuous bruit with systolic accentuation may be heard over the fistula in a peripheral arteriovenous fistula. A palpable thrill is also common.

Peripheral vascular disease. Peripheral vascular disease characteristically produces bruits over the femoral artery and other arteries in the legs. It can also cause diminished or absent femoral, popliteal, or pedal pulses; intermittent claudication; numbness, weakness, pain, and cramping in the legs, feet, and hips; and cool, shiny skin and hair loss on the affected extremity. It also predisposes the patient to lower-extremity ulcers that heal with difficulty.

Renal artery stenosis. With renal artery stenosis, systolic bruits are commonly heard over the abdominal midline and flank on the affected side. Hypertension commonly accompanies stenosis. Headache, palpitations, tachycardia, anxiety, dizziness, retinopathy, hematuria, and mental sluggishness may also appear.

Subclavian steal syndrome. With subclavian steal syndrome, systolic bruits may be heard over one or both subclavian arteries as a result of arterial lumen narrowing. They may be accompanied by decreased blood pressure and claudication in the affected arm, hemiparesis, vision disturbances, vertigo, and dysarthria.

Thyrotoxicosis. With thyrotoxicosis, a systolic bruit is commonly heard over the thyroid gland. Accompanying signs and symptoms appear in all body systems, but the most characteristic ones include thyroid enlargement, fatigue, nervousness, tachycardia, heat intolerance, sweating, tremor, diarrhea, and weight loss despite increased appetite. Exophthalmos may also be present.

Nursing considerations

- Frequently check the patient's vital signs, auscultate over the affected arteries, and monitor peripheral pulses.
- Check for bruits that become louder or develop a diastolic component.
- Administer prescribed drugs, such as a vasodilator, an anticoagulant, an antiplatelet drug, or an antihypertensive, as needed.
- Prepare the patient for diagnostic tests, such as blood studies, X-rays, an electrocardiogram, cardiac catheterization, and ultrasonography.

Patient teaching

- Teach the patient signs and symptoms of a stroke and to seek immediate medical attention if they occur.
- Discuss lifestyle changes, such as smoking cessation, exercising regularly, and eating a balanced diet.
- Teach the patient about the cause of the specific bruit and the treatment plan after a diagnosis is established.

Butterfly rash

The presence of a butterfly rash is typically a sign of systemic lupus erythematosus (SLE), but it can also signal a dermatologic disorder. Typically, butterfly rash appears in a malar distribution across the nose and cheeks. (See *Recognizing butterfly rash.*)

Similar rashes may appear on the neck, scalp, and other areas. Butterfly rash is sometimes mistaken for sunburn because it can be provoked or aggravated by ultraviolet rays, but it has more substance, is more sharply demarcated, and has a thicker feel in relation to surrounding skin.

History and physical examination

Ask the patient when he first noticed the butterfly rash and if he has recently been exposed to the sun. Has he noticed a rash elsewhere on his body? Ask about recent weight or hair loss. Does he have a family history of lupus? Is he taking hydralazine or procainamide (common causes of drug-induced lupus erythematosus)?

Inspect the rash, noting any macules, papules, pustules, or scaling. Is the rash edematous? Are areas of hypopigmentation or hyperpigmentation present? Look for blisters or ulcers in the mouth, and note any inflamed lesions. Check for rashes elsewhere on the body.

Medical causes

Discoid lupus erythematosus. With discoid lupus erythematosus, the patient may have a unilateral or butterfly rash that consists of erythematous, raised, sharply demarcated plaques with follicular plugging and central atrophy. The rash may also involve the scalp, ears, chest, or any part of the body exposed to the sun. Telangiectasia, scarring alopecia, and hypopigmentation or hy-

Recognizing butterfly rash

With classic butterfly rash, lesions appear on the cheeks and the bridge of the nose, creating a characteristic butterfly pattern. The rash may vary in severity from malar erythema to discoid lesions (plaques).

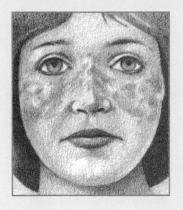

perpigmentation may occur later. Other accompanying signs include conjunctival redness, dilated capillaries of the nail fold, bilateral parotid gland enlargement, oral lesions, and mottled, reddish blue skin on the legs.

Erysipelas. Erysipelas causes rosy or crimson swollen lesions, mainly on the neck and head and commonly along the nasolabial fold. It may cause hemorrhagic pus-filled blisters. Other signs and symptoms include fever, chills, cervical lymphadenopathy, and malaise.

Polymorphous light eruption. A butterfly rash appears as erythema, vesicles, plaques, and multiple small papules that may later become eczematized, lichenified, and excoriated. Provoked by ultraviolet rays, the rash appears on the cheeks and bridge of the nose, the hands and arms, and other areas, beginning a few hours to several days after exposure. It may be accompanied by pruritus.

Rosacea. Initially, a butterfly rash may appear as a prominent, nonscaling, intermittent erythema limited to the lower half of the nose or including the chin, cheeks, and central forehead. As rosacea develops, the duration of the rash increases; instead of disappearing after each episode, the rash varies in intensity and is commonly accompanied by telangiectasia. With advanced rosacea, the skin is oily, with papules, pustules, nodules, and telangiectasis restricted to the central oval of the face. In men with severe rosacea, butterfly rash may be accompanied by rhinophyma—a thickened, lobulated overgrowth of sebaceous glands and epithelial connective tissue on the lower half of the nose and, possibly, the adjacent cheeks. This is more common in elderly patients.

Seborrheic dermatitis. A butterfly rash appears as greasy, scaling, slightly yellow macules and papules of varying size on the cheeks and the bridge of the nose, in a "butterfly" pattern. The scalp, beard, eyebrows, portions of the forehead above the bridge of the nose, nasolabial fold, or trunk may also be involved. Associated signs and symptoms include crusts and fissures (particularly when the external ear and scalp are involved), pruritus, redness, blepharitis, styes, severe acne, and oily skin. Severe seborrheic dermatitis of the face occurs in acquired immunodeficiency syndrome.

Systemic lupus erythematosus. Occurring in about 40% of patients with this connective tissue disorder, a butterfly rash appears as a red, usually scaly, sharply demarcated macular eruption. The rash may be transient in patients with acute SLE or may progress slowly to include the forehead, the chin, the area around the ears, and other exposed areas. Common associated skin findings include scaling, patchy alopecia, mucous membrane lesions, mottled erythema of the palms and fingers, periungual erythema with edema, reddish purple macular lesions on the volar surfaces of the fingers, telangiectasia of the base of the nails or eyelids, purpura, petechiae, and ecchymoses.

A butterfly rash may also be accompanied by joint pain, stiffness, and deformities, particularly ulnar deviation of the fingers and subluxation of the proximal interphalangeal joints. Related findings include periorbital and facial edema, dyspnea, a low-grade fever, malaise, weakness, fatigue, weight loss, anorexia, nausea, vomiting, lymphadenopathy, photosensitivity, and hepatosplenomegaly.

Other causes

Drugs. Hydralazine and procainamide can cause a lupuslike syndrome, producing a butterfly rash.

Nursing considerations

- Prepare the patient for immunologic studies, complete blood count and, possibly, liver studies.
- Obtain a urine specimen if needed.
- Withhold photosensitizing drugs, such as phenothiazines, sulfonamides, sulfonylureas, and thiazide diuretics.

Patient teaching

- Instruct the patient to avoid prolonged exposure to the sun and to use sunscreen whenever outside.
- Suggest that the patient use hypoallergenic makeup to help conceal facial lesions.
- Teach the patient about the cause of the butterfly rash and the treatment plan afetr a diagnosis is established.

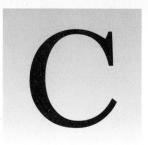

Capillary refill time, increased

Capillary refill time is the duration required for color to return to the nail bed of a finger or toe after application of slight pressure, which causes blanching. This duration reflects the quality of peripheral vasomotor function. Normal capillary refill time is less than 3 seconds.

Increased refill time isn't diagnostic of a disorder, but must be evaluated along with other signs and symptoms. This sign usually signals obstructive peripheral arterial disease or decreased cardiac output.

Capillary refill time is typically tested during a routine cardiovascular assessment. It isn't tested with suspected life-threatening disorders because other, more characteristic signs and symptoms appear earlier.

History and physical examination

If you detect increased capillary refill time, take the patient's vital signs and check pulses in the affected limb. Does the limb feel cold or look cyanotic? Does the patient report pain or unusual or decreased sensations in his fingers or toes, especially after exposure to cold?

Take a brief medical history, especially noting previous peripheral vascular disease. Find out which medications the patient is taking.

Medical causes

Aortic aneurysm (dissecting). Capillary refill time is increased in the fingers and toes with a dissecting aneurysm in the thoracic aorta, and is prolonged in just the toes with a dissecting aneurysm in the abdominal aorta. Common accompanying signs and symptoms include a pulsating abdominal mass, a systolic bruit, and substernal back or abdominal pain.

Aortic arch syndrome. Increased capillary refill time in the fingers occurs early in the patient with this syndrome. He displays absent carotid pulses and possibly unequal radial pulses. Other signs and symptoms usually precede loss of pulses and include fever, night sweats, arthralgia, weight loss, anorexia, nausea, malaise, a skin rash, splenomegaly, and pallor.

Arterial occlusion (acute). Increased capillary refill time occurs early in the affected limb. Arterial pulses are usually absent distal to the obstruction; the affected limb appears cool and pale or cyanotic. Intermittent claudication, moderate to severe pain, numbness, and paresthesia or paralysis of the affected limb may occur.

Buerger's disease. Capillary refill time is increased in the toes. Exposure to low temperatures turns the feet cold, cyanotic, and numb; later, they redden, become hot, and tingle. Other findings include intermittent claudication of the instep and weak peripheral pulses; in later stages, the patient may experience ulceration, muscle atrophy, and gangrene. If the disease affects the hands, increased capillary refill time may accompany painful fingertip ulcerations.

Cardiac tamponade. Increased capillary refill time represents a late sign of decreased cardiac output. Associated signs include paradoxical pulse, tachycardia, cyanosis, dyspnea, jugular vein distention, and hypotension.

Hypothermia. Increased capillary refill time may appear early as a compensatory response. Associated signs and symptoms depend on the degree of hypothermia and may include shivering, fatigue, weakness, a decreased level of consciousness (LOC), slurred speech, ataxia, muscle stiffness or rigidity, tachycardia or bradycardia, hyporeflexia or areflexia, diuresis, oliguria, bradypnea, decreased blood pressure, and cold, pale skin.

Peripheral arterial trauma. Trauma to a peripheral artery that reduces distal blood flow also increases capillary refill time in the affected extremity. Related findings in that extremity include bruising or pulsating bleeding, a weakened pulse, cyanosis, paresthesia, sensory loss, and cool, pale skin.

Peripheral vascular disease. Increased capillary refill time in the affected extremities is a late sign. Peripheral pulses gradually weaken and then disappear. Intermittent claudication, coolness, pallor, and decreased hair growth are associated signs. Impotence may accompany arterial occlusion in the descending aorta or femoral areas.

Raynaud's disease. Capillary refill time is prolonged in the fingers, the usual site of this disease's characteristic episodic arterial vasospasm. Exposure to cold or stress produces blanching in the fingers, then cyanosis, and then erythema before the fingers return to normal temperature. Warmth relieves the symptoms, which may include paresthesia. Chronic disease may produce trophic changes, such as sclerodactyly, ulcerations, or chronic paronychia.

Volkmann's contracture. Increased capillary refill time results from this contracture's characteristic vasospasm. Associated signs include the loss of mobility and loss of strength in the affected extremity.

Other causes

Diagnostic tests. Cardiac catheterization can cause arterial hematoma or clot formation and increased capillary refill time.

Drugs. Drugs that cause vasoconstriction (particularly alpha-adrenergic blockers) increase capillary refill time.

Treatments. Increased capillary refill time can result from an arterial or umbilical line (which can cause arterial hematoma and obstructed distal blood flow), or from an improperly fitting cast (which constricts circulation).

Nursing considerations

■ Frequently assess the patient's vital signs, LOC, and affected extremity, and report any changes, such as progressive cyanosis or loss of an existing pulse.
■ Prepare the patient for diagnostic tests, which may include arteriography or Doppler ultrasonography, to help confirm or rule out arterial occlusion.

Patient teaching

■ Explain the signs and symptoms that the patient should report.
■ Discuss ways to reduce the risk of aggravating or reintroducing the underlying disorder.

- Instruct the patient in ways to promote circulation, such as keeping the extremities warm and avoiding cold environments.
- Stress to the patient the importance of not smoking.

Carpopedal spasm

Carpopedal spasm is the violent, painful contraction of the muscles in the hands and feet. (See *Recognizing carpopedal spasm.*)

It's an important sign of tetany, a potentially life-threatening condition characterized by increased neuromuscular excitation and sustained muscle contraction and is commonly associated with hypocalcemia.

Carpopedal spasm requires prompt evaluation and intervention. If the primary event isn't treated promptly, the patient can also develop laryngospasm, seizures, cardiac arrhythmias, and cardiac and respiratory arrest.

ACTION STAT!

 If you detect carpopedal spasm, quickly examine the patient for signs of respiratory distress (such as laryngospasm, stridor, loud-crowing noises, and cyanosis) or cardiac arrhythmias, which indicate hypocalcemia. Obtain blood specimens for electrolyte analysis (especially calcium), and perform an electrocardiogram. Connect the patient to a cardiac monitor to watch for the appearance of arrhythmias. Administer an I.V. calcium preparation, and provide emergency respiratory and cardiac support. If calcium infusion doesn't control seizures, administer a sedative, such as chloral hydrate or phenobarbital.

Recognizing carpopedal spasm

In the hand, carpal carpopedal spasm involves adduction of the thumb over the palm, followed by flexion of the metacarpophalangeal joints, extension of the interphalangeal joints (fingers together), adduction of the hyperextended fingers, and flexion of the wrist and elbow joints. Similar effects occur in the joints of the feet.

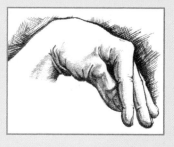

History and physical examination

If the patient isn't in distress, obtain a detailed history. Ask about the onset and duration of the spasms and ask for a description of pain they produce. Also ask about related signs and symptoms of hypocalcemia, such as numbness and tingling of the fingertips and feet, other muscle cramps or spasms, and nausea, vomiting, and abdominal pain. Check for previous neck surgery, calcium or magnesium deficiency, tetanus exposure, and hypoparathyroidism.

During the history, form a general impression of the patient's mental status and behavior. If possible, ask family members or friends if they've noticed changes in the patient's behavior. Mental confusion or even personality changes may occur with hypocalcemia.

Inspect the patient's skin and fingernails, noting dryness or scaling and ridged, brittle nails.

Medical causes

Hypocalcemia. Carpopedal spasm is an early sign of hypocalcemia. It's usually accompanied by paresthesia of the fingers, toes, and perioral area; muscle weakness, twitching, and cramping; hyperreflexia; chorea; fatigue; and palpitations. Positive Chvostek's and Trousseau's signs can be elicited. Laryngospasm, stridor, and seizures may appear in severe hypocalcemia.

Chronic hypocalcemia may be accompanied by mental status changes; cramps; dry, scaly skin; brittle nails; and thin, patchy hair and eyebrows.

Tetanus. With tetanus, the patient develops muscle spasms and painful seizures. Difficulty swallowing and a low-grade fever are also present. If the patient isn't treated or treatment is delayed, the mortality rate is very high.

Other causes

Treatments. Multiple blood transfusions and parathyroidectomy may cause hypocalcemia, resulting in carpopedal spasm. Surgical procedures that impair calcium absorption, such as ileostomy formation and gastric resection with gastrojejunostomy, may also cause hypocalcemia.

Nursing considerations

- If carpopedal spasm causes severe pain and anxiety, leading to hyperventilation, help the patient slow his breathing through your relaxing touch, reassuring attitude, and clear directions about what he should do.
- Provide a quiet, dark environment to reduce his anxiety.
- Prepare the patient for laboratory tests, such as complete blood count and serum calcium, phosphorus, and parathyroid hormone studies.
- Suspect tetanus in anyone with carpopedal spasm, difficulty swallowing, and seizures.

Patient teaching

- Explain the underlying disorder and treatment plan.
- Teach the patient the importance of receiving immunization against tetanus and of keeping a vaccination record.
- Explain that a tetanus toxoid booster shot should be given every 10 years prophylactically, after the patient has been properly immunized in childhood.

Cat's cry

Occurring during infancy, a mewing, kittenlike sound is the primary indicator of cat's cry syndrome (also known as *cri du chat*). This syndrome affects about 1 in 50,000 neonates and causes profound mental retardation and failure to thrive. Most of those affected can have a normal life span; however, a few have serious organ defects and other life-threatening medical conditions.

The chromosomal defect responsible (deletion of the short arm of chromosome 5) usually appears spontaneously, but may be inherited from a carrier parent. The characteristic cry is thought to result from abnormal laryngeal development.

ACTION STAT!

 Suspect cat's cry syndrome if you detect a kittenlike cry in a neonate. Be alert for signs of respiratory distress, such as nasal flaring; irregular, shallow respirations; cyanosis; and a respiratory rate over 60 breaths/minute. Be prepared to suction the neonate and to administer warmed oxygen. Keep emergency resuscitation equipment nearby because bradycardia may develop.

History and physical examination

Perform a physical examination, and note abnormalities. If you detect cat's cry in an older infant, ask the parents when it developed. The sudden onset of an abnormal cry in an infant with a previously normal, vigorous cry suggests other disorders. (See "Cry, high-pitched," page 172.)

Medical causes

Cat's cry syndrome. A kittenlike cry begins at birth or shortly thereafter. It's accompanied by profound mental retardation, microcephaly, low birth weight, hypotonia, failure to thrive, and feeding difficulties. Typically, the neonate has a round face with wide-set eyes; strabismus; a broad-based nose with oblique or down-sloping epicanthal folds; abnormally shaped, low-set ears; and an unusually small jaw. He may also have a short neck, webbed fingers, and a simian crease. Other abnormalities may include heart defects and GI abnormalities.

Nursing considerations

■ Connect the neonate to an apnea monitor, and check for signs of respiratory distress.
■ Keep suction equipment and warmed oxygen available.
■ Obtain a blood sample for chromosomal analysis.
■ Prepare the neonate for a computed tomography scan to rule out other causes of microcephaly and for an ear, nose, and throat examination to evaluate vocal cords.
■ Because the neonate with cat's cry syndrome is usually a poor eater, monitor his intake, output, and weight.

Patient teaching

■ Teach the parents about the child's disorder and treatment options.
■ Instruct the parents to offer the neonate small, frequent feedings.

■ Prepare the parents to work long-term with a team of specialists, such as those in genetics, neurology, cardiology, and speech and language.
■ Discuss counselors or support groups that are available for the parents and family.

■ Chest expansion, asymmetrical

Asymmetrical chest expansion is the uneven extension of portions of the chest wall during inspiration. During normal respiration, the thorax uniformly expands upward and outward, and then contracts downward and inward. When this process is disrupted, breathing becomes uncoordinated, resulting in asymmetrical chest expansion.

Asymmetrical chest expansion may develop suddenly or gradually and may affect one or both sides of the chest wall. It may occur as delayed expiration (chest lag), as abnormal movement during inspiration (for example, intercostal retractions, paradoxical movement, or chest-abdomen asynchrony), or as a unilateral absence of movement. This sign usually results from pleural disorders, such as life-threatening hemothorax or tension pneumothorax. (See *Recognizing life-threatening causes of asymmetrical chest expansion,* page 122.)

However, asymmetrical chest expansion can also result from a musculoskeletal or urologic disorder, airway obstruction, or trauma. Regardless of its underlying cause, asymmetrical chest expansion produces rapid and shallow or deep respirations that increase the work of breathing.

A C T I O N   S T A T !

 If you detect asymmetrical chest expansion, first consider traumatic injury to the patient's

Recognizing life-threatening causes of asymmetrical chest expansion

Asymmetrical chest expansion can result from several life-threatening disorders. Two common causes—bronchial obstruction and flail chest—produce distinctive chest wall movements that provide important clues about the underlying disorder.

With bronchial obstruction, only the unaffected portion of the chest wall expands during inspiration. Intercostal bulging during expiration may indicate that the air is trapped in the chest.

With flail chest—a disruption of the thorax due to multiple rib fractures—the unstable portion of the chest wall collapses inward at inspiration and balloons outward at expiration.

Inspiration

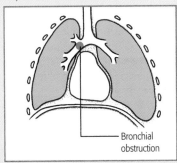

Bronchial obstruction

Inspiration

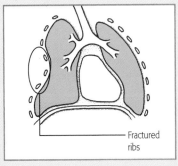

Fractured ribs

Expiration

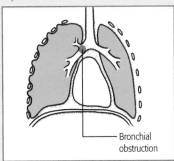

Bronchial obstruction

Expiration

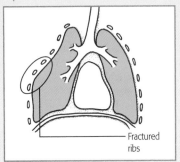

Fractured ribs

ribs or sternum, which can cause flail chest, a life-threatening emergency characterized by paradoxical chest movement. Quickly take the patient's vital signs and look for signs of acute respiratory distress—rapid and shallow respirations, tachycardia, and cyanosis. Use tape or sandbags to temporarily splint the unstable flail segment.

Depending on the severity of respiratory distress, administer oxygen by nasal cannula, mask, or mechanical ventilator. Insert an I.V. catheter to allow fluid replacement and administration of pain medication. Draw a blood sample from the patient for arterial blood gas analysis, and connect the patient to a cardiac monitor.

Although asymmetrical chest expansion may result from hemothorax, tension pneumothorax, bronchial obstruction, and other life-threatening causes, it isn't a cardinal sign of these disorders. Because any form of asymmetrical chest expansion can compromise the patient's respiratory status, don't leave the patient unattended, and be alert for signs of respiratory distress.

History and physical examination

If you don't suspect flail chest or tension pneumothorax and if the patient isn't experiencing acute respiratory distress, obtain a brief history. Asymmetrical chest expansion commonly results from mechanical airflow obstruction, so find out if the patient is experiencing dyspnea or pain during breathing. If so, does he feel short of breath constantly or intermittently? Does the pain worsen his feeling of breathlessness? Does repositioning, coughing, or other activity relieve or worsen the patient's dyspnea or pain? Is the pain more noticeable during inspiration or expiration? Can he inhale deeply?

Ask if the patient has a history of pulmonary or systemic illness, such as frequent upper respiratory tract infections, asthma, tuberculosis, pneumonia, or cancer. Has he had thoracic surgery? (This typically produces asymmetrical chest expansion on the affected side.) Also ask about blunt or penetrating chest trauma, which may have caused pulmonary injury. Obtain an occupational history to find out if the patient may have inhaled toxic fumes or aspirated a toxic substance.

Next, perform a physical examination. Begin by gently palpating the tra-

chea for midline positioning. (Deviation of the trachea usually indicates an acute problem requiring immediate intervention.) Then examine the posterior chest wall for areas of tenderness or deformity. To evaluate the extent of asymmetrical chest expansion, place your hands—fingers together and thumbs abducted toward the spine—flat on both sections of the lower posterior chest wall. Position your thumbs at the 10th rib, and grasp the lateral rib cage with your hands. As the patient inhales, note the uneven separation of your thumbs, and gauge the distance between them. Then repeat this technique on the upper posterior chest wall. Next, use the ulnar surface of your hand to palpate for vocal or tactile fremitus on both sides of the chest. To check for vocal fremitus, ask the patient to repeat "99" as you proceed. Note asymmetrical vibrations and areas of enhanced, diminished, or absent fremitus. Then percuss and auscultate to detect air and fluid in the lungs and pleural spaces. Finally, auscultate all lung fields for normal and adventitious breath sounds. Examine the patient's anterior chest wall, using the same assessment techniques.

Medical causes

Bronchial obstruction. With a bronchial obstruction, life-threatening loss of airway patency may occur gradually or suddenly. Typically, a lack of chest movement indicates complete obstruction; chest lag signals partial obstruction. If air is trapped in the chest, you may detect intercostal bulging during expiration and hyperresonance on percussion. You may also note dyspnea, accessory muscle use, decreased or absent breath sounds, and suprasternal, substernal, or intercostal retractions.

Flail chest. With flail chest, a life-threatening injury to the ribs or sternum, the unstable portion of the chest wall collapses inward during inspiration and balloons outward during expiration (paradoxical movement). The patient may have ecchymoses, severe localized pain, or other signs of traumatic injury to the chest wall. He may also exhibit rapid, shallow respirations, tachycardia, and cyanosis.

Hemothorax. Hemothorax is life-threatening bleeding into the pleural space that causes chest lag during inspiration. Other findings include signs of traumatic chest injury, stabbing pain at the injury site, anxiety, dullness on percussion, tachypnea, tachycardia, and hypoxemia. If hypovolemia occurs, you'll note signs of shock, such as hypotension and a rapid, weak pulse.

Kyphoscoliosis. Abnormal curvature of the thoracic spine in the anteroposterior direction (kyphosis) and the lateral direction (scoliosis) gradually compresses one lung and distends the other. This produces decreased chest wall movement on the compressed-lung side and expands the intercostal muscles during inspiration on the opposite side. It can also produce ineffective coughing, dyspnea, back pain, and fatigue.

Myasthenia gravis. With myasthenia gravis, progressive loss of ventilatory muscle function produces asynchrony of the chest and abdomen during inspiration ("abdominal paradox"), which can lead to the onset of acute respiratory distress. Typically, the patient's shallow respirations and increased muscle weakness cause severe dyspnea, tachypnea, and possible apnea.

Pleural effusion. Chest lag at end-inspiration occurs gradually in this life-threatening accumulation of fluid, blood, or pus in the pleural space. Usually, some combination of dyspnea, tachypnea, and tachycardia precedes chest lag; the patient may also have pleuritic pain that worsens with coughing or deep breathing. The area of the effusion is delineated by dullness on percussion and by egophony, bronchophony, whispered pectoriloquy, decreased or absent breath sounds, and decreased tactile fremitus. A fever appears if infection causes the effusion.

Pneumonia. Depending on whether fluid consolidation in the lungs develops unilaterally or bilaterally, asymmetrical chest expansion occurs with pneumonia, as inspiratory chest lag or as chest-abdomen asynchrony. The patient typically has a fever, chills, tachycardia, tachypnea, and dyspnea along with crackles, rhonchi, and chest pain that worsens during deep breathing. He may also be fatigued and anorexic and have a productive cough with rust-colored sputum.

Pneumothorax. Entrapment of air in the pleural space can cause chest lag at end-inspiration. Pneumothorax, a life-threatening condition, also causes sudden, stabbing chest pain that may radiate to the arms, face, back, or abdomen and dyspnea unrelated to the chest pain's severity. Other findings include tachypnea, decreased pulse oximetry, decreased tactile fremitus, tympany on percussion, decreased or absent breath sounds over the trapped air, tachycardia, restlessness, and anxiety.

With tension pneumothorax, the same signs and symptoms occur as in pneumothorax, but they're much more severe. Tension pneumothorax rapidly compresses the heart and great vessels, causing cyanosis, hypotension, decreased pulse oximetry, tachycardia, restlessness, and anxiety. The patient may also develop subcutaneous crepitation of the upper trunk, neck, and face and mediastinal and tracheal deviation away from the affected side. You may auscultate a crunching sound over the precordium with each heartbeat; this indicates pneumomediastinum.

Pulmonary embolism. Pulmonary embolism is an acute, life-threatening disorder that causes chest lag; sudden, stabbing chest pain; and tachycardia. The patient usually has severe dyspnea, blood-tinged sputum, a pleural friction rub, and acute anxiety.

Other causes

Treatments. Asymmetrical chest expansion can result from pneumonectomy and the surgical removal of several ribs. Chest lag or the absence of chest movement may also result from intubation of a mainstem bronchus, a serious complication typically due to the incorrect insertion of an endotracheal (ET) tube or movement of the tube while it's in the trachea.

Nursing considerations

▪ If you're caring for an intubated patient, regularly auscultate breath sounds in the lung peripheries to help detect a misplaced ET tube.
▪ If you detect a misplaced ET tube, prepare the patient for a chest X-ray to allow rapid repositioning of the tube.
▪ Because asymmetrical chest expansion increases the work of breathing, supplemental oxygen is usually given during acute events.
▪ If the patient is acutely hypoxic, prepare him for ET intubation.

Patient teaching

▪ Teach the patient to recognize early signs and symptoms of respiratory distress.
▪ Encourage coughing and deep-breathing exercises to promote oxygenation.
▪ With flail chest, show the patient how to splint his chest so he can perform breathing exercises more effectively.
▪ Teach the patient techniques that can help reduce anxiety.

▪ Once the patient is stable, explain the cause of his respiratory distress and the treatment plan.

▐ Chest pain

Chest pain usually results from disorders that affect thoracic or abdominal organs—the heart, pleurae, lungs, esophagus, rib cage, gallbladder, pancreas, or stomach. An important indicator of several acute and life-threatening cardiopulmonary and GI disorders, chest pain can also result from a musculoskeletal or hematologic disorder, anxiety, and drug therapy.

Chest pain can arise suddenly or gradually, and its cause may be difficult to ascertain initially. The pain can radiate to the arms, neck, jaw, or back. It can be steady or intermittent, mild or acute. It can range in character from a sharp shooting sensation to a feeling of heaviness, fullness, or even indigestion. It can be provoked or aggravated by stress, anxiety, exertion, deep breathing, or eating certain foods.

ACTION STAT!

 Ask the patient when his chest pain began. Did it develop suddenly or gradually? Is it more severe or frequent now than when it first started? Does anything relieve the pain? Does anything aggravate the pain? Ask the patient about associated symptoms. Sudden, severe chest pain requires prompt evaluation and treatment because it may herald a life-threatening disorder. (See *Managing severe chest pain,* pages 126 and 127.)

History and physical examination

If the chest pain isn't severe, proceed with the history. Ask if the patient feels diffuse pain or can point to the painful

Managing severe chest pain

Sudden, severe chest pain may result from any one of several life-threatening disorders. Your evaluation and interventions will vary, depending on the pain's location and character. This flowchart will help you establish priorities for managing this emergency successfully.

Ask the patient to characterize his chest pain.

Patient reports sudden onset of pleuritic chest pain, which he characterizes as crushing, shooting, and deep.	Patient reports sudden onset of tearing, ripping, stabbing chest pain, with syncope and hemiplegia.
Assess him for diaphoresis, dyspnea, tachypnea, hemoptysis, and tachycardia.	Assess for differences in blood pressure between legs and arms, as well as weak or absent femoral or pedal pulses.
If you detect these signs and symptoms, suspect *pulmonary embolism*.	If you detect these signs, suspect *dissecting aortic aneurysm*.

What to do: Quickly take the patient's vital signs. Obtain a 12-lead electrocardiogram. Insert an I.V. catheter to administer fluids and drugs, and give oxygen. Check the patient's vital signs frequently to detect changes from baseline. Begin cardiac monitoring to detect arrhythmias. As appropriate, prepare the patient for emergency surgery. Prepare the patient with pulmonary embolism or myocardial infarction (MI) for possible thrombolytic therapy.

area. Ask when the pain began and if the patient ever experienced this type of pain in the past. Sometimes a patient won't perceive the sensation he's feeling as pain, so ask whether he has any discomfort radiating to his neck, jaw, arms, or back. If he does, ask him to describe it. Is it a dull, aching, pressurelike sensation? A sharp, stabbing, knifelike pain? Does he feel it on the surface or deep inside? Ask him to rate the pain on a pain scale. Find out whether it's constant or intermittent. If it's intermittent, how long does it last? Ask if movement, exertion, breathing, position changes, or eating certain foods worsens or helps re-

lieve the pain. Does anything in particular seem to bring it on?

Review the patient's history for cardiac or pulmonary disease, chest trauma, intestinal disease, or sickle cell anemia. Find out which medications he's taking, if any, and ask about recent dosage or schedule changes.

Take the patient's vital signs, noting tachypnea, fever, tachycardia, oxygen saturation, paradoxical pulse, and hypertension or hypotension. Place the patient on a cardiac monitor and evaluate his heart rhythm. Also, look for jugular vein distention and peripheral edema. Note the feel of his skin. Is it cool and

| Patient reports sudden onset of severe substernal pain that radiates to his left arm, jaw, neck, or shoulder blades; he describes the pain as a squeezing, viselike, burning sensation. | Patient reports sudden onset of diffuse chest tightness. |

| Assess him for pallor, diaphoresis, nausea, vomiting, apprehension, anxiety, weakness, fatigue, and dyspnea. | Assess him for wheezing, dry cough, chest tightness, dyspnea, tachycardia, and hyperventilation. |

| If you detect these signs and symptoms, suspect an *MI*. | If you detect these signs and symptoms, suspect an *acute asthma attack*. |

What to do: Try to calm the patient to slow his respiratory rate. Ask the patient if he's ever had this pain before and, if so, what (if anything) eased it. Give oxygen and insert an I.V. catheter to administer fluids and drugs. Expect to give epinephrine and a bronchodilator and to begin respiratory therapy.

clammy or warm and diaphoretic? Auscultate his chest for extra heart sounds. Observe the patient's breathing pattern, and inspect his chest for asymmetrical expansion. Auscultate his lungs for pleural friction rub, crackles, rhonchi, wheezing, or diminished or absent breath sounds. Next, auscultate for murmurs, clicks, gallops, or pericardial friction rub. Palpate for lifts, heaves, thrills, gallops, tactile fremitus, and abdominal masses or tenderness.

Medical causes

Angina pectoris. With angina pectoris, the patient may experience a feeling of tightness or pressure in the chest that he describes as pain or a sensation of indigestion or expansion. The pain usually occurs in the retrosternal region over a palm-sized or larger area. It may radiate to the neck, jaw, and arms—classically, to the inner aspect of the left arm. Angina tends to begin gradually, build to its maximum, and then slowly subside. Provoked by exertion, emotional stress, or a heavy meal, the pain typically lasts 2 to 10 minutes (usually no longer than 20 minutes). Associated findings include dyspnea, nausea, vomiting, tachycardia, dizziness, diaphoresis, belching, and palpitations. You may hear an atrial gallop (a fourth heart sound) or murmur during an anginal episode.

With *Prinzmetal's angina,* caused by vasospasm of coronary vessels, chest pain typically occurs when the patient is at rest—or it may awaken him. It may be accompanied by shortness of breath, nausea, vomiting, dizziness, and palpitations. During an attack, you may hear an atrial gallop.

Anthrax (inhalation). Inhalation anthrax is caused by inhalation of aerosolized spores. Initial signs and symptoms are flulike and include a fever, chills, weakness, a cough, and chest pain. The disease generally occurs in two stages with a period of recovery after the initial signs and symptoms. The second stage develops abruptly with rapid deterioration marked by a fever, dyspnea, stridor, and hypotension, generally leading to death within 24 hours. Radiologic findings include mediastinitis and symmetric mediastinal widening.

Anxiety. Acute anxiety—or, more commonly, panic attacks—can produce intermittent, sharp, stabbing pain, commonly located behind the left breast. This pain isn't related to exertion and lasts only a few seconds, but the patient may experience a precordial ache or a sensation of heaviness that lasts for hours or days. Associated signs and symptoms include precordial tenderness, palpitations, fatigue, a headache, insomnia, breathlessness, nausea, vomiting, diarrhea, and tremors. Panic attacks may be associated with agoraphobia— fear of leaving home or being in open places with other people.

Aortic aneurysm (dissecting). The chest pain associated with a dissecting aortic aneurysm usually begins suddenly and is most severe at its onset. The patient describes an excruciating tearing, ripping, stabbing pain in his chest and neck that radiates to his upper back, ab-

domen, and lower back. He may also have abdominal tenderness, a palpable abdominal mass, tachycardia, murmurs, syncope, blindness, loss of consciousness, weakness or transient paralysis of the arms or legs, a systolic bruit, systemic hypotension, asymmetrical brachial pulses, a lower blood pressure in the legs than in the arms, and weak or absent femoral or pedal pulses. His skin is pale, cool, diaphoretic, and mottled below the waist. Capillary refill time is increased in the toes, and palpation reveals decreased pulsation in one or both carotid arteries.

Asthma. In a life-threatening asthma attack, diffuse and painful chest tightness arises suddenly along with a dry cough and mild wheezing, which progress to a productive cough, audible wheezing, and severe dyspnea. Related respiratory findings include rhonchi, crackles, prolonged expirations, intercostal and supraclavicular retractions on inspiration, accessory muscle use, flaring nostrils, and tachypnea. The patient may also experience anxiety, tachycardia, diaphoresis, flushing, and cyanosis.

Blast lung injury. Caused by a percussive shock wave after an explosion, blast lung injury can cause severe chest pain and possibly tearing, contusion, edema, and hemorrhage of the lungs of affected people. Worldwide terrorist activity has recently increased the incidence of this condition, which may also cause dyspnea, hemoptysis, wheezing, and cyanosis. Chest X-rays, arterial blood gas measurements, and computed tomography scans are common diagnostic tools. Although no definitive guidelines exist for caring for those with blast lung injury, treatment is based on the nature of the explosion, the environment in which it occurred, and any chemical or biological agents involved.

Bronchitis. In its acute form, bronchitis produces a burning chest pain or a sensation of substernal tightness. It also produces a cough, initially dry but later productive, that worsens the chest pain. Other findings include a low-grade fever, chills, a sore throat, tachycardia, muscle and back pain, rhonchi, crackles, and wheezing. Severe bronchitis causes a fever of 101° to 102° F (38.3° to 38.9° C) and possible bronchospasm with worsening wheezing and increased coughing.

Cholecystitis. Cholecystitis typically produces abrupt epigastric or right upper quadrant pain, which may be sharp or intensely aching. Steady or intermittent pain may radiate to the back or right shoulder. Commonly associated findings include nausea, vomiting, a fever, diaphoresis, and chills. Palpation of the right upper quadrant may reveal an abdominal mass, rigidity, distention, or tenderness. Murphy's sign—inspiratory arrest elicited when the examiner palpates the right upper quadrant as the patient takes a deep breath—may also occur.

Interstitial lung disease. As interstitial lung disease advances, the patient may experience pleuritic chest pain along with progressive dyspnea, cellophane-type crackles, a nonproductive cough, fatigue, weight loss, decreased exercise tolerance, clubbing, and cyanosis.

Lung abscess. Pleuritic chest pain develops insidiously with a lung abscess along with a pleural friction rub and a cough that raises copious amounts of purulent, foul-smelling, blood-tinged sputum. The affected side is dull to percussion, and decreased breath sounds and crackles may be heard. The patient also displays diaphoresis, anorexia, weight loss, a fever, chills, fatigue, weakness, dyspnea, and clubbing.

Lung cancer. The chest pain associated with lung cancer is commonly described as an intermittent aching felt deep within the chest. If the tumor metastasizes to the ribs or vertebrae, the pain becomes localized, continuous, and gnawing. Associated findings include cough (sometimes bloody), wheezing, dyspnea, fatigue, anorexia, weight loss, and a fever.

Mitral valve prolapse. Most patients with mitral valve prolapse are asymptomatic, but some may experience sharp, stabbing precordial chest pain or precordial ache. The pain can last for seconds or for hours and occasionally mimics the pain of ischemic heart disease. The characteristic sign of mitral prolapse is a midsystolic click followed by a systolic murmur at the apex. Patients may experience cardiac awareness, a migraine headache, dizziness, weakness, episodic severe fatigue, dyspnea, tachycardia, mood swings, and palpitations.

Myocardial infarction (MI). The chest pain during an MI lasts from 15 minutes to hours. Typically a crushing substernal pain unrelieved by rest or nitroglycerin, it may radiate to the patient's left arm, jaw, neck, or shoulder blades. Women are less likely to experience chest pain with an MI, but may complain of pain in the shoulder blade, jaw, and upper back. Other findings include pallor, clammy skin, dyspnea, diaphoresis, nausea, vomiting, anxiety, restlessness, a feeling of impending doom, hypotension or hypertension, an atrial gallop, murmurs, and crackles. Women also complain of fatigue, palpitations, and indigestion.

Pancreatitis. In the acute form, pancreatitis usually causes intense pain in the epigastric area that radiates to the back and worsens when the patient is in a supine position. Nausea, vomiting, a fever, abdominal tenderness and rigidity, diminished bowel sounds, and crackles at the lung bases may also occur. A patient with severe pancreatitis may be extremely restless and have mottled skin, tachycardia, and cold, sweaty extremities. Fulminant pancreatitis causes massive hemorrhage, resulting in shock and coma.

Peptic ulcer. With a peptic ulcer, sharp and burning pain usually arises in the epigastric region. This pain characteristically arises hours after food intake, commonly during the night. It lasts longer than angina-like pain and is relieved by food or an antacid. Other findings include nausea, vomiting (sometimes with blood), melena, and epigastric tenderness.

Pericarditis. Pericarditis produces precordial or retrosternal pain aggravated by deep breathing, coughing, position changes, and occasionally by swallowing. The pain is commonly sharp or cutting and radiates to the shoulder and neck. Associated signs and symptoms include a pericardial friction rub, a fever, tachycardia, and dyspnea. Pericarditis usually follows a viral illness, but several other causes should be considered.

Plague **(Yersinia pestis).** Signs and symptoms of the plague include fever, chills, and swollen, inflamed, and tender lymph nodes near the site of the flea bite. Septicemic plague develops as a fulminant illness generally with the bubonic form. The pneumonic form may be contracted from person-to-person through direct contact via the respiratory system or through biological warfare from aerosolization and inhalation of the organism. The onset is usually sudden with chills, a fever, a headache, and myalgia. Pulmonary signs and symptoms include a productive cough, chest pain, tachypnea, dyspnea, hemoptysis, increasing respiratory distress, and cardiopulmonary insufficiency.

Pleurisy. The chest pain of pleurisy arises abruptly and reaches maximum intensity within a few hours. The pain is sharp, even knifelike, usually unilateral, and located in the lower and lateral aspects of the chest. Deep breathing, coughing, or thoracic movement characteristically aggravates it. Auscultation over the painful area may reveal decreased breath sounds, inspiratory crackles, and a pleural friction rub. Dyspnea; rapid, shallow breathing; cyanosis; a fever; and fatigue may also occur.

Pneumonia. Pneumonia produces pleuritic chest pain that increases with deep inspiration and is accompanied by shaking chills and fever. The patient has a dry cough that later becomes productive. Other signs and symptoms include crackles, rhonchi, tachycardia, tachypnea, myalgia, fatigue, a headache, dyspnea, abdominal pain, anorexia, cyanosis, decreased breath sounds, and diaphoresis.

Pneumothorax. Spontaneous pneumothorax, a life-threatening disorder, causes sudden sharp chest pain that's severe, typically unilateral, and rarely localized; it increases with chest movement. When the pain is centrally located and radiates to the neck, it may mimic that of an MI. After the pain's onset, dyspnea and cyanosis progressively worsen. Breath sounds are decreased or absent on the affected side with hyperresonance or tympany, subcutaneous crepitation, and decreased vocal fremitus. Asymmetrical chest expansion, accessory muscle use, a nonproductive cough, tachypnea, tachycardia, anxiety, and restlessness also occur.

Pulmonary embolism. A pulmonary embolism produces chest pain or a choking sensation. Typically, the patient first experiences sudden dyspnea with intense angina-like or pleuritic pain aggravated by deep breathing and thoracic movement. Other findings include tachycardia, tachypnea, decreased pulse oximetry, a cough (nonproductive or producing blood-tinged sputum), a low-grade fever, restlessness, diaphoresis, crackles, a pleural friction rub, diffuse wheezing, dullness to percussion, signs of circulatory collapse (a weak, rapid pulse; hypotension), paradoxical pulse, signs of cerebral ischemia (transient unconsciousness, coma, seizures), signs of hypoxia (restlessness) and, particularly in the elderly, hemiplegia and other focal neurologic deficits. Less common signs include massive hemoptysis, chest splinting, and leg edema. A patient with a large embolus may have cyanosis and jugular vein distention.

Q fever. Signs and symptoms of Q fever include a fever, chills, a severe headache, malaise, chest pain, nausea, vomiting, and diarrhea. The fever may last up to 2 weeks. In severe cases, the patient may develop hepatitis or pneumonia.

Sickle cell crisis. Chest pain associated with sickle cell crisis typically has a bizarre distribution. It may start as a vague pain, commonly located in the back, hands, or feet. As the pain worsens, it becomes generalized or localized to the abdomen or chest, causing severe pleuritic pain. The presence of chest pain and difficulty breathing requires prompt intervention. The patient may also have abdominal distention and rigidity, dyspnea, a fever, and jaundice.

Thoracic outlet syndrome. Commonly causing paresthesia along the ulnar distribution of the arm, thoracic outlet syndrome can be confused with angina, especially when it affects the left arm. The patient usually experiences angina-like pain after lifting his arms above his head, working with his hands above his shoulders, or lifting a weight. The pain disappears as soon as he lowers his arms. Other signs and symptoms include pale skin and a difference in blood pressure between both arms.

Tuberculosis (TB). In a patient with TB, pleuritic chest pain and fine crackles occur after coughing. Associated signs and symptoms include night sweats, anorexia, weight loss, a fever, malaise, dyspnea, easy fatigability, a mild to severe productive cough, occasional hemoptysis, dullness to percussion, increased tactile fremitus, and amphoric breath sounds.

Tularemia. Signs and symptoms of tularemia following inhalation of the organism include the abrupt onset of a fever, chills, a headache, generalized myalgia, a nonproductive cough, dyspnea, pleuritic chest pain, and empyema.

Other causes
Chinese restaurant syndrome (CRS). CRS is a benign condition—a reaction to excessive ingestion of monosodium glutamate, a common additive in Chinese foods—that mimics the signs of an acute MI. The patient may complain of retrosternal burning, ache, or pressure; a burning sensation over his arms, legs, and face; a sensation of facial pressure; a headache; shortness of breath; and tachycardia.

Drugs. The abrupt withdrawal of a beta-adrenergic blocker can cause rebound angina if the patient has coronary heart disease—especially if he has received high doses for a prolonged period.

Nursing considerations
- Prepare the patient for cardiopulmonary studies, such as an electrocardiogram, chest X-ray, magnetic resonance imaging, and a lung perfusion scan.
- Collect a serum sample for cardiac enzyme and electrolyte levels.
- Provide emotional support because chest pain produces increased anxiety.

Patient teaching
- Explain the purpose and procedure of each diagnostic test to the patient to help alleviate his anxiety.

- Teach the patient about the cause of his chest pain once a diagnosis is established.
- Explain the purpose of any prescribed drugs, and make sure that the patient understands the dosage, schedule, and possible adverse effects.
- Stress the importance of reporting symptoms to allow for the adjustment of treatment.
- Teach the patient with coronary artery disease about the typical features of cardiac ischemia as well as the symptoms that should prompt him to seek immediate medical attention.
- Discuss lifestyle changes that can reduce the risk of coronary artery disease.

Cheyne-Stokes respirations

The most common pattern of periodic breathing, Cheyne-Stokes respirations are characterized by a waxing and waning period of hyperpnea that alternates with a shorter period of apnea. This pattern can occur normally in patients with heart or lung disease. It usually indicates increased intracranial pressure (ICP) from a deep cerebral or brain stem lesion, or a metabolic disturbance in the brain.

Cheyne-Stokes respirations may indicate a major change in the patient's condition—usually a deterioration. For example, in a patient who has had head trauma or brain surgery, Cheyne-Stokes respirations may signal increasing ICP. Cheyne-Stokes respirations can occur normally in a patient who lives at high altitudes.

ACTION STAT!

 If you detect Cheyne-Stokes respirations in a patient with a history of head trauma, recent brain surgery, or another brain insult, quickly take his vital signs. Keep his head

elevated 30 degrees, and perform a rapid neurologic examination to obtain baseline data. Reevaluate the patient's neurologic status frequently. If ICP continues to rise, you'll detect changes in the patient's level of consciousness (LOC), pupillary reactions, and ability to move his extremities. ICP monitoring is indicated.

Time the periods of hyperpnea and apnea for 3 or 4 minutes to evaluate respirations and to obtain baseline data. Be alert for prolonged periods of apnea. Frequently check the patient's blood pressure; also check his skin color to detect signs of hypoxemia. Maintain airway patency and administer oxygen as needed. If the patient's condition worsens, endotracheal intubation is necessary.

History and physical examination

If the patient can answer questions, take a complete history or gather information from the his family. Find out the patient's history of chronic illness. Ask about all drugs that the patient has been using. Ask if he has any difficulty breathing. Find out if the patient is having any chest pain. Does he complain of a headache? Ask him if he has any visual disturbances. If the patient is not conscious, ask the family if they have noticed breathing irregularities while patient slept.

During the physical examination, assess the patient's neurologic status. Check his pupils and motor coordination. Then, assess heart sounds and blood pressure. Check for jugular vein distention and peripheral edema. Auscultate the lungs for crackles or other adventitious breath sounds. Check his pulse oximetry and nail beds for cyanosis. Listen to the lungs for egophony, bronchophony, and whispered pectoriloquy. Palpate the abdomen for hepatomegaly.

Medical causes
Heart failure. With left-sided heart failure, Cheyne-Stokes respirations may occur with exertional dyspnea and orthopnea. Related findings include fatigue, weakness, tachycardia, tachypnea, and crackles. The patient may also have a cough, generally nonproductive but occasionally producing clear or blood-tinged sputum.

Hypertensive encephalopathy. Hypertensive encephalopathy is a life-threatening disorder in which severe hypertension precedes Cheyne-Stokes respirations. The patient's LOC is decreased, and he may experience vomiting, seizures, severe headaches, vision disturbances (including transient blindness), or transient paralysis.

Increased ICP. As ICP rises, Cheyne-Stokes respirations is the first irregular respiratory pattern to occur. It's preceded by a decreased LOC and accompanied by hypertension, headache, vomiting, impaired or unequal motor movement, and vision disturbances (blurring, diplopia, photophobia, and pupillary changes). In late stages of increased ICP, bradycardia and a widened pulse pressure occur.

Renal failure. With end-stage chronic renal failure, Cheyne-Stokes respirations may occur in addition to bleeding gums, oral lesions, ammonia breath odor, and marked changes in every body system.

Other causes
Drugs. Large doses of an opioid, a hypnotic, or a barbiturate can precipitate Cheyne-Stokes respirations.

Nursing considerations
■ When evaluating Cheyne-Stokes respirations, be careful not to mistake periods of hypoventilation or decreased tidal volume for complete apnea.
■ Discuss end-of-life issues with the patient's family, if appropriate.

Patient teaching
■ Teach the patient or his family to recognize the difference between sleep apnea and Cheyne-Stokes respirations.
■ Explain the causes and treatments of Cheyne-Stokes respirations.

Chills
[Rigors]
Chills are extreme, involuntary muscle contractions with characteristic paroxysms of violent shivering and teeth chattering. Commonly accompanied by a fever, chills tend to arise suddenly, usually heralding the onset of infection. Certain diseases, such as pneumococcal pneumonia, produce only a single, shaking chill. Other diseases, such as malaria, produce intermittent chills with recurring high fever. Still others produce continuous chills for up to 1 hour, precipitating a high fever. (See *Why chills accompany fever*, page 134.)

Chills can also result from lymphomas, blood transfusion reactions, and certain drugs. Chills without fever occur as a normal response to exposure to cold.

History and physical examination
Ask the patient when the chills began and whether they're continuous or intermittent. Because fever commonly accompanies or follows chills, take his rectal temperature to obtain a baseline reading. Then check his temperature often to monitor fluctuations and to determine his temperature curve. Typically, a localized infection produces a sudden onset of shaking chills, sweats, and high fever. A systemic infection produces in-

Why chills accompany fever

Fever usually occurs when exogenous pyrogens activate endogenous pyrogens to reset the body's thermostat to a higher level. At this higher set point, the body feels cold and responds through several compensatory mechanisms, including rhythmic muscle contractions or chills. These muscle contractions generate body heat and help produce fever. This flowchart outlines the events that link chills to fever.

```
┌─────────────────────────────────────┐
│ Exogenous pyrogens (infectious       │
│ organisms, immune complexes,         │
│ toxins) enter the body.              │
└─────────────────────────────────────┘
                  ▼
┌─────────────────────────────────────┐
│ Phagocytic leukocytes release        │
│ endogenous pyrogens.                 │
└─────────────────────────────────────┘
                  ▼
┌─────────────────────────────────────┐
│ Endogenous pyrogens—possibly         │
│ with prostaglandins—stimulate        │
│ temperature-sensitive receptors in   │
│ the hypothalamus and raise the       │
│ thermostatic set point to a higher   │
│ level.                               │
└─────────────────────────────────────┘
                  ▼
┌─────────────────────────────────────┐
│ Descending efferent pathways from    │
│ the hypothalamus innervate           │
│ effectors such as skeletal muscles,  │
│ and stimulate them to rhythmically   │
│ contract.                            │
└─────────────────────────────────────┘
                  ▼
┌─────────────────────────────────────┐
│ Rhythmic muscle contractions, or     │
│ chills, generate body heat, which    │
│ helps produce fever.                 │
└─────────────────────────────────────┘
```

termittent chills with recurring episodes of high fever or continuous chills that may last up to 1 hour and precipitate a high fever.

Ask about related signs and symptoms, such as headache, dysuria, diarrhea, confusion, abdominal pain, cough, sore throat, or nausea. Does the patient have any known allergies, an infection, or a recent history of an infectious disorder? Find out which medications he's taking and whether a drug has improved or worsened his symptoms. Has he received treatment that may predispose him to an infection (such as chemotherapy)? Ask about recent exposure to farm animals, guinea pigs, hamsters, dogs, and such birds as pigeons, parrots, and parakeets. Also ask about recent insect or animal bites, travel to foreign countries, and contact with persons who have an active infection.

Medical causes

Acquired immunodeficiency syndrome (AIDS). With AIDS, the patient usually develops lymphadenopathy and may also experience fatigue, anorexia and weight loss, diarrhea, diaphoresis, skin disorders, and signs of upper respiratory tract infection. Opportunistic infections can cause serious disease in the patient with AIDS.

Anthrax (inhalation). Inhalation anthrax is caused by inhalation of aerosolized spores. Initial signs and symptoms are flulike and include a fever, chills, weakness, a cough, and chest pain. The disease generally occurs in two stages with a period of recovery after the initial signs and symptoms. The second stage develops abruptly with rapid deterioration marked by a fever, dyspnea, stridor, and hypotension generally leading to death within 24 hours. Radiologic findings include mediastinitis and symmetric mediastinal widening.

Cholangitis. Charcot's triad—chills with spiking fever, abdominal pain, and jaundice—characterizes a sudden obstruction of the common bile duct. The patient may have associated pruritus, weakness, and fatigue.

Gram-negative bacteremia. Gram-negative bacteremia causes sudden chills and a fever, nausea, vomiting, diarrhea, and prostration.

Hemolytic anemia. With acute hemolytic anemia, fulminating chills occur with a fever and abdominal pain. The patient rapidly develops jaundice and hepatomegaly; he may develop splenomegaly.

Hepatic abscess. Hepatic abscess usually arises abruptly, with chills, a fever, nausea, vomiting, diarrhea, anorexia, and severe upper abdominal tenderness and pain that may radiate to the right shoulder.

Infective endocarditis. Infective endocarditis produces the abrupt onset of intermittent, shaking chills with a fever. Petechiae commonly develop. The patient may also have Janeway lesions on his hands and feet and Osler's nodes on his palms and soles. Associated findings include a murmur, hematuria, eye hemorrhage, Roth's spots, and signs of cardiac failure (such as dyspnea and peripheral edema).

Influenza. Initially, influenza causes an abrupt onset of chills, a high fever, malaise, a headache, myalgia, and a nonproductive cough. Some patients may also suddenly develop rhinitis, rhinorrhea, laryngitis, conjunctivitis, hoarseness, and a sore throat. Chills generally subside after the first few days, but an intermittent fever, weakness, and a cough may persist for up to 1 week.

Legionnaires' disease. Within 12 to 48 hours after the onset of Legionnaires' disease, the patient suddenly develops chills and a high fever. Prodromal signs and symptoms characteristically include malaise, a headache, and possibly diarrhea, anorexia, diffuse myalgia, and general weakness. An initially nonproductive cough progresses to a productive cough with mucoid or mucopurulent sputum and possibly hemoptysis. The patient usually also develops nausea and vomiting, confusion, mild temporary

amnesia, pleuritic chest pain, dyspnea, tachypnea, crackles, tachycardia, and flushed and mildly diaphoretic skin.

Malaria. The paroxysmal cycle of malaria begins with a period of chills lasting 1 or 2 hours. This is followed by a high fever lasting 3 or 4 hours and then 2 to 4 hours of profuse diaphoresis. Paroxysms occur every 48 to 72 hours when caused by *Plasmodium malariae* and every 40 to 42 hours when caused by *P. vivax* or *P. ovale*. With benign malaria, the paroxysms may be interspersed with periods of well-being. The patient also has a headache, muscle pain and, possibly, hepatosplenomegaly.

Monkeypox. Many individuals infected with the monkeypox virus experience chills. Other common initial symptoms of this rare virus include fever, lymphadenopathy, sore throat, dyspnea, muscle aches, and rash. Although monkeypox occurs primarily in central and western Africa, it was confirmed in the United States in 2003 when several humans contracted the virus from infected pet prairie dogs. There's no treatment for this virus; however, given its similarity to smallpox, the smallpox vaccine is used in certain circumstances to protect individuals against monkeypox.

Pelvic inflammatory disease. Pelvic inflammatory disease causes chills and fever with, typically, lower abdominal pain and tenderness; profuse, purulent vaginal discharge; or abnormal menstrual bleeding. The patient may also develop nausea and vomiting, an abdominal mass, and dysuria.

Plague (Yersinia pestis). Signs and symptoms of the plague include a fever, chills, and swollen, inflamed, and tender lymph nodes near the site of the flea bite. Septicemic plague develops as a fulminant illness generally with the bubonic form. The pneumonic form may be contracted from person-to-person through direct contact via the respiratory system or through biological warfare from aerosolization and inhalation of the organism. The onset is usually sudden with chills, a fever, a headache, and myalgia. Pulmonary signs and symptoms include a productive cough, chest pain, tachypnea, dyspnea, hemoptysis, increasing respiratory distress, and cardiopulmonary insufficiency.

Pneumonia. A single shaking chill usually heralds the sudden onset of pneumococcal pneumonia; other pneumonias characteristically cause intermittent chills. With any type of pneumonia, related findings may include a fever, a productive cough with bloody sputum, pleuritic chest pain, dyspnea, tachypnea, and tachycardia. The patient may be cyanotic and diaphoretic, with bronchial breath sounds and crackles, rhonchi, increased tactile fremitus, and grunting respirations. He may also experience achiness, anorexia, fatigue, and a headache.

Puerperal or postabortal sepsis. Chills and a high fever occur as early as 6 hours or as late as 10 days postpartum or postabortion. The patient may also have a purulent vaginal discharge, an enlarged and tender uterus, abdominal pain, backache and, possibly, nausea, vomiting, and diarrhea.

Pyelonephritis. With acute pyelonephritis, the patient develops chills, a high fever, and possibly nausea and vomiting over several hours to days. He generally also has anorexia, fatigue, myalgia, flank pain, costovertebral angle (CVA) tenderness, hematuria or cloudy urine, and urinary frequency, urgency, and burning.

Q fever. Signs and symptoms of Q fever include a fever, chills, a severe headache, malaise, chest pain, nausea, vomiting, and diarrhea. The fever may last up to 2 weeks. In severe cases, the patient may develop hepatitis or pneumonia.

Renal abscess. Renal abscess initially produces sudden chills and a fever. Later effects include flank pain, CVA tenderness, abdominal muscle spasm, and transient hematuria.

Rocky Mountain spotted fever. Rocky Mountain spotted fever begins with a sudden onset of chills, a fever, malaise, an excruciating headache, and muscle, bone, and joint pain. Typically, the patient's tongue is covered with a thick white coating that gradually turns brown. After 2 to 6 days of fever and occasional chills, a macular or maculopapular rash appears on the hands and feet and then becomes generalized; after a few days, the rash becomes petechial.

Septic arthritis. Chills and fever accompany the characteristic red, swollen, and painful joints caused by septic arthritis.

Septic shock. Initially, septic shock produces chills, a fever and, possibly, nausea, vomiting, and diarrhea. The patient's skin is typically flushed, warm, and dry; his blood pressure is normal or slightly low; and he has tachycardia and tachypnea. As septic shock progresses, the patient's arms and legs become cool and cyanotic, and he develops oliguria, thirst, anxiety, restlessness, confusion, and hypotension. Later, his skin becomes cold and clammy; his pulse, rapid and thready. He further develops severe hypotension, persistent oliguria or anuria, signs of respiratory failure, and coma.

Sinusitis. With acute sinusitis, chills occur along with a fever, a headache, and pain, tenderness, and swelling over the affected sinuses. Maxillary sinusitis produces pain over the cheeks and upper teeth; ethmoid sinusitis, pain over the eyes; frontal sinusitis, pain over the eyebrows; and sphenoid sinusitis, pain behind the eyes. The primary indicator of sinusitis is nasal discharge, which is commonly bloody for 24 to 48 hours before it gradually becomes purulent.

Snake bite. Most pit viper bites that result in envenomization cause chills, typically with a fever. Other systemic signs and symptoms include sweating, weakness, dizziness, fainting, hypotension, nausea, vomiting, diarrhea, and thirst. The area around the snake bite may be marked by immediate swelling and tenderness, pain, ecchymoses, petechiae, blebs, bloody discharge, and local necrosis. The patient may have difficulty speaking, blurred vision, and paralysis. He may also show bleeding tendencies and signs of respiratory distress and shock.

Tularemia. Signs and symptoms of tularemia following inhalation of the organism include the abrupt onset of a fever, chills, a headache, generalized myalgia, a nonproductive cough, dyspnea, pleuritic chest pain, and empyema.

Typhus. Initial signs and symptoms of typhus include a headache, myalgia, arthralgia, and malaise followed by an abrupt onset of chills, a fever, nausea, and vomiting. A maculopapular rash may be present in some cases.

Violin spider bite. The violin spider bite produces chills, a fever, malaise, weakness, nausea, vomiting, and joint pain within 24 to 48 hours. The patient may also develop a rash and delirium.

Other causes

Drugs. Amphotericin B is a drug associated with chills. Phenytoin is also a common cause of drug-induced fever that can produce chills. I.V. bleomycin and intermittent administration of an oral antipyretic can also cause chills.

I.V. therapy. Infection at the I.V. insertion site (superficial phlebitis) can cause chills, high fever, and local redness, warmth, induration, and tenderness.

Transfusion reaction. A hemolytic reaction may cause chills during the transfusion or immediately afterward. A nonhemolytic febrile reaction may also cause chills.

Nursing considerations

- Check the patient's vital signs often, especially if his chills result from a known or suspected infection.
- Be alert for signs of progressive septic shock, such as hypotension, tachycardia, and tachypnea.
- Obtain samples of blood, sputum, wound drainage, or urine for culture to determine the causative organism.
- Give the appropriate antibiotic.
- Prepare the patient for radiographic studies, as required.
- Keep the room temperature as even as possible.
- Provide adequate hydration and nutrients.
- Administer an antipyretic to help control a fever.

Patient teaching

- Explain the importance of documenting temperature readings and times to reveal patterns.
- Teach him about his diagnosis and treatment, especially about the importance of taking the full course of antibiotics.
- Explain the signs and symptoms of a worsening condition and when to seek medical attention.

■ Chvostek's sign

Chvostek's sign is an abnormal spasm of the facial muscles that's elicited by lightly tapping the patient's facial nerve near his lower jaw. (See *Eliciting Chvostek's sign,* page 138.)

This sign usually suggests hypocalcemia, but can occur normally in about 25% of cases. Typically, it precedes other

Eliciting Chvostek's sign

Begin by telling the patient to relax his facial muscles. Then stand directly in front of him, and tap the facial nerve either just anterior to the earlobe and below the zygomatic arch or between the zygomatic arch and the corner of his mouth. A positive response varies from twitching of the lip at the corner of the mouth to spasm of all facial muscles, depending on the severity of hypocalcemia.

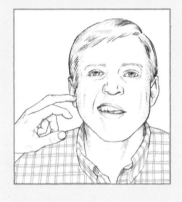

signs of hypocalcemia and persists until the onset of tetany. It can't be elicited during tetany because of strong muscle contractions.

Usually, eliciting Chvostek's sign is attempted only in patients with suspected hypocalcemic disorders. However, because the parathyroid gland regulates calcium balance, Chvostek's sign may also be tested in patients before neck surgery to obtain a baseline. Test the patient for Trousseau's sign, also a reliable indicator of hypocalcemia.

ACTION STAT!

Closely monitor the patient for signs of tetany, such as carpopedal spasms or circumoral and extremity paresthesia.

Be prepared to act quickly if a seizure occurs. Perform an electrocardiogram to check for changes associated with hypocalcemia that can predispose the patient to arrhythmias. Place the patient on a cardiac monitor.

History and physical examination

Obtain a brief history. Find out if the patient has had his parathyroid glands surgically removed or if he has a history of hypoparathyroidism, hypomagnesemia, or a malabsorption disorder. Ask him or his family if they have noticed changes in the patient's mental status, such as depression or slowed responses, which can accompany chronic hypocalcemia. Ask the patient if he has experienced any numbness and tingling in his fingers, toes, or around his mouth. Also ask him about muscle twitching or cramping.

Medical causes

Hypocalcemia. The degree of muscle spasm elicited reflects the patient's serum calcium level. Initially, hypocalcemia produces paresthesia in the fingers, toes, and circumoral area that progresses to muscle tension and carpopedal spasms. The patient may also complain of muscle weakness, fatigue, and palpitations. Muscle twitching, hyperactive deep tendon reflexes, choreiform movements, and muscle cramps may also occur. The patient with chronic hypocalcemia may have mental status changes; diplopia; difficulty swallowing; abdominal cramps; dry, scaly skin; brittle nails; and thin, patchy scalp and eyebrow hair.

Other causes

Blood transfusion. A massive blood transfusion can lower serum calcium levels and allow Chvostek's sign to be elicited.

Nursing considerations

- Collect blood samples for serial calcium studies to evaluate the severity of hypocalcemia and the effectiveness of therapy.
- Administer oral or I.V. calcium supplements.
- Assess for Chvostek's sign when evaluating a patient postoperatively.

Patient teaching

- Explain to the patient the early signs and symptoms of hypocalcemia that require immediate medical attention.

Clubbing

A nonspecific sign of pulmonary and cyanotic cardiovascular disorders, clubbing is the painless, usually bilateral increase in soft tissue around the terminal phalanges of the fingers or toes. It doesn't involve changes in the underlying bone. With early clubbing, the normal 160-degree angle between the nail and the nail base approximates 180 degrees. As clubbing progresses, this angle widens and the base of the nail becomes visibly swollen. With late clubbing, the angle where the nail meets the now-convex nail base extends more than halfway up the nail.

History and physical examination

You'll probably detect clubbing while evaluating other signs of known pulmonary or cardiovascular disease. Therefore, review the patient's current plan of treatment because clubbing may resolve with correction of the underlying disorder. Also, evaluate the extent of clubbing in the fingers and toes. (See *Checking for clubbed fingers.*)

Checking for clubbed fingers

To assess the patient for chronic tissue hypoxia, check his fingers for clubbing. Normally, the angle between the fingernail and the point where the nail enters the skin is about 160 degrees. Clubbing occurs when that angle increases to 180 degrees or more, as shown below.

Normal fingers

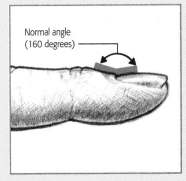

Normal angle (160 degrees)

Clubbed fingers

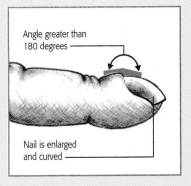

Angle greater than 180 degrees

Nail is enlarged and curved

Medical causes

Bronchiectasis. Clubbing commonly occurs in the late stage of bronchiectasis. Another classic sign is a cough that produces copious, foul-smelling, and mucopurulent sputum. Hemoptysis and coarse crackles over the affected area, heard during inspiration, are also characteristic. The patient may complain of weight loss, fatigue, weakness, and exertional dyspnea. He may also have rhonchi, fever, malaise, and halitosis.

Bronchitis. With chronic bronchitis, clubbing may occur as a late sign and is unrelated to the severity of the disease. The patient has a chronic productive cough and may display barrel chest, dyspnea, wheezing, increased use of accessory muscles, cyanosis, tachypnea, crackles, scattered rhonchi, and prolonged expiration.

Emphysema. Clubbing occurs late in emphysema. The patient may have anorexia, malaise, dyspnea, tachypnea, diminished breath sounds, peripheral cyanosis, and pursed-lip breathing. He may also display accessory muscle use, barrel chest, and a productive cough.

Endocarditis. With subacute infective endocarditis, clubbing may be accompanied by a fever, anorexia, pallor, weakness, night sweats, fatigue, tachycardia, and weight loss. The patient may also develop arthralgia, petechiae, Osler's nodes, splinter hemorrhages, Janeway lesions, splenomegaly, and Roth's spots. Cardiac murmurs are usually present.

Heart failure. Clubbing occurs as a late sign in heart failure along with wheezing, dyspnea, and fatigue. Other findings include jugular vein distention, hepatomegaly, tachypnea, palpitations, dependent edema, unexplained weight gain, nausea, anorexia, chest tightness, a slowed mental response, hypotension, diaphoresis, narrow pulse pressure, pallor, oliguria, a gallop rhythm (a third heart sound), and crackles on inspiration.

Interstitial fibrosis. Clubbing usually occurs in the patient with advanced interstitial fibrosis. Typically, he also develops intermittent chest pain, dyspnea, crackles, fatigue, weight loss, and possible cyanosis.

Lung abscess. Initially, a lung abscess produces clubbing, which may reverse with resolution of the abscess. It can also cause pleuritic chest pain; dyspnea; crackles; a productive cough with a lot of purulent, foul-smelling, usually bloody sputum; and halitosis. The patient may also experience weakness, fatigue, anorexia, a headache, malaise, weight loss, and a fever with chills. You may hear decreased breath sounds.

Lung and pleural cancer. Clubbing occurs commonly in lung and pleural cancers. Associated findings include hemoptysis, dyspnea, wheezing, chest pain, weight loss, anorexia, fatigue, and a fever.

Nursing considerations

■ Don't mistake curved nails—a normal variation—for clubbing; remember that the angle between the nail and its base remains normal in curved nails, but not in clubbed nails.

Patient teaching

■ Teach the patient about the cause of the clubbing.
■ Explain that clubbing may not disappear even if the cause has been removed.

▎Cogwheel rigidity

Cogwheel rigidity is a cardinal sign of Parkinson's disease, marked by muscle rigidity that reacts with superimposed ratchetlike movements when the muscle is passively stretched. This sign can be elicited by stabilizing the patient's forearm and then moving his wrist through the range of motion. (Cogwheel rigidity usually appears in the arms but can sometimes be elicited in the ankle.) The patient and examiner can see and feel these characteristic movements, thought to be a combination of rigidity and tremor.

History and physical examination

After you have elicited cogwheel rigidity, take the patient's history to determine when he first noticed associated signs of Parkinson's disease. For example, has he experienced tremors? Did he notice tremors of his hands first? Does he have "pill-rolling" hand movements? When did he first notice that his movements were becoming slower? How long has he been experiencing stiffness in his arms and legs? Has his handwriting gotten smaller? While taking the history, observe him for signs of pronounced parkinsonism, such as drooling, masklike facies, dysphagia, monotone speech, and an altered gait.

Find out which medications the patient is taking, and ask if they have helped relieve some of his symptoms. If he's taking levodopa and his symptoms have worsened, find out if he has exceeded the prescribed dosage. If you suspect an overdose, withhold the drug. If the patient has been taking a phenothiazine or another antipsychotic drug and has no history of Parkinson's disease, he may be having an adverse reaction. Withhold the drug, as appropriate.

Medical causes

Parkinson's disease. With Parkinson's disease, cogwheel rigidity occurs together with an insidious tremor, which usually begins in the fingers (unilateral pill-roll tremor), increases during stress or anxiety, and decreases with purposeful movement and sleep.

Bradykinesia (slowness of voluntary movements and speech) also occurs. The patient walks with short, shuffling steps; his gait lacks normal parallel motion and may be retropulsive or propulsive. He has a monotone way of speaking and a masklike facial expression. He may also experience drooling, dysphagia, dysarthria, and the loss of posture control, causing him to walk with his body bent forward. An oculogyric crisis (eyes fixed upward and involuntary tonic movements) or blepharospasm (complete eyelid closure) may also occur.

Other causes

Drugs. Phenothiazines and other antipsychotics (such as haloperidol, thiothixene, and loxapine) can cause cogwheel rigidity. Metoclopramide infrequently causes it.

Nursing considerations

- If the patient has associated muscular dysfunction, assist him with ambulation, bathing, feeding, and other activities of daily living as needed.
- Provide symptomatic care, for example, if the patient develops constipation, administer a stool softener; if he experiences dysphagia, offer a soft diet with small, frequent feedings.

Patient teaching

- Teach the patient about Parkinson's disease and its treatments.
- Refer the patient to the National Parkinson Foundation or the American Parkinson Disease Association for educational materials and support.

█ Confusion

An umbrella term for puzzling or inappropriate behavior or responses, confusion is the inability to think quickly and coherently. Depending on the cause, it may arise suddenly or gradually and may be temporary or irreversible. Aggravated by stress and sensory deprivation, confusion commonly occurs in hospitalized patients—especially the elderly, in whom it may be mistaken for senility.

When severe confusion arises suddenly and the patient also has hallucinations and psychomotor hyperactivity, his condition is classified as delirium. Long-term, progressive confusion with deterioration of all cognitive functions is classified as dementia.

Confusion can result from fluid and electrolyte imbalance or hypoxemia due to pulmonary disorders. It can also have a metabolic, neurologic, cardiovascular, cerebrovascular, or nutritional origin, or it can result from a severe systemic infection or the effects of toxins, drugs, or alcohol. Confusion may signal worsening of an underlying and perhaps irreversible disease.

History and physical examination

When you take his history, ask the patient to describe what's bothering him. He may not report confusion as his chief complaint, but may suffer from memory loss, persistent apprehension, or the inability to concentrate. He may be unable to respond logically to direct questions. Check with a family member or friend about its onset and frequency. Find out, too, if the patient has a history of head trauma or a cardiopulmonary, metabolic, cerebrovascular, or neurologic disorder. Which medications is he taking, if any? Ask about any changes in eating or sleeping habits and in drug or alcohol use.

Perform an assessment to determine the presence of systemic disorders. Check the patient's vital signs, and assess him for changes in blood pressure, temperature, and pulse.

Next, perform a neurologic assessment to establish the patient's level of consciousness.

Medical causes

Brain tumor. In the early stages of a brain tumor, confusion is usually mild and difficult to detect. As the tumor impinges on cerebral structures, however, confusion worsens and the patient may exhibit personality changes, bizarre behavior, sensory and motor deficits, visual field deficits, and aphasia.

Cerebrovascular disorders. Cerebrovascular disorders produce confusion due to tissue hypoxia and ischemia. Confusion may be insidious and fleeting, as in a transient ischemic attack, or acute and permanent, as in a stroke.

Decreased cerebral perfusion. Mild confusion is an early symptom of decreased cerebral perfusion. Associated findings usually include hypotension, tachycardia or bradycardia, an irregular pulse, ventricular gallop, edema, and cyanosis.

Fluid and electrolyte imbalance. The extent and type of fluid and electrolyte imbalance determines the severity of the patient's confusion. Typically, he'll show signs of dehydration, such as lassitude, poor skin turgor, dry skin and mucous membranes, and oliguria. He may also develop hypotension and a low-grade fever.

Head trauma. Concussion, contusion, and brain hemorrhage may produce confusion at the time of injury, shortly afterward, or months or even years afterward. The patient may be delirious, with periodic loss of consciousness. Vomiting, a severe headache, pupillary changes, and sensory and motor deficits are also common.

Heatstroke. Heatstroke causes pronounced confusion that gradually worsens as the patient's body temperature rises. Initially, he may be irritable and dizzy; later, he may become delirious, have seizures, and lose consciousness.

Hypothermia. Confusion may be an early sign of hypothermia. Typically, the patient displays slurred speech, cold and pale skin, hyperactive deep tendon reflexes, a rapid pulse, and decreased blood pressure and respirations. As his body temperature continues to drop, his confusion progresses to stupor and coma, his muscles become rigid, and his respiratory rate decreases.

Hypoxemia. Acute pulmonary disorders that result in hypoxemia produce confusion that can range from mild disorientation to delirium. Chronic pulmonary disorders produce persistent confusion.

Infection. Severe generalized infection, such as sepsis, typically produces delirium. Central nervous system (CNS) infections, such as meningitis, cause varying degrees of confusion along with a headache and nuchal rigidity.

Metabolic encephalopathy. Hyperglycemia and hypoglycemia can produce sudden confusion. A patient with hypoglycemia may also experience transient delirium and seizures. Uremic and hepatic encephalopathies produce gradual confusion that may progress to seizures and coma. Usually, the patient also experiences tremors and restlessness.

Nutritional deficiencies. Inadequate dietary intake of thiamine, niacin, or vitamin B_{12} produces insidious, progressive confusion and possible mental deterioration.

Seizure disorder. Mild to moderate confusion may immediately follow any type of seizure. The confusion usually disappears within several hours.

Other causes

Alcohol. Intoxication causes confusion and stupor, and alcohol withdrawal may cause delirium and seizures.

Drugs. Large doses of CNS depressants produce confusion that can persist for several days after the drug is discontinued. Opioid and barbiturate withdrawal also causes acute confusion, possibly with delirium. Other drugs that commonly cause confusion include lidocaine, a cardiac glycoside, indomethacin, cycloserine, chloroquine, atropine, cimetidine, and sleeping aids.

Nursing considerations
- Never leave a confused patient unattended, to prevent injury to himself and others.
- Take measures to ensure patient safety.
- Keep the patient calm and quiet, and plan uninterrupted rest periods.
- Correct the underlying cause of the patient's confusion.

Patient teaching
- To help the patient stay oriented, keep a large calendar and a clock visible, and make a list of his activities with specific dates and times.
- Always reintroduce yourself to the patient each time you enter his room.
- If possible, explain to the patient and his family the cause of his confusion.

Conjunctival injection

A common ocular sign associated with inflammation, conjunctival injection is nonuniform redness of the conjunctiva from hyperemia. This redness can be diffuse, localized, or peripheral, or it may encircle a clear cornea.

Conjunctival injection usually results from bacterial or viral conjunctivitis, but it can also signal a severe ocular disorder that, if untreated, may lead to permanent blindness. Conjunctival injection can also result from minor eye irritation due to inadequate sleep, overuse of contact lenses, environmental irritants, and excessive eye rubbing.

If the patient with conjunctival injection reports a chemical splash to the eye, quickly irrigate the eye with copious amounts of normal saline solution. (First, remove contact lenses.) Evert the lids and wipe the fornices with a cotton-tipped applicator to remove any foreign body particles and as much of the chemical as possible.

History and physical examination

When you take the patient's history, always ask if he has associated pain. If so, when did the pain begin, and where is it located? Is it constant or intermittent? Also, ask about itching, burning, photophobia, blurred vision, halo vision, excessive tearing, or a foreign body sensation in his eye. Does the patient have a history of eye disease or trauma? If he has suffered ocular trauma, avoid touching the affected eye. Does he wear contact lenses? If so, ask how often they're removed or changed if they're disposable. Test his visual acuity and intraocular pressure (IOP) only if his eyelids can be opened without applying pressure. Place a metal shield over the affected eye to protect it if needed.

If the patient's condition permits, examine the affected eye. First, determine the location and severity of conjunctival injection. Is it circumcorneal or localized? Peripheral or diffuse? Note any conjunctival or lid edema, ocular deviation, conjunctival follicles, ptosis, or exophthalmos. Also note the type and amount of any discharge.

Test the patient's visual acuity to establish a baseline. Note if the patient has had vision changes: Is his vision blurred or his visual acuity markedly decreased? Next, test pupillary reaction to light.

Perform IOP measurements. To gauge increased IOP without a tonometer, gently place your index finger over the closed eyelid; if the globe feels rock-hard, IOP is elevated.

Medical causes

Blepharitis. This disorder produces diffuse conjunctival injection. Ulcerations appear on the eyelids, which burn, itch, and have no lashes.

Chemical burns. Diffuse conjunctival injection occurs in this ocular emergency, but severe pain is the main symptom. The patient also displays photophobia, blepharospasm, and decreased visual acuity in the affected eye; the cornea may appear gray, and the pupil may be unilaterally smaller.

Conjunctival foreign bodies and abrasions. These conditions feature localized conjunctival injection with sudden, severe eye pain. The patient may have increased tearing and photophobia, but his visual acuity usually isn't impaired.

Conjunctivitis. Allergic conjunctivitis produces milky, diffuse peripheral conjunctival injection. Related findings include a watery, stringy eye discharge; increased tearing; itching; palpebral conjunctival follicles; and (with hay fever) conjunctival edema, photophobia, and a feeling of fullness around the eyes.

Bacterial conjunctivitis causes diffuse peripheral conjunctival injection along with a thick, purulent eye discharge that contains mucous threads. The patient's lids and lashes stick together, and he has excessive tearing, photophobia, burning, and itching. He may have pain and a foreign body sensation if the cornea is involved.

Besides diffuse peripheral conjunctival injection, the patient with *fungal conjunctivitis* complains of photophobia and increased tearing, itching, and burning. The discharge is thick and purulent, making his eyelids crusted, sticky, and swollen. Corneal involvement causes pain.

In *viral conjunctivitis,* the conjunctival injection is bright red, diffuse, and peripheral. The patient may also have conjunctival edema, follicles on the palpebral conjunctiva, and lid edema; a local viral rash; and signs of upper respiratory tract infection. He complains of itching, increased tearing and, possibly, a foreign body sensation.

Corneal abrasion. Diffuse conjunctival injection is extremely painful in this disorder, especially when the eyelids move over the abrasion. The patient may also report photophobia, excessive tearing, blurred vision, and a foreign body sensation.

Corneal erosion. Recurrent corneal erosion produces diffuse conjunctival injection; severe, continuous pain from rubbing of the eyelid over the eroded area of the cornea; and photophobia.

Corneal ulcer. Bacterial, viral, and fungal corneal ulcers produce diffuse conjunctival injection that increases in the circumcorneal area. Accompanying findings include severe photophobia, severe pain in and around the eye, markedly decreased visual acuity, and a copious amount of purulent eye discharge and crusting. If the patient develops associated iritis, a physical examination will also reveal corneal opacities and an abnormal pupillary response to light.

Dacryoadenitis. This disorder produces diffuse conjunctival injection, pain over the temporal part of the eye, considerable lid swelling and, possibly, a purulent eye discharge.

Episcleritis. Conjunctival injection is localized and raised and may be violet or purplish pink in patients with episcleritis. Associated signs and symptoms include an inflamed sclera, deep pain,

photophobia, increased tearing, and conjunctival edema.

Glaucoma. In acute angle-closure glaucoma, conjunctival injection is typically circumcorneal. Other signs and symptoms include severe eye pain, nausea and vomiting, severely elevated IOP, blurred vision, and the perception of rainbow-colored halos around lights. Corneas appear steamy because of corneal edema. The pupil of the affected eye is moderately dilated and completely unresponsive to light.

Hyphema. Depending on the type and extent of traumatic injury, a hyphema may produce diffuse conjunctival injection, possibly with lid and orbital edema. The patient may complain of pain in and around the eye. The extent of visual impairment depends on the hyphema's size and location.

Iritis. In acute iritis, marked conjunctival injection is found mainly around the cornea. Other findings include moderate to severe pain, photophobia, blurred vision, constricted pupils, and poor pupillary response to light.

Kawasaki syndrome. Conjunctival injection is a characteristic sign of Kawasaki syndrome and usually occurs bilaterally. This febrile illness, which primarily affects children younger than age 5, also causes erythema, lymphadenopathy, and swelling in the peripheral extremities. Treatment with I.V. gamma globulin is extremely effective if given immediately, so early detection is essential. Delaying treatment may cause coronary artery dilation and aneurysm, resulting in ischemic heart disease and, possibly, sudden death.

Keratoconjunctivitis sicca. This disorder produces severe diffuse conjunctival injection. The patient reports generalized eye pain along with burning, itching, a foreign body sensation, excessive mucus secretion from the eye, absence of tears, and photophobia.

Lyme disease. Spread by tick bites, Lyme disease may cause conjunctival injection, diffuse urticaria, malaise, fatigue, headache, fever, chills, aches, and lymphadenopathy.

Ocular lacerations and intraocular foreign bodies. Diffuse conjunctival injection may be increased in the area of injury. The patient experiences impaired visual acuity and moderate to severe pain that varies with the type and extent of injury. He may also develop lid edema, photophobia, excessive tearing, and an abnormal pupillary response to light.

Ocular tumors. A tumor located in the orbit behind the globe may produce conjunctival injection together with exophthalmos. Conjunctival edema, ocular deviation, and diplopia usually occur if muscles are involved.

Refractive error. An uncorrected or poorly corrected refractive error can produce conjunctival injection. The patient may complain of headache, eye pain, and eye fatigue.

Scleritis. In this relatively rare disorder, conjunctival injection can be diffuse or localized over the area of the scleritis nodule. The patient has severe pain on moving the eye, photophobia, tenderness, and tearing.

Stevens-Johnson syndrome. This disorder produces diffuse conjunctival injection, a purulent eye discharge, severe eye pain, photophobia, decreased tearing, entropion, and trichiasis.

Trachoma. Conjunctival injection is an early sign of trachoma, a leading cause of blindness in Third World countries and among Native Americans in the southwestern United States. Caused by a bacterial infection, trachoma may also produce eyelid swelling and corneal cloudiness.

Uveitis. Diffuse conjunctival injection, which may be increased in the circumcorneal area, characterizes this disorder. Accompanying signs and symptoms include constricted, irregularly shaped pupils; blurred vision; tenderness; photophobia; and possibly sudden, severe ocular pain.

Nursing considerations

- Prepare the patient for such diagnostic tests as orbital X-rays, ocular ultrasonography, and fluorescein staining.
- Obtain cultures of any eye discharge, and record its appearance, consistency, and amount.
- If the patient complains of photophobia, darken the room or recommend that he wear sunglasses.

Patient teaching

- If the patient's visual acuity is markedly decreased, orient him to his environment to ensure his comfort and safety.
- Because most forms of conjunctivitis are contagious, stress the importance of frequent hand washing and of not touching the affected eye.
- Teach the patient ways to reduce photophobia.
- Explain the cause of conjunctival injection and its treatment.

Constipation

Constipation is defined as small, infrequent, or difficult bowel movements. Because normal bowel movements can vary in frequency and from individual to individual, constipation is relative and must be determined in relation to the patient's normal elimination pattern. Constipation may be a minor annoyance or, uncommonly, a sign of a life-threatening disorder such as an acute intestinal obstruction. Untreated, constipation can lead to headache, anorexia, and abdominal discomfort and can adversely affect the patient's lifestyle and well-being.

Constipation usually occurs when the urge to defecate is suppressed and

How habits and stress cause constipation

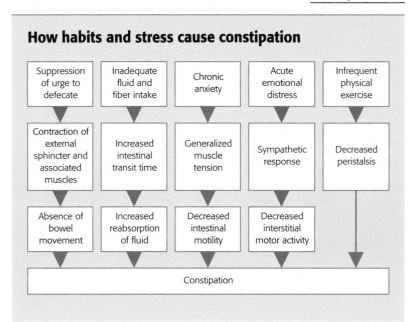

| Suppression of urge to defecate | Inadequate fluid and fiber intake | Chronic anxiety | Acute emotional distress | Infrequent physical exercise |

| Contraction of external sphincter and associated muscles | Increased intestinal transit time | Generalized muscle tension | Sympathetic response | Decreased peristalsis |

| Absence of bowel movement | Increased reabsorption of fluid | Decreased intestinal motility | Decreased interstitial motor activity | |

Constipation

the muscles associated with bowel movements remain contracted. Because the autonomic nervous system controls bowel movements—by sensing rectal distention from fecal contents and by stimulating the external sphincter—any factor that influences this system may cause bowel dysfunction. (See *How habits and stress cause constipation*.)

History and physical examination

Ask the patient to describe the frequency of his bowel movements and the size and consistency of his stools. How long has he had constipation? Acute constipation usually has a physiological cause such as an anal or rectal disorder. In a patient older than age 45, a recent onset of constipation may be an early sign of colorectal cancer. Conversely, chronic constipation typically has a functional cause and may be related to stress.

Does the patient have pain related to constipation? If so, when did he first notice the pain, and where is it located?

Cramping abdominal pain and distention suggest obstipation—extreme, persistent constipation due to intestinal tract obstruction. Ask the patient if defecation worsens or helps relieve the pain. Defecation usually worsens pain, but with such disorders as irritable bowel syndrome, it may relieve it.

Ask the patient to describe a typical day's diet; estimate his daily fiber and fluid intake. Ask him about recent changes in eating habits, medication or alcohol use, or physical activity. Has he experienced recent emotional distress? Has constipation affected his family life or social contacts? Also ask about his job and exercise pattern. A sedentary or stressful job can contribute to constipation.

Find out whether the patient has a history of GI, rectoanal, neurologic, or metabolic disorders; abdominal surgery; or radiation therapy. Then ask about the medications he's taking, including opioids and over-the-counter preparations, such as laxatives, mineral oil, stool softeners, and enemas.

Inspect the abdomen for distention or scars from previous surgery. Then auscultate for bowel sounds, and characterize their motility. Percuss all four quadrants, and gently palpate for abdominal tenderness, a palpable mass, and hepatomegaly. Next, examine the patient's rectum. Spread his buttocks to expose the anus, and inspect for inflammation, lesions, scars, fissures, and external hemorrhoids. Use a disposable glove and lubricant to palpate the anal sphincter for laxity or stricture. Also palpate for rectal masses and fecal impaction. Finally, obtain a stool sample and test it for occult blood.

As you assess the patient, remember that constipation can result from several life-threatening disorders, such as an acute intestinal obstruction and mesenteric artery ischemia, but it doesn't herald these conditions.

Medical causes

Anal fissure. A crack or laceration in the lining of the anal wall can cause acute constipation, usually due to the patient's fear of the severe tearing or burning pain associated with bowel movements. He may notice a few drops of blood streaking toilet tissue or his underwear.

Anorectal abscess. In anorectal abscess, constipation occurs together with severe, throbbing, localized pain and tenderness at the abscess site. The patient may also have localized inflammation, swelling, and purulent drainage and may complain of fever and malaise.

Cirrhosis. In the early stages of cirrhosis, the patient experiences constipation along with nausea and vomiting and a dull pain in the right upper quadrant. Other early findings include indigestion, anorexia, fatigue, malaise, flatulence, hepatomegaly and, possibly, splenomegaly and diarrhea.

Diabetic neuropathy. Diabetic neuropathy produces episodic constipation or diarrhea. Other signs and symptoms include dysphagia, orthostatic hypotension, syncope, and painless bladder distention with overflow incontinence. A male patient may also experience impotence and retrograde ejaculation.

Diverticulitis. In diverticulitis, constipation or diarrhea occurs with left lower quadrant pain and tenderness and possibly a palpable, tender, firm, fixed abdominal mass. The patient may develop mild nausea, flatulence, or a low-grade fever.

Hemorrhoids. Thrombosed hemorrhoids cause constipation as the patient tries to avoid the severe pain of defecation. The hemorrhoids may bleed during defecation.

Hepatic porphyria. Abdominal pain, which may be severe, colicky, localized, or generalized, precedes constipation in hepatic porphyria. The patient may also have a fever, sinus tachycardia, labile hypertension, excessive diaphoresis, severe vomiting, photophobia, urine retention, nervousness or restlessness, disorientation and, possibly, visual hallucinations. Deep tendon reflexes may be diminished or absent. He may also have skin lesions causing itching, burning, erythema, altered pigmentation, and edema in areas exposed to light. Severe hepatic porphyria can produce delirium, coma, seizures, paraplegia, or complete flaccid quadriplegia.

Hypercalcemia. With hypercalcemia, constipation usually occurs along with anorexia, nausea, vomiting, polyuria, and polydipsia. The patient may also display arrhythmias, bone pain, muscle weakness and atrophy, hypoactive deep tendon reflexes, and personality changes.

Hypothyroidism. Constipation occurs early and insidiously in patients with hypothyroidism, in addition to fatigue, sensitivity to cold, anorexia with weight gain, menorrhagia in women, decreased memory, hearing impairment, muscle cramps, and paresthesia.

Intestinal obstruction. Constipation associated with an intestinal obstruction varies in severity and onset, depending on the location and extent of the obstruction. With partial obstruction, constipation may alternate with leakage of liquid stools. With complete obstruction, obstipation may occur. Constipation can be the earliest sign of partial colon obstruction, but it usually occurs later if the level of the obstruction is more proximal. Associated findings include episodes of colicky abdominal pain, abdominal distention, nausea, or vomiting. The patient may also develop hyperactive bowel sounds, visible peristaltic waves, a palpable abdominal mass, and abdominal tenderness.

Irritable bowel syndrome (IBS). IBS commonly produces chronic constipation, although some patients have intermittent, watery diarrhea and others complain of alternating constipation and diarrhea. Stress may trigger nausea and abdominal distention and tenderness, but defecation usually relieves these signs and symptoms. Patients typically have an intense urge to defecate and feelings of incomplete evacuation. Typically, the stools are scybalous and contain visible mucus.

Mesenteric artery ischemia. Mesenteric artery ischemia is a life-threatening disorder that produces sudden constipation with failure to expel stool or flatus. Initially, the abdomen is soft and nontender, but soon severe abdominal pain, tenderness, vomiting, and anorexia occur. Later, the patient may develop abdominal guarding, rigidity, and distention; tachycardia; syncope; tachypnea; a fever; and signs of shock, such as cool, clammy skin and hypotension. A bruit may be heard.

Spinal cord lesion. Constipation may occur with a spinal cord lesion, in addition to urine retention, sexual dysfunction, pain and, possibly, motor weakness, paralysis, or sensory impairment below the level of the lesion.

Other causes

Diagnostic tests. Constipation can result from the retention of barium given during certain GI studies.

Drugs. Patients commonly experience constipation when taking an opioid analgesic or other drugs, including vinca alkaloids, calcium channel blockers, antacids containing aluminum or calcium, anticholinergics, and drugs with anticholinergic effects (such as tricyclic antidepressants). Patients may also experience constipation from excessive use of laxatives or enemas.

Surgery and radiation therapy. Constipation can result from rectoanal surgery, which may traumatize nerves, and abdominal irradiation, which may cause intestinal stricture.

Nursing considerations

- Prepare the patient for diagnostic tests, such as proctosigmoidoscopy, colonoscopy, barium enema, plain abdominal films, and an upper GI series.
- If the patient is on bed rest, reposition him frequently, and help him perform active or passive exercises, as indicated.

Patient teaching

- Teach the patient abdominal toning exercises if his abdominal muscles are weak.
- Teach relaxation techniques to help him reduce stress.
- Encourage the patient to avoid straining.

■ Stress the importance of a high fiber diet and encourage the patient to drink plenty of fluids.

■ Discuss the importance of regular exercise and avoidance of chronic use of laxatives or enemas.

■ Explain the cause of his constipation and the treatment plan.

Corneal reflex, absent

The corneal reflex is tested bilaterally by drawing a fine-pointed wisp of sterile cotton from a corner of each eye to the cornea. Normally, even though only one eye is tested at a time, the patient blinks bilaterally each time either cornea is touched—this is the corneal reflex. When this reflex is absent, neither eyelid closes when the cornea of one is touched. (See *Eliciting the corneal reflex.*)

The site of the afferent fibers for this reflex is in the ophthalmic branch of the trigeminal nerve (cranial nerve [CN] V);

Eliciting the corneal reflex

To elicit the corneal reflex, have the patient turn his eyes away from you to avoid involuntary blinking during the procedure. Then approach the patient from the opposite side, out of his line of vision, and brush the cornea lightly with a fine wisp of sterile cotton. Repeat the procedure on the other eye.

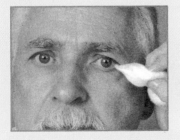

the efferent fibers are located in the facial nerve (CN VII). Unilateral or bilateral absence of the corneal reflex may result from damage to these nerves.

History and physical examination

If you can't elicit the corneal reflex, look for other signs of trigeminal nerve dysfunction. To test the three sensory portions of the nerve, touch each side of the patient's face on the brow, cheek, and jaw with a cotton wisp, and ask him to compare the sensations.

If you suspect facial nerve involvement, note if the upper face (brow and eyes) and lower face (cheek, mouth, and chin) are weak bilaterally. Lower motor neuron facial weakness affects the face on the same side as the lesion, whereas upper motor neuron weakness affects the side opposite the lesion—predominantly the lower facial muscles.

Because an absent corneal reflex may signify such progressive neurologic disorders as Guillain-Barré syndrome, ask the patient about associated symptoms—facial pain, dysphagia, and limb weakness.

Medical causes

Acoustic neuroma. Acoustic neuroma affects the trigeminal nerve, causing a diminished or absent corneal reflex, tinnitus, and unilateral hearing impairment. Facial palsy and anesthesia, palate weakness, and signs of cerebellar dysfunction (for example, ataxia or nystagmus) may result if the tumor impinges on the adjacent cranial nerves, brain stem, and cerebellum.

Bell's palsy. A common cause of diminished or absent corneal reflex, Bell's palsy causes paralysis of CN VII. It can also produce complete hemifacial weakness or paralysis and drooling on the affected side, which also sags and appears masklike. The eye on this side can't be shut and tears constantly.

Brain stem infarction or injury. An absent corneal reflex can occur on the side opposite the lesion when infarction or injury affects CN V or VII or their connection in the central trigeminal tract. Associated findings include a decreased level of consciousness, dysphagia, dysarthria, contralateral limb weakness, and early signs and symptoms of increased intracranial pressure, such as a headache and vomiting.

With massive brain stem infarction or injury, the patient also displays respiratory changes, such as apneustic breathing or periods of apnea; bilateral pupillary dilation or constriction with decreased responsiveness to light; rising systolic blood pressure; a widening pulse pressure; bradycardia; and coma.

Guillain-Barré syndrome. With this polyneuropathic disorder, a diminished or absent corneal reflex accompanies ipsilateral loss of facial muscle control. Muscle weakness, the dominant neurologic sign of this disorder, typically starts in the legs, and then extends to the arms and facial nerves within 72 hours. Other findings include dysarthria, dysphagia, paresthesia, respiratory muscle paralysis, respiratory insufficiency, orthostatic hypotension, incontinence, diaphoresis, and tachycardia.

Nursing considerations

- When the corneal reflex is absent, you'll need to take measures to protect the patient's affected eye from injury such as lubricating the eye with artificial tears to prevent drying.
- Cover the cornea with a shield and avoid excessive corneal reflex testing.
- Prepare the patient for cranial X-rays or a computed tomography scan.
- Discuss end-of-life issues with the patient's family, if appropriate.

Patient teaching

- Teach the patient how to protect his eye from injury.
- Demonstrate how to apply eye drops correctly.

Costovertebral angle tenderness

Costovertebral angle (CVA) tenderness indicates sudden distention of the renal capsule. It almost always accompanies unelicited, dull, constant flank pain in the CVA just lateral to the sacrospinalis muscle and below the 12th rib. This associated pain typically travels anteriorly in the subcostal region toward the umbilicus.

Percussing the CVA elicits tenderness, if present. (See *Eliciting CVA tenderness*, page 152.)

A patient who doesn't have this symptom will perceive a thudding, jarring, or pressurelike sensation when tested, but no pain. A patient with a disorder that distends the renal capsule will experience intense pain as the renal capsule stretches and stimulates the afferent nerves, which emanate from the spinal cord at levels T11 through L2 and innervate the kidney.

History and physical examination

After detecting CVA tenderness, determine the possible extent of renal damage. First, find out if the patient has other symptoms of renal or urologic dysfunction. Ask about voiding habits: How frequently does he urinate, and in what amounts? Has he noticed any change in intake or output? If so, when did he notice the change? (Ask about fluid intake before judging his output as abnormal.) Does he have nocturia? Ask about pain or burning during urination or difficulty starting a stream. Does the patient strain to urinate without being able to do so

Eliciting CVA tenderness

To elicit costovertebral angle (CVA) tenderness, have the patient sit upright facing away from you or have him lie in a prone position. Place the palm of your left hand over the left CVA, then strike the back of your left hand with the ulnar surface of your right fist (as shown below). Repeat this percussion technique over the right CVA. A patient with CVA tenderness will experience intense pain.

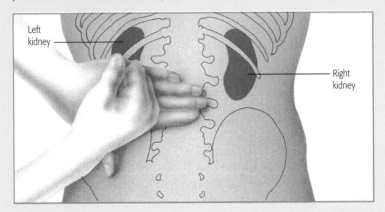

Left kidney

Right kidney

(tenesmus)? Ask about urine color; brown or bright red urine may contain blood.

Explore other signs and symptoms. For example, if the patient is experiencing pain in his flank, abdomen, or back, when did he first notice the pain? How severe is it, and where is it located? Find out if the patient or a family member has a history of urinary tract infections, congenital anomalies, calculi, or other obstructive nephropathies or uropathies. Also, ask about a history of renovascular disorders such as occlusion of the renal arteries or veins.

Perform a brief physical examination. Begin by taking the patient's vital signs. A fever and chills in a patient with CVA tenderness may indicate acute pyelonephritis. If the patient has hypertension and bradycardia, be alert for other autonomic effects of renal pain, such as diaphoresis and pallor. Inspect, auscultate, and gently palpate the abdomen for clues to the underlying cause of CVA tenderness. Be alert for abdominal distention, hypoactive bowel sounds, and palpable masses.

Medical causes

Calculi. Infundibular and ureteropelvic or ureteral calculi produce CVA tenderness and waves of waxing and waning flank pain that may radiate to the groin, testicles, suprapubic area, or labia. The patient may also develop nausea, vomiting, severe abdominal pain, abdominal distention, and decreased bowel sounds.

Perirenal abscess. Causing exquisite CVA tenderness, perirenal abscess may also produce severe unilateral flank pain, dysuria, a persistent high fever, chills, erythema of the skin and, sometimes, a palpable abdominal mass.

Pyelonephritis (acute). Perhaps the most common cause of CVA tenderness, acute pyelonephritis is commonly accompanied by a persistent high fever, chills, flank pain, anorexia, nausea and vomiting, weakness, dysuria, hematuria, nocturia, urinary urgency and frequency, and tenesmus.

Renal artery occlusion. With renal artery occlusion, the patient experiences flank pain as well as CVA tenderness. Other findings include severe, continuous upper abdominal pain; nausea; vomiting; decreased bowel sounds; and a high fever.

Renal vein occlusion. The patient with renal vein occlusion has CVA tenderness and flank pain. He may also have sudden, severe back pain; a fever; oliguria; edema; and hematuria.

Nursing considerations

- Assess for pain and administer pain medication as needed.
- Monitor the patient's vital signs and intake and output.
- Collect blood and urine samples as indicated.
- Prepare the patient for radiologic studies, such as excretory urography, renal arteriography, and a computed tomography scan.

Patient teaching

- Teach the patient with calculi about dietary restrictions.
- Tell the patient to drink at least 2 qt (2 L) of fluids each day.
- Explain signs and symptoms of kidney infection that should be reported immediately.
- Emphasize the importance of taking the full course of antibiotics.
- Explain to the patient his diagnosis and the treatment plan.

▌Cough, barking

Resonant, brassy, and harsh, a barking cough is part of a complex of signs and symptoms that characterize croup syndrome, a group of pediatric disorders marked by varying degrees of respiratory distress. It's most prevalent in the fall and may recur in the same child.

A barking cough indicates edema of the larynx and surrounding tissue. Because children's airways are smaller in diameter than those of adults, edema can rapidly lead to airway occlusion—a life-threatening emergency.

A CTION STAT!

 Quickly evaluate a child's respiratory status, and then take his vital signs. Be particularly alert for tachycardia and signs of hypoxemia. Also, check for a decreased level of consciousness. Try to determine if the child has been playing with any small object that he may have aspirated.

Check for cyanosis in the lips and nail beds. Observe the patient for sternal or intercostal retractions or nasal flaring. Next, note the depth and rate of his respirations; they may become increasingly shallow as respiratory distress increases. Observe the child's body position. Is he sitting up, leaning forward, and struggling to breathe? Observe his activity level and facial expression. As respiratory distress increases from airway edema, the child will become restless and have a frightened, wide-eyed expression. As air hunger continues, the child will become lethargic and difficult to arouse.

If the child shows signs of severe respiratory distress, try to calm him, maintain airway patency, and provide oxygen. Endotracheal intubation or a tracheotomy may be necessary.

History and physical examination

Ask the child's parents when the barking cough began and what other signs and symptoms accompanied it. When did the child first appear to be ill? Has he had previous episodes of croup syndrome? Did his condition improve upon exposure to cold air?

Spasmodic croup and epiglottiditis typically occur in the middle of the night. The child with spasmodic croup has no fever, but the child with epiglottiditis has a sudden high fever. An upper respiratory tract infection typically is followed by laryngotracheobronchitis.

Medical causes

Aspiration of foreign body. Partial obstruction of the upper airway first produces sudden hoarseness, and then a barking cough and inspiratory stridor. Other effects of this life-threatening condition include gagging, tachycardia, dyspnea, decreased breath sounds, wheezing and, possibly, cyanosis.

Epiglottiditis. Epiglottiditis is a life-threatening disorder that has become less common since the use of influenza vaccines. It occurs nocturnally, heralded by a barking cough and a high fever. The child is hoarse, dysphagic, dyspneic, and restless and appears extremely ill and panicky. The cough may progress to severe respiratory distress with sternal and intercostal retractions, nasal flaring, cyanosis, and tachycardia. The child will struggle to get sufficient air as epiglottic edema increases. Epiglottiditis is a true medical emergency.

Laryngotracheobronchitis (acute). Also known as *viral croup,* laryngotracheobronchitis initially produces a low to moderate fever, a runny nose, a poor appetite, and an infrequent cough. When the infection descends into the laryngotracheal area, a barking cough, hoarseness, and inspiratory stridor occur.

As respiratory distress progresses, substernal and intercostal retractions occur along with tachycardia and shallow, rapid respirations. Sleeping in a dry room worsens these signs. The patient becomes restless, irritable, pale, and cyanotic.

Spasmodic croup. Acute spasmodic croup usually occurs during sleep with the abrupt onset of a barking cough that awakens the child. Typically, he doesn't have a fever, but may be hoarse, restless, and dyspneic. As his respiratory distress worsens, the child may exhibit sternal and intercostal retractions, nasal flaring, tachycardia, cyanosis, and an anxious, frantic appearance. The signs usually subside within a few hours, but attacks tend to recur.

Nursing considerations

▪ Don't attempt to inspect the throat of a child with a barking cough unless intubation equipment is available. (See *Managing the patient with epiglottiditis.*)
▪ If the child isn't in severe respiratory distress, a lateral neck X-ray may be done to visualize epiglottal edema.
▪ A chest X-ray may be done to rule out lower respiratory tract infection.
▪ Depending on the child's age and degree of respiratory distress, oxygen may be administered.
▪ Rapid-acting epinephrine and a steroid may be administered.
▪ Observe the child frequently, and monitor pulse oximetry.
▪ Provide the child with periods of rest with minimal interruptions.
▪ Maintain a calm, quiet environment and offer reassurance.
▪ Encourage the parents to stay with the child to help alleviate stress.

Managing the patient with epiglottiditis

Acute epiglottiditis is an inflammation of the epiglottis that tends to cause airway obstruction. It typically strikes children ages 2 to 8. A critical emergency, epiglottiditis can prove fatal in 8% to 12% of victims unless it's recognized and treated promptly.

Do's

■ Keep the following equipment available in case the patient experiences complete airway obstruction: a tracheostomy tray, endotracheal tubes, a handheld resuscitation bag, oxygen equipment, and a laryngoscope with blades of various sizes.

■ Monitor arterial blood gas levels for hypoxia and hypercapnia and administer oxygen as needed.

■ Watch for increasing restlessness, rising heart rate, fever, dyspnea, and retractions, which may indicate the need for emergency tracheotomy.

■ Maintain fluid hydration with I.V. therapy or oral clear liquids or ice popsicles as tolerated.

■ Administer I.V. antibiotics and corticosteroid, as ordered.

Don'ts

■ If you suspect epiglottiditis, don't inspect the epiglottis unless team members are prepared to perform emergency intubation because inspection can produce laryngospasm, airway obstruction, and respiratory arrest.

■ Send someone else to call for help and get the resuscitation cart, don't leave the patient alone.

■ To avoid complete airway obstruction, don't lie the patient flat; keep him upright possibly on the lap of a parent to calm him.

Patient teaching

■ Teach the parents how to evaluate and treat recurrent episodes of croup syndrome.

■ Teach parents how to administer prescribed medications.

Cough, nonproductive

A nonproductive cough is a noisy, forceful expulsion of air from the lungs that doesn't yield sputum or blood. It's one of the most common complaints of patients with respiratory disorders.

Coughing is a necessary protective mechanism that clears airway passages. However, a nonproductive cough is ineffective and can cause damage, such as airway collapse or rupture of alveoli or blebs. A nonproductive cough that later becomes productive is a classic sign of progressive respiratory disease.

The cough reflex generally occurs when mechanical, chemical, thermal, inflammatory, or psychogenic stimuli activate cough receptors. (See *Reviewing the cough mechanism*, page 156.)

However, external pressure—for example, from subdiaphragmatic irritation or a mediastinal tumor—can also induce it, as well as voluntary expiration of air, which occasionally occurs as a nervous habit. Certain drugs, such as angiotensin-converting enzyme inhibitors, may also cause a nonproductive cough.

A nonproductive cough may occur in paroxysms and can worsen by becoming more frequent. An acute cough has a sudden onset and may be self-limiting; a cough that persists beyond 1 month is

Reviewing the cough mechanism

Cough receptors are thought to be located in the nose, sinuses, auditory canals, nasopharynx, larynx, trachea, bronchi, pleurae, diaphragm and, possibly, the pericardium and GI tract. When a cough receptor is stimulated, the vagus and glossopharyngeal nerves transmit the impulse to the "cough center" in the medulla. From there, the impulse is transmitted to the larynx and to the intercostal and abdominal muscles. Deep inspiration (1) is followed by closure of the glottis (2), relaxation of the diaphragm, and contraction of the abdominal and intercostal muscles. The resulting increased pressure in the lungs opens the glottis to release the forceful, noisy expiration known as a cough (3).

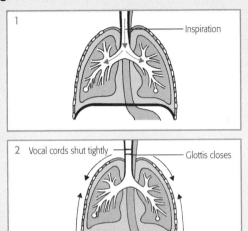

1 — Inspiration

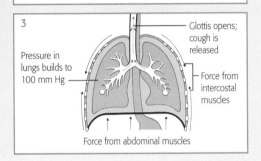

2 Vocal cords shut tightly — Glottis closes

Air becomes trapped in the lungs

3 — Glottis opens; cough is released

Pressure in lungs builds to 100 mm Hg — Force from intercostal muscles

Force from abdominal muscles

considered chronic and commonly results from cigarette smoking.

Someone with a chronic nonproductive cough may downplay or overlook it or accept it as normal. In fact, he generally won't seek medical attention unless he has other symptoms. A foreign body in a child's external auditory canal may result in a cough. Always examine the child's ears.

History and physical examination

Ask the patient when his cough began and whether body position, the time of day, or a specific activity affects it. How does the cough sound—harsh, brassy, dry, or hacking? Try to determine if the cough is related to smoking or a chemical irritant. If the patient smokes or has smoked, note the number of packs smoked daily multiplied by years ("pack-years"). Next, ask about the frequency and intensity of the coughing. If he has pain associated with coughing, breathing, or activity, when did it begin? Where is it located?

Ask the patient about recent illness (especially a cardiovascular or pulmonary disorder), surgery, or trauma.

Also ask about hypersensitivity to drugs, foods, pets, dust, or pollen. Find out which medications the patient takes, if any, and ask about recent changes in schedule or dosages. Ask about recent changes in his appetite, weight, exercise tolerance, or energy level and recent exposure to irritating fumes, chemicals, or smoke.

As you're taking his history, observe the patient's general appearance and manner: Is he agitated, restless, or lethargic; pale, diaphoretic, or flushed; anxious, confused, or nervous? Also, note whether he's cyanotic or has clubbed fingers or peripheral edema.

Next, perform a physical examination. Start by taking the patient's vital signs. Check the depth and rhythm of his respirations, and note if wheezing or "crowing" noises occur with breathing. Feel the patient's skin: Is it cold or warm; clammy or dry? Check his nose and mouth for congestion, inflammation, drainage, or signs of infection. Inspect his neck for distended jugular veins and tracheal deviation, and palpate for masses or enlarged lymph nodes.

Examine his chest, observing its configuration and looking for abnormal chest wall motion. Do you note any retractions or use of accessory muscles? Percuss for dullness, tympany, or flatness. Auscultate for wheezing, crackles, rhonchi, pleural friction rubs, and decreased or absent breath sounds. Finally, examine his abdomen for distention, tenderness, masses, or abnormal bowel sounds.

Medical causes

Airway occlusion. Partial occlusion of the upper airway produces a sudden onset of dry, paroxysmal coughing. The patient is gagging, wheezing, and hoarse, with stridor, tachycardia, and decreased breath sounds.

Anthrax (inhalation). Inhalation anthrax is caused by inhaling aerosolized spores. Initial signs and symptoms are flulike and include a fever, chills, weakness, a cough, and chest pain. The disease generally occurs in two stages, with a period of recovery after the initial signs and symptoms. The second stage develops abruptly with rapid deterioration marked by a fever, dyspnea, stridor, and hypotension generally leading to death within 24 hours. Radiologic findings include mediastinitis and symmetric mediastinal widening.

Aortic aneurysm (thoracic). Aortic aneurysm causes a brassy cough with dyspnea, hoarseness, wheezing, and a substernal ache in the shoulders, lower back, or abdomen. The patient may also have facial or neck edema, jugular vein distention, dysphagia, prominent veins over his chest, stridor and, possibly, paresthesia or neuralgia.

Asthma. Asthma attacks typically occur at night, starting with a nonproductive cough and mild wheezing; this progresses to severe dyspnea, audible wheezing, chest tightness, and a cough that produces thick mucus. Other signs include apprehension, rhonchi, prolonged expirations, intercostal and supraclavicular retractions on inspiration, accessory muscle use, flaring nostrils, tachypnea, tachycardia, diaphoresis, and flushing or cyanosis.

Atelectasis. As lung tissue deflates, it stimulates cough receptors, causing a nonproductive cough. The patient may also have pleuritic chest pain, anxiety, dyspnea, tachypnea, and tachycardia. His skin may be cyanotic and diaphoretic, his breath sounds may be decreased, his chest may be dull on percussion, and he may exhibit inspiratory lag, substernal or intercostal retractions, decreased vocal fremitus, and tracheal deviation toward the affected side.

Avian influenza. Individuals infected with avian influenza may initially have symptoms of conventional influenza, including a nonproductive cough, fever, sore throat, and muscle aches. The most virulent avian virus, influenza A (H5N1), may lead to severe and life-threatening complications, such as acute respiratory distress and pneumonia.

Bronchitis (chronic). Bronchitis starts with a nonproductive, hacking cough that later becomes productive. Other findings include prolonged expiration, wheezing, dyspnea, accessory muscle use, barrel chest, cyanosis, tachypnea, crackles, and scattered rhonchi. Clubbing can occur in late stages.

Bronchogenic carcinoma. The earliest indicators of bronchogenic carcinoma can be a chronic, nonproductive cough; dyspnea; and vague chest pain. The patient may also be wheezing.

Common cold. The common cold generally starts with a nonproductive, hacking cough and progresses to some mix of sneezing, headaches, malaise, fatigue, rhinorrhea, myalgia, arthralgia, nasal congestion, and a sore throat.

Esophageal achalasia. In esophageal achalasia, regurgitation and aspiration produce a dry cough. The patient may also have recurrent pulmonary infections and dysphagia.

Esophageal diverticula. The patient with esophageal diverticula has a nocturnal nonproductive cough, regurgitation and aspiration, dyspepsia, and dysphagia. His neck may appear swollen and have a gurgling sound. He may also exhibit halitosis and weight loss.

Esophageal occlusion. Esophageal occlusion is marked by immediate nonproductive coughing and gagging, with a sensation of something stuck in the throat. Other findings include neck or chest pain, dysphagia, and the inability to swallow.

Hantavirus pulmonary syndrome. A nonproductive cough is common in patients with *Hantavirus* pulmonary syndrome, which is marked by noncardiogenic pulmonary edema. Other findings include a headache, myalgia, fever, nausea, and vomiting.

Hypersensitivity pneumonitis. With hypersensitivity pneumonitis, an acute nonproductive cough, a fever, dyspnea, and malaise usually occur 5 or 6 hours after exposure to an antigen.

Interstitial lung disease. A patient with interstitial lung disease has a nonproductive cough and progressive dyspnea. He may also be cyanotic and have clubbing, fine crackles, fatigue, variable chest pain, and weight loss.

Laryngeal tumor. A mild, nonproductive cough is an early sign of a laryngeal tumor, in addition to minor throat discomfort and hoarseness. Later, dysphagia, dyspnea, cervical lymphadenopathy, stridor, and an earache may occur.

Laryngitis. In its acute form, laryngitis causes a nonproductive cough with localized pain (especially when the patient is swallowing or speaking) as well as fever and malaise. His hoarseness can range from mild to complete loss of voice.

Lung abscess. Lung abscess typically begins with a nonproductive cough, weakness, dyspnea, and pleuritic chest pain. The patient may also exhibit diaphoresis, a fever, a headache, malaise, fatigue, crackles, decreased breath sounds, anorexia, and weight loss. Later, his cough produces large amounts of purulent, foul-smelling and, possibly, bloody sputum.

Pleural effusion. A nonproductive cough along with dyspnea, pleuritic chest pain, and decreased chest motion are characteristic of pleural effusion. Other findings include a pleural friction rub, tachycardia, tachypnea, egophony, flatness on percussion, decreased or absent breath sounds, and decreased tactile fremitus.

Pneumonia. *Bacterial pneumonia* usually starts with a nonproductive, hacking, painful cough that rapidly becomes productive. Other findings include shaking chills, a headache, a high fever, dyspnea, pleuritic chest pain, tachypnea, tachycardia, grunting respirations, nasal flaring, decreased breath sounds, fine crackles, rhonchi, and cyanosis. The patient's chest may be dull on percussion.

With *mycoplasma pneumonia,* a nonproductive cough arises 2 or 3 days after the onset of malaise, a headache, and a sore throat. The cough can be paroxysmal, causing substernal chest pain. Fever commonly occurs, but the patient doesn't appear seriously ill.

Viral pneumonia causes a nonproductive, hacking cough and the gradual onset of malaise, headache, anorexia, and a low-grade fever.

Pneumothorax. Pneumothorax is a life-threatening disorder that causes a dry cough and signs of respiratory distress, such as severe dyspnea, tachycardia, tachypnea, and cyanosis. The patient experiences sudden, sharp chest pain that worsens with chest movement as well as subcutaneous crepitation, hyperresonance or tympany, decreased vocal fremitus, and decreased or absent breath sounds on the affected side.

Pulmonary edema. Pulmonary edema initially causes a dry cough, exertional dyspnea, paroxysmal nocturnal dyspnea, orthopnea, tachycardia, tachypnea, dependent crackles, a ventricular gallop, and anxiety and restlessness. If pulmonary edema is severe, the patient's respirations become more rapid and labored, with diffuse crackles and coughing that produces frothy, bloody sputum.

Pulmonary embolism. A life-threatening pulmonary embolism may suddenly produce a dry cough along with dyspnea and pleuritic or anginal chest pain. Typically, however, the cough produces blood-tinged sputum. Tachycardia and a low-grade fever are also common; less common signs and symptoms include massive hemoptysis, chest splinting, leg edema and, with a large embolus, cyanosis, syncope, and jugular vein distention. The patient may also have a pleural friction rub, diffuse wheezing, dullness on percussion, and decreased breath sounds.

Sarcoidosis. With sarcoidosis, a nonproductive cough is accompanied by dyspnea, substernal pain, and malaise. The patient may also develop fatigue, arthralgia, myalgia, weight loss, tachypnea, crackles, lymphadenopathy, hepatosplenomegaly, skin lesions, visual impairment, difficulty swallowing, and arrhythmias.

Severe acute respiratory syndrome (SARS). SARS generally begins with a fever (usually greater than 100.4° F [38° C]). Other symptoms include a headache; malaise; a dry, nonproductive cough; and dyspnea. The severity of the illness is highly variable, ranging from mild illness to pneumonia and, in some cases, progressing to respiratory failure and death.

Tracheobronchitis (acute). Initially, tracheobronchitis produces a dry cough that later becomes productive as secretions increase. Chills, a sore throat, a slight fever, muscle and back pain, and substernal tightness generally precede the cough's onset. Rhonchi and wheezes are usually heard. Severe illness causes a fever of 101° to 102° F (38.3° to 38.9° C) and, possibly, bronchospasm, with severe wheezing and increased coughing.

Tularemia. Signs and symptoms of tularemia following inhalation of the organism include the abrupt onset of a fever, chills, a headache, generalized myalgia, a nonproductive cough, dyspnea, pleuritic chest pain, and empyema.

Other causes

Diagnostic tests. Pulmonary function tests (PFTs) and bronchoscopy may stimulate cough receptors and trigger coughing.

Treatments. Irritation of the carina during suctioning or deep endotracheal or tracheal tube placement can trigger a paroxysmal or hacking cough. Intermittent positive-pressure breathing or spirometry can also cause a nonproductive cough. Some inhalants, such as pentamidine, may stimulate coughing.

Nursing considerations

▪ A nonproductive, paroxysmal cough may induce life-threatening bronchospasm; the patient may need a bronchodilator to relieve his bronchospasm and open his airways.
▪ Unless he has chronic obstructive pulmonary disease, you may have to give the patient an antitussive and a sedative to suppress the cough.
▪ To relieve mucous membrane inflammation and dryness, humidify the air in the patient's room.
▪ Prepare the patient for diagnostic tests, such as X-rays, a lung scan, bronchoscopy, and PFTs.

Patient teaching

▪ Teach the patient to use a humidifier if his home is dry.
▪ Tell him to avoid using aerosols, powders, or other respiratory irritants—especially cigarettes.
▪ If the patient smokes, stress the importance of smoking cessation, and refer him to appropriate resources, support groups, and information to help him quit smoking.

▪ Explain the importance of adequate fluids and nutrition.
▪ Explain to the patient the cause of his cough and the treatment plan.

▎Cough, productive

Productive coughing is the body's mechanism for clearing airway passages of accumulated secretions that normal mucociliary action doesn't remove. It's a sudden, forceful, noisy expulsion of air from the lungs that contains sputum, blood, or both. The sputum's color, consistency, and odor provide important clues about the patient's condition. A productive cough can occur as a single cough or as paroxysmal coughing, and it can be voluntarily induced, although it's usually a reflexive response to stimulation of the airway mucosa.

Usually due to a cardiovascular or respiratory disorder, productive coughing commonly results from an acute or chronic infection that causes inflammation, edema, and increased mucus production in the airways. However, this sign can also result from acquired immunodeficiency syndrome. Inhalation of antigenic or irritating substances or foreign bodies can also cause a productive cough. In fact, the most common cause of chronic productive coughing is cigarette smoking, which produces mucoid sputum ranging in color from clear to yellow to brown.

Many patients minimize or overlook a chronic productive cough or accept it as normal. Such patients may not seek medical attention until an associated problem—such as dyspnea, hemoptysis, chest pain, weight loss, or recurrent respiratory tract infections—develops. The delay can have serious consequences because productive coughing is associated with several life-threatening disorders and can also herald airway occlusion from excessive secretions.

A patient with a productive cough can develop acute respiratory distress from thick or excessive secretions, bronchospasm, or fatigue, so examine him before you take his history. Take his vital signs, measure oxygen saturation, and check the rate, depth, and rhythm of respirations. Keep his airway patent, and be prepared to provide supplemental oxygen if he becomes restless or confused or if his respirations become shallow, irregular, rapid, or slow. Look for stridor, wheezing, choking, or gurgling. Be alert for nasal flaring and cyanosis.

A productive cough may signal a severe, life-threatening disorder. For example, coughing due to pulmonary edema produces thin, frothy, pink sputum, and coughing due to an asthma attack produces thick, mucoid sputum. Assist the patient to clear excess mucous with tracheal suctioning if needed.

History and physical examination

When the patient's condition permits, ask when the cough began, and find out how much sputum he's coughing up each day. (The normal tracheobronchial tree can produce up to 3 oz [89 ml] of sputum per day.) At what time of day does he cough up the most sputum? Does his sputum production have any relationship to what or when he eats or to his activities or environment? Ask him if he has noticed an increase in sputum production since his coughing began. This may result from external stimuli or from such internal causes as chronic bronchial infection or a lung abscess. Also ask about the color, odor, and consistency of the sputum. Blood-tinged or rust-colored sputum may result from trauma due to coughing or from an underlying condition, such as a

pulmonary infection or a tumor. Foul-smelling sputum may result from an anaerobic infection, such as bronchitis or a lung abscess.

How does the cough sound? A hacking cough results from laryngeal involvement, whereas a "brassy" cough indicates major airway involvement. Does the patient feel pain associated with his productive cough? If so, ask about its location and severity and whether it radiates to other areas. Does coughing, changing body position, or inspiration increase or help relieve his pain?

Next, ask the patient about his cigarette, drug, and alcohol use and whether his weight or appetite has changed. Find out if he has a history of asthma, allergies, or respiratory disorders, and ask about recent illnesses, surgery, or trauma. What medications is he taking? Does he work around chemicals or respiratory irritants such as silicone?

Examine the patient's mouth and nose for congestion, drainage, or inflammation. Note his breath odor; halitosis can be a sign of pulmonary infection. Inspect his neck for distended veins, and palpate for tenderness and masses or enlarged lymph nodes. Observe his chest for accessory muscle use, retractions, and uneven chest expansion, and percuss for dullness, tympany, or flatness. Finally, auscultate for a pleural friction rub and abnormal breath sounds—rhonchi, crackles, or wheezes.

Medical causes

Actinomycosis. Actinomycosis begins with a cough that produces purulent sputum. A fever, weight loss, fatigue, weakness, dyspnea, night sweats, pleuritic chest pain, and hemoptysis may also occur.

Aspiration pneumonitis. Aspiration pneumonitis causes coughing that produces pink, frothy and, possibly, purulent sputum. The patient also has marked dyspnea, a fever, tachypnea, tachycardia, wheezing, and cyanosis.

Bronchiectasis. The chronic cough of bronchiectasis produces copious, mucopurulent sputum that has characteristic layering (top, frothy; middle, clear; bottom, dense with purulent particles). The patient has halitosis; his sputum may smell foul or sickeningly sweet. Other characteristic findings include hemoptysis, persistent coarse crackles over the affected lung area, occasional wheezing, rhonchi, exertional dyspnea, weight loss, fatigue, malaise, weakness, a recurrent fever, and late-stage finger clubbing.

Bronchitis (chronic). Bronchitis causes a cough that may be nonproductive initially. Eventually, however, it produces mucoid sputum that becomes purulent. Secondary infection can also cause mucopurulent sputum, which may become blood-tinged and foul-smelling. The coughing, which may be paroxysmal during exercise, usually occurs when the patient is recumbent or rises from sleep.

The patient also exhibits prolonged expirations, increased use of accessory muscles for breathing, barrel chest, tachypnea, cyanosis, wheezing, exertional dyspnea, scattered rhonchi, coarse crackles (which can be precipitated by coughing), and late-stage clubbing.

Chemical pneumonitis. Chemical pneumonitis causes a cough with purulent sputum. It can also cause dyspnea, wheezing, orthopnea, a fever, malaise, and crackles; mucous membrane irritation of the conjunctivae, throat, and nose; laryngitis; or rhinitis. Signs and symptoms may increase for 24 to 48 hours after exposure, then resolve; if severe, however, they may recur 2 to 5 weeks later.

Common cold. When the common cold causes productive coughing, the sputum is mucoid or mucopurulent.

Early indications include a dry hacking cough, sneezing, a headache, malaise, fatigue, rhinorrhea (watery to tenacious, mucopurulent secretions), nasal congestion, a sore throat, myalgia, and arthralgia.

Lung abscess (ruptured). The cardinal sign of a ruptured lung abscess is coughing that produces copious amounts of purulent, foul-smelling and, possibly, blood-tinged sputum. A ruptured abscess can also cause diaphoresis, anorexia, clubbing, weight loss, weakness, fatigue, a fever with chills, dyspnea, a headache, malaise, pleuritic chest pain, halitosis, inspiratory crackles, and tubular or amphoric breath sounds. The patient's chest is dull on percussion on the affected side.

Lung cancer. One of the earliest signs of bronchogenic carcinoma is a chronic cough that produces small amounts of purulent (or mucopurulent), blood-streaked sputum. In a patient with bronchoalveolar cancer, however, coughing produces large amounts of frothy sputum. Other signs and symptoms include dyspnea, anorexia, fatigue, weight loss, chest pain, a fever, diaphoresis, wheezing, and clubbing.

Nocardiosis. Nocardiosis causes a productive cough (with purulent, thick, tenacious, and possibly blood-tinged sputum) and fever that may last several months. Other findings include night sweats, pleuritic pain, anorexia, malaise, fatigue, weight loss, and diminished or absent breath sounds. The patient's chest is dull on percussion.

North American blastomycosis. North American blastomycosis is a chronic disorder that produces coughing that's dry and hacking or produces bloody or purulent sputum. Other findings include pleuritic chest pain, a fever, chills, anorexia, weight loss, malaise, fatigue, night sweats, cutaneous lesions (small, painless, nonpruritic macules or papules), and prostration.

Plague (Yersinia pestis). The pneumonic form of plague may be contracted from person-to-person through direct contact via the respiratory system or through biological warfare from aerosolization and inhalation of the organism. The onset is usually sudden with chills, a fever, a headache, and myalgia. Pulmonary signs and symptoms include a productive cough, chest pain, tachypnea, dyspnea, hemoptysis, increasing respiratory distress, and cardiopulmonary insufficiency.

Pneumonia. *Bacterial pneumonia* initially produces a dry cough that becomes productive. Associated signs and symptoms develop suddenly and include shaking chills, a high fever, myalgia, headache, pleuritic chest pain that increases with chest movement, tachypnea, tachycardia, dyspnea, cyanosis, diaphoresis, decreased breath sounds, fine crackles, and rhonchi.

Mycoplasma pneumonia may cause a cough that produces scant blood-flecked sputum. Typically, however, a nonproductive cough starts 2 or 3 days after the onset of malaise, a headache, a fever, and a sore throat. Paroxysmal coughing causes substernal chest pain. Patients may develop crackles, but generally don't appear seriously ill.

Psittacosis. As psittacosis progresses, the characteristic hacking cough, nonproductive at first, may later produce a small amount of mucoid, blood-streaked sputum. The infection may begin abruptly, with chills, a fever, a headache, myalgia, and prostration. Other signs and symptoms include tachypnea, fine crackles, chest pain (rare), epistaxis, photophobia, abdominal distention and tenderness, nausea, vomiting, and a faint macular rash. Severe infection may produce stupor, delirium, and coma.

Pulmonary coccidioidomycosis. Pulmonary coccidioidomycosis causes a nonproductive or slightly productive cough with a fever, occasional chills, pleuritic chest pain, a sore throat, a headache, backache, malaise, marked weakness, anorexia, hemoptysis, and an itchy macular rash. Rhonchi and wheezing may be heard. The disease may spread to other areas, causing arthralgia, swelling of the knees and ankles, and erythema nodosum or erythema multiforme.

Pulmonary edema. Severe, pulmonary edema, which is a life-threatening disorder, causes a cough that produces frothy, bloody sputum. Early signs and symptoms include exertional dyspnea; paroxysmal nocturnal dyspnea, followed by orthopnea; and coughing, which may be nonproductive initially. Others include a fever, fatigue, tachycardia, tachypnea, dependent crackles, and a ventricular gallop. As the patient's respirations become increasingly rapid and labored, he develops more diffuse crackles and a productive cough, anxiety, restlessness, worsening tachycardia and, possibly, arrhythmias. His skin becomes cold, clammy, and cyanotic; his blood pressure falls; and his pulse becomes thready.

Pulmonary embolism. Pulmonary embolism is a life-threatening disorder that causes a cough that may be nonproductive or may produce blood-tinged sputum. Usually, the first symptom of a pulmonary embolism is severe dyspnea, which may be accompanied by angina or pleuritic chest pain. The patient experiences marked anxiety, a low-grade fever, tachycardia, tachypnea, and diaphoresis. Less-common signs include massive hemoptysis, chest splinting, leg edema and, with a large embolus, cyanosis, syncope, and jugular vein distention. The patient may also have a pleural friction rub, diffuse wheezing, crackles, chest dullness on percussion, decreased breath sounds, and signs of circulatory collapse.

Pulmonary tuberculosis (TB). Pulmonary TB causes a mild to severe productive cough along with some combination of hemoptysis, malaise, dyspnea, and pleuritic chest pain. Sputum may be scant and mucoid or copious and purulent. Typically, the patient experiences night sweats, easy fatigability, and weight loss. His breath sounds are amphoric. He may have chest dullness on percussion and, after coughing, increased tactile fremitus with crackles.

Silicosis. A productive cough with mucopurulent sputum is the earliest sign of silicosis. The patient also has exertional dyspnea, tachypnea, weight loss, fatigue, general weakness, and recurrent respiratory infections. Auscultation reveals end-inspiratory, fine crackles at the lung bases.

Tracheobronchitis. Inflammation initially causes a nonproductive cough that later—following the onset of chills, a sore throat, a slight fever, muscle and back pain, and substernal tightness—becomes productive as secretions increase. Sputum is mucoid, mucopurulent, or purulent. The patient typically has rhonchi and wheezes; he may also develop crackles. Severe tracheobronchitis may cause a fever of 101° to 102° F (38.3° to 38.9° C) and bronchospasm.

Other causes

Diagnostic tests. Bronchoscopy and pulmonary function tests (PFTs) may increase productive coughing.

Drugs. Expectorants increase productive coughing. These include ammonium chloride, calcium iodide, guaifenesin, iodinated glycerol, potassium iodide, and terpin hydrate.

Respiratory therapy. Intermittent positive-pressure breathing, nebulizer therapy, and incentive spirometry can help loosen secretions and cause or increase productive coughing.

Nursing considerations

- Avoid taking measures to suppress a productive cough because retention of sputum may interfere with alveolar aeration or impair pulmonary resistance to infection.
- Expect to give a mucolytic and an expectorant.
- Increase the patient's intake of oral fluids to thin his secretions and increase their flow.
- Give a bronchodilator to relieve bronchospasms and open airways.
- Administer an antibiotic to treat any underlying infection.
- Humidify the air around the patient to relieve mucous membrane inflammation and help loosen dried secretions.
- Provide pulmonary physiotherapy, such as postural drainage with vibration and percussion, to loosen secretions.
- Administer aerosol therapy if necessary.
- Provide the patient with uninterrupted rest periods.
- If the patient is on bed rest, change his position often to promote the drainage of secretions.
- Prepare the patient for diagnostic tests, such as chest X-ray, imaging studies, bronchoscopy, a lung scan, and PFTs.
- Collect sputum samples for culture and sensitivity testing.

Patient teaching

- Encourage the patient to stop smoking and provide him with written resources and contact information for support groups.
- Teach him how to perform cough and deep-breathing exercises.
- Discuss ways to avoid respiratory irritants.
- Explain infection control techniques.

- Teach the patient and family how to use chest percussion to loosen secretions.
- Explain to the patient his diagnosis and the treatment plan.

Crackles
[Rales, crepitations]

A common finding in patients with certain cardiovascular and pulmonary disorders, crackles are nonmusical clicking or rattling noises heard during auscultation of breath sounds. They usually occur during inspiration and recur constantly from one respiratory cycle to the next. They can be unilateral or bilateral, moist or dry. They're characterized by their pitch, loudness, location, persistence, and occurrence during the respiratory cycle.

Crackles indicate abnormal movement of air through fluid-filled airways. They can be irregularly dispersed, as in pneumonia, or localized, as in bronchiectasis. (A few basilar crackles can be heard in normal lungs after prolonged shallow breathing. These normal crackles clear with a few deep breaths.) Usually, crackles indicate the degree of an underlying illness. When crackles result from a generalized disorder, they usually occur in the less distended and more dependent areas of the lungs, such as the lung bases, when the patient is standing. Crackles due to air passing through inflammatory exudate may not be audible if the involved portion of the lung isn't being ventilated because of shallow respirations. (See *How crackles occur*, page 166.)

ACTION STAT!

 If you discover the patient has crackles, quickly take his vital signs and examine him for signs of respiratory distress or airway obstruction. Check the depth and rhythm

of respirations. Is he struggling to breathe? Check for increased accessory muscle use and chest wall motion, retractions, stridor, or nasal flaring. Assess the patient for other signs and symptoms of fluid overload, such as jugular vein distention and edema. Provide supplemental oxygen and, if necessary, a diuretic. Endotracheal intubation may also be needed if the patient is experiencing respiratory distress.

History and physical examination

If the patient has a cough along with the crackles, ask when it began and if it's constant or intermittent. Find out what the cough sounds like and whether he's coughing up sputum or blood. If the cough is productive, determine the sputum's consistency, amount, odor, and color.

Ask the patient if he has pain. If so, where is it located? When did he first notice it? Does it radiate to other areas? Also ask the patient if movement, coughing, or breathing worsens or helps relieve his pain. Note the patient's position: Is he lying still or moving about restlessly?

Obtain a brief medical history. Does the patient have cancer or a known respiratory or cardiovascular problem? Ask about recent surgery, trauma, or illness. Does he smoke or drink alcohol? Is he experiencing hoarseness or difficulty swallowing? Find out which medications he's taking. Also, ask about recent weight loss, anorexia, nausea, vomiting, fatigue, weakness, vertigo, and syncope. Has the patient been exposed to irritants, such as vapors, fumes, or smoke?

Next, perform a physical examination. Examine the patient's nose and mouth for signs of infection, such as inflammation or increased secretions. Note his breath odor; halitosis could in-

How crackles occur

Crackles occur when air passes through fluid-filled airways, causing collapsed alveoli to pop open as the airway pressure equalizes. They can also occur when membranes lining the chest cavity and the lungs become inflamed. The illustrations below show a normal alveolus and two pathologic alveolar changes that cause crackles.

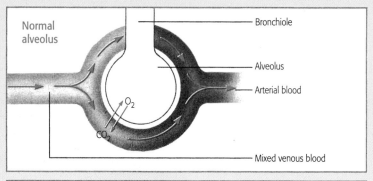

Normal alveolus

- Bronchiole
- Alveolus
- Arterial blood
- Mixed venous blood

O_2

CO_2

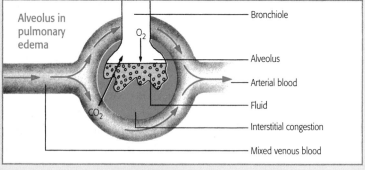

Alveolus in pulmonary edema

O_2

CO_2

- Bronchiole
- Alveolus
- Arterial blood
- Fluid
- Interstitial congestion
- Mixed venous blood

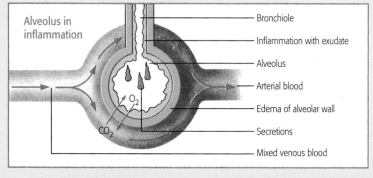

Alveolus in inflammation

O_2

CO_2

- Bronchiole
- Inflammation with exudate
- Alveolus
- Arterial blood
- Edema of alveolar wall
- Secretions
- Mixed venous blood

dicate pulmonary infection. Check his neck for masses, tenderness, swelling, lymphadenopathy, or venous distention.

Inspect the patient's chest for abnormal configuration or uneven expansion. Percuss for dullness, tympany, or flatness. Auscultate his lungs for other abnormal, diminished, or absent breath sounds. Listen to his heart for abnormal sounds, and check his hands and feet for edema or clubbing.

Medical causes

Acute respiratory distress syndrome (ARDS).
ARDS is a life-threatening disorder that causes diffuse, fine to coarse crackles usually heard in the dependent portions of the lungs. It also produces cyanosis, nasal flaring, tachypnea, tachycardia, grunting respirations, rhonchi, dyspnea, anxiety, and a decreased level of consciousness.

Bronchiectasis.
With bronchiectasis, persistent, coarse crackles are heard over the affected area of the lung. They're accompanied by a chronic cough that produces copious amounts of mucopurulent sputum. Other characteristics include halitosis, occasional wheezes, exertional dyspnea, rhonchi, weight loss, fatigue, malaise, weakness, a recurrent fever, and late-stage clubbing.

Bronchitis (chronic).
Bronchitis causes coarse crackles that are usually heard at the lung bases. Prolonged expirations, wheezing, rhonchi, exertional dyspnea, tachypnea, and a persistent, productive cough occur because of increased bronchial secretions. Clubbing and cyanosis may occur.

Legionnaires' disease.
Legionnaires' disease produces diffuse, moist crackles and a cough that produces scant mucoid, nonpurulent, and possibly blood-streaked sputum. Usually, prodromal signs and symptoms occur, including malaise, fatigue, weakness, anorexia, diffuse myalgia and, possibly, diarrhea. Within 12 to 48 hours, the patient develops a dry cough and a sudden high fever with chills. He may also have pleuritic chest pain, a headache, tachypnea, tachycardia, nausea, vomiting, dyspnea, mild temporary amnesia, confusion,

flushing, mild diaphoresis, and prostration.

Pneumonia.
Bacterial pneumonia produces diffuse fine crackles, a sudden onset of shaking chills, a high fever, tachypnea, pleuritic chest pain, cyanosis, grunting respirations, nasal flaring, decreased breath sounds, myalgia, a headache, tachycardia, dyspnea, cyanosis, diaphoresis, and rhonchi. The patient also has a dry cough that later becomes productive.

Mycoplasma pneumonia produces medium to fine crackles together with a nonproductive cough, malaise, a sore throat, a headache, and a fever. The patient may have blood-flecked sputum. Viral pneumonia causes gradually developing, diffuse crackles. The patient may also have a nonproductive cough, malaise, a headache, anorexia, a low-grade fever, and decreased breath sounds.

Pulmonary edema.
Moist, bubbling crackles on inspiration are one of the first signs of pulmonary edema, which is a life-threatening disorder. Other early findings include exertional dyspnea; paroxysmal nocturnal dyspnea, and then orthopnea; and coughing, which may be initially nonproductive but later produces frothy, bloody sputum. Related clinical effects include tachycardia, tachypnea, restlessness, anxiety, and a third heart sound (S_3 gallop). As the patient's respirations become increasingly rapid and labored, he develops more diffuse crackles, worsening tachycardia, hypotension, a rapid and thready pulse, cyanosis, and cold, clammy skin.

Pulmonary embolism.
Pulmonary embolism is a life-threatening disorder that can cause fine to coarse crackles and a cough that may be dry or produce blood-tinged sputum. Usually, the first sign of pulmonary embolism is severe dyspnea, which may be accompanied by angina or pleuritic chest pain. The patient has marked anxiety, a low-grade

fever, tachycardia, tachypnea, and diaphoresis. Less-common signs include massive hemoptysis, chest splinting, leg edema and, with a large embolus, cyanosis, syncope, and jugular vein distention. The patient may also have a pleural friction rub, diffuse wheezing, chest dullness on percussion, decreased breath sounds, and signs of circulatory collapse.

Pulmonary tuberculosis (TB). With pulmonary TB, fine crackles occur after coughing. The patient has some combination of hemoptysis, malaise, dyspnea, and pleuritic chest pain. Sputum may be scant and mucoid or copious and purulent. Typically, the patient is easily fatigued and experiences night sweats, weakness, and weight loss. His breath sounds are amphoric (hollow-sounding).

Tracheobronchitis. In its acute form, tracheobronchitis produces moist or coarse crackles along with a productive cough, chills, a sore throat, a slight fever, muscle and back pain, and substernal tightness. The patient typically has rhonchi and wheezes. Severe tracheobronchitis may cause a moderate fever and bronchospasm.

Nursing considerations

- Elevate the head of the patient's bed to keep his airway patent and facilitate his breathing.
- Administer fluids, humidified air, or oxygen to liquefy thick secretions and relieve mucous membrane inflammation.
- Administer a diuretic, if crackles result from cardiogenic pulmonary edema.
- Maintain a fluid restriction, if necessary, and monitor his intake and output.
- Turn the patient every 1 or 2 hours, and encourage him to breathe deeply.
- Plan rest periods to help the patient relax and sleep.

- Prepare the patient for diagnostic tests, such as chest X-rays, a lung scan, and sputum analysis.

Patient teaching

- Teach the patient to cough effectively.
- Teach him to avoid respiratory irritants.
- For the patient who smokes, stress the importance of quitting smoking, and refer him to appropriate resources to help him quit smoking.
- Explain to the patient his diagnosis and the treatment plan.

Crepitation, bony
[Bony crepitus]

Bony crepitation is a palpable vibration or an audible crunching sound that results when one bone grates against another. This sign commonly results from a fracture, but it can happen when bones that have been stripped of their protective articular cartilage grind against each other as they articulate— for example, in patients with advanced arthritic or degenerative joint disorders.

Eliciting bony crepitation can help confirm the diagnosis of a fracture, but it can also cause further soft tissue, nerve, or vessel injury. Always evaluate distal pulses and perform neurologic checks distal to the suspected fracture site before manipulating an extremity. In addition, rubbing fractured bone ends together can convert a closed fracture into an open one if a bone end penetrates the skin. Therefore, after the initial detection of crepitation in a patient with a fracture, avoid subsequent elicitation of this sign.

History and physical examination

If you detect bony crepitation in a patient with a suspected fracture, ask him if he feels pain and if he can point to the painful area. To prevent lacerating nerves, blood vessels, or other structures, immobilize the affected area by applying a splint that includes the joints above and below the affected area. Elevate the affected area, if possible, and apply cold packs. Inspect for abrasions or lacerations. Find out how and when the injury occurred. Palpate pulses distal to the injury site; check the skin for pallor or coolness. Test motor and sensory function distal to the injury site.

If the patient doesn't have a suspected fracture, ask about a history of osteoarthritis or rheumatoid arthritis. Which medications does he take? Has any medication helped ease arthritic discomfort? Take the patient's vital signs and test his joint range of motion (ROM).

Medical causes

Fracture. In addition to bony crepitation, a fracture causes acute local pain, hematoma, edema, and decreased ROM. Other findings may include deformity, point tenderness, discoloration of the limb, and loss of limb function. Neurovascular damage may cause increased capillary refill time, diminished or absent pulses, mottled cyanosis, paresthesia, and decreased sensation (all distal to the fracture site). An open fracture, of course, produces an obvious skin wound.

Osteoarthritis. In its advanced form, joint crepitation may be elicited during ROM testing. Soft fine crepitus on palpation may indicate roughening of the articular cartilage; coarse grating may indicate badly damaged cartilage. The cardinal symptom of osteoarthritis is joint pain, especially during motion and weight bearing. Other findings include joint stiffness that typically occurs after resting and subsides within a few minutes after the patient begins moving.

Rheumatoid arthritis. In its advanced form, bony crepitation is heard when the affected joint is rotated. However, rheumatoid arthritis usually develops insidiously, producing nonspecific signs and symptoms, such as fatigue, malaise, anorexia, a persistent low-grade fever, weight loss, lymphadenopathy, and vague arthralgia and myalgia. Later, more specific and localized articular signs develop, commonly at the proximal finger joints. These signs usually occur bilaterally and symmetrically and may extend to the wrists, knees, elbows, and ankles. The affected joints stiffen after inactivity. The patient also has increased warmth, swelling, and tenderness of affected joints as well as limited ROM.

Nursing considerations
- If a fracture is suspected, prepare the patient for X-rays of the affected area.
- Assess his neurovascular status frequently.
- Keep the affected part immobilized and elevated until treatment begins.
- Give an analgesic to relieve pain.

Patient teaching
- Teach the patient about activity limitations.
- Show the patient how to perform skin and foot care.
- Show the patient how to use ambulatory aids, such as walkers, canes, and crutches.
- Discuss the use of proper body mechanics to prevent injury.
- Encourage the patient to perform activities of daily living as much as possible to maintain independence, muscle strength, and joint ROM.
- If the patient has a cast, explain proper cast care and when to seek medical attention.

Crepitation, subcutaneous

[Subcutaneous crepitus, subcutaneous emphysema]

When bubbles of air or other gases (such as carbon dioxide) are trapped in subcutaneous tissue, palpating or stroking the skin produces a crackling sound called *subcutaneous crepitation* or *subcutaneous emphysema*. The bubbles feel like small, unstable nodules and aren't painful, even though subcutaneous crepitation is commonly associated with painful disorders. Usually, the affected tissue is visibly edematous; this can lead to life-threatening airway occlusion if the edema affects the neck or upper chest.

The air or gas bubbles enter the tissues through open wounds from the action of anaerobic microorganisms or from traumatic or spontaneous rupture or perforation of pulmonary or GI organs.

History and physical examination

Because subcutaneous crepitation can indicate a life-threatening disorder, you'll need to perform a rapid initial evaluation and intervene if necessary. (See *Managing subcutaneous crepitation.*)

When the patient's condition permits, palpate the affected skin to evaluate the location and extent of subcutaneous crepitation and to obtain baseline information. Delineate the borders of the area of crepitus with a marker. Palpate the area frequently to determine if the subcutaneous crepitation is increasing. Ask the patient if he's experiencing pain or having difficulty breathing. If he's in pain, find out where the pain is located, how severe it is, and when it began. Ask about recent thoracic surgery, diagnostic tests, and respiratory

therapy or a history of trauma or chronic pulmonary disease.

Medical causes

Gas gangrene. Subcutaneous crepitation is the hallmark of gas gangrene, a rare but commonly fatal infection that's caused by anaerobic microorganisms. It's accompanied by local pain, swelling, and discoloration, with the formation of bullae and necrosis. The skin over the wound may rupture, revealing dark red or black necrotic muscle and producing foul-smelling, watery, or frothy discharge. Related findings include tachycardia, tachypnea, a moderate fever, cyanosis, and lassitude.

Orbital fracture. An orbital fracture allows air from the nasal sinuses to escape into subcutaneous tissue, causing subcutaneous crepitation of the eyelid and orbit. The most common sign of this fracture is periorbital ecchymosis. Visual acuity is usually normal, although a swollen lid may prevent accurate testing. The patient has facial edema, diplopia, a hyphema and, occasionally, a dilated or unreactive pupil on the affected side. Extraocular movements may also be affected.

Pneumothorax. Severe pneumothorax produces subcutaneous crepitation in the upper chest and neck. In many cases, the patient has chest pain that's unilateral, rarely localized initially, and increased on inspiration. Dyspnea, anxiety, restlessness, tachypnea, cyanosis, tachycardia, accessory muscle use, asymmetrical chest expansion, and a nonproductive cough can also occur. On the affected side, breath sounds are absent or decreased, hyperresonance or tympany may be heard, and decreased vocal fremitus may be present.

Rupture of the esophagus. A ruptured esophagus usually produces subcutaneous crepitation in the neck, chest wall, or supraclavicular fossa, although

Managing subcutaneous crepitation

Subcutaneous crepitation occurs when air or gas bubbles escape into tissues. It may signal life-threatening rupture of an air-filled or gas-producing organ or a fulminating anaerobic infection.

Organ rupture

If the patient shows signs of respiratory distress—such as severe dyspnea, tachypnea, accessory muscle use, nasal flaring, air hunger, or tachycardia—quickly test for Hamman's sign to detect trapped air bubbles in the mediastinum.

To test for Hamman's sign, help the patient assume a left-lateral recumbent position. Then place your stethoscope over the precordium. If you hear a loud crunching sound that synchronizes with his heartbeat, the patient has a positive Hamman's sign.

Depending on which organ is ruptured, be prepared for endotracheal intu-bation, an emergency tracheotomy, or chest tube insertion. Start administering supplemental oxygen immediately. Insert an I.V. catheter to administer fluids and medication, and connect the patient to a cardiac monitor.

Anaerobic infection

If the patient has an open wound with a foul odor and local swelling and discoloration, you must act quickly. Take the patient's vital signs, checking especially for fever, tachycardia, hypotension, and tachypnea. Next, insert an I.V. catheter to administer fluids and medication, and provide supplemental oxygen.

In addition, be prepared for emergency surgery to drain and debride the wound. If the patient's condition is life-threatening, you may need to prepare him for transfer to a facility with a hyperbaric chamber.

this sign doesn't always occur. With a rupture of the cervical esophagus, the patient has excruciating pain in the neck or supraclavicular area, his neck is resistant to passive motion, and he has local tenderness, soft-tissue swelling, dysphagia, odynophagia, and orthostatic vertigo.

Life-threatening rupture of the intrathoracic esophagus can produce mediastinal emphysema confirmed by a positive Hamman's sign. The patient has severe retrosternal, epigastric, neck, or scapular pain and edema of the chest wall and neck. He may also display dyspnea, tachypnea, asymmetrical chest expansion, nasal flaring, cyanosis, diaphoresis, tachycardia, hypotension, dysphagia, and a fever.

Rupture of the trachea or major bronchus. Rupture of the trachea or major bronchus is a life-threatening injury that produces abrupt subcutaneous crepitation of the neck and anterior chest wall. The patient has severe dyspnea with nasal flaring, tachycardia, accessory muscle use, hypotension, cyanosis, extreme anxiety and, possibly, hemoptysis and mediastinal emphysema, with a positive Hamman's sign.

Other causes

Diagnostic tests. Endoscopic tests, such as bronchoscopy and upper GI tract endoscopy, can cause rupture or perforation of respiratory or GI organs, producing subcutaneous crepitation.

Respiratory treatments. Mechanical ventilation and intermittent positive-pressure breathing can rupture alveoli, producing subcutaneous crepitation.

Thoracic surgery. If air escapes into the tissue in the area of the incision, subcutaneous crepitation can occur.

Nursing considerations
- Monitor the patient's vital signs frequently, especially respirations.
- Because excessive edema from subcutaneous crepitation in the neck and upper chest can cause airway obstruction, be alert for signs of respiratory distress such as dyspnea.

Patient teaching
- Tell the patient that the affected tissues will eventually absorb the air or gas bubbles and the subcutaneous crepitation will decrease.
- Warn the patient with asthma or chronic bronchitis to be alert for subcutaneous crepitation, which can signal pneumothorax, a dangerous complication.
- Reassure the patient frequently to reduce anxiety.
- Explain the diagnosis and treatment plan.

Cry, high-pitched
[Cerebral cry]

A high-pitched cry is a brief, sharp, piercing vocal sound produced by a neonate or infant. Whether acute or chronic, this cry is a late sign of increased intracranial pressure (ICP). The acute onset of a high-pitched cry demands emergency treatment to prevent permanent brain damage or death.

A change in the volume of one of the brain's components—brain tissue, cerebrospinal fluid, and blood—may cause increased ICP. In neonates, increased ICP may result from intracranial bleeding associated with birth trauma or from congenital malformations, such as craniostenosis and Arnold-Chiari deformity. In fact, a high-pitched cry may be an early sign of a congenital malformation. In infants, increased ICP may result from meningitis, head trauma, or child abuse.

History and physical examination
Take the infant's vital signs, and then obtain a brief history from the parents. Did the infant fall recently or experience even minor head trauma? Make sure to ask the mother about changes in the infant's behavior during the past 24 hours. Has he been vomiting? Has he seemed restless or unlike himself? Has his sucking reflex diminished? Does he cry when he's moved? Suspect child abuse if the infant's history is inconsistent with physical findings.

Next, perform a neurologic examination. Remember that neurologic responses in a neonate or young infant are primarily reflex responses. Determine the infant's level of consciousness (LOC). Is he awake, irritable, or lethargic? Does he reach for an attractive object or turn toward the sound of a rattle? Observe his posture. Is he in the normal flexed position or in extension or opisthotonos? Examine muscle tone and observe the infant for signs of seizure, such as tremors and twitching.

Examine the size and shape of the infant's head. Is the anterior fontanel bulging? Measure the infant's head circumference, and check pupillary size and response to light. Unilateral or bilateral dilation and a sluggish response to light may accompany increased ICP. Finally, test the infant's reflexes; expect Moro's reflex to be diminished.

ACTION STAT!

 If the patient has bulging fontanels, elevate the infant's head to promote cerebral venous drainage and decrease ICP. Start an I.V. line, and give a diuretic and a corticosteroid to decrease ICP. Be sure to keep endotracheal (ET) intubation equipment close by to secure an airway.

Medical causes

Increased ICP. A high-pitched cry is a late sign of increased ICP. Typically, the infant also displays bulging fontanels, increased head circumference, and widened sutures. Signs and symptoms of increasing ICP include seizures, bradycardia, possible vomiting, dilated pupils, decreased LOC, increased systolic blood pressure, a widened pulse pressure, and an altered respiratory pattern.

Nursing considerations

- Monitor the infant's vital signs, ICP, and neurologic status to detect subtle changes in his condition.
- Monitor his intake and output.
- Restrict fluids and administer a diuretic.
- Increase the head of the bed 30 degrees, if the condition permits, and keep the head midline.
- Perform nursing care judiciously because procedures may cause a further increase in ICP.
- For an infant with severely increased ICP, prepare for ET intubation and mechanical hyperventilation to decrease serum carbon dioxide levels and constrict cerebral blood vessels.
- Institute hyperventilation, as ordered, for acute increases in ICP after the health care team has weighed the risks and benefits.
- Alternatively, prepare for barbiturate coma or hypothermia therapy, as ordered, to decrease the infant's metabolic rate.

Patient teaching

- Because the infant with increased ICP requires specialized care and monitoring in the intensive care unit, prepare his parents for the transfer.
- Tell the parents to avoid jostling the infant, which may aggravate increased ICP.
- Show the parents how to comfort the infant and maintain a calm, quiet environment to avoid increasing ICP.
- Explain the infant's diagnosis and the treatment plan to the parents.

Cyanosis

Cyanosis—a bluish or bluish black discoloration of the skin and mucous membranes—results from excessive concentration of unoxygenated hemoglobin in the blood. This common sign may develop abruptly or gradually. It can be classified as central or peripheral, although the two types may coexist.

Central cyanosis reflects inadequate oxygenation of systemic arterial blood caused by right-to-left cardiac shunting, pulmonary disease, or hematologic disorders. It may occur anywhere on the skin and also on the mucous membranes of the mouth, lips, and conjunctiva.

Peripheral cyanosis reflects sluggish peripheral circulation caused by vasoconstriction, reduced cardiac output, or vascular occlusion. It may be widespread or may occur locally in one extremity; however, it doesn't affect mucous membranes. Typically, peripheral cyanosis appears on exposed areas, such as the fingers, nail beds, feet, nose, and ears.

Although cyanosis is an important sign of cardiovascular and pulmonary disorders, it isn't always an accurate gauge of oxygenation. Several factors contribute to its development: hemoglobin concentration and oxygen saturation, cardiac output, and partial pressure of arterial oxygen (Pao_2). Cyanosis is usually undetectable until the oxygen saturation of hemoglobin falls below 80%. Severe cyanosis is quite obvious, whereas mild cyanosis is more difficult to detect, even in natural, bright light. In dark-skinned patients, cyanosis is most apparent in the mucous membranes and nail beds.

Transient, nonpathologic cyanosis may result from environmental factors. For example, peripheral cyanosis may result from cutaneous vasoconstriction following a brief exposure to cold air or water. Central cyanosis may result from reduced Pa_{O_2} at high altitudes.

History and physical examination

If cyanosis accompanies less-acute conditions, perform a thorough examination. Begin with a history, focusing on cardiac, pulmonary, and hematologic disorders. Ask about previous surgery. Then begin the physical examination by taking the patient's vital signs and pulse oximetry. Inspect the skin and mucous membranes to determine the extent of cyanosis. Ask the patient when he first noticed the cyanosis. Does it subside and recur? Is it aggravated by cold, smoking, or stress? Is it alleviated by massage or rewarming? Check the skin for coolness, pallor, redness, pain, and ulceration. Also note clubbing.

Next, evaluate the patient's level of consciousness. Ask about headaches, dizziness, or blurred vision. Then test his motor strength. Ask about pain in the arms and legs (especially with walking) and about abnormal sensations,

such as numbness, tingling, and coldness.

Ask about chest pain and its severity. Can the patient identify aggravating and alleviating factors? Palpate peripheral pulses, and test the capillary refill time. Also, note edema. Auscultate heart rate and rhythm, especially noting gallops and murmurs. Also auscultate the abdominal aorta and femoral arteries to detect any bruits.

Does the patient have a cough? Is it productive? If so, have the patient describe the sputum. Evaluate his respiratory rate and rhythm. Check for nasal flaring and use of accessory muscles. Ask about sleep apnea. Does the patient sleep with his head propped up on pillows? Inspect the patient for asymmetrical chest expansion or barrel chest. Percuss the lungs for dullness or hyperresonance, and auscultate for decreased or adventitious breath sounds.

Inspect the abdomen for ascites, and test for shifting dullness or fluid wave. Percuss and palpate for liver enlargement and tenderness. Also, ask about nausea, anorexia, and weight loss.

Medical causes

Arteriosclerotic occlusive disease (chronic). With arteriosclerotic occlusive disease, peripheral cyanosis occurs in the legs whenever they're in a dependent position. Associated signs and symptoms include intermittent claudication and burning pain at rest, paresthesia, pallor, muscle atrophy, weak leg pulses, and impotence. Late signs are leg ulcers and gangrene.

Blast lung injury. Cyanosis is a serious sign of blast lung injury. The impact of this condition on the lungs of affected individuals varies and may include tearing, contusion, edema, and hemorrhage. Other signs and symptoms may include chest pain, wheezing, hemoptysis, and dyspnea. Treatment for patients with blast lung injury typically involves high-flow oxygen, careful fluid management, possible intubation, and close observation in an intensive care setting.

Bronchiectasis. Bronchiectasis produces chronic central cyanosis. Its classic sign, however, is a chronic productive cough with copious, foul-smelling, mucopurulent sputum or hemoptysis. Auscultation reveals rhonchi and coarse crackles during inspiration. Other signs and symptoms include dyspnea, recurrent fever and chills, weight loss, malaise, clubbing, and signs of anemia.

Buerger's disease. With Buerger's disease, exposure to cold initially causes the feet to become cold, cyanotic, and numb; later, they redden, become hot, and tingle. Intermittent claudication of the instep is characteristic; it's aggravated by exercise and smoking and relieved by rest. Associated signs and symptoms include weak peripheral pulses and, in later stages, ulceration, muscle atrophy, and gangrene.

Chronic obstructive pulmonary disease (COPD). Chronic central cyanosis occurs in advanced stages of COPD and may be aggravated by exertion. Associated signs and symptoms include exertional dyspnea, a productive cough with thick sputum, anorexia, weight loss, pursed-lip breathing, tachypnea, and the use of accessory muscles. Examination reveals wheezing and hyperresonant lung fields. Barrel chest and clubbing are late signs. Tachycardia, diaphoresis, and flushing may also accompany COPD.

Deep vein thrombosis. With deep vein thrombosis, acute peripheral cyanosis occurs in the affected extremity associated with tenderness, painful movement, edema, warmth, and prominent superficial veins. Homans' sign can also be elicited.

Heart failure. Acute or chronic cyanosis may occur in patients with heart failure. Typically, it's a late sign and may be central, peripheral, or both. With left-sided heart failure, central cyanosis occurs with tachycardia, fatigue, dyspnea, cold intolerance, orthopnea, a cough, a ventricular or an atrial gallop, bibasilar crackles, and a diffuse apical impulse. With right-sided heart failure, peripheral cyanosis occurs with fatigue, peripheral edema, ascites, jugular vein distention, and hepatomegaly.

Lung cancer. Lung cancer causes chronic central cyanosis accompanied by a fever, weakness, weight loss, anorexia, dyspnea, chest pain, hemoptysis, and wheezing. Atelectasis causes mediastinal shift, decreased diaphragmatic excursion, asymmetrical chest expansion, a dull percussion note, and diminished breath sounds.

Peripheral arterial occlusion (acute). Peripheral arterial occlusion produces acute cyanosis of one arm or leg or, occasionally, both legs. The cyanosis is accompanied by sharp or aching pain that worsens when the patient moves. The affected extremity also exhibits paresthesia, weakness, and pale, cool skin. Examination reveals a decreased or an absent pulse and increased capillary refill.

Pneumonia. With pneumonia, acute central cyanosis is usually preceded by a fever, shaking chills, a cough with purulent sputum, crackles, rhonchi, and pleuritic chest pain that's exacerbated by deep inspiration. Associated signs and symptoms include tachycardia, dyspnea, tachypnea, diminished breath sounds, diaphoresis, myalgia, fatigue, a headache, and anorexia.

Pneumothorax. A cardinal sign of pneumothorax, acute central cyanosis is accompanied by sharp chest pain that's exacerbated by movement, deep breathing, and coughing; asymmetrical chest wall expansion; and shortness of breath. The patient may also exhibit rapid, shallow respirations; a weak, rapid pulse; pallor; jugular vein distention; anxiety; and the absence of breath sounds over the affected lobe.

Polycythemia vera. A ruddy complexion that can appear cyanotic is characteristic in polycythemia vera, which is a chronic myeloproliferative disorder. Other findings include hepatosplenomegaly, headache, dizziness, fatigue, aquagenic pruritus, blurred vision, chest pain, intermittent claudication, and coagulation defects.

Pulmonary edema. With pulmonary edema, acute central cyanosis occurs with dyspnea; orthopnea; frothy, blood-tinged sputum; tachycardia; tachypnea; dependent crackles; a ventricular gallop; cold, clammy skin; hypotension; a weak, thready pulse; and confusion.

Pulmonary embolism. Acute central cyanosis occurs when a large embolus causes significant obstruction of the pulmonary circulation. Syncope and jugular vein distention may also occur. Other common signs and symptoms include dyspnea, chest pain, tachycardia, a paradoxical pulse, a dry or productive cough with blood-tinged sputum, a low-grade fever, restlessness, anxiety, and diaphoresis.

Raynaud's disease. With Raynaud's disease, exposure to cold or stress causes the fingers or hands first to blanch and turn cold, then become cyanotic, and finally to redden with a return to a normal temperature. Numbness and tingling may also occur. Raynaud's phenomenon describes the same presentation when associated with other disorders, such as rheumatoid arthritis, scleroderma, or lupus erythematosus.

Shock. With shock, acute peripheral cyanosis develops in the hands and feet, which may also be cold, clammy, and pale. Other characteristic signs and symptoms include lethargy, confusion, an increased capillary refill time, and a rapid, weak pulse. Tachypnea, hyperpnea, and hypotension may also be present.

Sleep apnea. When chronic and severe, sleep apnea causes pulmonary hypertension and cor pulmonale (right-sided heart failure), which can produce chronic cyanosis.

Nursing considerations

- Provide supplemental oxygen to relieve shortness of breath, improve oxygenation, and decrease cyanosis.
- Deliver small doses of oxygen (2 L/ minute) in the patient with COPD and in the patient with mild COPD exacerbations.
- For acute situations, a high-flow oxygen rate may be needed initially; in working with a patient who has COPD, remember to be attentive to his respiratory drive and adjust the amount of oxygen accordingly.
- Position the patient comfortably to ease breathing.
- Administer a diuretic, bronchodilator, antibiotic, or cardiac drug as needed.
- Make sure that the patient gets sufficient rest between activities to prevent dyspnea.
- Prepare the patient for such tests as arterial blood gas analysis, complete blood count, and imaging studies and scans to determine the cause of cyanosis.

Patient teaching

- Instruct the patient to seek immediate medical attention if cyanosis occurs.
- Discuss the safe use of oxygen at home.
- Explain to the patient his diagnosis and the treatment plan.

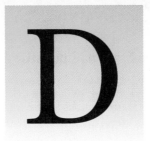

Decerebrate posture
[Decerebrate rigidity, abnormal extensor reflex]

Decerebrate posture is characterized by adduction (internal rotation) and extension of the arms, with the wrists pronated and the fingers flexed. The legs are stiffly extended, with forced plantar flexion of the feet. In severe cases, the back is acutely arched (opisthotonos). This sign indicates upper brain stem damage, which may result from primary lesions, such as infarction, hemorrhage, or tumor; metabolic encephalopathy; a head injury; or brain stem compression associated with increased intracranial pressure (ICP).

Decerebrate posture may be elicited by noxious stimuli or may occur spontaneously. It may be unilateral or bilateral. With concurrent brain stem and cerebral damage, decerebrate posture may affect only the arms, with the legs remaining flaccid. Alternatively, decerebrate posture may affect one side of the body and decorticate posture the other. The two postures may also alternate as the patient's neurologic status fluctuates. Generally, the duration of each posturing episode correlates with the severity of brain stem damage. (See *Comparing decerebrate and decorticate postures,* page 178.)

ACTION STAT!

 Your first priority is to ensure a patent airway. Insert an artificial airway and institute measures to prevent aspiration. (Don't disrupt spinal alignment if you suspect spinal cord injury.) Suction the patient as needed.

Next, examine spontaneous respirations. Give supplemental oxygen, and ventilate the patient with a handheld resuscitation bag if needed. Endotracheal intubation and mechanical ventilation may be indicated. Keep emergency resuscitation equipment handy. Monitor the patient's neurologic status, vital signs, and oxygen saturation.

History and physical examination

After taking the patient's vital signs, determine his level of consciousness (LOC). Use the Glasgow Coma Scale as a reference. Evaluate the pupils for size, equality, and response to light. Test deep tendon reflexes and cranial nerve reflexes, and check for doll's eye sign.

Next, explore the history of the patient's coma. If you can't obtain this information, look for clues to the causative disorder, such as hepatomegaly, cyanosis, diabetic skin changes, needle tracks, or obvious trauma. If a family member is available, find out when the

Comparing decerebrate and decorticate postures

Decerebrate posture results from damage to the upper brain stem. In this posture (shown below), the arms are adducted and extended, with the wrists pronated and the fingers flexed. The legs are stiffly extended, with plantar flexion of the feet.

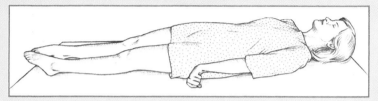

Decorticate posture results from damage to one or both corticospinal tracts. In this posture (shown below), the arms are adducted and flexed, with the wrists and fingers flexed on the chest. The legs are stiffly extended and internally rotated, with plantar flexion of the feet.

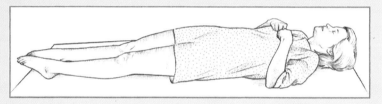

patient's LOC began deteriorating. Did it occur abruptly? What did the patient complain of before he lost consciousness? Does he have a history of diabetes, liver disease, cancer, blood clots, or aneurysm? Ask about any accident or trauma responsible for the coma.

Medical causes

Brain stem infarction. When brain stem infarction produces a coma, decerebrate posture may be elicited. Associated signs and symptoms vary with the severity of the infarct and may include cranial nerve palsies, bilateral cerebellar ataxia, and sensory loss. With deep coma, all normal reflexes are usually lost, resulting in the absence of doll's eye sign, a positive Babinski's reflex, and flaccidity.

Cerebral lesion. Whether the cause is trauma, a tumor, an abscess, or an in-

farction, any cerebral lesion that increases ICP may also produce decerebrate posture. Typically, this posture is a late sign. Associated findings vary with the lesion's site and extent, but commonly include coma, abnormal pupil size and response to light, and the classic triad of increased ICP—bradycardia, increasing systolic blood pressure, and a widening pulse pressure.

Hypoglycemic encephalopathy. Characterized by extremely low blood glucose levels, hypoglycemic encephalopathy may produce decerebrate posture and coma. It also causes dilated pupils, slow respirations, and bradycardia. Muscle spasms, twitching, and seizures eventually progress to flaccidity.

Hypoxic encephalopathy. Severe hypoxia may produce decerebrate posture—the result of brain stem compression associated with anaerobic metabolism and increased ICP. Other findings include coma, a positive Babinski's reflex, an absence of doll's eye sign, hypoactive deep tendon reflexes and, possibly, fixed pupils and respiratory arrest.

Pontine hemorrhage. Typically, pontine hemorrhage, a life-threatening disorder, rapidly leads to decerebrate posture with coma. Accompanying signs include total paralysis, the absence of doll's eye sign, a positive Babinski's reflex, and small, reactive pupils.

Posterior fossa hemorrhage. Posterior fossa hemorrhage is a subtentorial lesion that causes decerebrate posture. Its early signs and symptoms include vomiting, a headache, vertigo, ataxia, a stiff neck, drowsiness, papilledema, and cranial nerve palsies. The patient eventually slips into coma and may experience respiratory arrest.

Other causes

Diagnostic tests. Relief from high ICP by removing spinal fluid during a lumbar puncture may precipitate cerebral compression of the brain stem and cause decerebrate posture and coma.

Nursing considerations

- Prepare the patient and his family for diagnostic tests that will determine the cause of his decerebrate posture, such as skull X-rays, a computed tomography scan, magnetic resonance imaging, cerebral angiography, digital subtraction angiography, electroencephalography, a brain scan, and ICP monitoring.
- Monitor the patient's neurologic status and vital signs every 30 minutes or as indicated.
- Be alert for signs of increased ICP (such s bradycardia, increasing systolic blood pressure, and a widening pulse pressure) and neurologic deterioration (for example, an altered respiratory pattern and abnormal temperature).

Patient teaching

- Inform the patient's family that decerebrate posture is a reflex response—not a voluntary response to pain or a sign of recovery.
- Offer emotional support to the patient and his family.
- Explain the diagnosis and treatment plan.

▌Decorticate posture
[Decorticate rigidity, abnormal flexor response]

A sign of corticospinal damage, decorticate posture is characterized by adduction of the arms and flexion of the elbows, with wrists and fingers flexed on the chest. The legs are extended and internally rotated, with plantar flexion of the feet. This posture may occur unilaterally or bilaterally. It usually results from stroke or head injury. It may be elicited by noxious stimuli or may occur spontaneously. The intensity of the required stimulus, the duration of the posture, and the frequency of spontaneous episodes vary with the severity and location of cerebral injury.

Although a serious sign, decorticate posture carries a more favorable prognosis than decerebrate posture. However, if the causative disorder extends lower in the brain stem, decorticate posture may progress to decerebrate posture. (See *Comparing decerebrate and decorticate postures.*)

ACTION STAT!

 Obtain the patient's vital signs and evaluate his level of consciousness (LOC). If his consciousness is impaired, insert an oropharyngeal airway, and take measures to prevent aspiration (unless spinal cord injury is suspected). Evaluate the patient's respiratory rate, rhythm, and depth. Prepare to assist respirations with a handheld resuscitation bag or with endotracheal intubation and mechanical ventilation if necessary. Institute seizure precautions.

History and physical examination

Test the patient's motor and sensory functions. Evaluate pupil size, equality, and response to light. Then test cranial nerve function and deep tendon reflexes. Ask the patient about headache, dizziness, nausea, changes in vision, and numbness or tingling. When did the patient first notice these symptoms? Is his family aware of behavioral changes? Also ask about a history of cerebrovascular disease, cancer, meningitis, encephalitis, upper respiratory tract infection, bleeding or clotting disorders, or recent trauma.

Medical causes

Brain abscess. Decorticate posture may occur with brain abscess. Accompanying findings vary depending on the size and location of the abscess, but may include aphasia, hemiparesis, a headache, dizziness, seizures, nausea, and vomiting. The patient may also experience behavioral changes, altered vital signs, and a decreased LOC.

Brain tumor. A brain tumor may produce decorticate posture that's usually bilateral—the result of increased intracranial pressure (ICP) associated with tumor growth. Related signs and symptoms include a headache, behavioral changes, memory loss, diplopia, blurred vision or vision loss, seizures, ataxia, dizziness, apraxia, aphasia, paresis, sensory loss, paresthesia, vomiting, papilledema, and signs of hormonal imbalance.

Head injury. Decorticate posture may be among the variable features of a head injury, depending on the site and

severity of the injury. Associated signs and symptoms include a headache, nausea and vomiting, dizziness, irritability, a decreased LOC, aphasia, hemiparesis, unilateral numbness, seizures, and pupillary dilation.

Stroke. Typically, a stroke involving the cerebral cortex produces unilateral decorticate posture, also called *spastic hemiplegia*. Other signs and symptoms include hemiplegia (contralateral to the lesion), dysarthria, dysphagia, unilateral sensory loss, apraxia, agnosia, aphasia, memory loss, a decreased LOC, urine retention, urinary incontinence, and constipation. Ocular effects include homonymous hemianopsia, diplopia, and blurred vision.

Nursing considerations

■ Assess the patient frequently to detect subtle signs of neurologic deterioration.
■ Monitor his neurologic status and vital signs every 30 minutes to 2 hours.
■ Be alert for signs of increased ICP, including bradycardia, an increasing systolic blood pressure, and a widening pulse pressure.

Patient teaching

■ Explain the signs and symptoms of decreased LOC and seizures to the patient and his family.
■ Discuss the patient's and family's quality-of-life concerns.
■ Explain to the family how to keep the patient safe, especially during a seizure.
■ Explain to the patient or family his diagnosis and the treatment plan.

Deep tendon reflexes, hyperactive

A hyperactive deep tendon reflex (DTR) is an abnormally brisk muscle contraction that occurs in response to a sudden stretch induced by sharply tapping the muscle's tendon of insertion. This elicited sign may be graded as brisk or pathologically hyperactive. Hyperactive DTRs are commonly accompanied by clonus.

The corticospinal tract and other descending tracts govern the reflex arc—the relay cycle that produces any reflex response. A corticospinal lesion above the level of the reflex arc being tested may result in hyperactive DTRs. Abnormal neuromuscular transmission at the end of the reflex arc may also cause hyperactive DTRs. For example, a calcium or magnesium deficiency may cause hyperactive DTRs because these electrolytes regulate neuromuscular excitability. (See *Tracing the reflex arc,* pages 182 and 183.)

Although hyperactive DTRs typically accompany other neurologic findings, they usually lack specific diagnostic value. They're an early, cardinal sign of hypocalcemia.(See *Documenting deep tendon reflexes,* page 185.)

History and physical examination

After eliciting hyperactive DTRs, take the patient's history. Ask about spinal cord injury or other trauma and about prolonged exposure to cold, wind, or water. Could the patient be pregnant? A positive response to any of these questions requires prompt evaluation to rule out life-threatening autonomic hyperreflexia, tetanus, preeclampsia, or hypothermia. Ask about the onset and progression of associated signs and symptoms. Next, perform a neurologic examination. Evaluate the patient's level of consciousness, and test motor and sensory function in the limbs. Ask about paresthesia. Check for ataxia or tremors and for speech and visual deficits. Test for Chvostek's (an abnormal spasm of the facial muscles elicited by light taps on the facial nerve in a patient who has hypocalcemia) and Trousseau's (a carpal spasm induced by inflating a sphygmo-

manometer cuff on the upper arm to a pressure exceeding systolic blood pressure for 3 minutes in a patient who has hypocalcemia or hypomagnesemia) signs and for carpopedal spasm. Ask about vomiting or altered bladder habits. Be sure to take the patient's vital signs.

Medical causes
Amyotrophic lateral sclerosis (ALS). ALS produces generalized hyperactive DTRs accompanied by weakness of the hands and forearms and spasticity of the legs. Eventually, the patient develops atrophy of the neck and tongue muscles, fasciculations, weakness of the legs and, possibly, bulbar signs (for example, dysphagia, dysphonia, facial weakness, and dyspnea).

Brain tumor. A cerebral tumor causes hyperactive DTRs on the side opposite the lesion. Associated signs and symptoms develop slowly and may include unilateral paresis or paralysis, anesthesia, visual field deficits, spasticity, and a positive Babinski's reflex.

Hypocalcemia. Hypocalcemia may produce a sudden or gradual onset of generalized hyperactive DTRs with paresthesia, muscle twitching and cramping, positive Chvostek's and Trousseau's signs, carpopedal spasm, and tetany.

Hypomagnesemia. Hypomagnesemia results in the gradual onset of generalized hyperactive DTRs accompanied by muscle cramps, hypotension, tachycardia, paresthesia, ataxia, tetany and, possibly, seizures.

Hypothermia. Mild hypothermia (90° to 94° F [32.2° to 34.4° C]) produces generalized hyperactive DTRs. Other signs and symptoms include shivering, fatigue, weakness, lethargy, slurred speech, ataxia, muscle stiffness, tachycardia, diuresis, bradypnea, hypotension, and cold, pale skin.

(*Text continues on page 184.*)

Tracing the reflex arc

Sharply tapping a tendon initiates a sensory (afferent) impulse that travels along a peripheral nerve to a spinal nerve and then to the spinal cord. The impulse enters the spinal cord through the posterior root, synapses with a motor (efferent) neuron in the anterior horn on the same side of the spinal cord, and then is transmitted through a motor nerve fiber back to the muscle. When the impulse crosses the neuromuscular junction, the muscle contracts, completing the reflex arc.

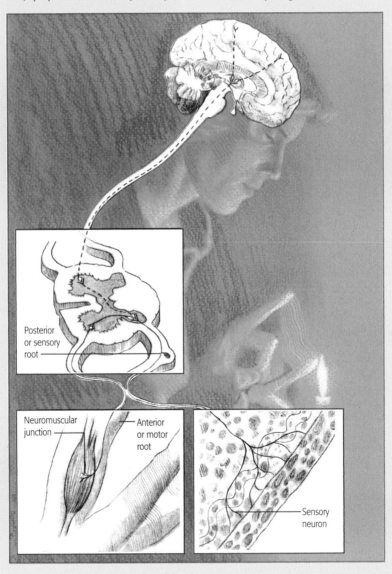

Posterior or sensory root

Neuromuscular junction

Anterior or motor root

Sensory neuron

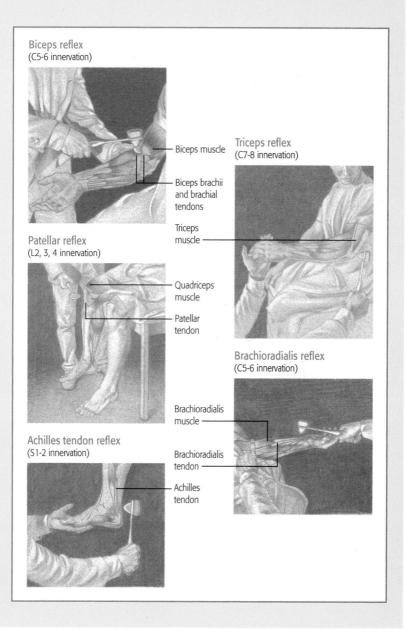

Biceps reflex
(C5-6 innervation)

Biceps muscle

Biceps brachii
and brachial
tendons

Triceps reflex
(C7-8 innervation)

Triceps
muscle

Patellar reflex
(L2, 3, 4 innervation)

Quadriceps
muscle

Patellar
tendon

Brachioradialis reflex
(C5-6 innervation)

Brachioradialis
muscle

Achilles tendon reflex
(S1-2 innervation)

Brachioradialis
tendon

Achilles
tendon

Preeclampsia. Occurring in pregnancy of at least 20 weeks' gestation, preeclampsia may cause a gradual onset of generalized hyperactive DTRs. Accompanying signs and symptoms include increased blood pressure; abnormal weight gain; edema of the face, fingers, and abdomen after bed rest; albuminuria; oliguria; a severe headache; blurred or double vision; epigastric pain; nausea and vomiting; irritability; cyanosis; shortness of breath; and crackles. If preeclampsia progresses to eclampsia, the patient develops seizures.

Spinal cord lesion. Incomplete spinal cord lesions cause hyperactive DTRs below the level of the lesion. In a traumatic lesion, hyperactive DTRs follow resolution of spinal shock. In a neoplastic lesion, hyperactive DTRs gradually replace normal DTRs. Other signs and symptoms are paralysis and sensory loss below the level of the lesion, urine retention and overflow incontinence, and alternating constipation and diarrhea. A lesion above T6 may also produce autonomic hyperreflexia with diaphoresis and flushing above the level of the lesion, a headache, nasal congestion, nausea, increased blood pressure, and bradycardia.

Stroke. A stroke that affects the origin of the corticospinal tracts causes the sudden onset of hyperactive DTRs on the side opposite the lesion. The patient may also have unilateral paresis or paralysis, anesthesia, visual field deficits, spasticity, and a positive Babinski's reflex.

Tetanus. With tetanus, the sudden onset of generalized hyperactive DTRs accompanies tachycardia, diaphoresis, a low-grade fever, painful and involuntary muscle contractions, trismus (lockjaw), and risus sardonicus (a masklike grin).

Nursing considerations

- Prepare the patient for diagnostic tests to evaluate hyperactive DTRs, such as laboratory tests for serum calcium, magnesium, and ammonia levels; spinal X-rays; magnetic resonance imaging; a computed tomography scan; lumbar puncture; and myelography.
- If motor weakness accompanies hyperactive DTRs, perform or encourage range-of-motion exercises to preserve muscle integrity and prevent deep vein thrombosis.
- Reposition the patient frequently, supply a special mattress, provide skin care, and ensure adequate nutrition to prevent skin breakdown.
- Administer a muscle relaxant and sedative to relieve severe muscle contractions.
- Keep emergency resuscitation equipment on hand.
- Provide a quiet, calm atmosphere to decrease neuromuscular excitability.
- Assist with activities of daily living, and provide emotional support.

Patient teaching

- Explain the diagnosis, procedures, and treatments to the family.
- Discuss measures necessary to keep the patient safe.
- Provide emotional support.

Deep tendon reflexes, hypoactive

A hypoactive deep tendon reflex (DTR) is an abnormally diminished muscle contraction that occurs in response to a sudden stretch induced by sharply tapping the muscle's tendon of insertion. It may be graded as minimal (+) or absent (0). Symmetrically reduced (+) reflexes may be normal.

Normally, a DTR depends on an intact receptor, an intact sensory-motor nerve fiber, an intact neuromuscular-

Documenting deep tendon reflexes

Record the patient's deep tendon reflex (DTR) scores by drawing a stick figure and entering the grades on this scale at the proper location. The figure shown here indicates hypoactive DTRs in the legs; other reflexes are normal.

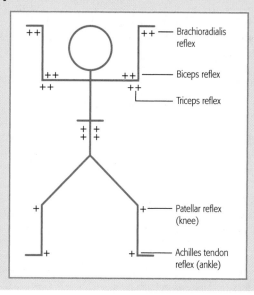

Key:

0	=	absent
+	=	hypoactive (diminished)
++	=	normal
+++	=	brisk (increased)
++++	=	hyperactive (clonus may be present)

glandular junction, and a functional synapse in the spinal cord. Hypoactive DTRs may result from damage to the reflex arc involving the specific muscle, the peripheral nerve, the nerve roots, or the spinal cord at that level. Hypoactive DTRs are an important sign of many disorders, especially when they appear with other neurologic signs and symptoms. (See *Documenting deep tendon reflexes.*)

History and physical examination

After eliciting hypoactive DTRs, obtain a thorough history from the patient or a family member. Have him describe current signs and symptoms in detail. Then take a family and drug history.

Next, evaluate the patient's level of consciousness. Test motor function in his limbs, and palpate for muscle atrophy or increased mass. Test sensory function, including pain, touch, temperature, and vibration sense. Ask about

paresthesia. To observe gait and coordination, have the patient take several steps. To check for Romberg's sign, ask him to stand with his feet together and his eyes closed. During conversation, evaluate speech. Check for signs of vision or hearing loss. Abrupt onset of hypoactive DTRs accompanied by muscle weakness may occur with life-threatening Guillain-Barré syndrome, botulism, or spinal cord lesions with spinal shock.

Look for autonomic nervous system effects by taking vital signs and monitoring for increased heart rate and blood pressure. Also, inspect the skin for pallor, dryness, flushing, or diaphoresis. Auscultate for hypoactive bowel sounds, and palpate for bladder distention. Ask about nausea, vomiting, constipation, and incontinence.

Medical causes

Botulism. With botulism, generalized hypoactive DTRs accompany progressive descending muscle weakness. Initially, the patient usually complains of blurred and double vision and, occasionally, anorexia, nausea, and vomiting. Other early bulbar findings include vertigo, hearing loss, dysarthria, and dysphagia. The patient may have signs of respiratory distress and severe constipation marked by hypoactive bowel sounds.

Eaton-Lambert syndrome. Eaton-Lambert syndrome produces generalized hypoactive DTRs. Early signs include difficulty rising from a chair, climbing stairs, and walking. The patient may complain of achiness, paresthesia, and muscle weakness that's most severe in the morning. Weakness improves with mild exercise and worsens with strenuous exercise.

Guillain-Barré syndrome. Guillain-Barré syndrome causes bilateral hypoactive DTRs that progress rapidly from hypotonia to areflexia in several days. This disorder typically causes muscle weakness that begins in the legs and then extends to the arms and, possibly, to the trunk and neck muscles. Occasionally, weakness may progress to total paralysis. Other signs and symptoms include cranial nerve palsies, pain, paresthesia, and signs of brief autonomic dysfunction, such as sinus tachycardia or bradycardia, flushing, fluctuating blood pressure, and anhidrosis or episodic diaphoresis.

Usually, muscle weakness and hypoactive DTRs peak in severity within 10 to 14 days, and then symptoms begin to clear. However, in severe cases, residual hypoactive DTRs and motor weakness may persist.

Peripheral neuropathy. Characteristic of end-stage diabetes mellitus, renal failure, and alcoholism and as an adverse effect of various medications, peripheral neuropathy results in progressive hypoactive DTRs. Other effects include motor weakness, sensory loss, paresthesia, tremors, and possible autonomic dysfunction, such as orthostatic hypotension and incontinence.

Polymyositis. With polymyositis, hypoactive DTRs accompany muscle weakness, pain, stiffness, spasms and, possibly, increased size or atrophy. These effects are usually temporary; their location varies with the affected muscles.

Spinal cord lesions. Spinal cord injury or complete transection produces spinal shock, resulting in hypoactive DTRs (areflexia) below the level of the lesion. Associated signs and symptoms include quadriplegia or paraplegia, flaccidity, a loss of sensation below the level of the lesion, and dry, pale skin. Also characteristic are urine retention with overflow incontinence, hypoactive bowel sounds, constipation, and genital reflex loss. Hypoactive DTRs and flaccidity are usually transient; reflex activity may return within several weeks.

Syringomyelia. Permanent bilateral hypoactive DTRs occur early in syringomyelia, which is a slowly progressive neurologic disorder. Other signs and symptoms include muscle weakness and atrophy; loss of sensation, usually extending in a capelike fashion over the arms, shoulders, neck, back, and occasionally the legs; deep, boring pain (despite analgesia) in the limbs; and signs of brain stem involvement (nystagmus, facial numbness, unilateral vocal cord paralysis or weakness, and unilateral tongue atrophy).

Other causes

Drugs. Barbiturates and paralyzing drugs, such as pancuronium and curare, may cause hypoactive DTRs.

Nursing considerations

■ Help the patient perform his daily activities, keeping a balance between promoting independence and ensuring his safety.

- Ambulate the patient with assistance.
- If the patient has sensory deficits, protect him from injury from heat, cold, or pressure.
- Reposition the patient frequently and perform or encourage range-of-motion exercises.
- Keep the skin clean and dry to prevent breakdown.
- Provide a balanced diet with plenty of protein and adequate hydration.

Patient teaching

- Teach skills to promote independence in daily life.
- Discuss safety measures with the patient and family, such as walking with assistance.
- Explain to the patient his diagnosis and the treatment plan.

Diaphoresis

Diaphoresis is profuse sweating—at times, amounting to more than 1 L of sweat per hour. This sign represents an autonomic nervous system response to physical or psychogenic stress or to a fever or high environmental temperature. When caused by stress, diaphoresis may be generalized or limited to the palms, soles, and forehead. When caused by a fever or high environmental temperature, it's usually generalized.

Diaphoresis usually begins abruptly and may be accompanied by other autonomic system signs, such as tachycardia and increased blood pressure. (See *When diaphoresis spells crisis,* page 188.)

However, this sign also varies with age because sweat glands function immaturely in infants and are less active in elderly patients. As a result, patients in these age-groups may fail to display diaphoresis associated with its common causes. Intermittent diaphoresis may accompany chronic disorders characterized by a recurrent fever; isolated di-

aphoresis may mark an episode of acute pain or fever. Night sweats may characterize intermittent fever because body temperature tends to return to normal between 2 a.m. and 4 a.m. before rising again. (Temperature is usually lowest around 6 a.m.)

When caused by a high external temperature, diaphoresis is a normal response. Acclimatization usually requires several days of exposure to high temperatures; during this process, diaphoresis helps maintain normal body temperature. Diaphoresis also commonly occurs during menopause, preceded by a sensation of intense heat (a hot flash). Other causes include exercise or exertion that accelerates metabolism, creating internal heat, and mild to moderate anxiety that helps initiate the fight-or-flight response. (See *Understanding diaphoresis,* pages 190 and 191.)

History and physical examination

If the patient is diaphoretic, quickly rule out the possibility of a life-threatening cause. Begin the history by having the patient describe his chief complaint. Then explore associated signs and symptoms. Note general fatigue and weakness. Does the patient have insomnia, headache, and changes in vision or hearing? Is he often dizzy? Does he have palpitations? Ask about chest pain, a cough, sputum, difficulty breathing, nausea, vomiting, abdominal pain, and altered bowel or bladder habits. Ask the female patient about amenorrhea and any changes in her menstrual cycle. Is she perimenopausal or menopausal? Ask about paresthesia, muscle cramps or stiffness, and joint pain. Has she noticed any changes in elimination habits? Note weight loss or gain. Has the patient had to change her glove or shoe size lately?

Complete the history by asking about travel to tropical countries. Note

When diaphoresis spells crisis

Diaphoresis is an early sign of certain life-threatening disorders. These guidelines will help you promptly detect such disorders and intervene to minimize harm to the patient.

Hypoglycemia

If you observe diaphoresis in a patient who complains of blurred vision, ask him about increased irritability and anxiety. Has he been unusually hungry lately? Does he have tremors? Take the patient's vital signs, noting hypotension and tachycardia. Then ask about a history of type 2 diabetes or antidiabetic therapy. If you suspect hypoglycemia, evaluate the patient's blood glucose level using a glucose reagent strip, or send a serum sample to the laboratory. Administer I.V. glucose 50%, as ordered, to return the patient's glucose level to normal. Monitor his vital signs and cardiac rhythm. Ensure a patent airway, and be prepared to assist with breathing and circulation if needed.

Heatstroke

If you observe profuse diaphoresis in a weak, tired, and apprehensive patient, suspect heatstroke, which can progress to circulatory collapse. Take his vital signs, noting a normal or subnormal temperature. Check for ashen gray skin and dilated pupils. Was the patient recently exposed to high temperatures and humidity? Was he wearing heavy clothing or performing strenuous physical activity at the time? Also ask if he takes a diuretic, which interferes with normal sweating.

Then take the patient to a cool room, remove his clothing, and use a fan to direct cool air over his body. Insert an I.V. catheter, and prepare for fluid and electrolyte replacement. Monitor him for signs of shock. Check his urine output carefully along with other sources of output (such as tubes, drains, and ostomies).

Autonomic hyperreflexia

If you observe diaphoresis in a patient with a spinal cord injury above T6 or T7, ask if he has a pounding headache, restlessness, blurred vision, or nasal congestion. Take the patient's vital signs, noting bradycardia and extremely elevated blood pressure. If you suspect autonomic hyperreflexia, quickly rule out its common complications. Examine the patient for eye pain associated with intraocular hemorrhage and for facial paralysis, slurred speech, or limb weakness associated with intracerebral hemorrhage.

Quickly reposition the patient to remove any pressure stimuli. Also, check for a distended bladder or fecal impaction. Remove any kinks from the urinary catheter if necessary, or administer a suppository or manually remove impacted feces. If you can't locate and relieve the causative stimulus, insert an I.V. catheter. Prepare to administer hydralazine for hypertension.

Myocardial infarction or heart failure

If the diaphoretic patient complains of chest pain and dyspnea or has arrhythmias or electrocardiogram changes, suspect a myocardial infarction or heart failure. Connect the patient to a cardiac monitor, ensure a patent airway, and administer supplemental oxygen. Insert an I.V. catheter, obtain a 12-lead electrocardiogram, and administer an analgesic. Be prepared to begin emergency resuscitation if cardiac or respiratory arrest occurs.

recent exposure to high environmental temperatures or pesticides. Did the patient recently experience an insect bite? Check for a history of partial gastrectomy or of drug or alcohol abuse. Finally, obtain a thorough drug history.

Next, perform a physical examination. First, determine the extent of diaphoresis by inspecting the trunk and extremities as well as the palms, soles, and forehead. Also, check the patient's clothing and bedding for dampness. Note whether diaphoresis occurs during the day or at night. Observe the patient for flushing, abnormal skin texture or lesions, and an increased amount of coarse body hair. Note poor skin turgor and dry mucous membranes. Check for splinter hemorrhages and Plummer's nails (separation of the fingernail ends from the nail beds).

Evaluate the patient's mental status and take his vital signs. Observe him for fasciculations and flaccid paralysis. Be alert for seizures. Note the patient's facial expression, and examine the eyes for pupillary dilation or constriction, exophthalmos, and excessive tearing. Test visual fields. Also, check for hearing loss and for tooth or gum disease. Percuss the lungs for dullness, and auscultate for crackles, diminished or bronchial breath sounds, and increased vocal fremitus. Look for decreased respiratory excursion. Palpate for lymphadenopathy and hepatosplenomegaly.

Medical causes

Acquired immunodeficiency syndrome (AIDS). Night sweats may be an early feature of AIDS, occurring either as a manifestation of the disease itself or secondary to an opportunistic infection. The patient also displays a fever, fatigue, lymphadenopathy, anorexia, dramatic and unexplained weight loss, diarrhea, and a persistent cough.

Acromegaly. With acromegaly, diaphoresis is a sensitive gauge of disease activity, which involves the hypersecretion of growth hormone and an increased metabolic rate. The patient has a hulking appearance with an enlarged supraorbital ridge and thickened ears and nose. Other signs and symptoms include warm, oily, thickened skin; enlarged hands, feet, and jaw; joint pain; weight gain; hoarseness; and increased coarse body hair. Increased blood pressure, a severe headache, and visual field deficits or blindness may also occur.

Anxiety disorders. Acute anxiety characterizes panic, whereas chronic anxiety characterizes phobias, conversion disorders, obsessions, and compulsions. Whether acute or chronic, anxiety may cause sympathetic stimulation, resulting in diaphoresis. The diaphoresis is most dramatic on the palms, soles, and forehead and is accompanied by palpitations, tachycardia, tachypnea, tremors, and GI distress. Psychological signs and symptoms—fear, difficulty concentrating, and behavior changes—also occur.

Autonomic hyperreflexia. Occurring after resolution of spinal shock in a spinal cord injury above T6, hyperreflexia causes profuse diaphoresis, a pounding headache, blurred vision, and dramatically elevated blood pressure. Diaphoresis occurs above the level of the injury, especially on the forehead, and is accompanied by flushing. Other findings include restlessness, nausea, nasal congestion, and bradycardia.

Drug and alcohol withdrawal syndromes. Withdrawal from alcohol or an opioid analgesic may cause generalized diaphoresis, dilated pupils, tachycardia, tremors, and an altered mental status (for example, confusion, delusions, hallucinations, and agitation). Associated signs and symptoms include severe muscle cramps, generalized paresthesia,

Understanding diaphoresis

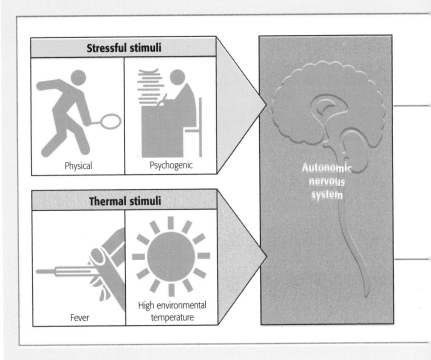

tachypnea, increased or decreased blood pressure and, possibly, seizures. Nausea and vomiting are common.

Empyema. Pus accumulation in the pleural space leads to drenching night sweats and fever. The patient also complains of chest pain, a cough, and weight loss. Examination reveals decreased respiratory excursion on the affected side and absent or distant breath sounds.

Heart failure. Typically, diaphoresis follows fatigue, dyspnea, orthopnea, and tachycardia in patients with left-sided heart failure and jugular vein distention and a dry cough in patients with right-sided heart failure. Other features include tachypnea, cyanosis, dependent edema, crackles, a ventricular gallop, and anxiety.

Heat exhaustion. Although heat exhaustion is marked by failure of heat to dissipate, it initially may cause profuse diaphoresis, fatigue, weakness, and anxiety. These signs and symptoms may progress to circulatory collapse and shock (for example, confusion, a thready pulse, hypotension, tachycardia, and cold, clammy skin). Other features include an ashen gray appearance, dilated pupils, and a normal or subnormal temperature.

Hodgkin's disease. Especially in elderly patients, early features of Hodgkin's disease may include night sweats, a fever, fatigue, pruritus, and weight loss. Usually, however, this disease initially causes painless swelling of a cervical lymph node. Occasionally, a Pel-Ebstein fever pattern is present—several days or

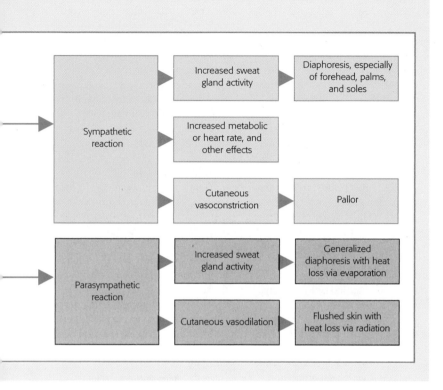

weeks of fever and chills alternating with afebrile periods with no chills. Systemic signs and symptoms—such as weight loss, a fever, and night sweats—indicate a poor prognosis. Progressive lymphadenopathy eventually causes widespread effects, such as hepatomegaly and dyspnea.

Hypoglycemia. Rapidly induced hypoglycemia may cause diaphoresis accompanied by irritability, tremors, hypotension, blurred vision, tachycardia, hunger, and loss of consciousness.

Infective endocarditis (subacute). Generalized night sweats occur early with infective endocarditis. Accompanying signs and symptoms include an intermittent low-grade fever, weakness, fatigue, weight loss, anorexia, and arthralgia. A sudden change in a murmur or

the discovery of a new murmur is a classic sign. Petechiae and splinter hemorrhages are also common.

Lung abscess. Drenching night sweats are common with lung abscess. Its chief sign, however, is a cough that produces copious purulent, foul-smelling, and typically bloody sputum. Associated findings include a fever with chills, pleuritic chest pain, dyspnea, weakness, anorexia, weight loss, a headache, malaise, clubbing, tubular or amphoric breath sounds, and dullness on percussion.

Malaria. Profuse diaphoresis marks the third stage of paroxysmal malaria; the first two stages are chills (first stage) and a high fever (second stage). A headache, arthralgia, and hepatosplenomegaly may also occur. In the benign form of malaria, these paroxysms alternate with periods of well-being. The severe form may progress to delirium, seizures, and coma.

Myocardial infarction (MI). Diaphoresis usually accompanies acute, substernal, radiating chest pain in MI, a life-threatening disorder. Associated signs and symptoms include anxiety, dyspnea, nausea, vomiting, tachycardia, an irregular pulse, blood pressure changes, fine crackles, pallor, and clammy skin.

Pheochromocytoma. Pheochromocytoma commonly produces diaphoresis, but its cardinal sign is persistent or paroxysmal hypertension. Other effects include a headache, palpitations, tachycardia, anxiety, tremors, pallor, flushing, paresthesia, abdominal pain, tachypnea, nausea, vomiting, and orthostatic hypotension.

Pneumonia. Intermittent, generalized diaphoresis accompanies a fever and chills in patients with pneumonia. They complain of pleuritic chest pain that increases with deep inspiration. Other features are tachypnea, dyspnea, a productive cough (with scant and mucoid or copious and purulent sputum), a headache, fatigue, myalgia, abdominal pain, anorexia, and cyanosis. Auscultation reveals bronchial breath sounds.

Tetanus. Tetanus commonly causes profuse sweating accompanied by a low-grade fever, tachycardia, and hyperactive deep tendon reflexes. Early restlessness and pain and stiffness in the jaw, abdomen, and back progress to spasms associated with lockjaw, risus sardonicus, dysphagia, and opisthotonos. Laryngospasm may result in cyanosis or sudden death by asphyxiation.

Thyrotoxicosis. Thyrotoxicosis commonly produces diaphoresis accompanied by heat intolerance, weight loss despite increased appetite, tachycardia, palpitations, an enlarged thyroid, dyspnea, nervousness, diarrhea, tremors, Plummer's nails and, possibly, exophthalmos. Gallops may also occur.

Tuberculosis (TB). Although many patients with primary infection are asymptomatic, TB may cause night sweats, a low-grade fever, fatigue, weakness, anorexia, and weight loss. In reactivation, a productive cough with mucopurulent sputum, occasional hemoptysis, and chest pain may be present.

Other causes

Drugs. Sympathomimetics, certain antipsychotics, thyroid hormones, corticosteroids, and antipyretics may cause diaphoresis. Aspirin and acetaminophen poisoning also cause this sign.

Dumping syndrome. The result of rapid emptying of gastric contents into the small intestine after partial gastrectomy, this syndrome causes diaphoresis, palpitations, profound weakness, epigastric distress, nausea, and explosive diarrhea. This syndrome occurs soon after eating.

Pesticide poisoning. Among the toxic effects of pesticides are diaphoresis, nausea, vomiting, diarrhea, blurred vision, miosis, and excessive lacrimation and salivation. The patient may display fasciculations, muscle weakness, and flaccid paralysis. Signs of respiratory depression and coma may also occur.

Nursing considerations

▪ After an episode of diaphoresis, sponge the patient's face and body and change wet clothes and sheets.
▪ To prevent skin irritation, dust skin folds in the groin and axillae and under pendulous breasts with cornstarch, or tuck gauze or cloth into the folds.
▪ Replace fluids and electrolytes.
▪ Monitor fluid intake and urine output.
▪ Keep the patient's room temperature moderate to prevent additional diaphoresis.

■ Prepare the patient for diagnostic tests, such as blood tests, cultures, chest X-rays, immunologic studies, biopsy, a computed tomography scan, and audiometry.

■ Monitor the patient's vital signs, including temperature.

Patient teaching

■ Explain proper skin care and the importance of good hygiene.

■ Discuss the importance of fluid replacement and encourage oral fluids high in electrolytes such as sports drinks.

■ Explain the underlying disease process and its treatments.

Diarrhea

Usually a chief sign of an intestinal disorder, diarrhea is an increase in the volume of stools compared with the patient's normal bowel habits. It varies in severity and may be acute or chronic. Acute diarrhea may result from acute infection, stress, fecal impaction, or the effect of a drug. Chronic diarrhea may result from chronic infection, obstructive and inflammatory bowel disease, malabsorption syndrome, an endocrine disorder, or GI surgery. Periodic diarrhea may result from food intolerance or from ingestion of spicy or high-fiber foods or caffeine.

One or more pathophysiologic mechanisms may contribute to diarrhea. (See *What causes diarrhea?* page 194.) The fluid and electrolyte imbalances it produces may precipitate life-threatening arrhythmias or hypovolemic shock.

ACTION STAT!

 If the patient's diarrhea is profuse, check for signs of shock—tachycardia, hypotension, and cool, pale, clammy skin. If you detect these signs, place the patient in the

supine position and elevate his legs 20 degrees. Insert an I.V. catheter for fluid replacement. Monitor him for electrolyte imbalances, and look for an irregular pulse, muscle weakness, anorexia, and nausea and vomiting. Keep emergency resuscitation equipment handy.

History and physical examination

If the patient isn't in shock, proceed with a physical examination. Evaluate hydration, check skin turgor and mucous membranes, and take blood pressure with the patient lying, sitting, and standing. Inspect the abdomen for distention, and palpate for tenderness. Auscultate bowel sounds. Check for tympany over the abdomen. Take the patient's temperature, and note any chills. Also, look for a rash. Conduct a rectal examination and a pelvic examination if indicated.

Explore signs and symptoms associated with diarrhea. Does the patient have abdominal pain and cramps? Difficulty breathing? Is he weak or fatigued? Find out his drug history. Has he had GI surgery or radiation therapy recently? Ask the patient to briefly describe his diet. Does he have any known food allergies? Last, find out if he's under unusual stress.

Medical causes

Anthrax (GI). Anthrax manifests after the patient has eaten contaminated meat from an animal infected with *Bacillus anthracis.* Early signs and symptoms include decreased appetite, nausea, vomiting, and a fever. Later signs and symptoms include severe bloody diarrhea, abdominal pain, and hematemesis.

Carcinoid syndrome. With carcinoid syndrome, severe diarrhea occurs with flushing—usually of the head and neck—that's commonly caused by emo-

What causes diarrhea?

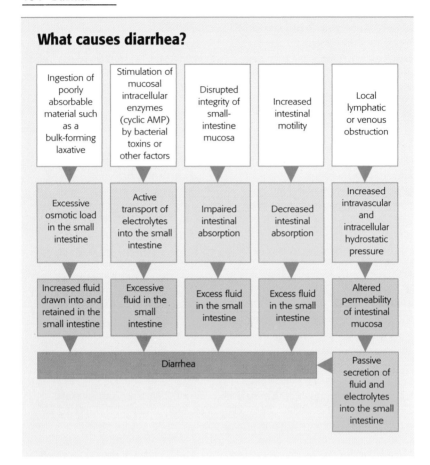

tional stimuli or the ingestion of food, hot water, or alcohol. Associated signs and symptoms include abdominal cramps, dyspnea, weight loss, anorexia, weakness, palpitations, valvular heart disease, and depression.

Cholera. After ingesting water or food contaminated by the bacterium *Vibrio cholerae,* the patient experiences abrupt watery diarrhea and vomiting. Other signs and symptoms include thirst (due to severe water and electrolyte loss), weakness, muscle cramps, decreased skin turgor, oliguria, tachycardia, and hypotension. Without treatment, death can occur within hours.

Clostridium difficile *infection.* The patient may be asymptomatic or may have soft, unformed stools or watery diarrhea that may be foul smelling or grossly bloody; abdominal pain, cramping, and tenderness; a fever; and a white blood cell count as high as 20,000/ml. In severe cases, the patient may develop toxic megacolon, colon perforation, or peritonitis.

Crohn's disease. Crohn's disease is a recurring inflammatory disorder that produces diarrhea accompanied by abdominal pain with guarding and tenderness and nausea. The patient may also display a fever, chills, weakness, anorexia, and weight loss.

Escherichia coli *O157:H7.* Watery or bloody diarrhea, nausea, vomiting, fever, and abdominal cramps occur after the patient eats undercooked beef or other foods contaminated with this particular strain of bacteria. Hemolytic uremic syndrome, which causes red blood cell destruction and eventually acute renal failure, is a complication of *E. coli* O157:H7 in children age 5 and younger and elderly people.

Infections. Acute viral, bacterial, and protozoal infections (such as cryptosporidiosis) cause the sudden onset of watery diarrhea as well as abdominal pain, cramps, nausea, vomiting, and a fever. Significant fluid and electrolyte loss may cause signs of dehydration and shock. Chronic tuberculosis and fungal and parasitic infections may produce a less severe but more persistent diarrhea, accompanied by epigastric distress, vomiting, weight loss and, possibly, passage of blood and mucus.

Intestinal obstruction. Partial intestinal obstruction increases intestinal motility, resulting in diarrhea, abdominal pain with tenderness and guarding, nausea and, possibly, distention.

Irritable bowel syndrome (IBS). With IBS, diarrhea alternates with constipation or normal bowel function. Related findings include abdominal pain, tenderness, and distention; dyspepsia; and nausea.

Ischemic bowel disease. Ischemic bowel disease is a life-threatening disorder that causes bloody diarrhea with abdominal pain. If severe, shock may occur, requiring surgery.

Lactose intolerance. With lactose intolerance, diarrhea occurs within several hours of ingesting milk or milk products. It's accompanied by cramps, abdominal pain, borborygmi, bloating, nausea, and flatus.

Listeriosis. With listeriosis, diarrhea occurs in conjunction with a fever, myalgia, abdominal pain, nausea, and vomiting. A fever, a headache, a nuchal rigidity, and an altered level of consciousness may occur if the infection spreads to the nervous system and causes meningitis.

Pseudomembranous enterocolitis. Pseudomembranous enterocolitis is a potentially life-threatening disorder that commonly follows antibiotic administration. It produces copious watery, green, foul-smelling, bloody diarrhea that rapidly precipitates signs of shock. Other signs and symptoms include colicky abdominal pain, distention, a fever, and dehydration.

Q fever. Q fever is caused by the bacterium *Coxiella burnetii* and causes diarrhea along with a fever, chills, a severe headache, malaise, chest pain, and vomiting. In severe cases, hepatitis or pneumonia may follow.

Rotavirus gastroenteritis. Rotavirus gastroenteritis commonly starts with a fever, nausea, and vomiting, followed by diarrhea. The illness can range from mild to severe and can last from 3 to 9 days. Diarrhea and vomiting may result in dehydration.

Thyrotoxicosis. With thyrotoxicosis, nervousness, tremors, diaphoresis, weight loss despite increased appetite, dyspnea, palpitations, tachycardia, an enlarged thyroid, heat intolerance and, possibly, exophthalmos accompany diarrhea.

Ulcerative colitis. The hallmark of ulcerative colitis is recurrent bloody diarrhea with pus or mucus. Other signs and symptoms include tenesmus, hyperactive bowel sounds, cramping lower abdominal pain, a low-grade fever, anorexia and, at times, nausea and vomiting. Weight loss, anemia, and weakness are late findings.

Other causes
Drugs. Many antibiotics—such as ampicillin, cephalosporins, tetracyclines,

and clindamycin—cause diarrhea. Other drugs that may cause diarrhea include magnesium-containing antacids, colchicine, guanethidine, lactulose, dantrolene, ethacrynic acid, mefenamic acid, methotrexate, metyrosine and, in high doses, cardiac glycosides and quinidine. Laxative abuse can cause acute or chronic diarrhea.

Treatments. Gastrectomy, gastroenterostomy, and pyloroplasty may produce diarrhea. High-dose radiation therapy may produce enteritis associated with diarrhea.

Nursing considerations

■ Administer an analgesic for pain and an opiate to decrease intestinal motility, unless the patient has a possible or confirmed stool infection.
■ Ensure the patient's privacy during defecation, and empty bedpans promptly.
■ Clean the perineum thoroughly, and apply ointment to prevent skin breakdown.
■ Note the amount and characteristics of the patient's stool.
■ Monitor intake and output.
■ Obtain serum samples for electrolytes and treat imbalances.
■ Provide fluid replacement orally or I.V., as appropriate.

Patient teaching

■ Stress the need for medical follow-up to patients with inflammatory bowel disease (particularly ulcerative colitis) who have an increased risk of developing colon cancer.
■ Emphasize the importance of maintaining adequate hydration.
■ Explain food or fluids that should be avoided.
■ Discuss stress reduction techniques.
■ Explain the diagnosis and treatment plan.

Diplopia

Diplopia is double vision—seeing one object as two. This symptom results when extraocular muscles fail to work together, causing images to fall on noncorresponding parts of the retinas. What causes this muscle incoordination? Orbital lesions, the effects of surgery, or impaired function of cranial nerves (CNs) that supply extraocular muscles (oculomotor, CN III; trochlear, CN IV; abducens, CN VI) may be responsible. (See *Testing extraocular muscles.*)

Diplopia usually begins intermittently and affects near or far vision exclusively. It can be classified as monocular or binocular. More common binocular diplopia may result from ocular deviation or displacement, extraocular muscle palsies, or psychoneurosis, or it may occur after retinal surgery. Monocular diplopia may result from an early cataract, retinal edema or scarring, iridodialysis, a subluxated lens, a poorly fitting contact lens, or an uncorrected refractive error such as astigmatism. Diplopia may also occur in hysteria or malingering.

History and physical examination

If the patient complains of double vision, first check his neurologic status. Evaluate his level of consciousness (LOC); pupil size, equality, and response to light; and motor and sensory function. Then take his vital signs. Briefly ask about associated symptoms, especially a severe headache. Find out about associated neurologic symptoms first because diplopia can accompany serious disorders.

Next, continue with a more detailed examination. Find out when the patient first noticed diplopia. Are the images side-by-side (horizontal), one above the other (vertical), or a combination? Does diplopia affect near or far vision? Does it

ASSESSMENT TIP

Testing extraocular muscles

The coordinated action of six muscles controls eyeball movements. To test the function of each muscle and the cranial nerve (CN) that innervates it, ask the patient to look in the direction controlled by that muscle. The six directions you can test make up the *cardinal fields of gaze*. The patient's inability to turn the eye in the designated direction indicates muscle weakness or paralysis.

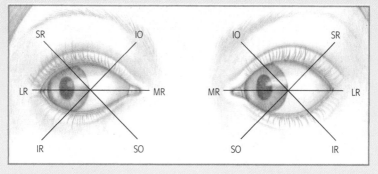

SR = superior rectus (CN III)	IR = inferior rectus (CN III)	MR = medial rectus (CN III)
LR = lateral rectus (CN VI)	IO = inferior oblique (CN III)	SO = superior oblique (CN IV)

affect certain directions of gaze? Ask if diplopia has worsened, remained the same, or subsided. Does its severity change throughout the day? Diplopia that worsens or appears in the evening may indicate myasthenia gravis. Find out if the patient can correct diplopia by tilting his head. If so, ask him to show you. (If the patient has a fourth nerve lesion, tilting of the head toward the opposite shoulder causes compensatory tilting of the unaffected eye. If he has incomplete sixth nerve palsy, tilting of the head toward the side of the paralyzed muscle may relax the affected lateral rectus muscle.)

Explore associated symptoms such as eye pain or limited eye movement. Ask about hypertension, diabetes mellitus, allergies, and thyroid, neurologic, or muscular disorders. Also, note a history of extraocular muscle disorders, trauma, or eye surgery.

Observe the patient for ocular deviation, ptosis, proptosis, lid edema, and conjunctival injection. Distinguish monocular from binocular diplopia by asking the patient to occlude one eye at a time. If he still sees double out of one eye, he has monocular diplopia. Test his visual acuity and extraocular muscles. Check his vital signs.

Medical causes

Alcohol intoxication. Diplopia is a common symptom of alcohol intoxication. It's accompanied by confusion, slurred speech, halitosis, a staggering gait, behavior changes, nausea, vomiting and, possibly, conjunctival injection.

Botulism. Hallmark signs of botulism include diplopia, dysarthria, dysphagia, and ptosis. Early findings include a dry mouth, a sore throat, vomiting, and diarrhea. Later, descending weakness or paralysis of extremity and trunk muscles causes hyporeflexia and dyspnea.

Brain tumor. Diplopia may be an early symptom of a brain tumor. Accompanying signs and symptoms vary with the tumor's size and location, but may include eye deviation, emotional lability, a decreased LOC, a headache, vomiting, absence or generalized tonic-clonic seizures, hearing loss, visual field deficits, abnormal pupillary responses, nystagmus, motor weakness, and paralysis.

Cavernous sinus thrombosis. Cavernous sinus thrombosis may produce diplopia and limited eye movement. Associated signs and symptoms include proptosis, orbital and lid edema, diminished or absent pupillary responses, impaired visual acuity, papilledema, and a fever.

Diabetes mellitus. Among the long-term effects of diabetes mellitus may be diplopia due to isolated CN III palsy. Diplopia typically begins suddenly and may be accompanied by pain.

Encephalitis. Initially, encephalitis may cause a brief episode of diplopia and eye deviation. However, it usually begins with the sudden onset of a high fever, a severe headache, and vomiting. As the inflammation progresses, the patient may display signs of meningeal irritation, a decreased LOC, seizures, ataxia, and paralysis.

Head injury. Potentially life-threatening head injuries may cause diplopia, depending on the site and extent of the injury. Associated signs and symptoms include eye deviation, pupillary changes, a headache, a decreased LOC, altered vital signs, nausea, vomiting, and motor weakness or paralysis.

Intracranial aneurysm. Intracranial aneurysm is a life-threatening disorder that initially produces diplopia and eye deviation, perhaps accompanied by ptosis and a dilated pupil on the affect-

ed side. The patient complains of a recurrent, severe, unilateral, frontal headache. After the aneurysm ruptures, the headache becomes violent. Associated signs and symptoms include neck and spinal pain and rigidity, a decreased LOC, tinnitus, dizziness, nausea, vomiting, and unilateral muscle weakness or paralysis.

Multiple sclerosis (MS). Diplopia, a common early symptom in MS, is usually accompanied by blurred vision and paresthesia. As MS progresses, signs and symptoms may include nystagmus, constipation, muscle weakness, paralysis, spasticity, hyperreflexia, intention tremor, gait ataxia, dysphagia, dysarthria, impotence, emotional lability, and urinary frequency, urgency, and incontinence.

Myasthenia gravis. Myasthenia gravis initially produces diplopia and ptosis, which worsen throughout the day. It then progressively involves other muscles, resulting in a blank facial expression; a nasal voice; difficulty chewing, swallowing, and making fine hand movements; and, possibly, signs of life-threatening respiratory muscle weakness.

Ophthalmologic migraine. Ophthalmologic migraine results in diplopia that persists for days after the headache. Accompanying signs and symptoms include severe, unilateral pain; ptosis; and extraocular muscle palsies. Irritability, depression, or slight confusion may also occur.

Orbital blowout fracture. An orbital blowout fracture usually causes monocular diplopia affecting the upward gaze. However, with marked periorbital edema, diplopia may affect other directions of gaze. This fracture commonly causes periorbital ecchymosis, but doesn't affect visual acuity, although eyelid edema may prevent accurate testing. Subcutaneous crepitation of the eyelid and orbit is typical. Occasionally, the patient's pupil is dilated and unreactive, and he may have a hyphema.

Orbital cellulitis. Inflammation of the orbital tissues and eyelids causes sudden diplopia. Other findings are eye deviation and pain, purulent drainage, lid edema, chemosis and redness, proptosis, nausea, and a fever.

Orbital tumor. An enlarging orbital tumor can cause diplopia. Proptosis and possibly blurred vision may also occur.

Stroke. Diplopia characterizes stroke when it affects the vertebrobasilar artery. Other signs and symptoms include unilateral motor weakness or paralysis, ataxia, a decreased LOC, dizziness, aphasia, visual field deficits, circumoral numbness, slurred speech, dysphagia, and amnesia.

Thyrotoxicosis. Diplopia occurs when exophthalmos characterizes the disorder. It usually begins in the upper field of gaze because of infiltrative myopathy involving the inferior rectus muscle. It's accompanied by impaired eye movement, excessive tearing, lid edema and, possibly, an inability to close the lids. Other cardinal findings include tachycardia, palpitations, weight loss, diarrhea, tremors, an enlarged thyroid, dyspnea, nervousness, diaphoresis, and heat intolerance.

Transient ischemic attack (TIA). TIA is generally accompanied by diplopia, dizziness, tinnitus, hearing loss, and numbness. It can last for a few seconds or up to 24 hours and may be a warning sign of a future stroke.

Other causes

Eye surgery. Fibrosis associated with eye surgery may restrict eye movement, resulting in diplopia.

Nursing considerations

■ Monitor the patient's vital signs and neurologic status.

■ Prepare the patient for neurologic tests such as a computed tomography scan.
■ Provide a safe environment and assist with ambulation.
■ Institute seizure precautions, if indicated.

Patient teaching

■ Explain safety measures to the patient.
■ Reinforce that the patient must not drive or operate heavy machinery upon discharge.
■ Explain to the patient his diagnosis and the treatment plan.

▉Dizziness

A common symptom, dizziness is a sensation of imbalance or faintness, sometimes associated with giddiness, weakness, confusion, and blurred or double vision. Episodes of dizziness are usually brief; they may be mild or severe with an abrupt or a gradual onset. Dizziness may be aggravated by standing up quickly and alleviated by lying down and by rest.

Dizziness typically results from inadequate blood flow and oxygen supply to the cerebrum and spinal cord. It may occur with anxiety, respiratory and cardiovascular disorders, and postconcussion syndrome. It's a key symptom in certain serious disorders, such as hypertension and vertebrobasilar artery insufficiency.

Dizziness is commonly confused with vertigo—a sensation of revolving in space or of surroundings revolving about oneself. However, unlike dizziness, vertigo is commonly accompanied by nausea, vomiting, nystagmus, a staggering gait, and tinnitus or hearing loss. Dizziness and vertigo may occur together, as in postconcussion syndrome.

If the patient complains of dizziness, first ensure his safety by assisting him back to bed and preventing falls. Then determine the severity and onset of the dizziness. Ask him to describe it. Is the dizziness associated with a headache or blurred vision? Next, take his blood pressure while he's lying down, sitting, and standing to check for orthostatic hypotension. Ask about a history of high blood pressure. Determine if he's at risk for hypoglycemia. Check his blood glucose level. Tell him to lie down, and recheck his vital signs every 15 minutes. Insert an I.V. catheter, and prepare to administer medications and fluids as ordered.

History and physical examination

Ask about a history of diabetes and cardiovascular disease. Is the patient taking drugs prescribed for high blood pressure? If so, when did he take his last dose?

If the patient's blood pressure is normal, obtain a more complete history. Ask about myocardial infarction, heart failure, kidney disease, or atherosclerosis, which may predispose the patient to cardiac arrhythmias, hypertension, and a transient ischemic attack. Does he have a history of anemia, chronic obstructive pulmonary disease, anxiety disorders, or head injury? Obtain a complete drug history.

Next, explore the patient's dizziness. How often does it occur? How long does each episode last? Does the dizziness abate spontaneously? Does it lead to loss of consciousness? Find out if dizziness is triggered by sitting or standing up suddenly or stooping over. Does being in a crowd make the patient feel dizzy? Ask about emotional stress. Has the patient been irritable or anxious lately? Does he

have insomnia or difficulty concentrating? Look for fidgeting and eyelid twitching. Does the patient startle easily? Also, ask about palpitations, chest pain, diaphoresis, shortness of breath, and chronic cough.

Next, perform a physical examination. Begin with a quick neurologic assessment, checking the patient's level of consciousness (LOC), motor and sensory functions, and reflexes. Then inspect for poor skin turgor and dry mucous membranes, signs of dehydration. Auscultate heart rate and rhythm. Inspect for barrel chest, clubbing, cyanosis, and use of accessory muscles. Also auscultate breath sounds. Take the patient's blood pressure while he's lying down, sitting, and standing to check for orthostatic hypotension. Test capillary refill time in the extremities, and palpate for edema.

Medical causes

Anemia. Typically, anemia causes dizziness that's aggravated by postural changes or exertion. Other signs and symptoms include pallor, dyspnea, fatigue, tachycardia, and a bounding pulse. The capillary refill time is increased.

Cardiac arrhythmias. Dizziness may occur for several seconds or longer and may precede fainting in arrhythmias. The patient may experience palpitations; irregular, rapid, or thready pulse; and, possibly, hypotension. He may also experience weakness, blurred vision, paresthesia, and confusion.

Emphysema. Dizziness may follow exertion or the chronic productive cough in patients with emphysema. Associated signs and symptoms include dyspnea, anorexia, weight loss, malaise, use of accessory muscles, pursed-lip breathing, tachypnea, peripheral cyanosis, and diminished breath sounds. Barrel chest and clubbing may be seen.

Generalized anxiety disorder. Generalized anxiety disorder produces continuous dizziness that may intensify as the disorder worsens. Associated signs and symptoms are persistent anxiety (for at least 1 month), insomnia, difficulty concentrating, and irritability. The patient may show signs of motor tension—for example, twitching or fidgeting, muscle aches, a furrowed brow, and a tendency to be startled. He may also display signs of autonomic hyperactivity, such as diaphoresis, palpitations, cold and clammy hands, dry mouth, paresthesia, indigestion, hot or cold flashes, frequent urination, diarrhea, a lump in the throat, pallor, and increased pulse and respiratory rates.

Hypertension. With hypertension, dizziness may precede fainting, but it may also be relieved by rest. Other common signs and symptoms include a headache and blurred vision. Retinal changes include hemorrhage, sclerosis of retinal blood vessels, exudate, and papilledema.

Hyperventilation syndrome. Episodes of hyperventilation cause dizziness that usually lasts a few minutes; however, if these episodes occur frequently, dizziness may persist between them. Other effects include apprehension, diaphoresis, pallor, dyspnea, chest tightness, palpitations, trembling, fatigue, and peripheral and circumoral paresthesia.

Hypovolemia. A lack of circulating blood volume may cause dizziness and may be accompanied by other signs of fluid volume deficit (dry mucous membranes, decreased blood pressure, increased heart rate).

Orthostatic hypotension. Orthostatic hypotension produces dizziness that may terminate in fainting or disappear with rest. Related findings include dim vision, spots before the eyes, pallor, diaphoresis, hypotension, tachycardia and, possibly, signs of dehydration.

Postconcussion syndrome. Occurring 1 to 3 weeks after a head injury, postconcussion syndrome is marked by dizziness, a headache (throbbing, aching, bandlike, or stabbing), emotional lability, alcohol intolerance, fatigue, anxiety and, possibly, vertigo. Dizziness and other symptoms are intensified by mental or physical stress. The syndrome may persist for years, but symptoms eventually abate.

Rift Valley fever. Typical signs and symptoms of Rift Valley fever include dizziness, a fever, myalgia, weakness, and back pain. A small percentage of patients may develop encephalitis or may progress to hemorrhagic fever that can lead to shock and hemorrhage. Inflammation of the retina may result in some permanent vision loss.

Transient ischemic attack (TIA). Lasting from a few seconds to 24 hours, a TIA commonly signals an impending stroke and may be triggered by turning the head to the side. Besides dizziness of varying severity, TIAs are accompanied by unilateral or bilateral diplopia, blindness or visual field deficits, ptosis, tinnitus, hearing loss, paresis, and numbness. Other findings include dysarthria, dysphagia, vomiting, hiccups, confusion, a decreased LOC, and pallor.

Other causes
Drugs. Anxiolytics, central nervous system depressants, opioids, decongestants, antihistamines, antihypertensives, and vasodilators commonly cause dizziness.

Nursing considerations
▪ Prepare the patient for diagnostic tests, such as blood studies, arteriography, a computed tomography scan, EEG, magnetic resonance imaging, and tilt-table studies.

■ Ensure safety measures.

Patient teaching

■ Teach the patient how to control dizziness.

■ Discuss safety measures.

■ Teach the patient about his underlying disorder and its treatment.

▌Doll's eye sign, absent

[Negative oculocephalic reflex]

An indicator of brain stem dysfunction, the absence of the doll's eye sign is detected by rapid, gentle turning of the patient's head from side to side. The eyes remain fixed in midposition, instead of the normal response of moving laterally toward the side opposite the direction the head is turned. (See *Testing for absent doll's eye sign.*)

The absence of doll's eye sign indicates injury to the midbrain or pons, involving cranial nerves III and VI. It typically accompanies coma caused by lesions of the cerebellum and brain stem. This sign usually can't be relied upon in a conscious patient because he can control eye movements voluntarily. Absent doll's eye sign is necessary for a diagnosis of brain death.

A variant of absent doll's eye sign that develops gradually is known as *abnormal doll's eye sign*. Because conjugate eye movement is lost, one eye may move laterally while the other remains fixed or moves in the opposite direction. An abnormal doll's eye sign usually accompanies metabolic coma or increased intracranial pressure (ICP). Associated brain stem dysfunction may be reversible or may progress to deeper coma with absent doll's eye sign.

History and physical examination

After detecting an absent doll's eye sign, perform a neurologic examination. First, evaluate the patient's level of consciousness, using the Glasgow Coma Scale. Note decerebrate or decorticate posture. Examine the pupils for size, equality, and response to light. Check for signs of increased ICP—increased blood pres-

A S S E S S M E N T   T I P

Testing for absent doll's eye sign

To evaluate the patient's oculocephalic reflex, hold her upper eyelids open and quickly (but gently) turn her head from side to side, noting eye movements with each head turn.

With absent doll's eye sign, the eyes remain fixed in midposition.

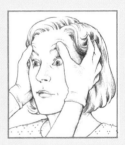 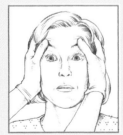 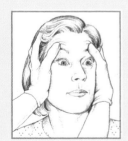

sure, increasing pulse pressure, and bradycardia.

Medical causes

Brain stem infarction. Brain stem infarction causes absent doll's eye sign with coma. It also causes limb paralysis, cranial nerve palsies (facial weakness, diplopia, blindness or visual field deficits, and nystagmus), bilateral cerebellar ataxia, variable sensory loss, a positive Babinski's reflex, decerebrate posture, and muscle flaccidity.

Brain stem tumor. Absent doll's eye sign accompanies coma with a brain stem tumor. This sign may be preceded by hemiparesis, nystagmus, extraocular nerve palsies, facial pain or sensory loss, facial paralysis, a diminished corneal reflex, tinnitus, hearing loss, dysphagia, drooling, vertigo, dizziness, ataxia, and vomiting.

Central midbrain infarction. With a central midbrain infarction, absent doll's eye sign is associated with coma, Weber's syndrome (oculomotor palsy with contralateral hemiplegia), contralateral ataxic tremor, nystagmus, and pupillary abnormalities.

Pontine hemorrhage. Absent doll's eye sign and coma develop within minutes with pontine hemorrhage, a life-threatening disorder. Other ominous signs—such as complete paralysis, decerebrate posture, a positive Babinski's reflex, and small, reactive pupils—may rapidly progress to death.

Posterior fossa hematoma. A subdural hematoma at the posterior fossa typically causes absent doll's eye sign and coma. These signs may be preceded by characteristic signs and symptoms, such as a headache, vomiting, drowsiness, confusion, unequal pupils, dysphagia, cranial nerve palsies, a stiff neck, and cerebellar ataxia.

Other causes

Drugs. Barbiturates may produce severe central nervous system depression, resulting in coma and absent doll's eye sign.

Nursing considerations

- Don't attempt to elicit doll's eye sign in a comatose patient with suspected cervical spine injury; doing so risks spinal cord damage.
- Monitor vital signs and neurologic status.
- Discuss end-of-life issues with the patient's family, if appropriate.
- Provide emotional support to the family.

Patient teaching

- Explain to the patient the underlying cause and its treatment.

▌Drooling

Drooling—the flow of saliva from the mouth—results from a failure to swallow or retain saliva or from excess salivation. It may stem from facial muscle paralysis or weakness that prevents mouth closure, from neuromuscular disorders or local pain that causes dysphagia or, less commonly, from the effects of drugs or toxins that induce salivation. Drooling may be scant or copious (up to 1 L daily) and may cause circumoral irritation. Because it signals an inability to handle secretions, drooling warns of potential aspiration.

History and physical examination

If you observe the patient drooling, first determine the amount. Is it scant or copious? When did it begin? Ask the patient if his pillow is wet in the morning. Also, inspect for circumoral irritation.

Then explore associated signs and symptoms. Ask about sore throat and difficulty swallowing, chewing, speaking, or breathing. Have the patient describe pain or stiffness in the face and neck and muscle weakness in the face and extremities. Has he noticed mental status changes, such as drowsiness or agitation? Ask about changes in vision, hearing, and sense of taste. Also ask about anorexia, weight loss, fatigue, nausea, vomiting, and altered bowel or bladder habits. Has the patient recently had a cold or other infection? Was he recently bitten by an animal or exposed to pesticides? Finally, obtain a complete drug history.

Next, perform a physical examination. Take the patient's vital signs. Inspect for signs of facial paralysis or abnormal expression. Examine the mouth and neck for swelling, the throat for edema and redness, and the tonsils for exudate. Note foul breath odor. Examine the tongue for bilateral furrowing (trident tongue). Look for pallor and skin lesions and for frontal baldness. Carefully assess any bite or puncture marks.

Assess cranial nerves II through VII, IX, and X. Then check pupillary size and response to light. Assess the patient's speech. Evaluate muscle strength, and palpate for tenderness or atrophy. Also, palpate for lymphadenopathy, especially in the cervical area. Observe the patient's ability to swallow, and assess his gag reflex. Test for poor balance, hyperreflexia, and a positive Babinski's reflex. Also, assess sensory function for paresthesia.

Medical causes

Bell's palsy. With Bell's palsy, drooling accompanies the gradual onset of facial hemiplegia. The affected side of the face sags and is expressionless, the nasolabial fold flattens, and the palpebral fissure (the distance between the upper and lower eyelids) widens. The patient usually complains of pain in or behind the ear. Other cardinal signs and symptoms include unilateral diminished or absent corneal reflex, decreased lacrimation, Bell's phenomenon (upward deviation of the eye with attempt at lid closure), and partial loss of taste or abnormal taste sensation.

Esophageal tumor. With an esophageal tumor, copious and persistent drooling is typically preceded by weight loss and progressively severe dysphagia. Other signs and symptoms include substernal, back, or neck pain and blood-flecked regurgitation.

Ludwig's angina. With Ludwig's angina, moderate to copious drooling stems from dysphagia and local swelling of the floor of the mouth, causing tongue displacement. Submandibular swelling of the neck and signs of respiratory distress may also occur.

Myotonic dystrophy. Facial weakness and a sagging jaw account for constant drooling with this disorder. Other characteristic findings include myotonia (inability to relax a muscle after its contraction), muscle wasting, cataracts, testicular atrophy, frontal baldness, ptosis, and a nasal, monotone voice.

Peritonsillar abscess. A severe sore throat causes dysphagia with moderate to copious drooling with this abscess. Accompanying signs and symptoms are a high fever, rancid breath, and enlarged, reddened, edematous tonsils that may be covered by a soft, gray exudate. Palpation may reveal cervical lymphadenopathy.

Pesticide poisoning. Toxic effects of pesticides may include excess salivation with drooling. Other effects are diaphoresis, nausea and vomiting, involuntary urination and defecation, blurred vision, miosis, increased lacrimation, fasciculations, weakness, flaccid paralysis, signs of respiratory distress, and coma.

Rabies. When this acute central nervous system infection advances to the brain stem, it causes drooling, or "foaming at the mouth." Drooling stems from excessive salivation, facial palsy, or extremely painful pharyngeal spasms that prohibit swallowing. Rabies is accompanied by hydrophobia in about 50% of cases. Seizures and hyperactive deep tendon reflexes may also occur before the patient develops generalized flaccid paralysis and coma.

Seizures (generalized). Generalized seizures are tonic-clonic muscular reactions that cause excessive salivation and frothing at the mouth accompanied by loss of consciousness and cyanosis. In the unresponsive postictal state, the patient may also drool.

Nursing considerations

- Be alert for aspiration in the drooling patient and position him upright or on his side.
- Provide frequent mouth care, and suction as necessary to control drooling.
- Assist with meticulous skin care, especially around the mouth and in the neck area, to prevent skin breakdown.
- Provide a covered, opaque collecting jar to decrease odor and prevent possible transmission of infection.
- Keep tissues handy and drape a towel across the patient's chest at mealtime.

Patient teaching

- Teach the patient good oral hygiene and skin care.
- Show the patient exercises to help strengthen facial muscles, if appropriate.
- Explain to the patient his diagnosis and the treatment plan.

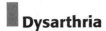

Dysarthria

Dysarthria, poorly articulated speech, is characterized by slurring and labored, irregular rhythm. It may be accompa-

nied by a nasal voice tone caused by palate weakness. Whether it occurs abruptly or gradually, dysarthria is usually evident in ordinary conversation. It's confirmed by asking the patient to produce a few simple sounds and words, such as "ba," "sh," and "cat." However, dysarthria is occasionally confused with aphasia, the loss of the ability to produce or comprehend speech.

Dysarthria results from damage to the brain stem that affects cranial nerves IX, X, or XII. Degenerative neurologic disorders and cerebellar disorders commonly cause dysarthria. In fact, dysarthria is a chief sign of olivopontocerebellar degeneration. It may also result from ill-fitting dentures.

ACTION STAT!

 If the patient displays dysarthria, ask him about associated difficulty swallowing. Then determine his respiratory rate and depth. Measure his vital capacity with a Wright respirometer, if available. Assess the patient's blood pressure and heart rate. Usually, tachycardia, slightly increased blood pressure, and shortness of breath are early signs of respiratory muscle weakness.

Ensure a patent airway. Place the patient in Fowler's position and suction him if necessary. Administer oxygen, and keep emergency resuscitation equipment nearby. Anticipate endotracheal intubation and mechanical ventilation in progressive respiratory muscle weakness. Withhold oral fluids in the patient with associated dysphagia.

History and physical examination

If dysarthria isn't accompanied by respiratory muscle weakness and dysphagia, assess for other neurologic deficits. Compare muscle strength and tone in the limbs. Then evaluate tactile sensation. Ask the patient about numbness or tingling. Test deep tendon reflexes (DTRs), and note gait ataxia. Assess cerebellar function by observing rapid alternating movement, which should be smooth and coordinated. Next, test visual fields and ask about double vision. Check for signs of facial weakness such as ptosis. Next, determine the patient's level of consciousness (LOC) and mental status.

Obtain a patient history. Explore dysarthria completely. When did it begin? Has it gotten better? Speech improves with resolution of a transient ischemic attack, but not in a completed stroke. Ask if dysarthria worsens during the day. Then obtain a drug and alcohol history. Also ask about a history of seizures. Check dentures for a proper fit.

Medical causes

Alcoholic cerebellar degeneration. Alcoholic cerebellar degeneration commonly causes chronic, progressive dysarthria along with ataxia, diplopia, ophthalmoplegia, hypotension, and an altered mental status.

Amyotrophic lateral sclerosis (ALS). Dysarthria occurs when ALS affects the bulbar nuclei; it may worsen as the disease progresses. Other signs and symptoms include dysphagia; difficulty breathing; muscle atrophy and weakness, especially of the hands and feet; fasciculations; spasticity; hyperactive DTRs in the legs; and, occasionally, excessive drooling. Progressive bulbar palsy may cause crying spells or inappropriate laughter.

Basilar artery insufficiency. Basilar artery insufficiency causes random, brief episodes of bilateral brain stem dysfunction, resulting in dysarthria. Accompanying it are diplopia, vertigo, facial numbness, ataxia, paresis, and visual field loss, all of which last for minutes to hours.

Botulism. The hallmark of botulism is acute cranial nerve dysfunction causing dysarthria, dysphagia, diplopia, and ptosis. Early findings include a dry mouth, a sore throat, weakness, vomiting, and diarrhea. Later, descending weakness or paralysis of muscles in the extremities and trunk causes hyporeflexia and dyspnea.

Mercury poisoning. Chronic mercury poisoning causes progressive dysarthria accompanied by weakness, fatigue, depression, lethargy, irritability, confusion, ataxia, and tremors.

Multiple sclerosis (MS). When demyelination affects the brain stem and cerebellum as with MS, the patient displays dysarthria accompanied by nystagmus, blurred or double vision, dysphagia, ataxia, and intention tremor. Exacerbations and remissions of these signs and symptoms are common. Other findings include paresthesia, spasticity, intention tremor, hyperreflexia, muscle weakness or paralysis, constipation, emotional lability, and urinary frequency, urgency, and incontinence.

Myasthenia gravis. Myasthenia gravis causes dysarthria associated with a nasal voice tone. Typically, the dysarthria worsens during the day and may temporarily improve with short rest periods. Other findings include dysphagia, drooling, facial weakness, diplopia, ptosis, dyspnea, and muscle weakness.

Olivopontocerebellar degeneration. Dysarthria, a major sign of olivopontocerebellar degeneration, accompanies cerebellar ataxia and spasticity.

Parkinson's disease. Parkinson's disease produces dysarthria and a monotone voice. It also produces muscle rigidity, bradykinesia, involuntary tremor usually beginning in the fingers, difficulty walking, muscle weakness, and a stooped posture. Other findings include masklike facies, dysphagia, and occasionally drooling.

Shy-Drager syndrome. Marked by chronic orthostatic hypotension, Shy-Drager syndrome eventually causes dysarthria as well as cerebellar ataxia, bradykinesia, masklike facies, dementia, impotence and, possibly, a stooped posture and incontinence.

Stroke (brain stem). A brain stem stroke is characterized by bulbar palsy, resulting in the triad of dysarthria, dysphonia, and dysphagia. Dysarthria is most severe at its onset; it may lessen or disappear with rehabilitation and training. Other findings include facial weakness, diplopia, hemiparesis, spasticity, drooling, dyspnea, and a decreased LOC.

Stroke (cerebral). A massive bilateral stroke causes pseudobulbar palsy. Bilateral weakness produces dysarthria that's most severe at onset. This sign is accompanied by dysphagia, drooling, dysphonia, bilateral hemianopsia, and aphasia. Sensory loss, spasticity, and hyperreflexia may also occur.

Other causes

Drugs. Dysarthria can occur when the anticonvulsant dosage is too high. Ingestion of large doses of barbiturates may also cause dysarthria.

Nursing considerations

- Consult with a speech pathologist, as needed.
- Administer medications and treatments as needed.
- Assess the patient's swallow and gag reflexes before feeding him.
- Give the patient time to express himself.
- Encourage the patient to express his feelings.

Patient teaching

- Encourage the patient with dysarthria to speak slowly so that he can be understood.
- Encourage him to use gestures to aid communication.
- Discuss different ways to communicate.
- Explain to the patient his diagnosis and the treatment plan.

■ Dysmenorrhea

Dysmenorrhea—painful menstruation—affects more than 50% of menstruating women; in fact, it's the leading cause of lost time from school and work among women of childbearing age. Dysmenorrhea may involve sharp, intermittent pain or dull, aching pain. It's usually characterized by mild to severe cramping or colicky pain in the pelvis or lower abdomen that may radiate to the thighs and lower sacrum. This pain may precede menstruation by several days or may accompany it. The pain gradually subsides as bleeding tapers off.

Dysmenorrhea may be idiopathic, as in premenstrual syndrome (PMS) and primary dysmenorrhea. It commonly results from endometriosis and other pelvic disorders. It may also result from structural abnormalities such as an imperforate hymen. Stress and poor health may aggravate dysmenorrhea; rest and mild exercise may relieve it.

History and physical examination

If the patient complains of dysmenorrhea, have her describe it fully. Is it intermittent or continuous? Sharp, cramping, or aching? Ask where the pain is located and whether it's bilateral. When does the pain begin and end, and when is it severe? Does it radiate to the back? How long has she been experiencing the pain? If it's a recent complaint, obtain a human chorionic gonadotropin level to determine if the patient is or was pregnant, because miscarriage can cause painful bleeding. Explore associated signs and symptoms, such as nausea and vomiting, altered bowel or urinary habits, bloating, water retention, pelvic or rectal pressure, and unusual fatigue, irritability, or depression.

Then obtain a menstrual and sexual history. Ask the patient if her menstrual flow is heavy or scant. Have her describe vaginal discharge between menses. Does she experience pain during sexual intercourse? Does it occur with menses? Find out what relieves her cramps. Does she take pain medication? Is it effective? Note her method of contraception, and ask about a history of pelvic infection. Does she have signs and symptoms of urinary system obstruction, such as pyuria, urine retention, or incontinence? Determine how she copes with stress. Determine her risk of sexually transmitted diseases.

Next, perform a focused physical examination. Take the patient's vital signs, noting fever and accompanying chills. Inspect the abdomen for distention, and palpate for tenderness and masses. Note costovertebral angle tenderness.

Medical causes

Adenomyosis. In adenomyosis, endometrial tissue invades the myometrium, resulting in severe dysmenorrhea with pain radiating to the back or rectum, menorrhagia, and a symmetrically enlarged, globular uterus that's usually softer on palpation than a uterine myoma.

Cervical stenosis. Cervical stenosis causes dysmenorrhea and scant or absent menstrual flow.

Endometriosis. Endometriosis typically produces steady, aching pain that begins before menses and peaks at the height of menstrual flow; however, the pain may also occur between menstrual periods. The pain may arise at the endometrial deposit site or may radiate to the perineum or rectum. Associated signs and symptoms include premenstrual spotting, dyspareunia, infertility, nausea and vomiting, painful defecation, and rectal bleeding and hematuria during menses. A tender, fixed adnexal mass is usually palpable on bimanual examination.

Pelvic inflammatory disease. Chronic uterine infection produces dysmenorrhea accompanied by a fever; malaise; foul-smelling, purulent vaginal discharge; menorrhagia; dyspareunia; severe abdominal pain; nausea and vomiting; and diarrhea. A pelvic examination may reveal cervical motion tenderness and bilateral adnexal tenderness.

PMS. The cramping pain of PMS usually begins with menstrual flow and persists for several hours or days, diminishing with decreasing flow. Common associated effects precede menses by several days to 2 weeks: abdominal bloating, breast tenderness, palpitations, diaphoresis, flushing, depression, and irritability. Other findings include nausea, vomiting, diarrhea, and a headache. Because PMS usually follows an ovulatory cycle, it rarely occurs during the first 12 months of menses, which may be anovulatory.

Primary (idiopathic) dysmenorrhea. Increased prostaglandin secretion intensifies uterine contractions, apparently causing mild to severe spasmodic cramping pain in the lower abdomen, which radiates to the sacrum and inner thighs. The cramping abdominal pain peaks a few hours before menses. Patients may also experience nausea and vomiting, fatigue, diarrhea, and a headache.

Uterine leiomyomas. If these tumors twist or degenerate after circulatory occlusion or infection or if the uterus con-

Relief for dysmenorrhea

To relieve cramping and other symptoms caused by primary dysmenorrhea or an intrauterine device, the patient may receive a prostaglandin inhibitor, such as aspirin, ibuprofen, indomethacin, or naproxen. These nonsteroidal anti-inflammatory drugs block prostaglandin synthesis early in the inflammatory reaction, thereby inhibiting prostaglandin action at receptor sites. These drugs also have analgesic and antipyretic effects.

Make sure that you and the patient are informed about the adverse effects and cautions associated with these drugs.

Adverse effects

Alert the patient to possible adverse effects of prostaglandin inhibitors. Central nervous system effects include dizziness, a headache, and vision disturbances. GI effects include nausea, vomiting, heartburn, and diarrhea. Advise the patient to take the drug with milk or after meals to reduce gastric irritation.

Contraindications

Because prostaglandin inhibitors are potentially teratogenic, make sure to rule out the possibility of pregnancy before starting therapy. Advise the patient who suspects she's pregnant to delay therapy until menses begins.

Other cautions

If the patient has cardiac decompensation, hypertension, renal dysfunction, an ulcer, or a coagulation defect (and receiving ongoing anticoagulant therapy), use caution when administering a prostaglandin inhibitor. Because a patient who's hypersensitive to aspirin may also be hypersensitive to other prostaglandin inhibitors, watch for signs of gastric ulceration and bleeding.

---

tracts in an attempt to expel them, the tumors may cause constant or intermittent lower abdominal pain that worsens with menses. Associated signs and symptoms include backache, constipation, menorrhagia, and urinary frequency or retention. Palpation may reveal the tumor mass and an enlarged uterus. The tumors are almost always nontender.

Other causes

Intrauterine devices (IUDs). IUDs may cause severe cramping and heavy menstrual flow.

Nursing considerations

- Assess the patient's level of discomfort and use pharmacologic and nonpharmacologic methods to relieve discomfort.

Patient teaching

- Encourage the patient to view dysmenorrhea as a medical problem—not as a sign of maladjustment—and explain her treatment options. (See *Relief for dysmenorrhea.*)
- Explain the cause of the patient's dysmenorrhea once a diagnosis is established.

 # Dyspepsia

Dyspepsia refers to an uncomfortable fullness after meals that's associated with nausea, belching, heartburn and, possibly, cramping and abdominal distention. Frequently aggravated by spicy, fatty, or high-fiber foods and by excess caffeine intake, dyspepsia without another disorder indicates impaired digestive function.

Dyspepsia is caused by GI disorders and, to a lesser extent, by cardiac, pulmonary, and renal disorders and the effects of drugs. It apparently results when altered gastric secretions lead to excess stomach acidity. This symptom may also result from emotional upset and overly rapid eating or improper chewing. It usually occurs a few hours after eating and lasts for a variable period. Its severity depends on the amount and type of food eaten and on GI motility. Additional food or an antacid may relieve the discomfort.

History and physical examination

If the patient complains of dyspepsia, begin by asking him to describe it in detail. How often and when does it occur, specifically in relation to meals? Do drugs or activities relieve or aggravate it? Has he had nausea, vomiting, melena, hematemesis, a cough, or chest pain? Ask if he's taking prescription drugs and if he has recently had surgery. Does he have a history of renal, cardiovascular, or pulmonary disease? Has he noticed a change in the amount or color of his urine?

Ask the patient if he's experiencing an unusual or overwhelming amount of emotional stress. Determine the patient's coping mechanisms and their effectiveness.

Focus the physical examination on the abdomen. Inspect for distention, ascites, scars, obvious hernias, jaundice, uremic frost, and bruising. Then auscultate for bowel sounds and characterize their motility. Palpate and percuss the abdomen, noting tenderness, pain, organ enlargement, or tympany.

Finally, examine other body systems. Ask about behavior changes, and evaluate the patient's level of consciousness. Auscultate for gallops and crackles. Percuss the lungs to detect consolidation.

Note peripheral edema and any swelling of the lymph nodes.

Medical causes

Cholelithiasis. Dyspepsia may occur with gallstones, usually after eating fatty foods. Biliary colic, a more common symptom of gallstones, causes acute pain that may radiate to the back, shoulders, and chest. The patient may also have diaphoresis, tachycardia, chills, a low-grade fever, petechiae, bleeding tendencies, jaundice with pruritus, dark urine, and clay-colored stools.

Cirrhosis. With cirrhosis, dyspepsia varies in intensity and duration and is relieved by taking an antacid. Other GI effects are anorexia, nausea, vomiting, flatulence, diarrhea, constipation, abdominal distention, and epigastric or right upper quadrant pain. Weight loss, jaundice, hepatomegaly, ascites, dependent edema, a fever, bleeding tendencies, and muscle weakness are also common. Skin changes include severe pruritus, extreme dryness, easy bruising, and lesions, such as telangiectasis and palmar erythema. Gynecomastia or testicular atrophy may also occur.

Duodenal ulcer. A primary symptom of a duodenal ulcer, dyspepsia ranges from a vague feeling of fullness or pressure to a boring or aching sensation in the middle or right epigastrium. It usually occurs $1\frac{1}{2}$ to 3 hours after a meal and is relieved by eating food or taking an antacid. The pain may awaken the patient at night with heartburn and fluid regurgitation. Abdominal tenderness and weight gain may occur; vomiting and anorexia are rare.

Gastric dilation (acute). Epigastric fullness is an early symptom of gastric dilation, a life-threatening disorder. Accompanying dyspepsia are nausea and vomiting, upper abdominal distention, succussion splash, and apathy. The patient may display signs and symptoms of dehydration, such as poor tissue turgor and dry mucous membranes, and of electrolyte imbalance, such as an irregular pulse and muscle weakness. Gastric bleeding may produce hematemesis and melena.

Gastric ulcer. Typically, dyspepsia and heartburn after eating occur early in gastric ulcer. The cardinal symptom, however, is epigastric pain that may occur with vomiting, fullness, and abdominal distention and may not be relieved by eating food. Weight loss and GI bleeding are also characteristic.

Gastritis (chronic). With chronic gastritis, dyspepsia is relieved by antacids; lessened by smaller, more frequent meals; and aggravated by spicy foods or excessive caffeine. It occurs with anorexia, a feeling of fullness, vague epigastric pain, belching, nausea, and vomiting.

GI cancer. GI cancer usually produces chronic dyspepsia. Other features include anorexia, fatigue, jaundice, melena, hematemesis, constipation, and abdominal pain.

Heart failure. Common with right-sided heart failure, transient dyspepsia may occur with chest tightness and a constant ache or sharp pain in the right upper quadrant. Heart failure also typically causes hepatomegaly, anorexia, nausea, vomiting, bloating, ascites, tachycardia, jugular vein distention, tachypnea, dyspnea, and orthopnea. Other findings include dependent edema, anxiety, fatigue, diaphoresis, hypotension, a cough, crackles, ventricular and atrial gallops, nocturia, diastolic hypertension, and cool, pale skin.

Hepatitis. Dyspepsia occurs in two of the three stages of hepatitis. The preicteric phase produces moderate to severe dyspepsia, a fever, malaise, arthralgia, coryza, myalgia, nausea, vomiting, an altered sense of taste or smell, and hepatomegaly. Jaundice marks the onset of the icteric phase, along with contin-

ued dyspepsia and anorexia, irritability, and severe pruritus. As jaundice clears, dyspepsia and other GI effects also diminish. In the recovery phase, only fatigue remains.

Hiatal hernia. Dyspepsia is a result of the lower portion of the esophagus and the upper portion of the stomach rising into the chest when abdominal pressure increases.

Pulmonary embolism. Sudden dyspnea characterizes pulmonary embolism, a potentially fatal disorder; however, dyspepsia may occur as an oppressive, severe, substernal discomfort. Other findings include anxiety, tachycardia, tachypnea, a cough, pleuritic chest pain, hemoptysis, syncope, cyanosis, jugular vein distention, and hypotension.

Pulmonary tuberculosis. Vague dyspepsia may occur along with anorexia, malaise, and weight loss. Common associated findings include a high fever, night sweats, palpitations on mild exertion, a productive cough, dyspnea, adenopathy, and occasional hemoptysis.

Uremia. Of the many GI complaints associated with uremia, dyspepsia may be the earliest and most important. Others include anorexia, nausea, vomiting, bloating, diarrhea, abdominal cramps, epigastric pain, and weight gain. As the renal system deteriorates, the patient may experience edema, pruritus, pallor, hyperpigmentation, uremic frost, ecchymoses, sexual dysfunction, poor memory, irritability, headache, drowsiness, muscle twitching, seizures, and oliguria.

Other causes

Drugs. Nonsteroidal anti-inflammatory drugs, especially aspirin, commonly cause dyspepsia. Diuretics, antibiotics, antihypertensives, corticosteroids, and many other drugs can cause dyspepsia, depending on the patient's tolerance of the dosage.

Surgery. After GI or other surgery, postoperative gastritis can cause dyspepsia, which usually disappears in a few weeks.

Nursing considerations

▪ Give an antacid 30 minutes before or 1 hour after a meal.
▪ Provide food to relieve dyspepsia.
▪ Because various drugs can cause dyspepsia, give these after meals or with food, if possible.
▪ Provide a calm environment to reduce stress, and make sure that the patient gets plenty of rest.
▪ Prepare the patient for endoscopy to evaluate the cause of dyspepsia.

Patient teaching

▪ Discuss stress reduction techniques, such as deep breathing and guided imagery.
▪ Discuss the importance of small, frequent meals.
▪ Explain to the patient his diagnosis and the treatment plan.

▌Dysphagia

Dysphagia—difficulty swallowing—is a common symptom that's usually easy to localize. It may be constant or intermittent and is classified by the phase of swallowing it affects. (See *Classifying dysphagia.*)

Among the factors that interfere with swallowing are severe pain, obstruction, abnormal peristalsis, an impaired gag reflex, and excessive, scanty, or thick oral secretions.

Dysphagia is the most common— and sometimes the *only*—symptom of esophageal disorders. However, it may also result from oropharyngeal, respiratory, neurologic, and collagen disorders or from the effects of toxins and treatments. Dysphagia increases the risk of

choking and aspiration and may lead to malnutrition and dehydration.

ACTION STAT!

 If the patient suddenly complains of dysphagia and displays signs of respiratory distress, such as dyspnea and stridor, suspect an airway obstruction and quickly perform abdominal thrusts. Prepare to administer oxygen by mask or nasal cannula, or to assist with endotracheal intubation.

History and physical examination

If the patient's dysphagia doesn't suggest an airway obstruction, begin a health history. Ask the patient if swallowing is painful. If so, is the pain constant or intermittent? Have the patient point to where dysphagia feels most intense. Does eating alleviate or aggravate the symptom? Are solids or liquids more difficult to swallow? If the answer is liquids, ask if hot, cold, and lukewarm fluids affect him differently. Does the symptom disappear after he tries to swallow a few times? Is swallowing easier if he changes position? Ask if he has recently experienced vomiting, regurgitation, weight loss, anorexia, hoarseness, dyspnea, or a cough.

To evaluate the patient's swallowing reflex, place your finger along his thyroid notch and instruct him to swallow. If you feel his larynx rise, the reflex is intact. Next, have him cough to assess his cough reflex. Check his gag reflex if you're sure he has a good swallow or cough reflex. Listen closely to his speech for signs of muscle weakness. Does he have aphasia or dysarthria? Is his voice nasal, hoarse, or breathy? Assess the patient's mouth carefully. Check for dry mucous membranes and thick, sticky secretions. Observe for tongue and facial

Classifying dysphagia

Because swallowing occurs in three distinct phases, dysphagia can be classified by the phase that it affects. Each phase suggests a specific disorder associated with dysphagia.

Phase 1
Swallowing begins in the transfer phase with chewing and moistening of food with saliva. The tongue presses against the hard palate to transfer the chewed food to the back of the throat; cranial nerve V then stimulates the swallowing reflex. Phase 1 dysphagia typically results from a neuromuscular disorder.

Phase 2
In the transport phase, the soft palate closes against the pharyngeal wall to prevent nasal regurgitation. At the same time, the larynx rises and the vocal cords close to keep food out of the lungs; breathing stops momentarily as the throat muscles constrict to move food into the esophagus. Phase 2 dysphagia usually indicates spasm or cancer.

Phase 3
Peristalsis and gravity work together in the entrance phase to move food through the esophageal sphincter and into the stomach. Phase 3 dysphagia results from lower esophageal narrowing by diverticula, esophagitis, and other disorders.

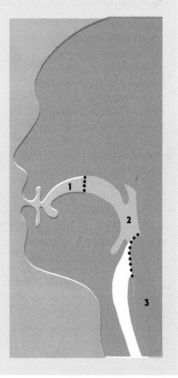

weakness and obvious obstructions (for example, enlarged tonsils). Assess the patient for disorientation, which may make him neglect to swallow.

Medical causes
Achalasia. Achalasia produces phase 3 dysphagia for solids and liquids. The dysphagia develops gradually and may be precipitated or exacerbated by stress. Occasionally, it's preceded by esophageal colic. Regurgitation of undigested food, especially at night, may cause wheezing, coughing, or choking as well as halitosis. Weight loss, cachexia, hematemesis and, possibly, heartburn are late findings.

Airway obstruction. Life-threatening upper airway obstruction is marked by signs of respiratory distress, such as crowing and stridor. Phase 2 dysphagia occurs with gagging and dysphonia. When hemorrhage obstructs the trachea, dysphagia is usually painless and rapid in onset. When inflammation causes the obstruction, dysphagia may be painful and develop slowly.

Amyotrophic lateral sclerosis (ALS). Besides dysphagia, ALS causes muscle weakness and atrophy, fasciculations, dysarthria, dyspnea, shallow respirations, tachypnea, slurred speech, hyperactive deep tendon reflexes (DTRs), and emotional lability.

Bulbar paralysis. Phase 1 dysphagia occurs along with drooling, difficulty chewing, dysarthria, and nasal regurgitation. Dysphagia for solids and liquids is painful and progressive. Accompanying features may include arm and leg spasticity, hyperreflexia, and emotional lability.

Esophageal cancer. Phases 2 and 3 dysphagia is the earliest and most common symptom of esophageal cancer. Typically, this painless, progressive symptom is accompanied by rapid weight loss. As the cancer advances, dysphagia becomes painful and constant. In addition, the patient complains of steady chest pain, a cough with hemoptysis, hoarseness, and a sore throat. He may also develop nausea and vomiting, a fever, hiccups, hematemesis, melena, and halitosis.

Esophageal compression (external). Usually caused by a dilated carotid or aortic aneurysm, esophageal compression—a rare condition—causes phase 3 dysphagia as the primary symptom. Other features depend on the cause of the compression.

Esophageal diverticulum. Esophageal diverticulum causes phase 3 dysphagia when the enlarged diverticulum obstructs the esophagus. Associated signs and symptoms include food regurgitation, a chronic cough, hoarseness, chest pain, and halitosis.

Esophageal obstruction by foreign body. Sudden onset of phase 2 or 3 dysphagia, gagging, coughing, and esophageal pain characterize this potentially life-threatening condition. Dyspnea may occur if the obstruction compresses the trachea.

Esophageal spasm. The most striking symptoms of esophageal spasm are phase 2 dysphagia for solids and liquids and a dull or squeezing substernal chest pain. The pain may last up to an hour and may radiate to the neck, arm, back, or jaw; however, it may be relieved by drinking a glass of water. Bradycardia may also occur.

Esophageal stricture. Usually caused by a chemical ingestion or scar tissue, esophageal stricture causes phase 3 dysphagia. Drooling, tachypnea, and gagging may also be evident.

Esophagitis. *Corrosive esophagitis,* resulting from ingestion of alkali or acids, causes severe phase 3 dysphagia. Accompanying it are marked salivation, hematemesis, tachypnea, a fever, and intense pain in the mouth and anterior chest that's aggravated by swallowing. Signs of shock, such as hypotension and tachycardia, may also occur.

Candidal esophagitis causes phase 2 dysphagia, a sore throat and, possibly, retrosternal pain on swallowing. With *reflux esophagitis,* phase 3 dysphagia is a late symptom that usually accompanies stricture development. The patient complains of heartburn, which is aggravated by strenuous exercise, bending over, or lying down and is relieved by sitting up or taking an antacid.

Other features of esophagitis include regurgitation; frequent, effortless vomiting; a dry, nocturnal cough; and substernal chest pain that may mimic angina pectoris. If the esophagus ulcerates, signs of bleeding, such as melena and hematemesis, may occur along with weakness and fatigue.

Gastric carcinoma. Infiltration of the cardia or esophagus by gastric carcinoma causes phase 3 dysphagia along with nausea, vomiting, and pain that may radiate to the neck, back, or retrosternum. In addition, perforation causes massive bleeding with coffee-ground vomitus or melena.

Laryngeal cancer (extrinsic). Phase 2 dysphagia and dyspnea develop late in laryngeal cancer. Accompanying features include a muffled voice, stridor, pain, halitosis, weight loss, ipsilateral otalgia, a chronic cough, and cachexia. Palpation reveals enlarged cervical nodes.

Lead poisoning. Painless, progressive dysphagia may result from lead poisoning. Related findings include a lead line on the gums, a metallic taste, papilledema, ocular palsy, footdrop or wristdrop, and signs of hemolytic anemia, such as abdominal pain and a fever. The patient may be depressed and display severe mental impairment and seizures.

Myasthenia gravis. Fatigue and progressive muscle weakness characterize myasthenia gravis and account for painless phase 1 dysphagia and possibly choking. Typically, dysphagia follows ptosis and diplopia. Other features include masklike facies, a nasal voice, frequent nasal regurgitation, and head bobbing. Shallow respirations and dyspnea may occur with respiratory muscle weakness. Signs and symptoms worsen during menses and with exposure to stress, cold, or infection.

Oral cavity tumor. Painful phase 1 dysphagia develops along with hoarseness and ulcerating lesions.

Plummer-Vinson syndrome. Plummer-Vinson syndrome causes phase 3 dysphagia for solids in some women with severe iron deficiency anemia. Related features include upper esophageal pain; atrophy of the oral or pharyngeal mucous membranes; tooth loss; a smooth, red, sore tongue; a dry mouth; chills; inflamed lips; spoon-shaped nails; pallor; and splenomegaly.

Rabies. Severe phase 2 dysphagia for liquids results from painful pharyngeal muscle spasms occurring late in this rare, life-threatening disorder. In fact, the patient may become dehydrated and possibly apneic. Dysphagia also causes drooling, and in 50% of cases it's responsible for hydrophobia. Eventually, rabies causes progressive flaccid paraly-sis that leads to peripheral vascular collapse, coma, and death.

Systemic lupus erythematosus (SLE). SLE may cause progressive phase 2 dysphagia. However, its primary signs and symptoms include nondeforming arthritis, a characteristic butterfly rash, and photosensitivity.

Tetanus. Phase 1 dysphagia usually develops about 1 week after the patient receives a puncture wound. Other characteristics include marked muscle hypertonicity, hyperactive DTRs, tachycardia, diaphoresis, drooling, and a low-grade fever. Painful, involuntary muscle spasms account for lockjaw (trismus), risus sardonicus, opisthotonos, board-like abdominal rigidity, and intermittent tonic seizures.

Other causes
Procedures. Recent tracheostomy or repeated or prolonged endotracheal intubation may cause temporary dysphagia.

Radiation therapy. When directed against oral cancer, this therapy may cause scant salivation and temporary dysphagia.

Nursing considerations
- Stimulate salivation by talking with the patient about food, adding a lemon slice or dill pickle to his tray, and providing mouth care before and after meals.
- Moisten his food with a little liquid if the patient has decreased salivation.
- Administer an anticholinergic or antiemetic to control excess salivation.
- If the patient has a weak or absent cough reflex, begin tube feedings.
- Consult with the dietitian to select foods with distinct temperatures and textures.
- Consult with a speech therapist to assess the patient for his aspiration risk and for swallowing exercises to help decrease his risk.

■ When feeding the patient, place him in an upright position, and have him flex his neck forward slightly and keep his chin at midline.

■ Instruct the patient to swallow multiple times before taking the next bite or sip.

■ Separate solids from liquids, which are harder to swallow.

■ Prepare the patient for diagnostic evaluation, including endoscopy, esophageal manometry, esophagography, and the esophageal acidity test, to pinpoint the cause of dysphagia.

Patient teaching

■ Tell the patient which foods and textures he should avoid.

■ Explain measures to take to reduce the risk of choking and aspiration.

■ Explain to the patient his diagnosis and the treatment plan.

Dyspnea

Typically a symptom of cardiopulmonary dysfunction, dyspnea is the sensation of difficult or uncomfortable breathing. It's usually reported as shortness of breath. Its severity varies greatly and is usually unrelated to the severity of the underlying cause. Dyspnea may arise suddenly or slowly and may subside rapidly or persist for years.

Most people normally experience dyspnea when they exert themselves, and its severity depends on their physical condition. In a healthy person, dyspnea is quickly relieved by rest. Pathologic causes of dyspnea include pulmonary, cardiac, neuromuscular, and allergic disorders. It may also be caused by anxiety.

<small>ACTION STAT!</small>

 If a patient complains of shortness of breath, quickly look for signs of respiratory distress, such as tachypnea, cyanosis, restlessness, and accessory muscle use. Prepare to administer oxygen by nasal cannula, mask, or endotracheal tube. Ensure patent I.V. access, and begin cardiac monitoring and oxygen saturation monitoring to detect arrhythmias and low oxygen saturation, respectively. Expect to insert a chest tube for severe pneumothorax.

History and physical examination

If the patient can answer questions without increasing his distress, take a complete history. Ask if the shortness of breath began suddenly or gradually. Is it constant or intermittent? Does it occur during activity or while at rest? If the patient has had dyspneic attacks before, ask if they're increasing in severity. Can he identify what aggravates or alleviates these attacks? Does he have a productive or nonproductive cough or chest pain? Ask about recent trauma, and note a history of upper respiratory tract infection, deep vein phlebitis, or other disorders. Ask the patient if he smokes or is exposed to toxic fumes or irritants on the job. Find out if he also has orthopnea, paroxysmal nocturnal dyspnea, or progressive fatigue.

During the physical examination, look for signs of chronic dyspnea such as accessory muscle hypertrophy (especially in the shoulders and neck). Also look for pursed-lip exhalation, clubbing, peripheral edema, barrel chest, diaphoresis, and jugular vein distention.

Check blood pressure and auscultate for crackles, abnormal heart sounds or rhythms, egophony, bronchophony, and whispered pectoriloquy. Finally, palpate the abdomen for hepatomegaly, and assess the patient for edema.

Medical causes

Acute respiratory distress syndrome (ARDS). ARDS is a life-threatening form of noncardiogenic pulmonary edema that usually produces acute dyspnea as the first complaint. Progressive respiratory distress then develops with restlessness, anxiety, decreased mental acuity, tachycardia, and crackles and rhonchi in both lung fields. Other findings include cyanosis, tachypnea, motor dysfunction, and intercostal and suprasternal retractions. Severe ARDS can produce signs of shock, such as hypotension and cool, clammy skin.

Amyotrophic lateral sclerosis (ALS). ALS causes the slow onset of dyspnea that worsens with time. Other features include dysphagia, dysarthria, muscle weakness and atrophy, fasciculations, shallow respirations, tachypnea, and emotional lability.

Anthrax (inhalation). Dyspnea is a symptom of the second stage of anthrax, along with a fever, stridor, and hypotension (the patient usually dies within 24 hours). Initial symptoms of this disorder, which are due to the inhalation of aerosolized spores (from infected animals or as a result of bioterrorism) from the bacterium *Bacillus anthracis,* are flulike and include a fever, chills, weakness, a cough, and chest pain.

Aspiration of a foreign body. Acute dyspnea marks this life-threatening condition, along with paroxysmal intercostal, suprasternal, and substernal retractions. The patient may also display accessory muscle use, inspiratory stridor, tachypnea, decreased or absent breath sounds, possibly asymmetrical chest expansion, anxiety, cyanosis, diaphoresis, and hypotension.

Asthma. Acute dyspneic attacks occur with asthma, along with audible wheezing, a dry cough, accessory muscle use, nasal flaring, intercostal and supraclavicular retractions, tachypnea,

tachycardia, diaphoresis, prolonged expiration, flushing or cyanosis, and apprehension. Medications that block beta receptors can exacerbate asthma attacks.

Avian influenza. These potentially life-threatening viruses are spread to humans through contact with infected poultry or surfaces contaminated with infected bird excretions. Within 1 to 5 days of exposure to avian influenza, the patient typically develops flulike symptoms, such as fever, sore throat, cough, and muscle aches. Those with severe forms of the virus may develop dyspnea caused by acute respiratory distress or pneumonia.

Blast lung injury. The result of a forceful percussive wave following an explosive detonation, blast lung injury is commonly characterized by dyspnea and hypoxia. Worldwide terrorist activity has recently increased the incidence of this condition, which may also cause cyanosis, chest pain, wheezing, and hemoptysis. Chest X-ray, the primary diagnostic tool, reveals a characteristic "butterfly" pattern. Many of these patients suffer concomitant injuries and require complex management, usually in an intensive care setting.

Cor pulmonale. With cor pulmonale, chronic dyspnea begins gradually with exertion and progressively worsens until it occurs even at rest. Underlying cardiac or pulmonary disease is usually present. The patient may have a chronic productive cough, wheezing, tachypnea, jugular vein distention, dependent edema, and hepatomegaly. He may also experience increasing fatigue, weakness, and light-headedness.

Emphysema. Emphysema is a chronic disorder that gradually causes progressive exertional dyspnea. A history of smoking, an alpha$_1$-antitrypsin deficiency, or exposure to an occupational or environmental irritant usually accompanies barrel chest, accessory muscle hypertrophy, diminished breath sounds, anorexia, weight loss, malaise, peripheral cyanosis, tachypnea, pursed-lip breathing, prolonged expiration and, possibly, a chronic productive cough. Clubbing is a late sign.

Flail chest. Sudden dyspnea results from multiple rib fractures and is accompanied by paradoxical chest movement, severe chest pain, hypotension, tachypnea, tachycardia, and cyanosis. Bruising and decreased or absent breath sounds occur over the affected side.

Heart failure. Dyspnea usually develops gradually in patients with heart failure. Chronic paroxysmal nocturnal dyspnea, orthopnea, tachypnea, tachycardia, palpitations, a ventricular gallop, fatigue, dependent peripheral edema, hepatomegaly, a dry cough, weight gain, and loss of mental acuity may occur. With acute onset, heart failure may produce jugular vein distention, bibasilar rates, oliguria, and hypotension.

Inhalation injury. Dyspnea may develop suddenly or gradually over several hours after the inhalation of chemicals or hot gases. Increasing hoarseness, a persistent cough, sooty or bloody sputum, and oropharyngeal edema may also be present. The patient may also exhibit thermal burns, singed nasal hairs, and orofacial burns as well as crackles, rhonchi, wheezing, and signs of respiratory distress.

Monkeypox. Dyspnea is one of the less common symptoms of this rare viral disease. Infected individuals may also experience fever, muscle aches, sore throat, chills, and lymphadenopathy. A papular rash appears 1 to 3 days after the fever begins. The virus is similar to smallpox; however, the symptoms are milder and the disease is rarely fatal in developed countries.

Myasthenia gravis. Myasthenia gravis causes bouts of dyspnea as the respiratory muscles weaken. With myas-

thenic crisis, acute respiratory distress may occur, with shallow respirations and tachypnea.

Myocardial infarction. Sudden dyspnea occurs with crushing substernal chest pain that may radiate to the back, neck, jaw, and arms. Other signs and symptoms include nausea, vomiting, diaphoresis, vertigo, hypertension or hypotension, tachycardia, anxiety, and pale, cool, clammy skin.

Plague (Yersinia pestis). Among the symptoms of the pneumonic form of plague are dyspnea, a productive cough, chest pain, tachypnea, hemoptysis, increasing respiratory distress, and cardiopulmonary insufficiency. The onset of this virulent infection is usually sudden and includes such signs and symptoms as chills, fever, headache, and myalgia. If untreated, plague is one of the most potentially lethal diseases known.

Pleural effusion. With pneumonia, yspnea develops slowly and becomes progressively worse with pleural effusion. Initial findings include a pleural friction rub accompanied by pleuritic pain that worsens with coughing or deep breathing. Other findings include a dry cough; dullness on percussion; egophony, bronchophony, and whispered pectoriloquy; tachycardia; tachypnea; weight loss; and decreased chest motion, tactile fremitus, and decreased breath sounds. With infection, a fever may occur.

Pneumonia. With pneumonia, dyspnea occurs suddenly, usually accompanied by a fever, shaking chills, pleuritic chest pain that worsens with deep inspiration, and a productive cough. Fatigue, a headache, myalgia, anorexia, abdominal pain, crackles, rhonchi, tachycardia, tachypnea, cyanosis, decreased breath sounds, and diaphoresis may also occur.

Pneumothorax. Pneumothorax is a life-threatening disorder that causes acute dyspnea unrelated to the severity of the pain. Sudden, stabbing chest pain may radiate to the arms, face, back, or abdomen. Other signs and symptoms include anxiety, restlessness, a dry cough, cyanosis, decreased vocal fremitus, tachypnea, tympany, decreased or absent breath sounds on the affected side, asymmetrical chest expansion, splinting, and accessory muscle use. In patients with tension pneumothorax, tracheal deviation occurs in addition to these typical findings. Decreased blood pressure and tachycardia may also occur.

Poliomyelitis (bulbar). Dyspnea develops gradually and progressively worsens. Additional signs and symptoms include a fever, facial weakness, dysphasia, hypoactive deep tendon reflexes, decreased mental acuity, dysphagia, nasal regurgitation, and hypopnea.

Pulmonary edema. Commonly preceded by signs of heart failure, such as jugular vein distention and orthopnea, pulmonary edema—a life-threatening disorder—causes acute dyspnea. Other features include tachycardia, tachypnea, crackles in both lung fields, a third heart sound (S₃ gallop), oliguria, a thready pulse, hypotension, diaphoresis, cyanosis, and marked anxiety. The patient's cough may be dry or may produce copious amounts of pink, frothy sputum.

Pulmonary embolism. Acute dyspnea that's usually accompanied by sudden pleuritic chest pain characterizes pulmonary embolism, a life-threatening disorder. Related findings include tachycardia, a low-grade fever, tachypnea, a nonproductive or productive cough with blood-tinged sputum, a pleural friction rub, crackles, diffuse wheezing, dullness on percussion, decreased breath sounds, diaphoresis, restlessness, and acute anxiety. A massive embolism may cause signs of shock, such as hypotension and cool, clammy skin.

Severe acute respiratory syndrome (SARS). SARS generally begins with a fever (usually greater than 100.4° F [38° C]). Other symptoms include a headache, malaise, a dry nonproductive cough, and dyspnea. The severity of the illness is highly variable, ranging from mild illness to pneumonia and, in some cases, progressing to respiratory failure and death.

Shock. Dyspnea arises suddenly and worsens progressively with shock, a life-threatening disorder. Related findings include severe hypotension, tachypnea, tachycardia, decreased peripheral pulses, decreased mental acuity, restlessness, anxiety, and cool, clammy skin.

Tuberculosis. Dyspnea commonly occurs with chest pain, crackles, and a productive cough. Other findings are night sweats, a fever, anorexia and weight loss, vague dyspepsia, palpitations on mild exertion, and dullness on percussion.

Tularemia. Also known as *rabbit fever,* tularemia causes dyspnea along with a fever, chills, a headache, generalized myalgia, a nonproductive cough, pleuritic chest pain, and empyema.

Nursing considerations

- Monitor the patient with dyspnea closely.
- Be calm and reassuring to reduce the patient's anxiety.
- Position the patient comfortably, usually high Fowler's or the forward-leaning position.
- Administer oxygen if needed and monitor pulse oximetry.
- Prepare the patient for diagnostic studies, such as arterial blood gas analysis, chest X-rays, and pulmonary function tests.
- Administer a bronchodilator, an antiarrhythmic, a diuretic, and an analgesic, as needed, to dilate bronchioles,

correct cardiac arrhythmias, promote fluid excretion, and relieve pain.

Patient teaching

- Teach the patient pursed-lip breathing, diaphragmatic breathing, and chest splinting.
- Instruct the patient to avoid chemical irritants, pollutants, and people with respiratory infections.
- Explain the underlying causes of his dyspnea and the treatment plan.

Dysuria

Dysuria—painful or difficult urination—is commonly accompanied by urinary frequency, urgency, or hesitancy. This symptom usually reflects lower urinary tract infection (UTI)—a common disorder, especially in women.

Dysuria results from lower urinary tract irritation or inflammation, which stimulates nerve endings in the bladder and urethra. The onset of pain provides clues to its cause. For example, pain just before voiding usually indicates bladder irritation or distention, whereas pain at the start of urination typically results from bladder outlet irritation. Pain at the end of voiding may signal bladder spasms; in women, it may indicate vaginal candidiasis.

History and physical examination

If the patient complains of dysuria, have him describe its severity and location. When did he first notice it? Did anything precipitate it? Does anything aggravate or alleviate it?

Next, ask about previous urinary or genital tract infections. Has the patient recently undergone an invasive procedure, such as cystoscopy or urethral dilatation, or had a urinary catheter placed? Also ask if he has a history of intestinal disease. Ask the female patient about menstrual disorders and the use of products that irritate the urinary tract, such as bubble bath salts, feminine deodorants, contraceptive gels, or perineal lotions. Also ask her about vaginal discharge or pruritus.

During the physical examination, inspect the urethral meatus for discharge, irritation, or other abnormalities. A pelvic or rectal examination may be necessary.

Medical causes

Appendicitis. Occasionally, appendicitis causes dysuria that persists throughout voiding and is accompanied by bladder tenderness. Appendicitis is characterized by periumbilical abdominal pain that shifts to McBurney's point, anorexia, nausea, vomiting, constipation, a slight fever, abdominal rigidity and rebound tenderness, and tachycardia.

Bladder cancer. Bladder cancer, a predominantly male disorder, causes dysuria throughout voiding—a late symptom associated with urinary frequency and urgency, nocturia, hematuria, and perineal, back, or flank pain.

Cystitis. Dysuria throughout voiding is common in all types of cystitis, as are urinary frequency, nocturia, straining to void, and hematuria. Bacterial cystitis, the most common cause of dysuria in women, may also produce urinary urgency, perineal and lower back pain, suprapubic discomfort, fatigue and, possibly, a low-grade fever. With chronic interstitial cystitis, dysuria is accentuated at the end of voiding. In tubercular cystitis, symptoms may also include urinary urgency, flank pain, fatigue, and anorexia. With viral cystitis, severe dysuria occurs with gross hematuria, urinary urgency, and a fever.

Paraurethral gland inflammation. Dysuria throughout voiding occurs with urinary frequency and urgency, a diminished urine stream, mild perineal pain and, occasionally, hematuria.

Prostatitis. Acute prostatitis commonly causes dysuria throughout or toward the end of voiding as well as a diminished urine stream, urinary frequency and urgency, hematuria, suprapubic fullness, a fever, chills, fatigue, myalgia, nausea, vomiting, and constipation. With chronic prostatitis, urethral narrowing causes dysuria throughout voiding. Related effects are urinary frequency and urgency; a diminished urine stream; perineal, back, and buttock pain; urethral discharge; nocturia; and, at times, hematospermia and ejaculatory pain.

Pyelonephritis (acute). Pyelonephritis causes dysuria throughout voiding. Other features include a persistent high fever with chills, costovertebral angle tenderness, unilateral or bilateral flank pain, weakness, urinary urgency and frequency, nocturia, straining on urination, and hematuria. Nausea, vomiting, and anorexia may also occur.

Reiter's syndrome. Reiter's syndrome is a disorder in which dysuria occurs 1 or 2 weeks after sexual contact. Initially, the patient has a mucopurulent discharge, urinary urgency and frequency, meatal swelling and redness, suprapubic pain, anorexia, weight loss, and a low-grade fever. Hematuria, conjunctivitis, arthritic symptoms, a papular rash, and oral and penile lesions may follow.

Urinary obstruction. Outflow obstruction by urethral strictures or calculi produces dysuria throughout voiding. (With complete obstruction, bladder distention develops and dysuria precedes voiding.) Other features are a diminished urine stream, urinary frequency and urgency, and a sensation of fullness or bloating in the lower abdomen or groin.

Vaginitis. Characteristically, dysuria occurs throughout voiding as urine touches inflamed or ulcerated labia with vaginitis. Other findings include urinary frequency and urgency, nocturia, hematuria, perineal pain, and vaginal discharge and odor.

Other causes

Chemical irritants. Dysuria may result from irritating substances, such as bubble bath salts and feminine deodorants; it's usually most intense at the end of voiding. Spermicides may cause dysuria in both sexes. Other findings include urinary frequency and urgency, a diminished urine stream and, possibly, hematuria.

Drugs. Dysuria can result from monoamine oxidase inhibitors. Metyrosine can also cause transient dysuria.

Nursing considerations

- Monitor the patient's vital signs and intake and output.
- Administer prescribed drugs.
- Prepare the patient for such tests as urinalysis and cystoscopy.

Patient teaching

- Explain the importance of increased fluid intake.
- Emphasize the importance of frequent urination.
- Teach the patient to perform perineal care.
- Discourage the use of bubble baths and vaginal deodorants.
- Discuss the importance of taking prescribed drugs as instructed.
- Explain to the patient his diagnosis and the treatment plan.

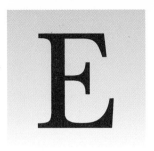

Earache
[Otalgia]

Earaches usually result from disorders of the external and middle ear associated with infection, obstruction, or trauma. Their severity ranges from a feeling of fullness or blockage to deep, boring pain. At times, it may be difficult to determine the precise location of the earache. Earaches can be intermittent or continuous and may develop suddenly or gradually.

History and physical examination

Ask the patient to characterize his earache. How long has he had it? Is it intermittent or continuous? Is it painful or slightly annoying? Can he localize the site of ear pain? Does he have pain in other areas such as the jaw? Does he experience any associated hearing loss?

Ask about recent ear injury or other trauma. Does swimming or showering trigger ear discomfort? Is discomfort associated with itching? If so, find out where the itching is most intense and when it began. Ask about ear drainage and, if present, have the patient characterize it. Does he hear ringing, "swishing," or other noise in his ears? Ask about dizziness or vertigo. Does it worsen when the patient changes position? Does he have difficulty swallowing, hoarseness, neck pain, or pain when he opens his mouth?

Find out if the patient has recently had a head cold or problems with his eyes, mouth, teeth, jaws, sinuses, or throat. Disorders in these areas may refer pain to the ear along the cranial nerves.

Find out if the patient has flown, been to a high-altitude location, or been scuba diving.

Begin your physical examination by inspecting the external ear for redness, drainage, swelling, or deformity. Then apply pressure to the mastoid process and tragus to elicit tenderness. Using an otoscope, examine the external auditory canal for lesions, bleeding or discharge, impacted cerumen, foreign bodies, tenderness, or swelling. Examine the tympanic membrane: Is it intact? Is it pearly gray (normal)? Look for tympanic membrane landmarks: the cone of light, umbo, pars tensa, and the handle and short process of the malleus. (See *Using an otoscope correctly*.) Perform the watch tick, whispered voice, Rinne, and Weber's tests to assess for hearing loss.

Medical causes

Abscess (extradural). Severe earache accompanied by a persistent ipsilateral headache, malaise, and a recurrent mild fever characterizes an abscess, which is a

Using an otoscope correctly

When the patient reports an earache, use an otoscope to inspect ear structures closely. Follow these techniques to obtain the best view and ensure patient safety.

Child younger than age 3

To inspect an infant's or a young child's ear, grasp the *lower part* of the auricle and pull it *down and back* to straighten the upward S curve of the external canal. Then gently insert the speculum into the canal no more than ½″ (1.2 cm).

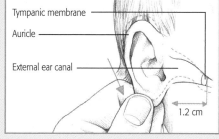

Tympanic membrane
Auricle
External ear canal
1.2 cm

Adult

To inspect an adult's ear, grasp the *upper part* of the auricle and pull it *up and back* to straighten the external canal. Then insert the speculum about 1″ (2.5 cm). Also, use this technique for children ages 3 and older.

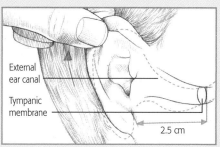

External ear canal
Tympanic membrane
2.5 cm

serious complication of middle ear infection.

Barotrauma (acute). Earache associated with barotrauma ranges from mild pressure to severe pain. Tympanic membrane ecchymosis or bleeding into the tympanic cavity may occur, producing a blue drumhead; the eardrum usually isn't perforated.

Cerumen impaction. Impacted cerumen (earwax) may cause a sensation of blockage or fullness in the ear. Additional features include partial hearing loss, itching and, possibly, dizziness.

Herpes zoster oticus (Ramsay Hunt syndrome). Herpes zoster oticus causes burning or stabbing ear pain, commonly associated with ear vesicles. The patient also complains of hearing loss and vertigo. Associated signs and symptoms include transitory, ipsilateral, facial paralysis; partial loss of taste; tongue vesicles; and nausea and vomiting.

Keratosis obturans. Mild ear pain is common with keratosis obturans, along with otorrhea and tinnitus. Inspection reveals a white glistening plug obstructing the external meatus.

Mastoiditis (acute). Mastoiditis causes a dull ache behind the ear accompanied by a low-grade fever (99° to 100° F [37.2° to 37.8° C]). The eardrum appears dull and edematous and may perforate, and soft tissue near the eardrum may sag. A purulent discharge is seen in the external canal.

Ménière's disease. Ménière's disease is an inner ear disorder that can produce a sensation of fullness in the affected ear. Its classic effects, however, include severe vertigo, tinnitus, and sensorineural hearing loss. The patient may also experience nausea and vomiting, diaphoresis, and nystagmus.

Otitis externa. An earache characterizes acute and malignant otitis externa. *Acute otitis externa* begins with mild to moderate ear pain that occurs with tragus manipulation. The pain may be accompanied by a low-grade fever, sticky yellow or purulent ear discharge, partial hearing loss, and a feeling of blockage. Later, ear pain intensifies, causing the entire side of the head to ache and throb. Fever may reach 104° F (40° C). Examination reveals swelling of the tragus, external meatus, and external canal; eardrum erythema; and lymphadenopathy. The patient also complains of dizziness and malaise.

Malignant otitis externa abruptly causes ear pain that's aggravated by moving the auricle or tragus. The pain is accompanied by intense itching, purulent ear discharge, a fever, parotid gland swelling, and trismus. Examination reveals a swollen external canal with exposed cartilage and temporal bone. Cranial nerve palsy may occur.

Otitis media (acute). Otitis media is middle ear inflammation that may be serous or suppurative. *Acute serous otitis media* may cause a feeling of fullness in the ear, hearing loss, and a vague sensation of top-heaviness. The eardrum may be slightly retracted, amber, and marked by air bubbles and a meniscus, or it may be blue-black from hemorrhage.

Severe, deep, throbbing ear pain; hearing loss; and a fever that may reach 102° F (38.9° C) characterize acute suppurative otitis media. The pain increases steadily over several hours or days and may be aggravated by pressure on the mastoid antrum. Perforation of the eardrum is possible. Before rupture, the eardrum appears bulging and fiery red.

Rupture causes purulent drainage and relieves the pain.

Chronic otitis media usually isn't painful except during exacerbations. Persistent pain and discharge from the ear suggest osteomyelitis of the skull base or cancer.

Nursing considerations
- Administer an analgesic.
- Apply heat to relieve discomfort.
- Instill eardrops if necessary.

Patient teaching
- Teach the patient or the parents how to instill drops if they're prescribed for home use.
- Explain the importance of taking prescribed antibiotics correctly.
- Explain ways to avoid vertigo.
- Instruct the patient and family about ways to avoid ear trauma.
- Explain the cause of the earache once a diagnosis has been established.

Edema, generalized

A common sign in severely ill patients, generalized edema is the excessive accumulation of interstitial fluid throughout the body. Its severity varies widely; slight edema may be difficult to detect, especially if the patient is obese, whereas massive edema is immediately apparent.

Generalized edema is typically chronic and progressive. It may result from cardiac, renal, endocrine, or hepatic disorders as well as from severe burns, malnutrition, or the effects of certain drugs and treatments.

Common factors responsible for edema are hypoalbuminemia and excess sodium ingestion or retention, both of which influence plasma osmotic pressure. (See *Understanding fluid balance.*) Cyclic edema associated with increased aldosterone secretion may occur in premenopausal women.

Understanding fluid balance

Normally, fluid moves freely between the interstitial and intravascular spaces to maintain homeostasis. Four basic pressures control fluid shifts across the capillary membrane that separates these spaces:

■ capillary hydrostatic pressure (the internal fluid pressure on the capillary membrane)

■ interstitial fluid pressure (the external fluid pressure on the capillary membrane)

■ osmotic pressure (the fluid-attracting pressure from protein concentration within the capillary)

■ interstitial osmotic pressure (the fluid-attracting pressure from protein concentration outside the capillary).

Here's how these pressures maintain homeostasis. Normally, capillary hydrostatic pressure is greater than plasma osmotic pressure at the capillary's arterial end, forcing fluid out of the capillary. At the capillary's venous end, the reverse is true: The plasma osmotic pressure is greater than the capillary hydrostatic pressure, drawing fluid into the capillary. Normally, the lymphatic system transports excess interstitial fluid back to the intravascular space.

Edema results when this balance is upset by increased capillary permeability, lymphatic obstruction, persistently increased capillary hydrostatic pressure, decreased plasma osmotic or interstitial fluid pressure, or dilation of precapillary sphincters.

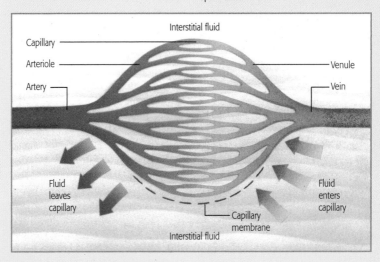

ACTION STAT!

Quickly determine the extent and severity of edema, including the degree of pitting. (See *Edema: Pitting or nonpitting?* page 226.) If the patient has severe edema, promptly take his vital signs, oxygen saturation, and check for jugular vein distention and cyanotic lips. Auscultate the lungs and heart. Be alert for signs of cardiac failure or pulmonary congestion, such as crackles, muffled heart sounds, or a ventricular gallop. Unless the patient is hypotensive, place him in Fowler's position to promote lung expansion. Prepare to administer oxygen and an I.V. diuretic. Have emergency resuscitation equipment nearby.

Edema: Pitting or nonpitting?

To differentiate pitting from nonpitting edema, press your finger against a swollen area for 5 seconds and then quickly remove it.

With pitting edema, pressure forces fluid into the underlying tissues, causing an indentation that slowly fills. To determine the severity of pitting edema, estimate the indentation's depth in centimeters: 1+ (1 cm), 2+ (2 cm), 3+ (3 cm), or 4+ (4 cm).

With nonpitting edema, pressure leaves no indentation because fluid has coagulated in the tissues. Typically, the skin feels unusually tight and firm.

Pitting edema (4+)

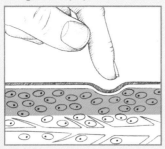

Nonpitting edema

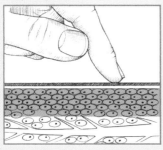

History and physical examination

When the patient's condition permits, obtain a complete medical history. First, note when the edema began. Does it move throughout the course of the day— for example, from the upper extremities to the lower, periorbitally, or within the sacral area? Is the edema worse in the morning or at the end of the day? Is it affected by position changes? Is it accompanied by shortness of breath or pain in the arms or legs? Find out how much weight the patient has gained. Has his urine output changed in quantity or quality?

Next, ask about previous burns or cardiac, renal, hepatic, endocrine, or GI disorders. Have the patient describe his diet so you can determine whether he suffers from protein malnutrition. Explore his drug history, and note recent I.V. therapy.

Begin the physical examination by comparing the patient's arms and legs for symmetrical edema. Also, note ecchymoses and cyanosis. Assess the back, sacrum, and hips of the bedridden patient for dependent edema. Palpate peripheral pulses, noting whether hands and feet feel cold. Finally, perform a complete cardiac and respiratory assessment.

Medical causes

Angioneurotic edema or angioedema. Recurrent attacks of acute, painless, nonpitting edema involving the skin and mucous membranes—especially those of the respiratory tract, face, neck, lips, larynx, hands, feet, genitalia, or viscera—may be the result of a food or drug allergy or emotional stress or they may be hereditary. Abdominal pain, nausea, vomiting, and diarrhea accompany visceral edema; dyspnea and stridor accompany life-threatening laryngeal edema.

Burns. Edema and associated tissue damage vary with the severity of the burn. Severe generalized edema (4+) may occur within 2 days of a major burn; localized edema may occur with a less severe burn.

Heart failure. Severe, generalized pitting edema—occasionally anasarca—may follow leg edema late in this disorder. The edema may improve with exercise or elevation of the limbs and is typically worse at the end of the day. Among other classic late findings are hemoptysis, cyanosis, marked hepatomegaly, clubbing, crackles, and a ventricular gallop. Typically, the patient has tachypnea, palpitations, hypotension, weight gain despite anorexia, nausea, a slowed mental response, diaphoresis, and pallor. Dyspnea, orthopnea, tachycardia, and fatigue typify leftsided heart failure; jugular vein distention, enlarged liver, and peripheral edema typify right-sided heart failure.

Malnutrition. Anasarca in malnutrition may mask dramatic muscle wasting. Malnutrition also typically causes muscle weakness; lethargy; anorexia; diarrhea; apathy; dry, wrinkled skin; and signs of anemia, such as dizziness and pallor.

Myxedema. With myxedema, which is a severe form of hypothyroidism, generalized nonpitting edema is accompanied by dry, flaky, inelastic, waxy, pale skin; a puffy face; and an upper eyelid droop. Observation also reveals mask-like facies, hair loss or coarsening, and psychomotor slowing. Associated findings include hoarseness, weight gain, fatigue, cold intolerance, bradycardia, hypoventilation, constipation, abdominal distention, menorrhagia, impotence, and infertility.

Nephrotic syndrome. Although nephrotic syndrome is characterized by generalized pitting edema, it's initially localized around the eyes. With severe cases, anasarca develops, increasing body weight by up to 50%. Other common signs and symptoms are ascites, anorexia, fatigue, malaise, depression, and pallor.

Pericardial effusion. With pericardial effusion, generalized pitting edema may be most prominent in the arms and legs. It may be accompanied by chest pain, dyspnea, orthopnea, a nonproductive cough, a pericardial friction rub, jugular vein distention, dysphagia, and a fever.

Pericarditis (chronic constrictive). Resembling right-sided heart failure, pericarditis usually begins with pitting edema of the arms and legs that may progress to generalized edema. Other signs and symptoms include ascites, Kussmaul's sign, dyspnea, fatigue, weakness, abdominal distention, and hepatomegaly.

Renal failure. With acute renal failure, generalized pitting edema occurs as a late sign. With chronic renal failure, edema is less likely to become generalized; its severity depends on the degree of fluid overload. Both forms of renal failure cause oliguria, anorexia, nausea and vomiting, drowsiness, confusion, hypertension, dyspnea, crackles, dizziness, and pallor.

Other causes

Drugs. Any drug that causes sodium retention may aggravate or cause generalized edema. Examples include antihypertensives, corticosteroids, androgenic and anabolic steroids, estrogens, and nonsteroidal anti-inflammatory drugs, such as phenylbutazone, ibuprofen, and naproxen.

Treatments. I.V. saline solution infusions and internal feedings may cause sodium and fluid overload, resulting in generalized edema, especially in patients with cardiac or renal disease.

Nursing considerations

■ Position the patient with his limbs above heart level to promote drainage, if the patient can tolerate it.
■ Periodically reposition him to avoid pressure ulcers.
■ If the patient develops dyspnea, lower his limbs, elevate the head of the bed, and administer oxygen.
■ Prevent skin breakdown by placing a pressure mattress on the patient's bed.
■ Restrict fluids and sodium, and administer a diuretic.
■ Monitor the patient's intake and output and daily weight.
■ Monitor serum electrolyte levels—especially sodium and albumin.
■ Prepare the patient for blood and urine tests, X-rays, echocardiography, or an electrocardiogram.

Patient teaching

■ Explain signs and symptoms of edema that the patient should report.
■ Discuss food or fluid restrictions.
■ Explain the underlying cause of the patient's edema and its treatment.

▌Edema of the arm

The result of excess interstitial fluid in the arm, arm edema may be unilateral or bilateral and may develop gradually or abruptly. It may be aggravated by immobility and alleviated by arm elevation and exercise.

Arm edema signals a localized fluid imbalance between the vascular and interstitial spaces. (See *Understanding fluid balance,* page 225.) It commonly results from trauma, venous disorders, toxins, or certain treatments.

A CTION STAT!

 Remove rings, bracelets, and watches from the patient's affected arm. These items may act as a tourniquet. Make sure that the patient's sleeves don't inhibit fluid drainage or blood flow. Elevate the affected extremity.

History and physical examination

When taking the patient's history, one of the first questions to ask is, "How long has your arm been swollen?" Then find out if the patient also has arm pain, numbness, or tingling. Does exercise or arm elevation decrease the edema? Ask about recent arm injury, such as burns or insect stings. Also, note recent I.V. therapy, surgery, or radiation therapy for breast cancer.

Determine the edema's severity by comparing the size and symmetry of both arms. Use a tape measure to determine the exact girth, and mark the location where the measurement was obtained in order to make comparative measurements later. Make sure to note whether the edema is unilateral or bilateral, and test for pitting. (See *Edema: Pitting or nonpitting?* page 226.) Next, examine and compare the color and temperature of both arms. Look for erythema and ecchymoses and for wounds that suggest injury. Palpate and compare radial and brachial pulses. Finally, look for arm tenderness and decreased sensation or mobility. If you detect signs of neurovascular compromise, elevate the arm.

Medical causes

Angioneurotic edema. Angioneurotic edema is a common reaction that's characterized by the sudden onset of painless, nonpruritic edema affecting the hands, feet, eyelids, lips, face, neck, genitalia, or viscera. Although swelling usually doesn't itch, it may burn and tingle. If edema spreads to the larynx, signs of respiratory distress may occur.

Arm trauma. Shortly after a crush injury, severe edema may affect the entire arm. Ecchymoses or superficial bleeding, pain or numbness, and paralysis may occur.

Burns. Two days or less after injury, arm burns may cause mild to severe edema, pain, and tissue damage.

Envenomation. Envenomation by snakes, aquatic animals, or insects initially may cause edema around the bite or sting that quickly spreads to the entire arm. Pain, erythema, and pruritus at the site are common; paresthesia occurs occasionally. Later, the patient may develop generalized signs and symptoms, such as nausea, vomiting, weakness, muscle cramps, a fever, chills, hypotension, a headache and, in severe cases, dyspnea, seizures, and paralysis.

Superior vena cava syndrome. Bilateral arm edema usually progresses slowly and is accompanied by facial and neck edema. Dilated veins mark these edematous areas. The patient also complains of a headache, vertigo, and vision disturbances.

Thrombophlebitis. Thrombophlebitis, which can result from peripherally inserted central catheters and arm portocaths, may cause arm edema, pain, and warmth. Deep vein thrombophlebitis can also produce cyanosis, a fever, chills, and malaise; superficial thrombophlebitis also causes redness, tenderness, and induration along the vein.

Other causes

Treatments. Localized arm edema may result from infiltration of I.V. fluid into the interstitial tissue. A radical or modified radical mastectomy that disrupts lymphatic drainage may cause edema of the entire arm, as can axillary lymph node dissection. Also, radiation therapy for breast cancer may produce arm edema immediately after treatment or months later.

Nursing considerations
- Elevate the arm and frequently reposition the patient.
- Use bandages and dressings as needed to promote drainage.
- Provide meticulous skin care to prevent breakdown and formation of pressure ulcers.
- Administer an analgesic and anticoagulant as needed.

Patient teaching
- Instruct the patient in postoperative arm care.
- Teach the patient arm exercises to prevent lymphedema.
- Explain the underlying cause of the patient's arm edema and its treatment.

■ Edema of the face

Facial edema refers to either localized swelling—around the eyes, for example—or more generalized facial swelling that may extend to the neck and upper arms. Occasionally painful, this sign may develop gradually or abruptly. Sometimes it precedes the onset of peripheral or generalized edema. Mild edema may be difficult to detect; the patient or someone who's familiar with his appearance may report it before it's noticed during assessment.

Facial edema results from disruption of the hydrostatic and osmotic pressures that govern fluid movement between the arteries, veins, and lymphatics. (See *Understanding fluid balance,* page 225.) It may result from venous, inflammatory, and certain systemic disorders; trauma; allergy; malnutrition; or the effects of certain drugs, tests, and treatments.

If the patient has facial edema associated with burns or if he reports recent exposure to an allergen, quickly evaluate his respiratory status. Edema may also affect his upper airway, causing life-threatening obstruction. If you detect audible wheezing, inspiratory stridor, or other signs of respiratory distress, administer epinephrine. For the patient in severe distress—with absent breath sounds and cyanosis—tracheal intubation, cricothyroidotomy, or tracheotomy may be required. Always administer oxygen.

History and physical examination

If the patient isn't in severe distress, take his health history. Ask if facial edema developed suddenly or gradually. Is it more prominent in early morning, or does it worsen throughout the day? Has the patient gained weight? If so, how much and over what length of time? Has he noticed a change in his urine color or output? In his appetite? Take a drug history and ask about recent facial trauma.

Begin the physical examination by characterizing the edema. Is it localized to one part of the face, or does it affect the entire face or other parts of the body? Determine if the edema is pitting or nonpitting, and grade its severity. (See *Edema: Pitting or nonpitting?* page 226.) Next, take the patient's vital signs, and assess his neurologic status. Examine the oral cavity to evaluate dental hygiene and look for signs of infection. Visualize the oropharynx and look for soft-tissue swelling.

Medical causes

Allergic reaction. Facial edema may characterize local allergic reactions and anaphylaxis. With life-threatening anaphylaxis, angioneurotic facial edema may occur with urticaria and flushing. (See *Recognizing angioneurotic edema.*) Airway edema causes hoarseness, stridor, and bronchospasm with dyspnea and tachypnea. Signs of shock, such as hypotension and cool, clammy skin, may also occur. A localized reaction produces facial edema, erythema, and urticaria.

Chalazion. A chalazion causes localized swelling and tenderness of the affected eyelid, accompanied by a small red lump on the conjunctival surface.

Conjunctivitis. Conjunctivitis causes eyelid edema, excessive tearing, and itchy, burning eyes. Inspection reveals a thick purulent discharge, crusty eyelids, and conjunctival injection. Corneal involvement causes photophobia and pain.

Dacryoadenitis. Severe periorbital swelling characterizes dacryoadenitis, which may also cause conjunctival injection, purulent discharge, and temporal pain.

Dacryocystitis. Lacrimal sac inflammation causes prominent eyelid edema and constant tearing. With acute cases, pain and tenderness near the tear sac accompany purulent discharge.

Facial burns. Burns may cause extensive edema that impairs respiration. Additional findings include singed nasal hairs, red mucosa, sooty sputum, and signs of respiratory distress such as inspiratory stridor.

Facial trauma. The extent of edema varies with the type of injury. For example, a contusion may cause localized edema, whereas a nasal or maxillary fracture causes more generalized edema. Associated features also depend on the type of injury.

Herpes zoster ophthalmicus (shingles). With shingles, edematous and red eyelids are usually accompanied by excessive tearing and a serous discharge.

Severe unilateral facial pain may occur several days before vesicles erupt.

Myxedema. Myxedema eventually causes generalized facial edema; waxy, dry skin; hair loss or coarsening; and other signs of hypothyroidism.

Nephrotic syndrome. Commonly the first sign of nephrotic syndrome, periorbital edema precedes dependent and abdominal edema. Associated findings include weight gain, nausea, anorexia, lethargy, fatigue, and pallor.

Orbital cellulitis. The sudden onset of periorbital edema marks orbital cellulitis. It may be accompanied by a unilateral purulent discharge, hyperemia, exophthalmos, conjunctival injection, impaired extraocular movements, a fever, and extreme orbital pain.

Periodontal abscess. A periodontal abscess can cause swelling or edema of the gums and can progress to cause facial edema, ear and jaw pain, as well as tooth pain.

Preeclampsia. Edema of the face, hands, and ankles is an early sign of preeclampsia. Other characteristics include excessive weight gain, a severe headache, blurred vision, hypertension, and midepigastric pain.

Rhinitis (allergic). With rhinitis, red and edematous eyelids are accompanied by paroxysmal sneezing, itchy nose and eyes, and profuse, watery rhinorrhea. The patient may also develop nasal congestion, excessive tearing, a headache, sinus pain and, sometimes, malaise and a fever.

Sinusitis. Frontal sinusitis causes edema of the forehead and eyelids. Maxillary sinusitis produces edema in the maxillary area as well as malaise, gingival swelling, and trismus. Both types are also accompanied by facial pain, a fever, nasal congestion, purulent nasal discharge, and red, swollen nasal mucosa.

Superior vena cava syndrome. Superior vena cava syndrome gradually

Recognizing angioneurotic edema

Most dramatic in the lips, eyelids, and tongue, angioneurotic edema commonly results from an allergic reaction. It's characterized by the rapid onset of painless, nonpitting, subcutaneous swelling that usually resolves in 1 or 2 days. This type of edema may also involve the hands, feet, genitalia, and viscera; laryngeal edema may cause life-threatening airway obstruction.

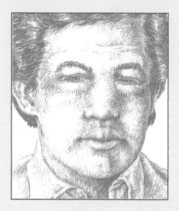

produces facial and neck edema accompanied by thoracic or jugular vein distention. It also causes central nervous system symptoms, such as a headache, vision disturbances, and vertigo.

Trachoma. With trachoma, edema affects the eyelid and conjunctiva and is accompanied by eye pain, excessive tearing, photophobia, and eye discharge. Examination reveals an inflamed preauricular node and visible conjunctival follicles.

Trichinosis. Trichinosis is a relatively rare infectious disorder that causes the sudden onset of eyelid edema with a fever (102° to 104° F [38.9° to 40° C]), conjunctivitis, muscle pain, itching and burning skin, sweating, skin lesions, and delirium.

Other causes

Diagnostic tests. An allergic reaction to contrast media used in radiologic tests may produce facial edema.

Drugs. Long-term use of glucocorticoids may produce facial edema (described as "moon face"). Any drug that causes an allergic reaction (aspirin, antipyretics, penicillin, and sulfa preparations, for example) may also cause edema.

Surgery and transfusion. Cranial, nasal, or jaw surgery may cause facial edema, as may a blood transfusion that causes an allergic reaction.

Nursing considerations

- Administer an analgesic for pain.
- Unless contraindicated, apply cold compresses to the patient's eyes to decrease edema.
- Elevate the head of the bed to help drain the accumulated fluid.

Patient teaching

- Explain the risks of delayed allergy symptoms.
- Explain which signs and symptoms the patient or family should report.
- Emphasize the importance of having an anaphylaxis kit and medical identification bracelet.
- Explain to the patient the underlying cause of edema and its treatment.

▌Edema of the leg

Leg edema is a common sign that results when excess interstitial fluid accumulates in one or both legs. It may affect just the foot and ankle or extend to the thigh, and may be slight or dramatic, pitting or nonpitting.

Leg edema may result from venous disorders, trauma, and certain bone and cardiac disorders that disturb normal fluid balance. (See *Understanding fluid balance,* page 225.) It may result from nephrotic syndrome, cirrhosis, acute and chronic thrombophlebitis, chronic venous insufficiency (most common), cellulitis, lymphedema, and drugs. However, several nonpathologic mechanisms may also cause leg edema. For example, prolonged sitting, standing, or immobility may cause bilateral orthostatic edema. This pitting edema usually affects the foot and disappears with rest and leg elevation. Increased venous pressure late in pregnancy may cause ankle edema. Constricting garters or pantyhose may mechanically cause lower-extremity edema.

History and physical examination

To evaluate the patient, first ask how long he has had the edema. Did it develop suddenly or gradually? Does it decrease if he elevates his legs? Is it painful when touched or when he walks? Is it worse in the morning, or does it get progressively worse during the day? Ask about a recent leg injury or recent surgery or illness that may have immobilized the patient. Does he have a history of cardiovascular disease? Finally, obtain a drug history.

Begin the physical examination by examining each leg for pitting edema. (See *Edema: Pitting or nonpitting?* page 226.) Because leg edema may compromise arterial blood flow, palpate or use a Doppler to auscultate peripheral pulses to detect an insufficiency. Observe leg color and look for unusual vein patterns. Then palpate for warmth, tenderness, and cords, and gently squeeze the calf muscle against the tibia to check for deep pain. If leg edema is unilateral, dorsiflex the foot to look for Homans' sign, which is indicated by calf pain. Finally, note skin thickening or ulceration in edematous areas.

Medical causes

Burns. Two days or less after injury, leg burns may cause mild to severe edema, pain, and tissue damage.

Cellulitis. Pitting edema and orange peel skin are caused by a streptococcal or staphylococcal infection that most commonly occurs in the lower extremities. Cellulitis is also associated with erythema, warmth, and tenderness in the infected area.

Envenomation. Mild to severe localized edema may develop suddenly at the site of a bite or sting, along with erythema, pain, urticaria, pruritus, and a burning sensation.

Heart failure. Bilateral leg edema is an early sign of right-sided heart failure. Other signs and symptoms include weight gain despite anorexia, nausea, chest tightness, hypotension, pallor, tachypnea, exertional dyspnea, orthopnea, paroxysmal nocturnal dyspnea, palpitations, a ventricular gallop, and inspiratory crackles. Pitting ankle edema, hepatomegaly, hemoptysis, and cyanosis signal more advanced heart failure.

Leg trauma. Mild to severe localized edema may form around the trauma site.

Osteomyelitis. When osteomyelitis— a bone infection—affects the lower leg, it usually produces localized, mild to moderate edema, which may spread to the adjacent joint. Edema typically follows a fever, localized tenderness, and pain that increases with leg movement.

Thrombophlebitis. Deep and superficial vein thrombosis may cause unilateral mild to moderate leg edema. Deep vein thrombophlebitis may be asymptomatic or may cause mild to severe pain, warmth, and cyanosis in the affected leg as well as a fever, chills, and malaise. Superficial thrombophlebitis typically causes pain, warmth, redness, tenderness, and induration along the affected vein.

Venous insufficiency (chronic). Moderate to severe, unilateral or bilateral leg edema occurs in patients with venous insufficiency. Initially, the edema is soft and pitting; later, it becomes hard as tissues thicken. Other signs include darkened skin and painless, easily infected stasis ulcers around the ankle. Venous insufficiency generally occurs in females.

Other causes

Coronary artery bypass surgery. Unilateral venous insufficiency may follow saphenous vein retrieval.

Diagnostic tests. Venography is a rare cause of leg edema.

Nursing considerations

- Provide an analgesic and antibiotic as needed.
- Prepare the patient for the application of a compression boot (Unna's boot), if indicated, to help reduce edema.
- Monitor the patient's intake and output, and check his weight and leg circumference daily to detect any change in the edema.
- Prepare the patient for diagnostic tests, such as blood and urine studies and X-rays.
- Monitor the affected extremity for skin breakdown.
- Elevate the affected extremity.

Patient teaching

- Tell the patient avoid prolonged sitting or standing, to elevate his legs as necessary, and not to cross his legs.
- Teach the application of antiembolism stockings or bandages.
- Instruct the patient in appropriate leg exercises.
- Explain food or fluid restrictions.

- Explain the underlying cause of the edema and its treatment.

Enuresis

Enuresis usually refers to nighttime urinary incontinence in girls age 5 and older and boys age 6 and older. This sign rarely continues into adulthood, but may occur in some adults with sleep apnea. It's classified as primary or secondary. Primary enuresis describes a child who has never achieved bladder control; secondary enuresis describes a child who achieved bladder control for at least 3 months but has lost it.

Among factors that may contribute to enuresis are delayed development of detrusor muscle control, unusually deep or sound sleep, organic disorders (such as a urinary tract infection [UTI] or obstruction), and psychological stress. Psychological stress, probably the most important factor, commonly results from the birth of a sibling, the death of a parent or loved one, divorce, or premature, rigorous toilet training. The child may be too embarrassed or ashamed to discuss his bed-wetting, which intensifies psychological stress and makes enuresis more likely—thus creating a vicious circle.

History and physical examination

When taking a history, include the parents as well as the child. First, determine the number of nights each week or month that the child wets the bed. Is there a family history of enuresis? Ask about the child's daily fluid intake. Does he drink much after dinner? What are his typical sleep and voiding patterns? Find out if the child has ever had control of his bladder. If so, try to pinpoint what may have precipitated enuresis, such as an organic disorder or psychological stress. Does the bed-wetting occur at home and away from home? Ask the parents how they've tried to manage the problem, and have them describe the child's toilet training. Observe the child's and parents' attitudes toward bed-wetting. Finally, ask the child if it hurts when he urinates.

Next, perform a physical examination to detect signs of neurologic or urinary tract disorders. Observe the child's gait to check for motor dysfunction, and test sensory function in the legs. Inspect the urethral meatus for erythema, and obtain a urine specimen. A rectal examination to evaluate sphincter control may be required.

Medical causes

Detrusor muscle hyperactivity. Involuntary detrusor muscle contractions may cause primary or secondary enuresis associated with urinary urgency, frequency, and incontinence. Signs and symptoms of a UTI are also common.

Urinary tract obstruction. Although daytime incontinence is more common, urinary tract obstruction may produce primary or secondary enuresis. It may also cause flank and lower back pain; upper abdominal distention; urinary frequency, urgency, hesitancy, and dribbling; dysuria; a diminished urine stream; hematuria; and variable urine output.

UTI. In children, most UTIs produce secondary enuresis. Associated features include urinary frequency and urgency, dysuria, straining to urinate, and hematuria. Lower back pain, fatigue, and suprapubic discomfort may also occur.

Nursing considerations

- Administer medications, such as imipramine, desmopressin, or an anticholinergic, as indicated.
- Provide emotional support to the child and his family.

Patient teaching

■ Encourage the parents to accept and support the child.
■ Teach the parents and child how to manage enuresis at home.
■ Discuss bladder training if the child has detrusor muscle hyperactivity.
■ Teach the use of an alarm device, if appropriate, for the child age 8 and older.
■ Explain any underlying causes of the enuresis and its treatment.

Epistaxis

A common sign, epistaxis (nosebleed) can be spontaneous or induced from the front or back of the nose. Most nosebleeds occur in the anterior-inferior nasal septum (Kiesselbach's plexus), but they may also occur at the point where the inferior turbinates meet the nasopharynx. Usually unilateral, they seem bilateral when blood runs from the bleeding side behind the nasal septum and out the opposite side. Epistaxis ranges from mild oozing to severe—possibly life-threatening—blood loss.

A rich supply of fragile blood vessels makes the nose particularly vulnerable to bleeding. Air moving through the nose can dry and irritate the mucous membranes, forming crusts that bleed when they're removed; dry mucous membranes are also more susceptible to infection, which can produce epistaxis as well. Trauma is another common cause of epistaxis. Additional causes include septal deviations; hematologic, coagulation, renal, and GI disorders; and certain drugs and treatments.

A<small>CTION</small> S<small>TAT</small>!

 If the patient has severe epistaxis, quickly take his vital signs. Be alert for tachypnea, hypotension, and other signs of hypovolemic shock. Insert a large-gauge I.V. line for rapid fluid and blood replacement, and

attempt to control bleeding by pinching the nares closed. (However, if you suspect a nasal fracture, don't pinch the nares. Instead, place gauze under the patient's nose to absorb the blood.)

Have a hypovolemic patient lie down and turn his head to the side to prevent blood from draining down the back of his throat, which could cause aspiration or vomiting of swallowed blood. If the patient isn't hypovolemic, have him sit upright and tilt his head forward. Constantly check airway patency. If the patient's condition is unstable, begin cardiac monitoring and give supplemental oxygen by mask.

History and physical examination

If the patient isn't in distress, take a history. Does he have a history of recent trauma? How often has he had nosebleeds in the past? Have the nosebleeds been long or unusually severe? Has the patient recently had surgery in the sinus area? Ask about a history of hypertension, bleeding or liver disorders, and other recent illnesses. Ask if the patient bruises easily. Find out what drugs he uses, especially anti-inflammatories, such as aspirin, and anticoagulants such as warfarin. Ask about a history of cocaine use.

Begin the physical examination by inspecting the patient's skin for other signs of bleeding, such as ecchymoses and petechiae, and noting jaundice, pallor, or other abnormalities. When examining a trauma patient, look for associated injuries, such as eye trauma or facial fractures.

Medical causes

Aplastic anemia. Aplastic anemia develops insidiously, eventually producing nosebleeds as well as ecchymoses, retinal hemorrhages, menorrhagia, petechiae, bleeding from the mouth, and signs of GI bleeding. Fatigue, dyspnea, a headache, tachycardia, and pallor may also occur.

Barotrauma. Commonly seen in airline passengers and scuba divers, barotrauma may cause severe, painful epistaxis when the patient has an upper respiratory tract infection.

Coagulation disorders. Such coagulation disorders as hemophilia and thrombocytopenic purpura can cause epistaxis along with ecchymoses, petechiae, and bleeding from the gums, mouth, and I.V. puncture sites. Menorrhagia and signs of GI bleeding, such as melena and hematemesis, can also occur.

Glomerulonephritis (chronic). Glomerulonephritis produces nosebleeds as well as hypertension, proteinuria, hematuria, a headache, edema, oliguria, hemoptysis, nausea, vomiting, pruritus, dyspnea, malaise, and fatigue.

Hepatitis. When hepatitis interferes with the clotting mechanism, epistaxis and abnormal bleeding tendencies can result. Associated signs and symptoms typically include jaundice, clay-colored stools, pruritus, hepatomegaly, abdominal pain, a fever, fatigue, weakness, dark amber urine, anorexia, nausea, and vomiting.

Hereditary hemorrhagic telangiectasia (HHT or Rendu-Osler-Weber syndrome). An inherited disorder, HHT causes frequent nosebleeds in children and may be an early sign of the disorder. Other signs include characteristic vascular lesions of the tongue, lips, ears, fingers, and skin. Shortness of breath may occur, along with GI bleeding and signs of neurologic impairment from intracranial bleeding.

Hypertension. Severe hypertension can produce extreme epistaxis, usually in the posterior nose, with pulsation above the middle turbinate. It may be accompanied by dizziness, a throbbing headache, anxiety, peripheral edema, nocturia, nausea, vomiting, drowsiness, and mental impairment.

Leukemia. With *acute leukemia,* sudden epistaxis is accompanied by a high fever and other types of abnormal bleeding, such as bleeding gums, ecchymoses, petechiae, easy bruising, and prolonged menses. These may follow less-noticeable signs and symptoms, such as weakness, lassitude, pallor, chills, recurrent infections, and a low-grade fever. Acute leukemia may also cause dyspnea, fatigue, malaise, tachycardia, palpitations, a systolic ejection murmur, and abdominal or bone pain.

With *chronic leukemia,* epistaxis is a late sign that may be accompanied by other types of abnormal bleeding, extreme fatigue, weight loss, hepatosplenomegaly, bone tenderness, edema, macular or nodular skin lesions, pallor, weakness, dyspnea, tachycardia, palpitations, and headache.

Maxillofacial injury. With a maxillofacial injury, a pumping arterial bleed usually causes severe epistaxis. Associated signs and symptoms include facial pain, numbness, swelling, asymmetry, open-bite malocclusion or an inability to open the mouth, diplopia, conjunctival hemorrhage, lip edema, and buccal, mucosal, and soft palate ecchymoses.

Nasal fracture. Unilateral or bilateral epistaxis occurs with nasal swelling, periorbital ecchymoses and edema, pain, nasal deformity, and crepitation of the nasal bones.

Nasal tumor. Blood may ooze from the nose when a tumor disrupts the nasal vasculature. Benign tumors usually bleed when touched, but malignant tumors produce spontaneous unilateral epistaxis, along with a foul discharge, cheek swelling, and—in the late stage—pain.

Polycythemia vera. A common sign of polycythemia vera, spontaneous epistaxis may be accompanied by bleeding gums; ecchymoses; ruddy cyanosis of the face, nose, ears, and lips; and congestion of the conjunctiva, retina, and oral mucous membranes. Other signs and symptoms vary according to the affected body system, but may include a headache, dizziness, tinnitus, vision disturbances, hypertension, chest pain, intermittent claudication, early satiety and fullness, marked splenomegaly, epigastric pain, pruritus, and dyspnea.

Sarcoidosis. Oozing epistaxis may occur in sarcoidosis, along with a nonproductive cough, substernal pain, malaise, and weight loss. Related findings include tachycardia, arrhythmias, parotid enlargement, cervical lymphadenopathy, skin lesions, hepatosplenomegaly, and arthritis in the ankles, knees, and wrists.

Scleroma. With scleroma, oozing epistaxis occurs with a watery nasal discharge that becomes foul-smelling and crusty. Progressive anosmia and turbinate atrophy may also occur.

Sinusitis (acute). With sinusitis, a bloody or blood-tinged nasal discharge may become purulent and copious after 24 to 48 hours. Associated signs and symptoms include nasal congestion, pain, tenderness, malaise, a headache, a low-grade fever, and red, edematous nasal mucosa.

Skull fracture. Depending on the type of fracture, epistaxis can be direct (when blood flows directly down the nares) or indirect (when blood drains through the eustachian tube and into the nose). Abrasions, contusions, lacerations, or avulsions are common. A *severe skull fracture* may cause a severe headache, a decreased level of consciousness, hemiparesis, dizziness, seizures, projec-

tile vomiting, and decreased pulse and respiratory rates.

A *basilar fracture* may also cause bleeding from the pharynx, ears, and conjunctiva as well as raccoon eyes and Battle's sign. Cerebrospinal fluid or even brain tissue may leak from the nose or ears. A *sphenoid fracture* may also cause blindness, whereas a temporal fracture may also cause unilateral deafness or facial paralysis.

Typhoid fever. Oozing epistaxis and a dry cough are common. Typhoid fever may also cause an abrupt onset of chills and a high fever, vomiting, abdominal distention, constipation or diarrhea, splenomegaly, hepatomegaly, "rose-spot" rash, jaundice, anorexia, weight loss, and profound fatigue.

Other causes
Chemical irritants. Some chemicals—including phosphorus, sulfuric acid, ammonia, printer's ink, and chromates—irritate the nasal mucosa, producing epistaxis.

Drugs. Anticoagulants, such as warfarin, and anti-inflammatories, such as aspirin, can cause epistaxis. Cocaine use, especially if frequent, can also cause epistaxis.

Surgery and procedures. Rarely, epistaxis results from facial and nasal surgery, including septoplasty, rhinoplasty, antrostomy, endoscopic sinus procedures, orbital decompression, and dental extraction.

Nursing considerations
▪ Until the bleeding is completely under control, continue to monitor the patient for signs of hypovolemic shock, such as tachycardia and clammy skin.
▪ If external pressure doesn't control the bleeding, insert cotton that has been impregnated with a vasoconstrictor and local anesthetic into the patient's nose.

Controlling epistaxis with nasal packing

When direct pressure and cautery fail to control epistaxis, nasal packing may be required. Anterior packing may be used if the patient has severe bleeding in the anterior nose. Horizontal layers of petroleum jelly gauze strips are inserted into the nostrils near the turbinates.

Posterior packing may be needed if the patient has severe bleeding in the posterior nose or if blood from anterior bleeding starts flowing backward. This type of packing consists of a gauze pack secured by three strong silk sutures. After the nose is anesthetized, sutures are pulled through the nostrils with a soft catheter and the pack is positioned behind the soft palate. Two of the sutures are tied to a gauze roll under the patient's nose, which keeps the pack in place. The third suture is taped to his cheek. Instead of a gauze pack, an indwelling urinary or nasal epistaxis catheter may be inserted through the nose into the area behind the soft palate and inflated with 10 ml of water to compress the bleeding point.

Precautions

If the patient has nasal packing, follow these guidelines:
■ Watch for signs of respiratory distress, such as dyspnea, which may occur if the packing slips and obstructs the airway.
■ Keep emergency equipment (flashlights, scissors, and a hemostat) at the patient's bedside. Expect to cut the cheek suture (or deflate the catheter) and remove the pack at the first sign of airway obstruction.
■ Avoid tension on the cheek suture, which could cause the posterior pack to slip out of place.
■ Keep the call bell within easy reach.
■ Monitor the patient's vital signs frequently. Watch for signs of hypoxia, such as tachycardia and restlessness.
■ Elevate the head of the patient's bed, and remind him to breathe through his mouth.
■ Administer humidified oxygen as needed.
■ Instruct the patient not to blow his nose for 48 hours after the packing is removed.

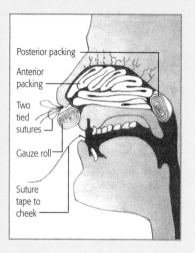

Posterior packing
Anterior packing
Two tied sutures
Gauze roll
Suture tape to cheek

■ If bleeding persists, expect to insert anterior or posterior nasal packing. (See *Controlling epistaxis with nasal packing*.)
■ Administer humidified oxygen by face mask to a patient with posterior packing.
■ Anticipate laboratory tests, such as a complete blood count to evaluate blood loss and detect anemia and clotting studies, such as prothrombin time and partial thromboplastin time, to test coagulation time.
■ Prepare the patient for X-rays if he has had a recent trauma.

Patient teaching
■ Teach the patient pinching pressure techniques.
■ Discuss ways to prevent nosebleeds.

- Tell the patient to sit upright and lean forward when a nosebleed occurs.
- Explain the underlying cause of the patient's epistaxis and its treatment.

Erythema
[Erythroderma]

Dilated or congested blood vessels produce red skin, or erythema, the most common sign of skin inflammation or irritation. Erythema may be localized or generalized and may occur suddenly or gradually. Skin color can range from bright red in patients with acute conditions to pale violet or brown in those with chronic problems. Erythema must be differentiated from purpura, which causes redness from bleeding into the skin. When pressure is applied directly to the skin, erythema blanches momentarily, but purpura doesn't.

Erythema usually results from changes in the arteries, veins, and small vessels that lead to increased small-vessel perfusion. Drugs and neurogenic mechanisms can allow extra blood to enter the small vessels. Erythema can also result from trauma and tissue damage; changes in supporting tissues, which increase vessel visibility; and many rare disorders.

A C T I O N   S T A T !

 If the patient has sudden progressive erythema with a rapid pulse, dyspnea, hoarseness, and agitation, quickly take his vital signs. These may be indications of anaphylactic shock. Provide emergency respiratory support and give epinephrine.

History and physical examination

If erythema isn't associated with anaphylaxis, obtain a detailed health history. Find out how long the patient has had the erythema and where it first began. Has he had associated pain or itching? Has he recently had a fever, upper respiratory tract infection, or joint pain? Does he have a history of skin disease or other illness? Does he or anyone in his family have allergies, asthma, or eczema? Find out if he has been exposed to someone who has had a similar rash or who's now ill. Did he have a recent fall or injury in the area of erythema?

Obtain a complete drug history, including recent immunizations. Ask about food intake and exposure to chemicals.

Begin the physical examination by assessing the extent, distribution, and intensity of erythema. Look for edema and other skin lesions, such as hives, scales, papules, and purpura. Examine the affected area for warmth, and gently palpate it to check for tenderness or crepitus.

Medical causes

Allergic reaction. Foods, drugs, chemicals, and other allergens can cause an allergic reaction and erythema. A localized allergic reaction also produces hivelike eruptions and edema.

Anaphylaxis, a life-threatening condition, produces relatively sudden erythema in the form of urticaria. It also produces flushing; facial edema; diaphoresis; weakness; sneezing; bronchospasm with dyspnea and tachypnea; shock with hypotension and cool, clammy skin; and, possibly, airway edema with hoarseness and stridor.

Burns. With thermal burns, erythema and swelling appear first, possibly followed by deep or superficial blisters and other signs of damage that vary with the burn's severity. Burns from ultraviolet rays, such as sunburn, cause delayed erythema and tenderness on exposed areas of the skin.

Candidiasis. When candidiasis—a fungal infection—affects the skin, it produces erythema and a scaly, papular rash under the breasts and at the axillae, neck, umbilicus, and groin, also known as *intertrigo.* Small pustules commonly occur at the periphery of the rash (satellite pustulosis).

Cellulitis. Erythema, tenderness, and edema are a result of a bacterial infection of the skin and subcutaneous tissue.

Dermatitis. Erythema commonly occurs in this family of inflammatory disorders. With *atopic dermatitis,* erythema and intense pruritus precede the development of small papules that may redden, weep, scale, and lichenify. These occur most commonly at skin folds of the extremities, neck, and eyelids.

Contact dermatitis occurs after exposure to an irritant. It quickly produces erythema and vesicles, blisters, or ulcerations on exposed skin.

With *seborrheic dermatitis,* erythema appears with dull red or yellow lesions. Sharply marginated, these lesions are sometimes ring shaped and covered with greasy scales. They usually occur on the scalp, eyebrows, ears, and nasolabial folds, but they may form a butterfly rash on the face or move to the chest or to skin folds on the trunk. This disorder is common in patients infected with human immunodeficiency virus and in infants (cradle cap).

Dermatomyositis. Dermatomyositis produces a dusky lilac rash on the face, neck, upper torso, and nail beds. Gottron's papules (violet, flat-topped lesions) may appear on finger joints.

Erythema annulare centrifugum. Small, pink infiltrated papules appear on the trunk, buttocks, and inner thighs, slowly spreading at the margins and clearing in the center. Itching, scaling, and tissue hardening may occur.

Erythema marginatum rheumaticum. Associated with rheumatic fever, erythema marginatum rheumaticum causes erythematous lesions that are superficial, flat, and slightly hardened. They shift, spread rapidly, and may last for hours or days, recurring after a time.

Erythema multiforme. Erythema multiforme minor has typical urticarial red-pink iris-shaped localized lesions with little or no mucous membrane involvement. Most lesions occur on flexor surfaces of the extremities. Burning or itching may occur before or in conjunction with lesion development. Lesions appear in crops and last 2 or 3 weeks. After 1 week, individual lesions become flat or hyperpigmented. Early signs and symptoms may include a mild fever, cough, and sore throat.

Erythema multiforme major usually occurs as a drug reaction; has widespread symmetrical, bullous lesions that may become confluent; and includes erosions of the mucous membranes. Erythema is characteristically preceded by blisters on the lips, tongue, and buccal mucosa and a sore throat. Additional signs and symptoms that manifest early in the course of the disease include a cough, vomiting, diarrhea, coryza, and epistaxis. Later signs and symptoms include a fever, prostration, difficulty with oral intake due to mouth and lip lesions, conjunctivitis due to ulceration, vulvitis, and balanitis. The maximal variant of this disease is considered by many to be Stevens-Johnson syndrome, a multisystem disorder that can occasionally be fatal. In addition to all signs and symptoms mentioned above, the patient develops exfoliation of the skin from disruptions of bullae, although less than 10% of the body surface area is affected. These areas resemble second-degree thermal burns and should be cared for as such. Fever may rise to 102° F to

104° F (38.9° C to 40° C). The patient may also experience tachypnea; a weak, rapid pulse; chest pain; malaise; and muscle or joint pain.

Erythema nodosum. Sudden bilateral eruption of tender erythematous nodules characterizes erythema nodosum. These firm, round, protruding lesions usually appear in crops on the shins, knees, and ankles, but may occur on the buttocks, arms, calves, and trunk as well. Other effects include a mild fever, chills, malaise, muscle and joint pain and, possibly, swollen feet and ankles. Erythema nodosum is associated with various diseases, most notably inflammatory bowel disease, sarcoidosis, tuberculosis, and streptococcal and fungal infections.

Gout. Gout is characterized by tight and erythematous skin over an inflamed, edematous joint.

Kawasaki syndrome. This acute illness of unknown cause commonly produces a rash or erythema. No test is available for Kawasaki syndrome, which can cause serious heart damage and death if not detected and treated immediately. Additional characteristic signs include fever, conjunctival injection, and lymphadenopathy.

Lupus erythematosus. Discoid and systemic lupus erythematosus (SLE) can produce a characteristic butterfly rash. This erythematous eruption may range from a blush with swelling to a scaly, sharply demarcated, macular rash with plaques that may spread to the forehead, chin, ears, chest, and other sun-exposed parts of the body.

With *discoid lupus erythematosus,* telangiectasia, hyperpigmentation, ear and nose deformity, and mouth, tongue, and eyelid lesions may occur.

With *SLE,* an acute onset of erythema may also be accompanied by photosensitivity and mucous membrane ul-

cers, especially in the nose and mouth. Mottled erythema may occur on the hands, with edema around the nails and macular reddish purple lesions on the fingers. Telangiectasia occurs at the base of the nails or eyelids, along with purpura, petechiae, ecchymoses, and urticaria. Joint pain and stiffness are common. Other findings vary according to the body systems affected, but typically include a low-grade fever, malaise, weakness, a headache, arthralgia, arthritis, depression, lymphadenopathy, fatigue, weight loss, anorexia, nausea, vomiting, diarrhea, and constipation.

Psoriasis. Silvery white scales over a thickened erythematous base usually affect the elbows, knees, chest, scalp, and intergluteal folds. The fingernails may become thick and pitted.

Raynaud's disease. Typically, the skin on the hands and feet blanches and cools after exposure to cold and stress. Later, it becomes warm and purplish red.

Rosacea. Scattered erythema initially develops across the center of the face, followed by superficial telangiectases, papules, pustules, and nodules. Rhinophyma may occur on the lower half of the nose.

Rubella. Typically, flat solitary lesions join to form a blotchy pink erythematous rash that spreads rapidly to the trunk and extremities in this disorder. Occasionally, small red lesions (Forschheimer spots) occur on the soft palate. Lesions clear in 4 or 5 days. The rash usually follows a fever (up to 102° F [38.9° C]), a headache, malaise, a sore throat, a gritty eye sensation, lymphadenopathy, pain in the joints, and coryza.

Other causes
Drugs. Many drugs commonly cause erythema. (See *Drugs associated with erythema,* page 242.)

Drugs associated with erythema

Suspect drug-induced erythema in a patient who develops this sign within 1 week of starting a drug. Erythematous lesions can vary in size, shape, type, and amount, but they almost always appear suddenly and symmetrically on the trunk and inner arms. These drugs can produce erythematous lesions:

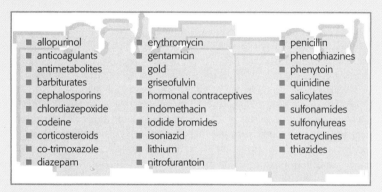

- allopurinol
- anticoagulants
- antimetabolites
- barbiturates
- cephalosporins
- chlordiazepoxide
- codeine
- corticosteroids
- co-trimoxazole
- diazepam

- erythromycin
- gentamicin
- gold
- griseofulvin
- hormonal contraceptives
- indomethacin
- iodide bromides
- isoniazid
- lithium
- nitrofurantoin

- penicillin
- phenothiazines
- phenytoin
- quinidine
- salicylates
- sulfonamides
- sulfonylureas
- tetracyclines
- thiazides

Some drugs—particularly barbiturates, hormonal contraceptives, salicylates, sulfonamides, and tetracycline—can cause a "fixed" drug eruption. In this type of reaction, lesions can appear on any body part and flake off after a few days, leaving a brownish purple pigmentation. Repeated drug administration causes the original lesions to recur and new ones to develop.

Radiation and other treatments. Radiation therapy may produce dull erythema and edema within 24 hours. As the erythema fades, the skin becomes light brown and mildly scaly. Any treatment that causes an allergic reaction can also cause erythema.

Nursing considerations

- Monitor and replace fluids and electrolytes, especially in patients with burns or widespread erythema.
- Withhold all medications until the cause of the erythema has been identified.
- Administer an antibiotic and a topical or systemic corticosteroid as ordered.
- For the patient with itching skin, give soothing baths or apply open wet dressings containing starch, bran, or sodium bicarbonate.
- Administer an antihistamine and analgesic as needed.
- For a burn patient with erythema, immerse the affected area in cold water, or apply a sheet soaked in cold water to reduce pain, edema, and erythema.
- Prepare the patient for diagnostic tests, such as skin biopsy to detect cancerous lesions, cultures to identify infectious organisms, and sensitivity studies to confirm allergies.
- Have the patient with leg erythema keep his legs elevated above heart level.

Patient teaching

- Stress the avoidance of sun exposure and use of sunblock.
- Teach the patient methods to relieve itching.
- Explain the underlying cause of the patient's erythema and its treatment.

Exophthalmos
[Proptosis]

Exophthalmos—the abnormal protrusion of one or both eyeballs—may result from hemorrhage, edema, or inflammation behind the eye; extraocular muscle relaxation; or space-occupying intraorbital lesions and metastatic tumors. This sign may occur suddenly or gradually, causing mild to dramatic protrusion. Occasionally, the affected eye also pulsates. The most common cause of exophthalmos in adults is dysthyroid eye disease.

Exophthalmos is usually easily observed. However, lid retraction may mimic exophthalmos even when protrusion is absent. Similarly, ptosis in one eye may make the other eye appear exophthalmic by comparison. An exophthalmometer can differentiate these signs by measuring ocular protrusion.

History and physical examination

Begin by asking when the patient first noticed exophthalmos. Is it associated with pain in or around the eye? If so, ask him how severe it is and how long he has had it. Then ask about recent sinus infection or vision problems. Take the patient's vital signs, noting a fever, which may accompany eye infection. Next, evaluate the severity of exophthalmos with an exophthalmometer. (See *Detecting unilateral exophthalmos*.) If the eyes bulge severely, look for cloudiness on the cornea, which may indicate ulcer formation. Describe any eye discharge and observe for ptosis. Then check visual acuity, with and without correction, and evaluate extraocular movements. Palpate the patient's thyroid for enlargement or goiter.

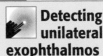
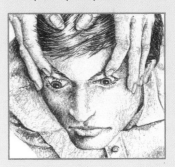
Medical causes

Cavernous sinus thrombosis. Usually, cavernous sinus thrombosis causes the sudden onset of pulsating, unilateral exophthalmos. Accompanying it may be eyelid edema, decreased or absent pupillary reflexes, and impaired extraocular movement and visual acuity. Other features include a high fever with chills, papilledema, a headache, nausea, vomiting, somnolence and, rarely, seizures.

Dacryoadenitis. Unilateral, slowly progressive exophthalmos is the most common sign of dacryoadenitis. Assessment may also reveal limited extraocular movements (especially on elevation and abduction), ptosis, eyelid edema and erythema, conjunctival injection, eye pain, and diplopia.

Foreign body in the eye. When a foreign body enters the eye, exophthalmos may accompany other signs and symptoms of ocular trauma, such as eye pain, redness, and tearing.

Hemangioma. This orbital tumor produces progressive exophthalmos, which may be mild or severe, unilateral or bilateral. Other signs and symptoms include ptosis, limited extraocular movements, and blurred vision.

Lacrimal gland tumor. Exophthalmos usually develops slowly in one eye, causing its downward displacement toward the nose. The patient may also have ptosis and eye deviation and pain.

Leiomyosarcoma. Leiomyosarcoma is characterized by slowly developing, unilateral exophthalmos. Other effects include diplopia, impaired vision, and intermittent eye pain.

Orbital cellulitis. Commonly the result of sinusitis, this ocular emergency causes the sudden onset of unilateral exophthalmos, which may be mild or severe. Orbital cellulitis may also produce a fever, eye pain, a headache, malaise, conjunctival injection, tearing, eyelid edema and erythema, purulent discharge, and impaired extraocular movements.

Orbital choristoma. A common sign of this benign tumor, progressive exophthalmos may be associated with diplopia and blurred vision.

Orbital emphysema. Air leaking from the sinus into the orbit usually causes unilateral exophthalmos. Palpation of the globe elicits crepitation.

Parasite infestation. Usually, parasite infestation causes painless, progressive exophthalmos in one eye that may spread to the other eye. Associated findings include limited extraocular movement, diplopia, eye pain, and impaired visual acuity.

Scleritis (posterior). The gradual onset of mild to severe unilateral exoph-

thalmos is common with scleritis. Other signs and symptoms include severe eye pain, diplopia, papilledema, limited extraocular movement, and impaired visual acuity.

Thyrotoxicosis. Although a classic sign of thyrotoxicosis, exophthalmos is absent in many patients. It's usually bilateral, progressive, and severe. Associated ocular features include ptosis, increased tearing, lid lag and edema, photophobia, conjunctival injection, diplopia, and decreased visual acuity. Other findings include an enlarged thyroid, nervousness, heat intolerance, weight loss despite increased appetite, sweating, diarrhea, tremors, palpitations, and tachycardia.

Nursing considerations
▪ Because exophthalmos usually makes the patient self-conscious, provide privacy and emotional support.
▪ Protect the affected eye from trauma, especially drying of the cornea.
▪ Don't place a gauze eye pad or other object over the affected eye; removal could damage the corneal epithelium.
▪ If necessary, refer him to an ophthalmologist for a complete examination.
▪ Prepare the patient for blood tests, such as a thyroid panel and a white blood cell count.

Patient teaching
▪ Teach ways to protect the eye from trauma, wind, and dust.
▪ Discuss the proper application of lubricants to the eye.
▪ Explain the underlying cause of the patient's exophthalmos and its treatment.

Eye discharge
Usually associated with conjunctivitis, eye discharge is the excretion of a substance other than tears. This common

sign may occur in one or both eyes, producing scant to copious discharge. The discharge may be purulent, frothy, mucoid, cheesy, serous, or clear or a stringy white discharge. Sometimes, the discharge can be expressed by applying pressure to the tear sac, punctum, meibomian glands, or canaliculus.

Eye discharge commonly results from inflammatory and infectious eye disorders, but may also occur in certain systemic disorders. (See *Sources of eye discharge*.) Because this sign may accompany a disorder that threatens vision, it must be assessed and treated immediately.

History and physical examination

Begin your evaluation by finding out when the discharge began. Does it occur at certain times of the day or in connection with certain activities? If the patient complains of pain, ask him to show you its exact location and to describe its character. Is the pain dull, continuous, sharp, or stabbing? Do his eyes itch or burn? Do they tear excessively? Are they sensitive to light? Does he feel like something is in them?

After taking the patient's vital signs, carefully inspect the eye discharge. Note its amount, color, and consistency. Then test visual acuity, with and without correction. Examine external eye structures, beginning with the unaffected eye to prevent cross-contamination. Observe for eyelid edema, entropion, crusts, lesions, and trichiasis. Next, ask the patient to blink as you watch for impaired lid movement. If the eyes seem to bulge, measure them with an exophthalmome-

---

ASSESSMENT TIP

Sources of eye discharge

Eye discharge can come from the tear sac, punctum, meibomian glands, or canaliculi. If the patient reports a discharge that isn't immediately apparent, you can express a sample by pressing your fingertip lightly over these structures. Then characterize the discharge, and note its source.

Punctum (visible without special manipulation)

Meibomian glands (behind and perpendicular to eyelids)

Punctum

Inferior canaliculus

Superior canaliculus

Tear sac (within bony orbit)

ter. Test the six cardinal fields of gaze. Examine for conjunctival injection and follicles and for corneal cloudiness or white lesions.

Medical causes

Conjunctivitis. Five types of conjunctivitis may cause an eye discharge with redness, hyperemia, foreign-body sensation, periocular edema, and tearing.

With *allergic conjunctivitis,* a bilateral ropey discharge is accompanied by itching and tearing.

Bacterial conjunctivitis causes a moderate purulent or mucopurulent discharge that may form sticky crusts on the eyelids during sleep. The discharge is commonly greenish white and usually occurs in one eye. The patient may also experience itching, burning, excessive tearing, and the sensation of a foreign body in the eye. Eye pain indicates corneal involvement. Preauricular adenopathy is uncommon.

Viral conjunctivitis is generally more common than the bacterial form. A serous, clear discharge and preauricular adenopathy are usually present. The history includes a runny nose, an upper respiratory tract infection, or recent contact with a person who had these signs. The onset is usually unilateral.

Fungal conjunctivitis produces a copious, thick, purulent discharge that makes the eyelids crusty and sticky. Also characteristic are eyelid edema, itching, burning, and tearing. Pain and photophobia occur only with corneal involvement.

Inclusion conjunctivitis causes scant mucoid discharge—especially in the morning—in both eyes, accompanied by pseudoptosis and conjunctival follicles.

Corneal ulcers. Bacterial and fungal corneal ulcers produce a copious, purulent unilateral eye discharge. Related findings are crusty, sticky eyelids and, possibly, severe pain, photophobia, and impaired visual acuity.

Bacterial corneal ulcers are also characterized by an irregular gray-white area on the cornea, blurred vision, unilateral pupil constriction, and conjunctival injection.

Fungal corneal ulcers are also characterized by conjunctival injection and eyelid edema and erythema. A painless, dense, whitish gray central ulcer develops slowly and may be surrounded by progressively clearer rings.

Erythema multiforme major (Stevens-Johnson syndrome). A purulent discharge characterizes Stevens-Johnson syndrome. Other ocular effects may include severe eye pain, entropion, trichiasis, photophobia, and decreased tear formation. Also typical are erythematous, urticarial, bullous lesions that suddenly erupt over the skin.

Herpes zoster ophthalmicus. Herpes zoster ophthalmicus yields a moderate to copious serous eye discharge accompanied by excessive tearing. Examination reveals eyelid edema and erythema, conjunctival injection, and a white, cloudy cornea. The patient also complains of eye pain and severe unilateral facial pain that occurs several days before vesicles erupt.

Keratoconjunctivitis sicca. Better known as *dry eye syndrome,* keratoconjunctivitis sicca typically causes excessive, continuous mucoid discharge and insufficient tearing. Accompanying signs and symptoms include eye pain, itching, burning, a foreign-body sensation, and dramatic conjunctival injection. The patient may also have difficulty closing his eyes.

Meibomianitis. Meibomianitis may produce a continuous frothy eye discharge. Applying pressure on the meibomian glands yields a soft, foul-smelling, cheesy yellow discharge. The eyes also appear chronically red, with inflamed lid margins.

Orbital cellulitis. Although exophthalmos is the most obvious sign of this disorder, a unilateral purulent eye discharge may also be present. Related findings include eyelid edema, conjunctival injection, a headache, orbital pain, impaired visual acuity, limited extraocular movement, and a fever.

Psoriasis vulgaris. Usually, psoriasis vulgaris causes a substantial mucus discharge in both eyes, accompanied by redness. The characteristic lesions it produces on the eyelids may extend into the conjunctiva, causing irritation, excessive tearing, and a foreign-body sensation.

Trachoma. A bilateral eye discharge occurs in trachoma along with severe pain, excessive tearing, photophobia, eyelid edema, redness, and visible conjunctival follicles.

Nursing considerations

▪ Apply warm soaks to soften crusts on the eyelids and lashes, then gently wipe the eyes with a soft gauze pad.
▪ Carefully dispose of all used dressings, tissues, and cotton swabs to prevent the spread of infection.

Patient teaching

▪ Teach the patient to avoid contaminating the unaffected eye and to refrain from sharing pillows, wash cloths, eyedrops, or eye makeup with others.
▪ Discuss ordered diagnostic tests, including culture and sensitivity studies to identify infectious organisms.
▪ Explain the underlying cause of the patient's eye discharge and its treatment.

▪ Eye pain
[Ophthalmalgia]

Eye pain may be described as a burning, throbbing, aching, or stabbing sensation in or around the eye. It may also be characterized as a foreign-body sensation. This sign varies from mild to severe; its duration and exact location provide clues to the causative disorder.

Eye pain usually results from corneal abrasion, but it may also be due to glaucoma or other eye disorders, trauma, and neurologic or systemic disorders. Any of these may stimulate nerve endings in the cornea or external eye, producing pain.

A CTION STAT!

 If the patient's eye pain results from a chemical burn, remove contact lenses, if present, and irrigate the eye with at least 1 L of normal saline solution over 10 minutes. Evert the lids and wipe the fornices with a cotton-tipped applicator to remove any particles or chemicals. Eye pain from acute angle-closure glaucoma is an ocular emergency requiring immediate intervention to reduce intraocular pressure (IOP). If drug treatment doesn't reduce IOP, the patient will need laser iridotomy or surgical peripheral iridectomy to save his vision.

History and physical examination

If the patient's eye pain doesn't result from a chemical burn, take a complete history. Have the patient describe the pain fully. Is it an ache or a sharp pain? How long does it last? Is it accompanied by burning, itching, or discharge? Find out when it began. Is it worse in the morning or late in the evening? Ask about recent trauma or surgery, especially if the patient complains of sudden, severe pain. Does the patient wear contact lenses? How often are they removed or replaced if they're disposable? Does he have headaches? If so, find out how often and at what time of day they occur.

Examining the external eye

For patients with eye pain or other ocular symptoms, examination of the external eye forms an important part of the ocular assessment. Here's how to examine the external eye.

First, inspect the eyelids for ptosis and incomplete closure. Also, observe the lids for edema, erythema, cyanosis, hematoma, and masses. Evaluate skin lesions, growths, swelling, and tenderness by gross palpation. Are the lids everted or inverted? Do the eyelashes turn inward? Have some of them been lost? Do the lashes adhere to one another or contain a discharge? Next, examine the lid margins, noting especially any debris, scaling, lesions, or unusual secretions. Also, watch for eyelid spasms.

Now gently retract the eyelid with your thumb and forefinger, and assess the conjunctiva for redness, cloudiness, follicles, and blisters or other lesions. Check for chemosis by pressing the lower lid against the eyeball and noting any bulging above this compression point. Observe the sclera, noting any change from its normal white color.

Next, shine a light across the cornea to detect scars, abrasions, or ulcers. Note color changes, dots, or opaque or cloudy areas. Also, assess the anterior eye chamber, which should be clean, deep, shadow-free, and filled with clear aqueous humor.

Inspect the color, shape, texture, and pattern of the iris. Then assess the pupils' size, shape, and equality. Finally, evaluate their response to light. Are they sluggish, fixed, or unresponsive? Does pupil dilation or constriction occur only on one side?

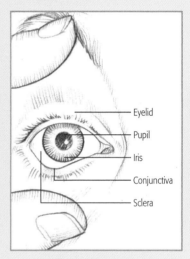

During the physical examination, *don't* manipulate the eye if you suspect trauma. Carefully assess the lids and conjunctiva for redness, inflammation, and swelling. Then examine the eyes for ptosis or exophthalmos. Finally, test visual acuity with and without correction, and assess extraocular movements. Characterize any discharge. (See *Examining the external eye.*)

Medical causes

Acute angle-closure glaucoma.
Blurred vision and sudden, excruciating pain in and around the eye characterize acute angle-closure glaucoma; the pain may be so severe that it causes nausea, vomiting, and abdominal pain. Other findings are halo vision, rapidly decreasing visual acuity, and a fixed, nonreactive, moderately dilated pupil.

Blepharitis. Burning pain in both eyelids is accompanied by itching, sticky discharge, and conjunctival injection. Related findings include a foreign-body sensation, lid ulcerations, and loss of eyelashes.

Burns. With chemical burns, sudden and severe eye pain may occur with erythema and blistering of the face and lids, photophobia, miosis, conjunctival injection, blurring, and an inability to keep the eyelids open. With ultraviolet radiation burns, moderate to severe pain occurs about 12 hours after exposure along with photophobia and vision changes.

Chalazion. A chalazion causes localized tenderness and swelling on the upper or lower eyelid. Eversion of the lid reveals conjunctival injection and a small red lump.

Conjunctivitis. Some degree of eye pain and excessive tearing occurs with four types of conjunctivitis. *Allergic conjunctivitis* causes mild, burning, bilateral pain accompanied by itching, conjunctival injection, and a characteristic ropey discharge. Bacterial conjunctivitis causes pain only when it affects the cornea. Otherwise, it produces burning and a foreign-body sensation. A purulent discharge and conjunctival injection are also typical.

If the cornea is affected, fungal conjunctivitis may cause pain and photophobia. Even without corneal involvement, it produces itching, burning eyes; a thick, purulent discharge; and conjunctival injection.

Viral conjunctivitis produces itching, red eyes, a foreign-body sensation, visible conjunctival follicles, and eyelid edema.

Corneal abrasions. With this type of injury, eye pain is characterized by a foreign-body sensation. Excessive tearing, photophobia, and conjunctival injection are also common.

Corneal ulcers. Bacterial and fungal corneal ulcers cause severe eye pain. They may also cause a purulent eye discharge, sticky eyelids, photophobia, and impaired visual acuity. In addition, bacterial corneal ulcers produce a grayish white, irregularly shaped ulcer on the cornea; unilateral pupil constriction; and conjunctival injection. Fungal corneal ulcers produce conjunctival injection, eyelid edema and erythema, and a dense, cloudy, central ulcer surrounded by progressively clearer rings.

Dacryocystitis. Pain and tenderness near the tear sac characterize acute dacryocystitis. Additional signs include excessive tearing, a purulent discharge, eyelid erythema, and swelling in the lacrimal punctum area.

Episcleritis. Deep eye pain occurs as tissues over the sclera become inflamed. Related effects include photophobia, excessive tearing, conjunctival edema, and a red or purplish sclera.

Erythema multiforme major. Erythema multiforme major commonly produces severe eye pain, entropion, trichiasis, purulent conjunctivitis, photophobia, and decreased tear formation.

Foreign bodies in the cornea and conjunctiva. Sudden severe pain is common, but vision usually remains intact. Other findings include excessive tearing, photophobia, miosis, a foreign-body sensation, a dark speck on the cornea, and dramatic conjunctival injection.

Hordeolum (stye). Hordeolum usually produces localized eye pain that increases as the stye grows. Eyelid erythema and edema are also common.

Iritis (acute). Moderate to severe eye pain occurs with severe photophobia, dramatic conjunctival injection, and blurred vision. The constricted pupil may respond poorly to light.

Lacrimal gland tumor. A lacrimal gland tumor is a neoplastic lesion that usually produces unilateral eye pain, impaired visual acuity, and some degree of exophthalmos.

Migraine headache. Migraines can produce pain so severe that the eyes also ache. Additionally, nausea, vomiting, blurred vision, and light and noise sensitivity may occur.

Ocular laceration and intraocular foreign bodies. Penetrating eye injuries usually cause mild to severe unilateral eye pain and impaired visual acuity. Eyelid edema, conjunctival injection, and an abnormal pupillary response may also occur.

Optic neuritis. With optic neuritis, pain in and around the eye occurs with eye movement. Severe vision loss and tunnel vision develop but improve in 2 to 3 weeks. Pupils respond sluggishly to direct light but normally to consensual light.

Scleritis. Scleritis produces severe eye pain and tenderness, along with conjunctival injection, a bluish purple sclera and, possibly, photophobia and excessive tearing.

Sclerokeratitis. Inflammation of the sclera and cornea causes pain, burning, irritation, and photophobia.

Subdural hematoma. Following head trauma, a subdural hematoma commonly causes severe eye ache and headache. Related neurologic signs depend on the hematoma's location and size.

Trachoma. Along with pain in the affected eye, trachoma causes excessive tearing, photophobia, eye discharge, eyelid edema and redness, and visible conjunctival follicles.

Uveitis. *Anterior uveitis* causes the sudden onset of severe pain, dramatic conjunctival injection, photophobia, and a small, nonreactive pupil.

Posterior uveitis causes an insidious onset of similar features as well as gradual blurring of vision and distorted pupil shape.

Lens-induced uveitis causes moderate eye pain, conjunctival injection, pupil constriction, and severely impaired visual acuity. In fact, the patient usually can perceive only light.

Other causes
Treatments and surgery. Contact lenses may cause eye pain and a foreign-body sensation. Ocular surgery may also produce eye pain, ranging from a mild ache to a severe pounding or stabbing sensation.

Nursing considerations
- To help ease eye pain, have the patient lie down in a darkened, quiet environment and close his eyes.
- Prepare the patient for diagnostic studies, including tonometry and orbital X-rays.

Patient teaching
- Stress the importance of following instructions for drug therapy.
- Teach the patient about ways to protect the eyes.
- Tell that the patient that he should seek medical attention for any eye pain.
- Explain the underlying cause of the patient's eye pain and its treatment.

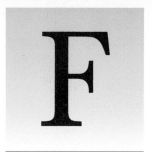

Fasciculations

Fasciculations, or *muscle twitches,* are local muscle contractions caused by the spontaneous discharge of a muscle fiber bundle supplied by a single motor nerve cell. These contractions cause visible dimpling or wavelike twitching of the skin, but aren't strong enough to cause a joint to move. Fasciculations occur irregularly, ranging from once every several seconds to two or three times per second; infrequently, myokymia—continuous, rapid fasciculations that cause a rippling effect—may occur. Because fasciculations are brief and painless, they commonly go undetected or are ignored.

Benign, nonpathologic fasciculations are common and normal. They typically occur in tense, anxious, or overtired people and typically affect the eyelid, thumb, or calf. However, fasciculations may also indicate a severe neurologic disorder, particularly a diffuse motor neuron disorder that causes loss of control over muscle fiber discharge. They're also an early sign of pesticide poisoning.

ACTION STAT!

 Begin by asking the patient about the nature, onset, and duration of the fasciculations. If the onset was sudden, ask about precipitating events such as exposure to pesticides. Pesticide poisoning, although uncommon, is a medical emergency requiring prompt and vigorous intervention. You may need to maintain airway patency, monitor the patient's vital signs, give oxygen, and perform gastric lavage or induce vomiting.

History and physical examination

If the patient isn't in severe distress, find out if he has experienced sensory changes, such as paresthesia, or any difficulty speaking, swallowing, breathing, or controlling bowel or bladder function. Ask him if he's in pain.

Explore the patient's medical history for neurologic disorders, cancer, and recent infections. Also, ask him about his lifestyle, especially stress at home, on the job, or at school.

Ask the patient about his dietary habits and for a recall of his food and fluid intake in the recent past because electrolyte imbalances may also cause muscle twitching.

Perform a physical examination, looking for fasciculations while the affected muscle is at rest. Observe and test for motor and sensory abnormalities, particularly muscle atrophy and weakness, and decreased deep tendon reflexes. If you note these signs and symptoms, suspect motor neuron disease, and perform a comprehensive neurologic examination.

Medical causes

Amyotrophic lateral sclerosis (ALS).
With ALS, coarse fasciculations usually begin in the small muscles of the hands and feet, and then spread to the forearms and legs. Widespread, symmetrical muscle atrophy and weakness may result in dysarthria; difficulty chewing, swallowing, and breathing; and, occasionally, choking and drooling.

Bulbar palsy.
Fasciculations of the face and tongue commonly appear early with bulbar palsy. Progressive signs and symptoms include dysarthria, dysphagia, hoarseness, and drooling. Eventually, weakness spreads to the respiratory muscles.

Poliomyelitis (spinal paralytic).
With poliomyelitis, coarse fasciculations, usually transient but occasionally persistent, accompany progressive muscle weakness, spasms, and atrophy. The patient may also exhibit decreased reflexes, paresthesia, coldness and cyanosis in the affected limbs, bladder paralysis, dyspnea, elevated blood pressure, and tachycardia.

Spinal cord tumors.
With spinal cord tumors, fasciculations may develop along with muscle atrophy and cramps, asymmetrically at first and then bilaterally as cord compression progresses. Motor and sensory changes distal to the tumor include weakness or paralysis, areflexia, paresthesia, and a tightening band of pain. Bowel and bladder control may be lost.

Other causes

Pesticide poisoning.
Ingestion of organophosphate or carbamate pesticides commonly produces an acute onset of long, wavelike fasciculations and muscle weakness that rapidly progresses to flaccid paralysis. Other common effects include nausea, vomiting, diarrhea, loss of bowel and bladder control, hyperactive bowel sounds, and abdominal cramping. Cardiopulmonary findings include bradycardia, dyspnea or bradypnea, and pallor or cyanosis. Seizures, vision disturbances (pupillary constriction or blurred vision), and increased secretions (tearing, salivation, pulmonary secretions, or diaphoresis) may also occur.

Nursing considerations
- Prepare the patient for diagnostic studies, such as spinal X-rays, myelography, a computed tomography scan, magnetic resonance imaging, and electromyography with nerve conduction velocity tests.
- Prepare the patient for laboratory tests such as serum electrolyte levels.
- Help the patient with progressive neuromuscular degeneration to cope with activities of daily living.

Patient teaching
- Teach the patient how to use assistive devices.
- Teach him about his underlying disorder, its progression, and treatment.
- Refer him to support groups, as indicated.

▌Fatigue

Fatigue is a feeling of excessive tiredness, a lack of energy, or exhaustion accompanied by a strong desire to rest or sleep. This common symptom is distinct from weakness, which involves the muscles, but may occur with it.

Fatigue is a normal and important response to physical overexertion, prolonged emotional stress, and sleep deprivation. However, it can also be a nonspecific symptom of a psychological or physiologic disorder—especially viral or bacterial infection and endocrine, cardiovascular, or neurologic disease.

Fatigue reflects hypermetabolic and hypometabolic states in which nutrients needed for cellular energy and growth are lacking because of overly rapid depletion, impaired replacement mechanisms, insufficient hormone production, or inadequate nutrient intake or metabolism.

History and physical examination

Obtain a careful history to identify the patient's fatigue pattern. Fatigue that worsens with activity and improves with rest generally indicates a physical disorder; the opposite pattern, a psychological disorder. Fatigue lasting longer than 4 months, constant fatigue that's unrelieved by rest, and transient exhaustion that quickly gives way to bursts of energy are other findings associated with psychological disorders.

Ask about related symptoms and recent viral or bacterial illness or stressful changes in lifestyle. Explore nutritional habits and appetite or weight changes. Carefully review the patient's medical and psychiatric history for chronic disorders that commonly produce fatigue. Ask about a family history of such disorders.

Obtain a thorough drug history, noting the use of any drug with fatigue as an adverse effect. Ask about alcohol and drug use patterns. Determine the patient's risk of carbon monoxide poisoning, and inquire as to whether the patient has a carbon monoxide detector in the home.

Observe the patient's general appearance for overt signs of depression or organic illness. Is he unkempt or expressionless? Does he appear tired or sickly, or have a slumped posture? If warranted, evaluate his mental status, noting especially mental clouding, attention deficits, agitation, or psychomotor retardation.

Medical causes

Acquired immunodeficiency syndrome (AIDS). In addition to fatigue, AIDS may cause a fever, night sweats, weight loss, diarrhea, and a cough, followed by several concurrent opportunistic infections.

Adrenocortical insufficiency. Mild fatigue, the hallmark of adrenocortical insufficiency, initially appears after exertion and stress, but later becomes more severe and persistent. Weakness and weight loss typically accompany GI disturbances, such as nausea, vomiting, anorexia, abdominal pain, and chronic diarrhea; hyperpigmentation; orthostatic hypotension; and a weak, irregular pulse.

Anemia. Fatigue following mild activity is commonly the first symptom of anemia. Associated findings vary, but generally include pallor, tachycardia, and dyspnea.

Anxiety. Chronic, unremitting anxiety invariably produces fatigue, typically characterized as nervous exhaustion. Other persistent findings include apprehension, indecisiveness, restlessness, insomnia, trembling, and increased muscle tension.

Cancer. Unexplained fatigue is commonly the earliest sign of cancer. Related findings reflect the type, location, and stage of the tumor and typically include pain, nausea, vomiting, anorexia, weight loss, abnormal bleeding, and a palpable mass.

Chronic fatigue syndrome. Chronic fatigue syndrome, whose cause is unknown, is characterized by incapacitating fatigue. Other findings are a sore throat, myalgia, and cognitive dysfunction. Diagnostic criteria have been determined, but research and data collection continue. These findings may alter the diagnostic criteria.

Chronic obstructive pulmonary disease (COPD). The earliest and most persistent symptoms of COPD are progressive fatigue and dyspnea. The patient may also experience a chronic and usually productive cough, weight loss, barrel chest, cyanosis, slight dependent edema, and poor exercise tolerance.

Depression. Persistent fatigue unrelated to exertion nearly always accompanies chronic depression. Associated somatic complaints include a headache, anorexia (occasionally, increased appetite), constipation, and sexual dysfunction. The patient may also experience insomnia, slowed speech, agitation or bradykinesia, irritability, loss of concentration, feelings of worthlessness, and persistent thoughts of death.

Diabetes mellitus. Fatigue, the most common symptom in diabetes mellitus, may begin insidiously or abruptly. Related findings include weight loss, blurred vision, polyuria, polydipsia, and polyphagia.

Heart failure. Persistent fatigue and lethargy characterize heart failure. Left-sided heart failure produces exertional and paroxysmal nocturnal dyspnea, orthopnea, and tachycardia. Right-sided heart failure produces jugular vein distention and, possibly, a slight but persistent nonproductive cough. In both types, mental status changes accompany later signs and symptoms, including nausea, anorexia, weight gain and, possibly, oliguria. Cardiopulmonary findings include tachypnea, inspiratory crackles, palpitations and chest tightness, hypotension, a narrowed pulse pressure, a ventricular gallop, pallor, diaphoresis, clubbing, and dependent edema.

Hypercortisolism. Hypercortisolism typically causes fatigue, related in part to accompanying sleep disturbances. Unmistakable signs include truncal obesity with slender extremities, buffalo hump, moon face, purple striae, acne, and hirsutism; increased blood pressure and muscle weakness are other findings.

Hypothyroidism. Fatigue occurs early in hypothyroidism, along with forgetfulness, cold intolerance, weight gain, metrorrhagia, and constipation.

Infection. With *chronic infection,* fatigue is commonly the most prominent symptom—and sometimes the only one. A low-grade fever and weight loss may accompany signs and symptoms that reflect the type and location of infection, such as burning upon urination or swollen, painful gums. Subacute bacterial endocarditis is an example of a chronic infection that causes fatigue and acute hemodynamic decompensation.

With *acute infection,* brief fatigue typically accompanies a headache, anorexia, arthralgia, chills, a high fever, and such infection-specific signs as a cough, vomiting, or diarrhea.

Lyme disease. In addition to fatigue and malaise, signs and symptoms of Lyme disease include an intermittent headache, a fever, chills, an expanding red rash, and muscle and joint aches. In later stages, patients may suffer arthritis, fluctuating meningoencephalitis, and cardiac abnormalities, such as a brief, fluctuating atrioventricular heart block.

Malnutrition. Easy fatigability is common in patients with protein-calorie malnutrition, along with lethargy and apathy. Patients may also exhibit weight loss, muscle wasting, sensations of coldness, pallor, edema, and dry, flaky skin.

Myasthenia gravis. The cardinal symptoms of myasthenia gravis are easy fatigability and muscle weakness, which worsen as the day progresses. They also worsen with exertion and abate with rest. Related findings depend on the specific muscles affected. (See *Managing the patient with myasthenia gravis.*)

Renal failure. *Acute renal failure* commonly causes sudden fatigue, drowsiness, and lethargy. Oliguria, an

Managing the patient with myasthenia gravis

Myasthenia gravis produces sporadic but progressive weakness and abnormal fatigability of striated (skeletal) muscles, which are exacerbated by exercise and repeated
movement but improved by anticholinesterase therapy. Usually, this disorder affects
muscles innervated by the cranial nerves (face, lips, tongue, neck, and throat), but it
can affect any muscle group. When the disease affects the respiratory system, it may
be life-threatening.

Do's

■ Help the patient plan daily activities to
coincide with energy peaks.
■ Stress the need for frequent rest periods through the day.
■ Establish an accurate neurologic and
respiratory baseline.
■ Be alert for impending crisis (increased muscle weakness, respiratory
distress, difficulty in talking or chewing).
■ Be prepared to give atropine for anticholinesterase overdose or toxicity.
■ Teach the patient how to recognize
adverse reactions and signs and symptoms of toxic reaction to an anticholinesterase (headaches, weakness,
sweating, abdominal cramps, nausea,
vomiting, diarrhea, excessive saliva, and
bronchospasm) and to a corticosteroid
(cushingoid symptoms [swelling of the
face, buffalo hump], adrenal insufficiency [fatigue, muscle weakness, dyspnea,
anorexia, nausea, fainting]).

Don'ts

■ Warn the patient to avoid strenuous
exercise, stress, infection, and needless
exposure to sun or cold weather.
■ To prevent relapses, warn the patient
not to delay or skip taking any ordered
drugs and to space them evenly.
■ To lessen the risk of choking when
swallowing is difficult, avoid liquids and
give the patient soft, solid food.

---

early sign, is followed by severe systemic effects: an ammonia breath odor, nausea, vomiting, diarrhea or constipation, and dry skin and mucous membranes. Neurologic findings include muscle twitching and changes in the patient's personality and level of consciousness, possibly progressing to seizures and coma.

With *chronic renal failure,* insidious fatigue and lethargy occur with marked changes in all body systems, including GI disturbances, an ammonia breath odor, Kussmaul's respirations, bleeding tendencies, poor skin turgor, severe pru-

ritus, paresthesia, vision disturbances, confusion, seizures, and coma.

Systemic lupus erythematosus (SLE). Fatigue usually occurs with SLE along with generalized aching, malaise, a low-grade fever, a headache, and irritability. Primary signs and symptoms include joint pain and stiffness, a butterfly rash, and photosensitivity. Also common are Raynaud's phenomenon, patchy alopecia, and mucous membrane ulcers.

Valvular heart disease. All types of valvular heart disease commonly produce progressive fatigue and a cardiac murmur. Additional signs and symptoms vary, but generally include exertional dyspnea, a cough, and hemoptysis.

Other causes

Carbon monoxide poisoning. Fatigue occurs with carbon monoxide poisoning along with a headache, dyspnea, and confusion and can eventually progress to unconsciousness and apnea.

Drugs. Fatigue may result from various drugs, notably antihypertensives and sedatives. In those receiving cardiac glycoside therapy, fatigue may indicate toxicity.

Surgery. Most types of surgery cause temporary fatigue, probably due to the combined effects of hunger, anesthesia, and sleep deprivation.

Nursing considerations

- Help the patient determine which daily activities he may need help with and how he should pace himself to ensure sufficient rest.
- Take measures to reduce pain and nausea.
- If fatigue results from a psychogenic cause, refer him for psychological counseling.

Patient teaching

- Educate the patient about lifestyle modifications, including diet and exercise.
- Stress the importance of pacing activities and planning rest periods.
- Discuss stress management techniques.

Fecal incontinence

Fecal incontinence, the involuntary passage of feces, follows a loss or an impairment of external anal sphincter control. It can result from many GI, neurologic, and psychological disorders; the effects of drugs; or surgery. In some patients, it

may even be a purposeful manipulative behavior.

Fecal incontinence may be temporary or permanent; its onset may be gradual, as in dementia, or sudden, as in spinal cord trauma. Although usually not a sign of severe illness, it can greatly affect the patient's physical and psychological well-being.

History and physical examination

Ask the patient with fecal incontinence about its onset, duration, and severity and about any discernible pattern—for example, does it occur at night or only with episodes of diarrhea? Note the frequency, consistency, and volume of stools passed within the past 24 hours and obtain a stool specimen. Focus your history taking on GI, neurologic, and psychological disorders.

Let the history guide your physical examination. If you suspect a brain or spinal cord lesion, perform a complete neurologic examination. (See *Neurologic control of defecation.*) If a GI disturbance seems likely, inspect the abdomen for distention, auscultate for bowel sounds, and percuss and palpate for a mass. Inspect the anal area for signs of excoriation or infection. If not contraindicated, check for fecal impaction, which may be associated with incontinence.

Medical causes

Dementia. Any chronic degenerative brain disease can produce fecal as well as urinary incontinence. Associated signs and symptoms include impaired judgment and abstract thinking, amnesia, emotional lability, hyperactive deep tendon reflexes, aphasia or dysarthria and, possibly, diffuse choreoathetoid movements.

Head trauma. Disruption of the neurologic pathways that control defecation can cause fecal incontinence. Addi-

Neurologic control of defecation

Three neurologic mechanisms normally regulate defecation: the intrinsic defecation reflex in the colon, the parasympathetic defecation reflex involving sacral segments of the spinal cord, and voluntary control. Here's how they interact.

Fecal distention of the rectum activates the relatively weak intrinsic reflex, causing afferent impulses to spread through the myenteric plexus, initiating peristalsis in the descending and sigmoid colon and rectum. Subsequent movement of feces toward the anus causes receptive relaxation of the internal anal sphincter.

To ensure defecation, the parasympathetic reflex magnifies the intrinsic reflex. Stimulation of afferent nerves in the rectal wall propels impulses through the spinal cord and back to the descending and sigmoid colon, rectum, and anus to intensify peristalsis (see illustration).

However, fecal movement and internal sphincter relaxation cause immediate contraction of the external anal sphincter and temporary fecal retention. At this point, conscious control of the external sphincter either prevents or permits defecation. Except in infants or neurologically impaired patients, this voluntary mechanism further contracts the sphincter to prevent defecation at inappropriate times, or relaxes it and allows defecation to occur.

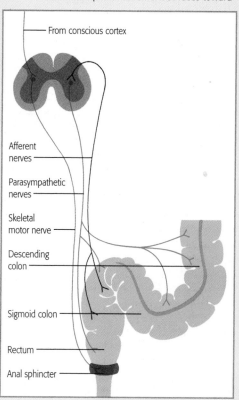

From conscious cortex

Afferent nerves

Parasympathetic nerves

Skeletal motor nerve

Descending colon

Sigmoid colon

Rectum

Anal sphincter

---

tional findings depend on the location and severity of the injury and may include a decreased level of consciousness, seizures, vomiting, and a wide range of motor and sensory impairments.

Inflammatory bowel disease. Nocturnal fecal incontinence occurs occasionally with diarrhea in inflammatory bowel disease. Related findings include abdominal pain, anorexia, weight loss,

blood in the stools, and hyperactive bowel sounds.

Rectovaginal fistula. With a rectovaginal fistula, fecal incontinence occurs in tandem with uninhibited passage of flatus.

Spinal cord lesions. Any lesion that causes compression or transsection of sensorimotor spinal tracts can lead to fecal incontinence. Incontinence may be permanent, especially with severe lesions of the sacral segments. Other signs and symptoms reflect motor and sensory disturbances below the level of the lesion, such as urinary incontinence, weakness or paralysis, paresthesia, analgesia, and thermanesthesia.

Other causes
Drugs. Chronic laxative abuse may cause insensitivity to a fecal mass or loss of the colonic defecation reflex.

Surgery. Pelvic, prostate, or rectal surgery occasionally produces temporary fecal incontinence. Colostomy or ileostomy causes permanent or temporary fecal incontinence.

Nursing considerations
- Maintain proper hygienic care, including control of foul odors.
- Provide meticulous skin care.
- For the neurologically capable patient with chronic incontinence, provide bowel retraining.
- Take measures to allay the patient's embarrassment.
- Provide emotional support for the patient.

Patient teaching
- Teach the patient to perform Kegel exercises to strengthen abdominal and perirectal muscles.
- Discuss how to maintain proper hygiene.

Fetor hepaticus

Fetor hepaticus—a distinctive musty, sweet breath odor—characterizes hepatic encephalopathy, a life-threatening complication of severe liver disease. The odor results from the damaged liver's inability to metabolize and detoxify mercaptans produced by bacterial degradation of methionine, a sulfurous amino acid. These substances circulate in the blood, are expelled by the lungs, and flavor the breath.

ACTION STAT!

 If you detect fetor hepaticus, quickly determine the patient's level of consciousness (LOC). If he's comatose, evaluate his respiratory status. Prepare to intubate and provide ventilatory support if necessary. Insert a peripheral I.V. catheter for fluid administration, begin cardiac monitoring, and insert an indwelling urinary catheter to monitor output. Obtain arterial and venous samples for analysis of blood gases, ammonia, and electrolytes.

History and physical examination
If the patient is conscious, closely observe him for signs of impending coma. Evaluate deep tendon reflexes, and test for asterixis and Babinski's sign. Be alert for signs of GI bleeding and shock, common complications of end-stage liver failure. Also, watch for increased anxiety, restlessness, tachycardia, tachypnea, hypotension, oliguria, hematemesis, melena, or cool, moist, pale skin. Place the patient in a supine position with the head of the bed at 30 degrees or greater. Administer oxygen if necessary, and determine the patient's need for I.V. fluids or albumin replacement. Draw blood samples for liver function tests, serum electrolyte levels, hepatitis panel, blood alcohol content, a complete blood count, typing and crossmatching, a clotting profile, and ammonia level. Intubation, ventilation, or cardiopulmonary resuscitation may be necessary. Evaluate the degree of jaundice and abdominal distention and palpate the liver to assess the degree of enlargement.

Obtain a complete medical history, relying on information from the patient's family if necessary. Focus on factors that may have precipitated hepatic disease or coma, such as a recent severe infection; overuse of sedatives, analgesics (especially acetaminophen), alcohol, or diuretics; excessive protein intake; or recent blood transfusion, surgery, or GI bleeding.

Medical causes

Hepatic encephalopathy. Fetor hepaticus usually occurs in the final, comatose stage of this disorder, but may occur earlier. Tremors progress to asterixis in the impending stage; lethargy, aberrant behavior, and apraxia also occur. Hyperventilation and stupor mark the stuporous stage, during which the patient acts agitated when aroused. Seizures and coma herald the final stage, along with decreased pulse and respiratory rates, a positive Babinski's sign, hyperactive reflexes, decerebrate posture, and opisthotonos.

Nursing considerations

- Administer neomycin or lactulose to suppress bacterial production of ammonia, sorbitol solution to induce osmotic diarrhea, and potassium supplements to correct alkalosis, as ordered.
- Provide continuous gastric aspiration of blood, as necessary.
- Maintain the patient on a low-protein diet, if indicated.
- If these methods prove unsuccessful, prepare the patient for hemodialysis or plasma exchange transfusions.
- Monitor the patient's LOC, intake and output, and fluid and electrolyte balance.

Patient teaching

- Advise the patient to restrict his intake of protein, as necessary.
- Teach the patient about any treatments as well as signs and symptoms that should be reported.

Fever
[Pyrexia]

A fever is a common sign that can arise from many disorders. Because these disorders can affect virtually any body system, a fever in the absence of other signs usually has little diagnostic significance. A persistent high fever, though, represents an emergency.

A fever can be classified as low (oral reading of 99° to 100.4° F [37.2° to 38° C]), moderate (100.5° to 104° F [38° to 40° C]), or high (above 104° F). A fever greater than 106° F (41.1° C) causes unconsciousness and, if sustained, leads to permanent brain damage.

A fever may also be classified as remittent, intermittent, sustained, relapsing, or undulant. Remittent fever, the most common type, is characterized by daily temperature fluctuations above the normal range. Intermittent fever is marked by a daily temperature drop into the normal range and then a rise back to above normal. An intermittent fever that fluctuates widely, typically producing chills and sweating, is called *hectic,* or *septic,* fever. Sustained fever involves persistent temperature elevation with little fluctuation. Relapsing fever consists of alternating feverish and afebrile periods. Undulant fever refers to a gradual increase in temperature that stays high for a few days and then decreases gradually.

Further classification involves duration—either brief (less than 3 weeks) or prolonged. Prolonged fevers include fever of unknown origin, a classification used when careful examination fails to detect an underlying cause.

ACTION STAT!

 If you detect a fever higher than 106° F, take the patient's other vital signs and determine his level of consciousness (LOC). Administer an antipyretic and begin rapid cooling measures: Apply ice packs to the axillae and groin, give tepid sponge baths, or apply a hypothermia blanket. These methods may evoke a cooling response; to prevent this, continually monitor the patient's rectal temperature.

History and physical examination

If the patient's fever is only mild to moderate, ask him when it began and how high his temperature reached. Did the fever disappear, only to reappear later? Did he experience other symptoms, such as chills, fatigue, or pain?

Obtain a complete medical history, noting especially immunosuppressive treatments or disorders, infection, trauma, surgery, diagnostic testing, and the use of anesthesia or other medications. Ask about recent travel because certain diseases are endemic.

Let the history findings direct your physical examination. Because a fever can accompany diverse disorders, the examination may range from a brief evaluation of one body system to a comprehensive review of all systems. (See *How fever develops.*)

Medical causes

Anthrax, cutaneous. The patient with cutaneous anthrax may experience a fever along with lymphadenopathy, malaise, and a headache. After the bacterium *Bacillus anthracis* enters a cut or abrasion on the skin, the infection begins as a small, painless, or pruritic macular or papular lesion resembling an insect bite. Within 1 to 2 days, the lesion develops into a vesicle and then into a painless ulcer with a characteristic black, necrotic center.

Anthrax, GI. Following the ingestion of contaminated meat from an animal infected with the bacterium *B. anthracis,*

the patient experiences a fever, a loss of appetite, nausea, and vomiting. The patient may also experience abdominal pain, severe bloody diarrhea, and hematemesis.

Anthrax, inhalation. The initial signs and symptoms of inhalation anthrax are flulike, including a fever, chills, weakness, a cough, and chest pain. The disease generally occurs in two stages, with a period of recovery after the initial symptoms. The second stage develops abruptly with rapid deterioration marked by a fever, dyspnea, stridor, and hypotension, generally leading to death within 24 hours.

Avian influenza. Fever is commonly an initial symptom of avian influenza along with other conventional influenza symptoms, such as muscle aches, sore throat, and cough. Individuals infected with the most virulent avian virus, influenza A (H5N1), may develop pneumonia, acute respiratory distress, and other life-threatening complications.

Escherichia coli O157:H7. A fever, bloody diarrhea, nausea, vomiting, and abdominal cramps occur after eating undercooked beef or other foods contaminated with this strain of bacteria. In children younger than age 5 and in elderly patients, hemolytic uremic syndrome may develop (in which the red blood cells are destroyed), and this may ultimately lead to acute renal failure.

Immune complex dysfunction. With immune complex dysfunction, a fever, when present, usually remains low, although moderate elevations may accompany erythema multiforme. Fever may be remittent or intermittent, as in acquired immunodeficiency syndrome (AIDS) or systemic lupus erythematosus, or sustained, as in polyarteritis. As one of several vague, prodromal complaints (such as fatigue, anorexia, and weight loss), a fever produces nocturnal diaphoresis and accompanies such asso-

How fever develops

Body temperature is regulated by the hypothalamic thermostat, which has a specific set point under normal conditions. A fever can result from a resetting of this set point or from an abnormality in the thermoregulatory system itself, as shown in this flowchart.

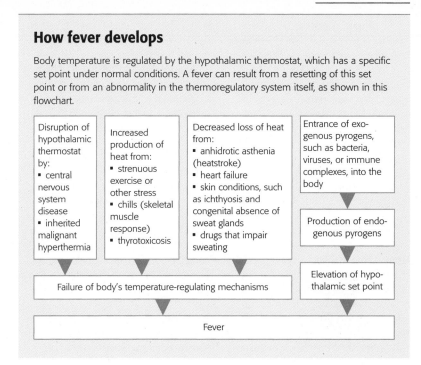

Disruption of hypothalamic thermostat by: • central nervous system disease • inherited malignant hyperthermia	Increased production of heat from: • strenuous exercise or other stress • chills (skeletal muscle response) • thyrotoxicosis	Decreased loss of heat from: • anhidrotic asthenia (heatstroke) • heart failure • skin conditions, such as ichthyosis and congenital absence of sweat glands • drugs that impair sweating	Entrance of exogenous pyrogens, such as bacteria, viruses, or immune complexes, into the body

Production of endogenous pyrogens

Failure of body's temperature-regulating mechanisms	Elevation of hypothalamic set point

Fever

---

ciated signs and symptoms as diarrhea and a persistent cough (with AIDS) or morning stiffness (with rheumatoid arthritis). Other disease-specific findings include a headache and vision loss (temporal arteritis); pain and stiffness in the neck, shoulders, back, or pelvis (ankylosing spondylitis and polymyalgia rheumatica); skin and mucous membrane lesions (erythema multiforme); and urethritis with urethral discharge and conjunctivitis (Reiter's syndrome).

Infectious and inflammatory disorders. With these disorders fever ranges from low (in patients with Crohn's disease or ulcerative colitis) to extremely high (in those with bacterial pneumonia, necrotizing fasciitis, or *Ebola* or *Hantavirus*). It may be remittent, as in those with infectious mononucleosis or otitis media; hectic (recurring daily with sweating, chills, and flushing), as in those with lung abscess, influenza, or

endocarditis; sustained, as in those with meningitis; or relapsing, as in those with malaria. A fever may arise abruptly, as in those with toxic shock syndrome or Rocky Mountain spotted fever, or insidiously, as in those with mycoplasmal pneumonia. In patients with hepatitis, a fever may represent a disease prodrome; in those with appendicitis, it follows the acute stage. Its sudden late appearance with tachycardia, tachypnea, and confusion heralds life-threatening septic shock in patients with peritonitis or gram-negative bacteremia.

Associated signs and symptoms involve every body system. The cyclic variations of hectic fever typically produce alternating chills and diaphoresis. General systemic complaints include weakness, anorexia, and malaise.

Kawasaki syndrome. Fever, typically high and spiking, is the primary characteristic of this acute illness. The diagnosis of Kawasaki syndrome is confirmed when fever persists for 5 or more days (or until administration of I.V. gamma globulin if given before the fifth day) and is accompanied by other clinical signs, including conjunctival injection, erythema, lymphadenopathy, and peripheral extremity swelling. This syndrome occurs worldwide, with the highest incidence in Japan. It primarily affects children under age 5, is more prevalent in boys, and can cause serious heart damage and death without prompt treatment with I.V. gamma globulin.

Listeriosis. Signs and symptoms of listeriosis include a fever, myalgia, abdominal pain, nausea, vomiting, and diarrhea. If the infection spreads to the nervous system, meningitis may develop; symptoms include a fever, a headache, nuchal rigidity, and a change in the LOC.

Monkeypox. Fever is one of the initial symptoms that occurs in almost all patients infected with this rare viral disease. A papular rash that may be localized or generalized appears within 1 to 3 days after the fever begins. Additional symptoms commonly include sore throat, chills, and lymphadenopathy. No treatment is available for monkeypox, but the disease is rarely fatal in developed countries and usually lasts 2 to 4 weeks.

Neoplasms. Primary neoplasms and metastasis can produce a prolonged fever of varying elevations. For instance, acute leukemia may present insidiously with a low-grade fever, pallor, and bleeding tendencies or more abruptly with a high fever, frank bleeding, and prostration. Occasionally, Hodgkin's disease produces an undulant fever or Pel-Ebstein fever, an irregularly relapsing fever.

In addition to a fever and nocturnal diaphoresis, neoplastic disease typically causes anorexia, fatigue, malaise, and weight loss. Examination may reveal lesions, lymphadenopathy, palpable masses, and hepatosplenomegaly.

Plague (Yersinia pestis). The bubonic form of plague (transmitted to man when bitten by infected fleas) causes a fever, chills, and swollen, inflamed, and tender lymph nodes near the bite site. The septicemic form develops as a fulminant illness generally with the bubonic form. The pneumonic form manifests as a sudden onset of chills, a fever, a headache, and myalgia after person-to-person transmission via the respiratory tract. Other signs and symptoms of the pneumonic form include a productive cough, chest pain, tachypnea, dyspnea, hemoptysis, increasing respiratory distress, and cardiopulmonary insufficiency.

Q fever. Q fever causes a fever, chills, a severe headache, malaise, chest pain, nausea, vomiting, and diarrhea. The fever may last up to 2 weeks. In severe cases, the patient may develop hepatitis or pneumonia.

Respiratory syncytial virus (RSV). Fever is one of the initial symptoms of this common illness that affects most children by age 2. Healthy adults and children older than age 3 usually develop a low-grade fever along with other common coldlike symptoms of runny nose, cough, and wheezing. Many children younger than age 3 have a high-grade fever that may be accompanied by a severe cough, rapid breathing, and high-pitched expiratory wheezing. Infants with RSV typically exhibit lethargy, poor eating, irritability, and difficulty breathing; severe cases may require hospitalization. To avoid repeated RSV infection, individuals should practice infection-control techniques, such as proper hand-washing and avoiding contact with contaminated surfaces.

Rhabdomyolysis. Rhabdomyolysis results in muscle breakdown and release of the muscle cell contents (myoglobin) into the bloodstream, with signs and symptoms that include a fever, muscle weakness or pain, nausea, vomiting, malaise, or dark urine. Acute renal failure is the most commonly reported complication of the disorder. It results from renal structure obstruction and injury during the kidney's attempt to filter myoglobin from the bloodstream.

Rift Valley fever. Typical signs and symptoms of Rift Valley fever include fever, myalgia, weakness, dizziness, and back pain. A small percentage of patients may develop encephalitis or may progress to hemorrhagic fever that can lead to shock and hemorrhage. Inflammation of the retina may result in some permanent vision loss.

Severe acute respiratory syndrome (SARS). SARS generally begins with a fever (usually greater than 100.4° F [38° C]). Other signs and symptoms include a headache, malaise, a dry nonproductive cough, and dyspnea. The severity of the illness is highly variable, ranging from mild illness to pneumonia and, in some cases, progressing to respiratory failure and death.

Smallpox (variola major). Initial signs and symptoms of smallpox include a high fever, malaise, prostration, a severe headache, a backache, and abdominal pain. A maculopapular rash develops on the mucosa of the mouth, pharynx, face, and forearms and then spreads to the trunk and legs. Within 2 days, the rash becomes vesicular and later pustular. The lesions develop at the same time, appear identical, and are more prominent on the face and extremities. The pustules are round, firm, and deeply embedded in the skin. After 8 to 9 days, the pustules form a crust, and later the scab separates from the skin, leaving a pitted scar. In fatal cases, death results from encephalitis, extensive bleeding, or secondary infection.

Thermoregulatory dysfunction. Thermoregulatory dysfunction is marked by a sudden onset of fever that rises rapidly and remains as high as 107° F (41.7° C). It occurs in such life-threatening disorders as heatstroke, thyroid storm, neuroleptic malignant syndrome, and malignant hyperthermia and in lesions of the central nervous system (CNS). A low or moderate fever appears in dehydrated patients.

A prolonged high fever commonly produces vomiting, anhidrosis, a decreased LOC, and hot, flushed skin. Related cardiovascular effects may include tachycardia, tachypnea, and hypotension. Other disease-specific findings include skin changes, such as dry skin and mucous membranes, poor skin turgor, and oliguria with dehydration; mottled cyanosis with malignant hyperthermia; diarrhea with thyroid storm; and ominous signs of increased intracranial pressure (a decreased LOC with bradycardia, a widened pulse pressure, and an increased systolic pressure) with CNS tumor, trauma, or hemorrhage.

Tularemia. Tularemia, also known as *rabbit fever*, causes an abrupt onset of a fever, chills, a headache, generalized myalgia, a nonproductive cough, dyspnea, pleuritic chest pain, and empyema.

Typhus. Typhus is a rickettsial disease in which the patient initially experiences a headache, myalgia, arthralgia, and malaise. These signs and symptoms are followed by an abrupt onset of a fever, chills, nausea, and vomiting. A maculopapular rash may be present in some cases.

West Nile encephalitis. Signs and symptoms of West Nile encephalitis include fever, headache, and body aches, usually with a skin rash and swollen lymph glands. More severe infection is marked by a high fever, headache, neck stiffness, stupor, disorientation, coma, tremors, occasional seizures, paralysis and, rarely, death.

Other causes

Diagnostic tests. Immediate or delayed fever uncommonly follows radiographic tests that use contrast medium.

Drugs. A fever and rash commonly result from hypersensitivity to antifungals, sulfonamides, penicillins, cephalosporins, tetracyclines, barbiturates, phenytoin, quinidine, iodides, phenolphthalein, methyldopa, procainamide, and some antitoxins. A fever can accompany chemotherapy, especially with bleomycin, vincristine, and asparaginase. It can result from drugs that impair sweating, such as anticholinergics, phenothiazines, and monoamine oxidase inhibitors. A drug-induced fever typically disappears after the involved drug is discontinued. A fever can also stem from toxic doses of salicylates, amphetamines, and tricyclic antidepressants.

Inhaled anesthetics and muscle relaxants can trigger malignant hyperthermia in patients with this inherited trait.

Treatments. Remittent or intermittent low fever may occur for several days after surgery. Transfusion reactions characteristically produce an abrupt onset of a fever and chills.

Nursing considerations

▪ Regularly monitor and record the patient's temperature.
▪ Provide increased fluid and nutritional intake.
▪ When administering a prescribed antipyretic, minimize chills and diaphoresis by following a regular dosage schedule.
▪ Promote patient comfort by maintaining a stable room temperature and providing frequent changes of bedding and clothing.

▪ For high fevers, initiate treatment with a hypothermia blanket.
▪ Prepare the patient for laboratory tests, such as complete blood count and cultures of blood, urine, sputum, and wound drainage.

Patient teaching

▪ Instruct the patient about the proper way to take an oral temperature at home.
▪ Emphasize the importance of increased fluid intake.
▪ Discuss the proper use of antipyretics and antibiotics.
▪ Teach signs and symptoms that require immediate medical attention.

Flank pain

Pain in the flank, the area extending from the ribs to the ilium, is a leading indicator of renal and upper urinary tract disease or trauma. Depending on the cause, this symptom may vary from a dull ache to severe stabbing or throbbing pain, and may be unilateral or bilateral and constant or intermittent. It's aggravated by costovertebral angle (CVA) percussion and, in patients with renal or urinary tract obstruction, by increased fluid intake and ingestion of alcohol, caffeine, or diuretics. Unaffected by position changes, flank pain typically responds only to analgesics or to treatment of the underlying disorder.

ACTION STAT!

 If the patient has suffered trauma, quickly look for a visible or palpable flank mass, associated injuries, CVA pain, hematuria, Turner's sign, and signs of shock, such as tachycardia and cool, clammy skin. If one or more is present, insert an I.V. catheter to allow fluid or drug infusion. Insert an indwelling urinary catheter to monitor urine output and evaluate hematuria.

Obtain blood samples for typing and crossmatching, a complete blood count, and electrolyte levels.

History and physical examination

If the patient's condition isn't critical, take a thorough history. Ask about the onset of his pain and apparent precipitating events. Have him describe the pain's location, intensity, pattern, and duration. Find out if anything aggravates or alleviates it.

Ask the patient about changes in his normal pattern of fluid intake and urine output. Explore his history for a urinary tract infection (UTI) or obstruction, renal disease, or recent streptococcal infection.

During the physical examination, palpate the patient's flank area and percuss the CVA to determine the extent of pain.

Medical causes

Calculi. Renal and ureteral calculi produce intense unilateral, colicky flank pain. Typically, initial CVA pain radiates to the flank, suprapubic region, and perhaps the genitalia; abdominal and lower back pain are also possible. Nausea and vomiting commonly accompany severe pain. Associated findings include CVA tenderness, hematuria, hypoactive bowel sounds and, possibly, signs and symptoms of a UTI (urinary frequency and urgency, dysuria, nocturia, fatigue, a low-grade fever, and tenesmus).

Cortical necrosis (acute). Unilateral flank pain is usually severe with corticol necrosis. Accompanying findings include gross hematuria, anuria, leukocytosis, and a fever.

Obstructive uropathy. With acute obstruction, flank pain may be excruciating; with gradual obstruction, it's typically a dull ache. With both, the pain

may also localize in the upper abdomen and radiate to the groin. Nausea and vomiting, abdominal distention, anuria alternating with periods of oliguria and polyuria, and hypoactive bowel sounds may also occur. Additional findings—a palpable abdominal mass, CVA tenderness, and bladder distention—vary with the site and cause of the obstruction.

Papillary necrosis (acute). Intense bilateral flank pain occurs with papillary necrosis along with renal colic, CVA tenderness, and abdominal pain and rigidity. Urinary signs and symptoms include oliguria or anuria, hematuria, and pyuria, with associated high fever, chills, vomiting, and hypoactive bowel sounds.

Perirenal abscess. With perirenal abscess, intense unilateral flank pain and CVA tenderness accompany dysuria, a persistent high fever, chills and, in some patients, a palpable abdominal mass.

Polycystic kidney disease. Dull, aching, bilateral flank pain is commonly the earliest symptom of polycystic kidney disease. The pain can become severe and colicky if cysts rupture and clots migrate or cause obstruction. Nonspecific early findings include polyuria, increased blood pressure, and signs of a UTI. Later findings include hematuria and perineal, low back, and suprapubic pain.

Pyelonephritis (acute). Intense, constant, and unilateral or bilateral flank pain develops over a few hours or days with acute pyelonephritis along with typical urinary features: dysuria, nocturia, hematuria, urgency, frequency, and tenesmus. Other common findings include a persistent high fever, chills, anorexia, weakness, fatigue, generalized myalgia, abdominal pain, and marked CVA tenderness.

Renal cancer. Unilateral flank pain, gross hematuria, and a palpable flank mass form the classic clinical triad in renal cancer. Flank pain is usually dull and vague, although severe colicky pain can occur during bleeding or passage of clots. Associated signs and symptoms include a fever, increased blood pressure, and urine retention. Weight loss, leg edema, nausea, and vomiting are indications of advanced disease.

Renal infarction. Unilateral, constant, severe flank pain and tenderness typically accompany persistent, severe upper abdominal pain with renal infarction. The patient may also develop CVA tenderness, anorexia, nausea and vomiting, a fever, hypoactive bowel sounds, hematuria, and oliguria or anuria.

Renal trauma. Variable bilateral or unilateral flank pain is a common symptom of renal trauma. A visible or palpable flank mass may also exist, along with CVA or abdominal pain—which may be severe and radiate to the groin. Other findings include hematuria, oliguria, abdominal distention, Turner's sign, hypoactive bowel sounds, and nausea or vomiting. Severe injury may produce signs of shock, such as tachycardia and cool, clammy skin.

Renal vein thrombosis. Severe unilateral flank and lower back pain with CVA and epigastric tenderness typify the rapid onset of venous obstruction. Other features include a fever, hematuria, and leg edema. Bilateral flank pain, oliguria, and other uremic signs and symptoms (nausea, vomiting, and uremic fetor) typify bilateral obstruction.

Nursing considerations

- Administer pain medication and evaluate effect.
- Monitor the patient's vital signs.
- Maintain a precise record of his intake and output.
- Prepare the patient for tests, such as serial urine and serum analysis, excretory urography, flank ultrasonography, a computed tomography scan, voiding cystourethrography, cystoscopy, and retrograde ureteropyelography, urethrography, and cystography.

Patient teaching

- Teach the patient about the underlying cause of flank pain.
- Describe the treatment plan and the need for follow-up care.

Fontanel, bulging

In a normal infant, the anterior fontanel, or "soft spot," is flat, soft yet firm, and well demarcated against surrounding skull bones. The posterior fontanel shouldn't be fused at birth, but may be overriding following the birthing process. This fontanel usually closes by age 3 months. (See *Locating fontanels.*) Subtle pulsations may be visible, reflecting the arterial pulse.

A bulging fontanel—widened, tense, and with marked pulsations—is a cardinal sign of meningitis associated with increased intracranial pressure (ICP), a medical emergency. It can also be an indication of encephalitis or fluid overload. Because prolonged coughing, crying, or lying down can cause transient, physiologic bulging, the infant's head should be observed and palpated while he's upright and relaxed to detect pathologic bulging.

ACTION STAT!

 If you detect a bulging fontanel, measure its size and the head circumference, and note the overall shape of the head. Take the infant's vital signs, and determine his level of consciousness (LOC) by observing spontaneous activity, postural reflex activity, and sensory responses. Note whether the infant assumes a normal, flexed posture or one of extreme extension, opisthotonos, or hypotonia. Observe arm and leg movements; exces-

Locating fontanels

The anterior fontanel lies at the junction of the sagittal, coronal, and frontal sutures. It normally measures about 2.5 × 4 to 5 cm at birth and usually closes by age 18 to 20 months.

The posterior fontanel lies at the junction of the sagittal and lambdoidal sutures. It measures 1 to 2 cm around and normally closes by age 3 months.

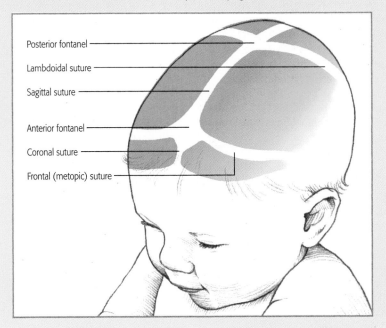

sive tremulousness or frequent twitching may herald the onset of a seizure. Look for other signs of increased ICP: abnormal respiratory patterns and a distinctive, high-pitched cry.

Ensure airway patency, and have size-appropriate emergency equipment on hand. Provide oxygen, establish I.V. access, and if the infant is having a seizure, stay with him to prevent injury and administer an anticonvulsant. Administer an antibiotic, antipyretic, and osmotic diuretic to help reduce cerebral edema and decrease ICP. If these measures fail to reduce ICP, neuromuscular blockade, intubation, mechanical ventilation and, in rare cases, barbiturate coma and total body hypothermia may be necessary.

History and physical examination

When the infant's condition is stabilized, you can begin investigating the underlying cause of increased ICP. Obtain the child's medical history from a parent or caretaker, paying particular attention to a recent infection or trauma, including birth trauma. Has the infant or a family member had a recent rash or fever? Ask about changes in the infant's behavior, such as frequent vomiting, lethargy, or disinterest in feeding. Then perform a complete physical examination focusing on neurologic signs and symptoms.

Medical causes

Increased ICP. Besides a bulging fontanel and increased head circumference, other early signs and symptoms of increased ICP are usually subtle and difficult to discern. They may include behavioral changes, irritability, fatigue, and vomiting. As ICP rises, the infant's pupils may dilate and his LOC may decrease to drowsiness and eventual coma. Seizures commonly occur.

Nursing considerations

- Closely monitor the infant's condition, including urine output (via an indwelling urinary catheter, if necessary).
- Observe the infant for seizures.
- Restrict fluids, and place the infant in the supine position, with his body tilted 30 degrees and his head up, to enhance cerebral venous drainage and reduce intracranial blood volume.
- Prepare the infant for diagnostic tests, such as an intracranial computed tomography scan or skull X-ray, cerebral angiography, and a full sepsis workup, including blood studies and urine cultures.

Patient teaching

- Explain the purpose and procedure of diagnostic tests to the infant's parents.
- Explain all treatments to the parents.
- Provide emotional support.
- Tell the parents how they can be involved in their infant's care.

Fontanel depression

Depression of the anterior fontanel below the surrounding bony ridges of the skull is a sign of dehydration. A common disorder of infancy and early childhood, dehydration can result from insufficient fluid intake, but typically reflects excessive fluid loss from severe vomiting or diarrhea. It may also reflect insensible water loss, pyloric stenosis, or tracheoesophageal fistula. It's best to assess the fontanel when the infant is in an upright position and isn't crying.

ACTION STAT!

 If you detect a markedly depressed fontanel, take the infant's vital signs, weigh him, and check for signs of shock—tachycardia, tachypnea, and cool, clammy skin. If these signs are present, insert an I.V. catheter and administer fluids. Have size-appropriate emergency equipment on hand. Anticipate oxygen administration. Monitor urine output by weighing wet diapers.

History and physical examination

Obtain a thorough patient history from a parent or caretaker, focusing on recent fever, vomiting, diarrhea, and behavioral changes. Monitor the infant's fluid intake and urine output over the past 24 hours, including the number of wet diapers during that time. Ask about the child's preillness weight, and compare it with his current weight; weight loss in an infant reflects water loss. Then perform a complete physical examination.

Medical causes

Dehydration. With *mild dehydration* (5% weight loss), the anterior fontanel appears slightly depressed. The infant has pale, dry skin and mucous membranes; decreased urine output; a normal or slightly elevated pulse rate; and, possibly, irritability.

Moderate dehydration (10% weight loss) causes slightly more pronounced fontanel depression, along with gray skin with poor turgor, dry mucous membranes, decreased tears, and decreased urine output. The infant has normal or decreased blood pressure, an increased pulse rate and, possibly, lethargy.

Severe dehydration (15% or greater weight loss) may result in a markedly sunken fontanel, along with extremely poor skin turgor, parched mucous membranes, marked oliguria or anuria, lethargy, and signs of shock, such as a rapid, thready pulse; very low blood pressure; and obtundation.

Nursing considerations
- Monitor the infant's vital signs and level of consciousness.
- Monitor intake and output and watch for signs of worsening dehydration.
- Obtain serum electrolyte values to check for an increased or decreased sodium, chloride, or potassium level.
- If the infant has mild dehydration, provide small amounts of clear fluids frequently or provide an oral rehydration solution.
- If the infant can't ingest sufficient fluid, begin I.V. parenteral nutrition.
- If the patient has moderate to severe dehydration, provide rapid restoration of extracellular fluid volume to treat or prevent shock.
- Continue to administer I.V. solution with sodium bicarbonate added to combat acidosis. As renal function improves, administer I.V. potassium replacements.
- When the infant's fluid status stabilizes, begin to replace depleted fat and protein stores through diet.
- Obtain urinalysis for specific gravity and, possibly, blood tests to determine blood urea nitrogen and serum creatinine levels, osmolality, and acid-base status.

Patient teaching
- Explain all procedures and treatments to the infant's parents.
- Provide emotional support.
- Explain ways to prevent dehydration.

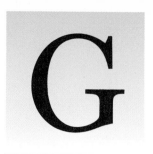

Gag reflex abnormalities
[Pharyngeal reflex abnormalities]

The gag reflex—a protective mechanism that prevents aspiration of food, fluid, and vomitus—normally can be elicited by touching the posterior wall of the oropharynx with a tongue blade or by suctioning the throat. Prompt elevation of the palate, constriction of the pharyngeal musculature, and a sensation of gagging indicate a normal gag reflex. An abnormal gag reflex—either decreased or absent—interferes with the ability to swallow and, more important, increases susceptibility to life-threatening aspiration.

An impaired gag reflex can result from a lesion that affects its mediators—cranial nerves (CNs) IX (glossopharyngeal) and X (vagus) or the pons or medulla. It can also occur during a coma, in muscle diseases such as severe myasthenia gravis, or as a temporary result of anesthesia.

A CTION STAT !

 If you detect an abnormal gag reflex, immediately stop the patient's oral intake to prevent aspiration. Quickly evaluate his level of consciousness (LOC). If it's decreased, place him in a side-lying position to prevent aspiration; if not, place him in Fowler's position. Have suction equipment at hand.

History and physical examination

Ask the patient (or a family member if the patient can't communicate) about the onset and duration of swallowing difficulties, if any. Are liquids more difficult to swallow than solids? Is swallowing more difficult at certain times of the day (as occurs in the bulbar palsy associated with myasthenia gravis)? If the patient also has trouble chewing, suspect more widespread neurologic involvement because chewing involves different CNs.

Explore the patient's medical history for vascular and degenerative disorders. Then assess his respiratory status for evidence of aspiration, and perform a neurologic examination.

Medical causes

Basilar artery occlusion. Basilar artery occlusion may suddenly diminish or obliterate the gag reflex. It also causes diffuse sensory loss, dysarthria, facial weakness, extraocular muscle palsies, quadriplegia, and a decreased LOC.

Brain stem glioma. Brain stem glioma causes a gradual loss of the gag reflex. Related symptoms reflect bilateral brain stem involvement and include diplopia and facial weakness. Common involvement of the corticospinal pathways causes spasticity and paresis of the arms and legs as well as gait disturbances.

Bulbar palsy. Loss of the gag reflex reflects temporary or permanent paralysis of muscles supplied by CNs IX and X. Other indicators of bulbar palsy include jaw and facial muscle weakness, dysphagia, loss of sensation at the base of the tongue, increased salivation, possible difficulty articulating and breathing, and fasciculations.

Wallenberg's syndrome. Paresis of the palate and an impaired gag reflex usually develop within hours to days of thrombosis. The patient may experience analgesia and thermanesthesia, occurring ipsilaterally on the face and contralaterally on the body, and vertigo. He may also display nystagmus, ipsilateral ataxia of the arm and leg, and signs of Horner syndrome (unilateral ptosis and miosis, hemifacial anhidrosis).

Other causes

Anesthesia. General and local (throat) anesthesia can produce temporary loss of the gag reflex.

Nursing considerations

- Frequently assess the patient's ability to swallow.
- If his gag reflex is absent, provide tube feedings.
- If the gag reflex is diminished, provide pureed foods.
- Stay with him while he eats and observe for choking.
- Keep suction equipment handy in case of aspiration.
- Maintain accurate intake and output records.
- Assess the patient's nutritional status daily.

- Refer the patient to a speech therapist to determine his aspiration risk and develop an exercise program to strengthen specific muscles.
- Prepare the patient for diagnostic studies, such as swallow studies, a computed tomography scan, magnetic resonance imaging, EEG, lumbar puncture, and arteriography.

Patient teaching

- Advise the patient to eat small amounts slowly while sitting or in high Fowler's position.
- Teach him techniques for safe swallowing.
- Discuss the types and textures of foods that reduce the risk of choking.

Gait, bizarre
[Hysterical gait]

A bizarre gait has no obvious organic basis; rather, it's produced unconsciously by a person with a somatoform disorder (hysterical neurosis) or consciously by a malingerer. The gait has no consistent pattern. It may mimic an organic impairment, but characteristically has a more theatrical or bizarre quality with key elements missing, such as a spastic gait without hip circumduction, or leg "paralysis" with normal reflexes and motor strength. Its manifestations may include wild gyrations, exaggerated stepping, leg dragging, or mimicking unusual walks such as that of a tightrope walker.

History and physical examination

If you suspect that the patient's gait impairment has no organic cause, begin to investigate other possibilities. Ask the patient when he first developed the impairment and whether it coincided with a stressful period or event, such as the death of a loved one or loss of a job. Ask about associated symptoms, and explore reports of frequent unexplained illnesses and multiple physician's visits. Subtly try to determine if the patient will gain anything from malingering, for instance, added attention or an insurance settlement.

Begin the physical examination by testing the patient's reflexes and sensorimotor function, noting abnormal response patterns. To quickly check his reports of leg weakness or paralysis, perform a test for Hoover's sign: Place the patient in the supine position and stand at his feet. Cradle a heel in each of your palms, and rest your hands on the table. Ask the patient to raise the affected leg. In true motor weakness, the heel of the other leg will press downward; in hysteria, this movement will be absent. As a further check, observe the patient for normal movements when he's unaware of being watched.

Medical causes

Conversion disorder. Conversion disorder is a rare somatoform disorder in which a bizarre gait or paralysis may develop after severe stress and isn't accompanied by other symptoms. The patient typically shows indifference toward his impairment.

Malingering. Malingering is a rare cause of bizarre gait, in which the patient may also complain of a headache and chest and back pain.

Somatization disorder. Bizarre gait is one of many possible somatic complaints. The patient may exhibit any combination of pseudoneurologic signs and symptoms—fainting, weakness, memory loss, dysphagia, vision problems (diplopia, vision loss, blurred vision), loss of voice, seizures, and bladder dysfunction. He may also report pain in the back, joints, and extremities (most commonly the legs) and complaints in almost any body system. For example, characteristic GI complaints include pain, bloating, nausea, and vomiting.

The patient's reflexes and motor strength remain normal, but peculiar contractures and arm or leg rigidity may occur. His reputed sensory loss doesn't conform to a known sensory dermatome. In some cases, he won't stand or walk (astasia or abasia), remaining bedridden although still able to move his legs in bed.

Nursing considerations

■ Prepare the patient for a full neurologic workup to completely rule out an organic cause of the patient's abnormal gait.
■ Remember, even though bizarre gait has no organic basis, it's real to the patient (unless, of course, he's malingering).
■ Avoid expressing judgment on the patient's actions or motives.
■ Be supportive and reinforce positive progress.
■ Encourage ambulation and resumption of normal activities because muscle atrophy and bone demineralization can develop in a bedridden patient.
■ Consider a referral for psychiatric counseling as appropriate.

Patient teaching

■ Instruct the patient in the use of assistive devices, as necessary.
■ Review safety measures such as wearing proper footwear.

Gait, propulsive
[Festinating gait]

Propulsive gait is characterized by a stooped, rigid posture—the patient's head and neck are bent forward; his flexed, stiffened arms are held away from the body; his fingers are extended; and his knees and hips are stiffly bent.

During ambulation, this posture results in a forward shifting of the body's center of gravity and consequent impairment of balance, causing increasingly rapid, short, shuffling steps with involuntary acceleration (festination) and lack of control over forward motion (propulsion) or backward motion (retropulsion). (See *Identifying gait abnormalities*, page 274.)

Propulsive gait is a cardinal sign of advanced Parkinson's disease; it results from progressive degeneration of the ganglia, which are primarily responsible for smooth-muscle movement. Because this sign develops gradually and its accompanying effects are usually wrongly attributed to aging, propulsive gait commonly goes unnoticed or unreported until severe disability results.

History and physical examination

Ask the patient when his gait impairment first developed and whether it has recently worsened. Because he may have difficulty remembering, having attributed the gait to "old age" or disease processes, you may be able to gain information from family members or friends, especially those who see the patient only sporadically.

Also, obtain a thorough drug history, including medication type and dosage. Ask the patient if he has been taking tranquilizers, especially phenothiazines. If he knows he has Parkinson's disease and has been taking levodopa, pay particular attention to the dosage because an overdose can cause an acute exacerbation of signs and symptoms. If Parkinson's disease isn't a known or suspected diagnosis, ask the patient if he has been acutely or routinely exposed to carbon monoxide or manganese.

Begin the physical examination by testing the patient's reflexes and sensorimotor function, noting abnormal response patterns.

Medical causes

Parkinson's disease. The characteristic and permanent propulsive gait begins early as a shuffle in Parkinson's disease. As the disease progresses, the gait slows. Cardinal signs of the disease are progressive muscle rigidity, which may be uniform (lead-pipe rigidity) or jerky (cogwheel rigidity); akinesia; and an insidious tremor that begins in the fingers, increases during stress or anxiety, and decreases with purposeful movement and sleep. Besides the gait, akinesia also typically produces a monotone voice, drooling, masklike facies, a stooped posture, and dysarthria, dysphagia, or both. Occasionally, it also causes oculogyric crises or blepharospasm.

Other causes

Carbon monoxide poisoning. A propulsive gait commonly appears several weeks after acute carbon monoxide intoxication. Earlier effects include muscle rigidity, choreoathetoid movements, generalized seizures, myoclonic jerks, masklike facies, and dementia.

Drugs. Propulsive gait and possibly other extrapyramidal effects can result from the use of phenothiazines, other antipsychotics (notably haloperidol, thiothixene, and loxapine) and, less commonly, metoclopramide and metyrosine. Such effects are usually temporary, disappearing within a few weeks after therapy is discontinued.

Manganese poisoning. Chronic overexposure to manganese can cause an insidious, usually permanent, propulsive gait. Typical early findings include fatigue, muscle weakness and rigidity, dystonia, resting tremor, choreoathetoid movements, masklike facies, and personality changes. Those at risk for manganese poisoning are welders,

Identifying gait abnormalities

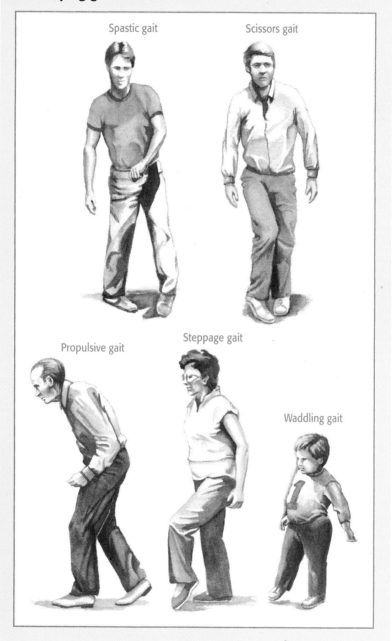

Spastic gait

Scissors gait

Propulsive gait

Steppage gait

Waddling gait

railroad workers, miners, steelworkers, and workers who handle pesticides.

Nursing considerations

- If the patient has problems performing activities of daily living, assist him as appropriate, while at the same time encouraging his independence, self-reliance, and confidence.
- Maintain a safe environment.
- Assist with ambulation, as needed.
- Refer the patient to a physical therapist for exercise therapy and gait retraining.

Patient teaching

- Advise the patient and his family to allow plenty of time for walking to avoid falls.
- Instruct the patient on the use of assistive devices, if appropriate.

Gait, scissors

Resulting from bilateral spastic paresis (diplegia), scissors gait affects both legs and has little or no effect on the arms. The patient's legs flex slightly at the hips and knees, so he looks as if he's crouching. With each step, his thighs adduct and his knees hit or cross in a scissors-like movement. (See *Identifying gait abnormalities*.) His steps are short, regular, and laborious, as if he were wading through waist-deep water. His feet may be plantar flexed and turned inward, with a shortened Achilles tendon; as a result, he walks on his toes or on the balls of his feet and may scrape his toes on the ground.

History and physical examination

Ask the patient (or a family member, if the patient can't answer) about the onset and duration of the gait. Has it progressively worsened or remained constant? Ask about a history of trauma, including birth trauma, and neurologic disorders.

Thoroughly evaluate motor and sensory function and deep tendon reflexes (DTRs) in the legs.

Medical causes

Cerebral palsy. In the spastic form of cerebral palsy, patients walk on their toes with a scissors gait. Other features include hyperactive DTRs, increased stretch reflexes, rapid alternating muscle contraction and relaxation, muscle weakness, underdevelopment of affected limbs, and a tendency toward contractures.

Cervical spondylosis with myelopathy. Scissors gait develops in the late stages of cervical spondylosis with myelopathy and steadily worsens. Related findings mimic those of a herniated disk: severe low back pain, which may radiate to the buttocks, legs, and feet; muscle spasms; sensorimotor loss; and muscle weakness and atrophy.

Multiple sclerosis. In multiple sclerosis, progressive scissors gait usually develops gradually, with infrequent remissions. Characteristic muscle weakness, usually in the legs, ranges from minor fatigability to paraparesis with urinary urgency and constipation. Related findings include facial pain, vision disturbances, paresthesia, incoordination, and loss of proprioception and vibration sensation in the ankle and toes.

Spinal cord tumor. Scissors gait can develop gradually from a thoracic or lumbar tumor. Other findings reflect the location of the tumor and may include radicular, subscapular, shoulder, groin, leg, or flank pain; muscle spasms or fasciculations; muscle atrophy; sensory deficits, such as paresthesia and a girdle sensation of the abdomen and chest; hyperactive DTRs; a bilateral Babinski's reflex; spastic neurogenic bladder; and sexual dysfunction.

Syringomyelia. Scissors gait usually occurs late in syringomyelia, along with analgesia and thermanesthesia, muscle atrophy and weakness, and Charcot's joint. Other effects may include the loss of fingernails, fingers, or toes; Dupuytren's contracture of the palms; scoliosis; and clubfoot. Skin in the affected areas is commonly dry, scaly, and grooved.

Nursing considerations

- Because of the sensory loss associated with scissors gait, provide meticulous skin care to prevent skin breakdown and pressure ulcer formation.
- Provide active and passive range-of-motion exercises.
- Refer the patient to a physical therapist for gait retraining and for possible in-shoe splints or leg braces to maintain proper foot alignment for standing and walking.
- Assist with ambulation.

Patient teaching

- Advise the patient and his family on complete skin care.
- Teach them about bladder and bowel retraining, if appropriate.
- Reinforce the proper use of splints or braces, if appropriate.

Gait, spastic
[Hemiplegic gait]

Spastic gait—sometimes referred to as *paretic* or *weak* gait—is a stiff, foot-dragging walk caused by unilateral leg muscle hypertonicity. This gait indicates focal damage to the corticospinal tract. The affected leg becomes rigid, with a marked decrease in flexion at the hip and knee and possibly plantar flexion and equinovarus deformity of the foot. Because the patient's leg doesn't swing normally at the hip or knee, his foot tends to drag or shuffle, scraping his toes on the ground. (See *Identifying gait abnormalities,* page 274.) To compensate, the pelvis of the affected side tilts up-

ward in an attempt to lift the toes, causing the patient's leg to abduct and circumduct. Also, arm swing is hindered on the same side as the affected leg.

Spastic gait usually develops after a period of flaccidity (hypotonicity) in the affected leg. Whatever the cause, the gait is usually permanent after it develops.

History and physical examination

Find out when the patient first noticed the gait impairment and whether it developed suddenly or gradually. Ask him if it waxes and wanes, or if it has worsened progressively. Does fatigue, hot weather, or warm baths or showers worsen the gait? Such exacerbation typically occurs in multiple sclerosis. Focus your medical history questions on neurologic disorders, recent head trauma, and degenerative diseases.

During the physical examination, test and compare strength, range of motion (ROM), and sensory function in all limbs. Also, observe and palpate for muscle flaccidity or atrophy.

Medical causes

Brain abscess. In brain abscess, spastic gait generally develops slowly after a period of muscle flaccidity and fever. Early signs and symptoms of abscess reflect increased intracranial pressure (ICP): a headache, nausea, vomiting, and focal or generalized seizures. Later, site-specific features may include hemiparesis, tremors, vision disturbances, nystagmus, and pupillary inequality. The patient's level of consciousness may range from drowsiness to stupor.

Brain tumor. Depending on the site and type of tumor, spastic gait usually develops gradually and worsens over time. Accompanying effects may include signs of increased ICP (a headache, nausea, vomiting, and focal or generalized seizures), papilledema, sensory loss on the affected side, dysarthria, ocular palsies, aphasia, and personality changes.

Head trauma. Spastic gait typically follows the acute stage of head trauma. The patient may also experience focal or generalized seizures, personality changes, a headache, and focal neurologic signs, such as aphasia and visual field deficits.

Multiple sclerosis. Spastic gait begins insidiously and follows multiple sclerosis' characteristic cycle of remission and exacerbation. The gait, as well as other signs and symptoms, commonly worsens in warm weather or after a warm bath or shower. Characteristic weakness, usually affecting the legs, ranges from minor fatigability to paraparesis with urinary urgency and constipation. Other effects include facial pain, paresthesia, incoordination, loss of proprioception and vibration sensation in the ankle and toes, and vision disturbances.

Stroke. With a stroke, spastic gait usually appears after a period of muscle weakness and hypotonicity on the affected side. Associated effects may include unilateral muscle atrophy, sensory loss, and footdrop; aphasia; dysarthria; dysphagia; visual field deficits; diplopia; and ocular palsies.

Nursing considerations

- Provide the patient with daily exercise and active and passive ROM exercises.
- Refer the patient to a physical therapist for gait retraining and possible in-shoe splints or leg braces to maintain proper foot alignment for standing and walking.
- Assist the patient with ambulation.

Patient teaching

- Reinforce the importance of ambulating with assistance.

- Teach the patient to use a cane or a walker, as indicated.

Gait, steppage
[Equine gait, paretic gait, prancing gait, weak gait]

Steppage gait typically results from foot-drop caused by weakness or paralysis of pretibial and peroneal muscles, usually from lower motor neuron lesions. Foot-drop causes the foot to hang with the toes pointing down, causing the toes to scrape the ground during ambulation. To compensate, the hip rotates outward and the hip and knee flex in an exaggerated fashion to lift the advancing leg off the ground. The foot is thrown forward and the toes hit the ground first, producing an audible slap. (See *Identifying gait abnormalities,* page 274.) The rhythm of the gait is usually regular, with even steps and normal upper body posture and arm swing. Steppage gait can be unilateral or bilateral and permanent or transient, depending on the site and type of neural damage.

History and physical examination

Begin by asking the patient about the onset of the gait and recent changes in its character. Does a family member have a similar gait? Find out if the patient has had a traumatic injury to the buttocks, hips, legs, or knees. Ask about a history of chronic disorders that may be associated with polyneuropathy, such as diabetes mellitus, polyarteritis nodosa, and alcoholism. While you're taking the history, observe whether the patient crosses his legs while sitting because this may put pressure on the peroneal nerve.

Inspect and palpate the patient's calves and feet for muscle atrophy and wasting. Using a pin, test for sensory deficits along the entire length of both legs.

Medical causes

Guillain-Barré syndrome. Typically occurring after recovery from the acute stage of Guillain-Barré syndrome, steppage gait can be mild or severe and unilateral or bilateral; it's invariably permanent. Muscle weakness usually begins in the legs, extends to the arms and face within 72 hours, and can progress to total motor paralysis and respiratory failure. Other effects include footdrop, transient paresthesia, hypernasality, dysphagia, diaphoresis, tachycardia, orthostatic hypotension, and incontinence.

Herniated lumbar disk. Unilateral steppage gait and footdrop commonly occur with late-stage weakness and atrophy of leg muscles that occur with a herniated lumbar disk. However, the most pronounced symptom is severe low back pain, which may radiate to the buttocks, legs, and feet, usually unilaterally. Sciatic pain follows, commonly accompanied by muscle spasms and sensorimotor loss. Paresthesia and fasciculations may occur.

Multiple sclerosis. Steppage gait and footdrop typically fluctuate in severity with multiple sclerosis' characteristic cycle of periodic exacerbation and remission. Muscle weakness, usually affecting the legs, can range from minor fatigability to paraparesis with urinary urgency and constipation. Related findings include facial pain, vision disturbances, paresthesia, incoordination, and sensory loss in the ankle and toes.

Peroneal muscle atrophy. Bilateral steppage gait and footdrop begin insidiously in peroneal muscle atrophy. Foot, peroneal, and ankle dorsiflexor muscles are affected first. Other early signs and symptoms include paresthesia, aching, and cramping in the feet and legs along with coldness, swelling, and cyanosis. As the disorder progresses, all leg muscles become weak and atrophic, with hypoactive or absent deep tendon reflexes. Later, atrophy and sensory losses spread to the hands and arms.

Peroneal nerve trauma. Temporary ipsilateral steppage gait occurs suddenly but resolves with the release of peroneal nerve pressure. The gait is associated with footdrop and muscle weakness and sensory loss over the lateral surface of the calf and foot.

Nursing considerations

- Because the patient may tire rapidly due to the extra effort needed to lift his feet off the ground, assess him for fatigue, which may cause him to stub his toes and fall.
- Take appropriate safety measures to reduce the risk of falls.
- Refer him to a physical therapist, if appropriate, for gait retraining and possible application of in-shoe splints or leg braces to maintain correct foot alignment.
- Assist the patient with ambulation.

Patient teaching

- Help the patient recognize his exercise limits and encourage him to get adequate rest.
- Teach the patient how to use splints and braces.

Gait, waddling

Waddling gait, a distinctive ducklike walk, is an important sign of muscular dystrophy, spinal muscle atrophy or, rarely, congenital hip displacement. It may be present when the child begins to walk or may appear only later in life. The gait results from deterioration of the pelvic girdle muscles—primarily the gluteus medius, hip flexors, and hip extensors. Weakness in these muscles hinders stabilization of the weight-bearing hip during walking, causing the opposite hip to drop and the trunk to lean toward that side in an attempt to maintain balance. (See *Identifying gait abnormalities,* page 274.)

Typically, the legs assume a wide stance and the trunk is thrown back to further improve stability, exaggerating lordosis and abdominal protrusion. In severe cases, leg and foot muscle contractures may cause equinovarus deformity of the foot combined with circumduction or bowing of the legs.

History and physical examination

Ask the patient (or a family member, if the patient is a young child) when the gait first appeared and if it has recently worsened. To determine the extent of pelvic girdle and leg muscle weakness, ask if the patient falls frequently or has difficulty climbing stairs, rising from a chair, or walking. Also, find out if he was late in learning to walk or holding his head upright. Obtain a family history, focusing on problems of muscle weakness and gait and on congenital motor disorders.

Inspect and palpate leg muscles, especially the calves, for size and tone. Check for a positive Gowers' sign, which indicates pelvic muscle weakness. (See *Identifying Gowers' sign.*) Next, assess motor strength and function in the shoulders, arms, and hands, looking for weakness or asymmetrical movements.

Identifying Gowers' sign

To check for Gowers' sign, place the patient in the supine position and ask him to rise. A positive Gowers' sign—an inability to lift the trunk without using the hands and arms to brace and push—indicates pelvic muscle weakness, as occurs in muscular dystrophy and spinal muscle atrophy.

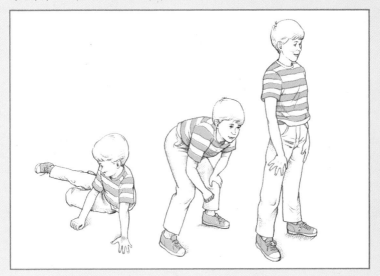

Medical causes

Developmental dysplasia of the hip.
Bilateral hip dislocation produces a waddling gait with lordosis and pain.

Muscular dystrophy. With *Duchenne's muscular dystrophy,* waddling gait becomes clinically evident between ages 3 and 5. The gait worsens as the disease progresses, until the child loses the ability to walk and requires the use of a wheelchair, usually between ages 10 and 12. Early signs are usually subtle: a delay in learning to walk, frequent falls, gait or posture abnormalities, and intermittent calf pain. Common later findings include lordosis with abdominal protrusion, a positive Gowers' sign, and equinovarus foot position. As the disease progresses, its effects become more prominent; they commonly include rapid muscle wasting beginning in the legs and spreading to the arms (although calf and upper arm muscles may become hypertrophied, firm, and rubbery), muscle contractures, limited dorsiflexion of the feet and extension of the knees and elbows, obesity and, possibly, mild mental retardation. Serious complications result when kyphoscoliosis develops, leading to respiratory dysfunction and, eventually, death from cardiac or respiratory failure.

With *Becker's muscular dystrophy,* waddling gait typically becomes apparent in late adolescence, slowly worsens during the third decade, and culminates in total loss of ambulation. Muscle weakness first appears in the pelvic and upper arm muscles. Progressive wasting with selected muscle hypertrophy produces lordosis with abdominal protrusion, poor balance, a positive Gowers' sign and, possibly, mental retardation.

With *facioscapulohumeral muscular dystrophy,* which usually occurs late in childhood and during adolescence, waddling gait appears after muscle wasting has spread downward from the face and shoulder girdle to the pelvic girdle and legs. Earlier effects include progressive weakness and atrophy of facial, shoulder, and arm muscles; slight lordosis; and pelvic instability.

Spinal muscle atrophy. With *Kugelberg-Welander syndrome,* waddling gait occurs early (usually after age 2) and typically progresses slowly, culminating in the total loss of ambulation up to 20 years later. Related findings may include muscle atrophy in the legs and pelvis, progressing to the shoulders; a positive Gowers' sign; ophthalmoplegia; and tongue fasciculations.

With *Werdnig-Hoffmann disease,* waddling gait typically begins when the child learns to walk. Reflexes may be absent. The gait progressively worsens, culminating in complete loss of ambulation by adolescence. Associated findings include lordosis with abdominal protrusion and muscle weakness in the hips and thighs.

Nursing considerations

■ Perform passive and active muscle-stretching exercises to the arms and legs.
■ Encourage the patient to walk at least 3 hours each day (with leg braces, if necessary) to maintain muscle strength, reduce contractures, and delay further gait deterioration, if possible.
■ Stay near the patient during ambulation, to provide support if necessary.
■ Provide a balanced diet to maintain energy levels and prevent obesity.
■ Because of the grim prognosis associated with muscular dystrophy and spinal muscle atrophy, provide emotional support for the patient and his family.

Patient teaching

■ Caution the patient about long, unbroken periods of bed rest, which accelerate muscle deterioration.

■ Refer the patient to a local Muscular Dystrophy Association chapter, as indicated.

■ Suggest genetic counseling for parents, if they're considering having more children.

Gallop, atrial
[S₄]

An atrial or presystolic gallop is an extra heart sound (known as S_4) that's heard or typically palpated immediately before the first heart sound (S_1), late in diastole. This low-pitched sound is heard best with the bell of the stethoscope pressed lightly against the cardiac apex. Some clinicians say that an S_4 has the cadence of the "Ten" in Tennessee (Ten = S_4; nes = S_1; see = S_2).

This gallop typically results from hypertension, conduction defects, valvular disorders, or other problems such as ischemia. Occasionally, it helps differentiate angina from other causes of chest pain. It results from abnormal forceful atrial contraction caused by augmented ventricular filling or by decreased left ventricular compliance. An atrial gallop usually originates from left atrial contraction, is heard at the apex, and doesn't vary with inspiration. A left-sided S_4 can occur in hypertensive heart disease, coronary artery disease, aortic stenosis, and cardiomyopathy. It may also originate from right atrial contraction. A right-sided S_4 is indicative of pulmonary hypertension and pulmonary stenosis. In that case, it's heard best at the lower left sternal border and intensifies with inspiration.

An atrial gallop seldom occurs in normal hearts; however, it may occur in elderly people and in athletes with physiologic hypertrophy of the left ventricle.

ACTION STAT!

 Suspect myocardial ischemia if you auscultate an atrial gallop in a patient with chest pain. (See *Locating heart sounds*, page 282, and *Interpreting heart sounds*, pages 284 and 285.) Take the patient's vital signs and quickly assess for signs of heart failure, such as dyspnea, crackles, and jugular vein distention. If you detect these signs, connect the patient to a cardiac monitor and obtain an electrocardiogram (ECG). Administer an antianginal and oxygen. If the patient has dyspnea, elevate the head of the bed. Then auscultate for abnormal breath sounds. If you detect coarse crackles, ensure patent I.V. access and give oxygen and diuretics as needed. If the patient has bradycardia, he may require atropine and a pacemaker.

History and physical examination

When the patient's condition permits, ask about a history of hypertension, angina, valvular stenosis, or cardiomyopathy. If appropriate, have him describe the frequency and severity of anginal attacks. Then perform a complete physical examination with special focus on the cardiovascular system.

Medical causes

Angina. An intermittent atrial gallop characteristically occurs during an anginal attack and disappears when angina subsides. This gallop may be accompanied by a paradoxical S_2 or a new murmur. Typically, the patient complains of anginal chest pain—a feeling of tightness, pressure, achiness, or burning that usually radiates from the retrosternal area to the neck, jaws, left shoulder, and arm. He may also exhibit dyspnea, tachycardia, palpitations, increased

Locating heart sounds

When auscultating heart sounds, remember that certain sounds are heard best in specific areas. Use the auscultatory points shown below to locate heart sounds quickly and accurately. Then expand your auscultation to nearby areas. Note that the numbers indicate pertinent intercostal spaces.

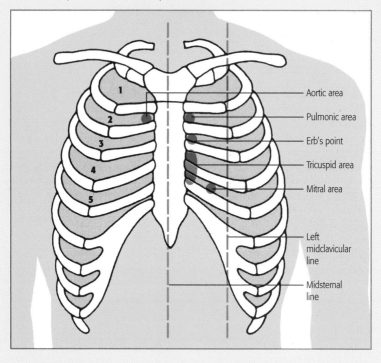

blood pressure, dizziness, diaphoresis, belching, nausea, and vomiting.

Aortic insufficiency (acute). Acute aortic insufficiency causes an atrial gallop accompanied by a soft, short diastolic murmur along the left sternal border. S_2 may be soft or absent. Sometimes a soft, short midsystolic murmur may be heard over the second right intercostal space. Related cardiopulmonary findings may include tachycardia, S_3, dyspnea, jugular vein distention, crackles and,

possibly, angina. The patient may also be fatigued and have cool extremities.

Aortic stenosis. Aortic stenosis usually causes an atrial gallop, especially when valvular obstruction is severe. Auscultation reveals a harsh, crescendo-decrescendo, systolic ejection murmur that's loudest at the right sternal border near the second intercostal space. Dyspnea, anginal chest pain, and syncope are cardinal associated findings. The patient may also display crackles, palpitations, fatigue, and diminished carotid pulses.

Atrioventricular (AV) block. First-degree AV block may cause an atrial gallop accompanied by a faint S_1. Although the patient may have bradycardia, he's usually asymptomatic. In second-degree AV block, an atrial gallop is easily heard. If bradycardia develops, the patient may also experience hypotension, light-headedness, dizziness, and fatigue. An atrial gallop is also common in third-degree AV block. It varies in intensity with S_1 and is loudest when atrial systole coincides with early, rapid ventricular filling during diastole. The patient may be asymptomatic or have hypotension, light-headedness, dizziness, or syncope, depending on the ventricular rate. Bradycardia may also aggravate or provoke angina or symptoms of heart failure such as dyspnea.

Cardiomyopathy. An atrial gallop is a sign associated with cardiomyopathy, regardless of the type—dilated (most common), hypertrophic, or restrictive (least common). Additional findings may include dyspnea, orthopnea, crackles, fatigue, syncope, chest pain, palpitations, edema, jugular vein distention, S_3, and transient or sustained bradycardia usually associated with tachycardia.

Hypertension. One of the earliest findings in systemic arterial hypertension is an atrial gallop. The patient may be asymptomatic, or he may experience a headache, weakness, epistaxis, tinnitus, dizziness, and fatigue.

Myocardial infarction (MI). An atrial gallop is a classic sign of a life-threatening MI; in fact, it may persist even after the infarction heals. Typically, the patient reports crushing substernal chest pain that may radiate to the back, neck, jaw, shoulder, and left arm. Associated signs and symptoms include dyspnea, restlessness, anxiety, a feeling of impending doom, diaphoresis, pallor, clammy skin, nausea, vomiting, and increased or decreased blood pressure.

Pulmonary embolism. Pulmonary embolism is a life-threatening disorder that causes a right-sided atrial gallop that's usually heard along the lower left sternal border with a loud pulmonic closure sound. Other features include tachycardia, tachypnea, fever, chest pain, dyspnea, decreased breath sounds, crackles, a pleural chest rub, apprehension, diaphoresis, syncope, and cyanosis. The patient may have a productive cough with blood-tinged sputum or a nonproductive cough.

Thyrotoxicosis. An atrial gallop and an S_3 may be auscultated in thyroid hormone overproduction. Other cardinal features include tachycardia, a bounding pulse, wide pulse pressure, palpitations, weight loss despite increased appetite, diarrhea, tremors, an enlarged thyroid, dyspnea, nervousness, difficulty concentrating, diaphoresis, heat intolerance, exophthalmos, weakness, fatigue, and muscle atrophy.

Nursing considerations

■ Prepare the patient for diagnostic tests, such as an electrocardiogram, echocardiography, cardiac catheterization, such laboratory tests as CK-MB and troponin and, possibly, a lung scan.
■ Monitor the patient for signs and symptoms of heart failure.
■ Administer medications and oxygen as ordered.

Patient teaching

■ Discuss lifestyle modifications to reduce the patient's risk of heart disease.
■ Teach the patient how to take his pulse and parameters that require medical attention.
■ Emphasize signs and symptoms that require prompt medical attention.

Interpreting heart sounds

Detecting subtle variations in heart sounds requires concentration and practice. When you can recognize normal heart sounds, the abnormal heart sounds become more obvious.

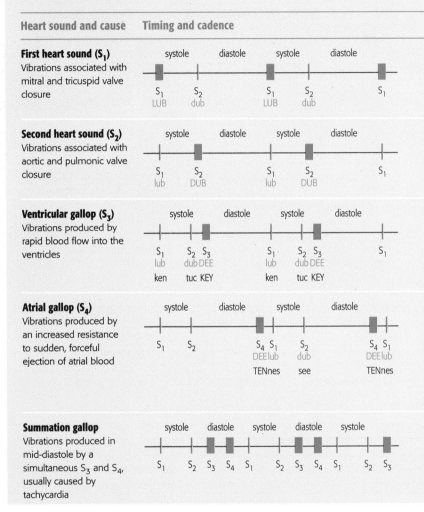

Heart sound and cause	Timing and cadence
First heart sound (S_1) Vibrations associated with mitral and tricuspid valve closure	systole / diastole / systole / diastole. S_1 S_2 S_1 S_2 S_1 / LUB dub LUB dub
Second heart sound (S_2) Vibrations associated with aortic and pulmonic valve closure	systole / diastole / systole / diastole. S_1 S_2 S_1 S_2 S_1 / lub DUB lub DUB
Ventricular gallop (S_3) Vibrations produced by rapid blood flow into the ventricles	systole / diastole / systole / diastole. S_1 S_2 S_3 S_1 S_2 S_3 S_1 / lub dub DEE lub dub DEE / ken tuc KEY ken tuc KEY
Atrial gallop (S_4) Vibrations produced by an increased resistance to sudden, forceful ejection of atrial blood	systole / diastole / systole / diastole. S_1 S_2 S_4 S_1 S_2 S_4 S_1 / DEE lub dub DEE lub / TENnes see TENnes
Summation gallop Vibrations produced in mid-diastole by a simultaneous S_3 and S_4, usually caused by tachycardia	systole / diastole / systole / diastole / systole. S_1 S_2 S_3 S_4 S_1 S_2 S_3 S_4 S_1 S_2 S_3

■ Stress the importance of keeping follow-up appointments.

■ Gallop, ventricular [S_3]

A ventricular gallop is a heart sound (known as S_3) associated with rapid ventricular filling in early diastole. Usu-

lower left sternal border or over the xiphoid region. A left-sided gallop usually sounds louder on expiration and is heard best at the apex.

Ventricular gallops are easily overlooked because they're usually faint. Fortunately, certain techniques make their detection more likely. These include auscultating in a quiet environment; examining the patient in the supine, left lateral, and semi-Fowler's positions; and having the patient cough or raise his legs to augment the sound.

A physiologic ventricular gallop normally occurs in children and adults younger than age 40; however, most people lose this third heart sound by age 40. This gallop may also occur during the third trimester of pregnancy. Abnormal S_3 (in adults older than age 40) can be a sign of decreased myocardial contractility, myocardial failure, and volume overload of the ventricle, as in mitral and tricuspid valve insufficiency. Although the physiologic S_3 has the same timing as the pathologic S_3, its intensity waxes and wanes with respiration. It's also heard more faintly if the patient is sitting or standing.

A pathologic ventricular gallop may be one of the earliest signs of ventricular failure. It may result from one of two mechanisms: rapid deceleration of blood entering a stiff, noncompliant ventricle or rapid acceleration of blood associated with increased flow into the ventricle. A gallop that persists despite therapy indicates a poor prognosis.

Patients with cardiomyopathy or heart failure may develop a ventricular and an atrial gallop—a condition known as a *summation gallop*. (See *Summation gallop: Two gallops in one,* page 286.)

History and physical examination

After auscultating a ventricular gallop, focus your history and examination on

Auscultation tips

Best heard with the diaphragm of the stethoscope at the apex (mitral area)

Best heard with the diaphragm of the stethoscope in the second or third right and left parasternal intercostal spaces with the patient sitting or in a supine position

Best heard through the bell of the stethoscope at the apex with the patient in the left lateral position; may be visible and palpable during early diastole at the midclavicular line between the fourth and fifth intercostal spaces

Best heard through the bell of the stethoscope at the apex with the patient in the left semilateral position; may be visible in late diastole at the midclavicular line between the fourth and fifth intercostal spaces; may also be palpable in the midclavicular area with the patient in the left lateral decubitus position

Best heard through the bell of the stethoscope at the apex with the patient in the left lateral position; may be louder than S_1 or S_2; may be visible and palpable during diastole

ally palpable, this low-frequency sound occurs about 0.15 second after the second heart sound (S_2). It may originate in either the left or right ventricle. A right-sided gallop usually sounds louder on inspiration and is heard best along the

Summation gallop: Two gallops in one

When atrial and ventricular gallops occur simultaneously, they produce a short, low-pitched sound known as a *summation gallop*. This relatively uncommon sound occurs during mid-diastole (between S_2 and S_1) and is best heard with the bell of the stethoscope pressed lightly against the cardiac apex. It may be louder than either S_1 or S_2 and may cause visible apical movement during diastole.

Causes

A summation gallop may result from tachycardia or from delayed or blocked atrioventricular (AV) conduction. Tachycardia shortens ventricular filling time during diastole, causing it to coincide with atrial contraction. When the heart rate slows, the summation gallop is replaced by separate atrial and ventricular gallops, producing a quadruple rhythm much like the canter of a horse. Delayed AV conduction also brings atrial contraction closer to ventricular filling, creating a summation gallop.

A summation gallop usually results from heart failure or dilated congestive cardiomyopathy. It may also accompany other cardiac disorders. Occasionally, it signals further cardiac deterioration. For example, consider the hypertensive patient with a chronic atrial gallop who develops tachycardia and a superimposed ventricular gallop. If this patient abruptly displays a summation gallop, heart failure is the likely cause.

---

the cardiovascular system. Begin the history by asking the patient if he has had chest pain. If so, have him describe its character, location, frequency, duration, and alleviating or aggravating factors. Also, ask about palpitations, dizziness, or syncope. Does the patient have difficulty breathing after exertion? While lying down? At rest? Does he have a cough? Ask about a history of cardiac disorders. Is the patient currently receiving treatment for heart failure? If so, which medications is he taking?

During the physical examination, carefully auscultate for murmurs or abnormalities in the first and second heart sounds. Then listen for pulmonary crackles. Next, assess peripheral pulses, noting an alternating strong and weak pulse. Finally, palpate the liver to detect enlargement or tenderness, and assess for jugular vein distention and peripheral edema.

Medical causes

Aortic insufficiency. Aortic insufficiency occurs secondary to reduced ejection fraction and elevated end-systolic volume. Acute and chronic aortic insufficiency may produce an S_3. Typically, *acute aortic insufficiency* also causes an atrial gallop and a soft, short diastolic murmur over the left sternal border. S_2 may be soft or absent. At times, a soft, short midsystolic murmur may be heard over the second right intercostal space. Related findings include tachycardia, dyspnea, jugular vein distention, and crackles.

Chronic aortic insufficiency produces a ventricular gallop and a high-pitched, blowing, decrescendo diastolic murmur that's best heard over the second or third right intercostal space or the left sternal border. An Austin Flint murmur—an apical, rumbling, mid- to late-diastolic murmur—may also occur. Typical related findings include palpitations, tachycardia, anginal chest pain, fatigue, dyspnea, orthopnea, and crackles.

Cardiomyopathy. A ventricular gallop is characteristic in cardiomyopathy. When accompanied by an alternating pulse and altered S_1 and S_2, this gallop usually signals advanced heart disease. Other effects may include fatigue, dyspnea, orthopnea, chest pain, palpitations, syncope, crackles, peripheral edema, jugular vein distention, and an atrial gallop.

Heart failure. A cardinal sign of heart failure is a ventricular gallop. When it's loud and accompanied by sinus tachycardia, this gallop may indicate severe heart failure. The patient with left-sided heart failure also exhibits fatigue, exertional dyspnea, paroxysmal nocturnal dyspnea, orthopnea and, possibly, a dry cough; with right-sided heart failure, jugular vein distention occurs. Other late features include tachypnea, chest tightness, palpitations, anorexia, nausea, dependent edema, weight gain, a slowed mental response, diaphoresis, pallor, hypotension, narrowed pulse pressure and, possibly, oliguria. In some cases, inspiratory crackles, clubbing, and a tender, palpable liver may be present. As heart failure progresses, hemoptysis, cyanosis, severe pitting edema, and marked hepatomegaly may develop.

Mitral insufficiency. Acute and chronic mitral insufficiency may produce a ventricular gallop. In *acute mitral insufficiency,* auscultation may also reveal an early or holosystolic decrescendo murmur at the apex, an atrial gallop, and a widely split S_2. Typically, the patient displays sinus tachycardia, tachypnea, orthopnea, dyspnea, crackles, jugular vein distention, and fatigue.

In *chronic mitral insufficiency,* a progressively severe ventricular gallop is typical. Auscultation also reveals a holosystolic, blowing, high-pitched apical murmur. The patient may report fatigue, exertional dyspnea, and palpitations or he may be asymptomatic.

Thyrotoxicosis. Thyrotoxicosis may produce ventricular and atrial gallops, but its cardinal features are an enlarged thyroid gland, weight loss despite increased appetite, heat intolerance, diaphoresis, nervousness, tremors, tachycardia, palpitations, diarrhea, and dyspnea.

Nursing considerations
- Assess the patient for tachycardia, dyspnea, crackles, and jugular vein distention.
- Give oxygen, diuretics, and other drugs, such as digoxin and angiotensin-converting enzyme inhibitors, to prevent pulmonary edema.
- Prepare the patient for electrocardiography, echocardiography, gated blood pool imaging, and cardiac catheterization.

Patient teaching
- Discuss lifestyle modifications to reduce the patient's risk of heart disease.
- Teach the patient about the signs and symptoms that require prompt medical attention.

Genital lesions, male

Among the diverse lesions that may affect the male genitalia are warts, papules, ulcers, scales, and pustules. These common lesions may be painful or painless, singular or multiple. They may be limited to the genitalia or may also occur elsewhere on the body. (See *Recognizing common male genital lesions,* page 288.)

Genital lesions may result from infection, neoplasms, parasites, allergy, or the effects of drugs. These lesions can profoundly affect the patient's self-image and personal relationships. In fact, the patient may hesitate to seek medical at-

Recognizing common male genital lesions

Many lesions may affect the male genitalia. Some of the more common ones and their causes appear below.

Penile cancer causes a painless ulcerative lesion on the glans or foreskin, possibly accompanied by a foul-smelling discharge.

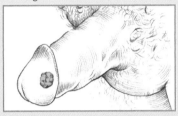

Genital warts are marked by clusters of flesh-colored papillary growths that may be barely visible or several inches in diameter.

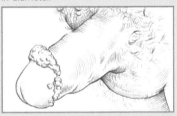

Tinea cruris (commonly known as *jock itch*) produces itchy patches of well-defined, slightly raised, scaly lesions that usually affect the inner thighs and groin.

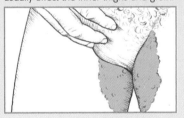

A fixed drug eruption causes a bright red to purplish lesion on the glans penis.

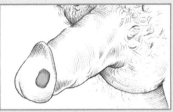

Genital herpes begins as a swollen, slightly pruritic wheal and later becomes a group of small vesicles or blisters on the foreskin, glans, or penile shaft.

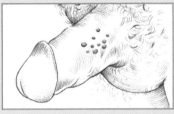

Chancroid causes a painful ulcer that's usually less than 2 cm in diameter and bleeds easily. The lesion may be deep and covered by a gray or yellow exudate at its base.

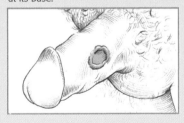

tention because he fears cancer or a sexually transmitted disease (STD).

Genital lesions that arise from an STD could mean that the patient is at risk for human immunodeficiency virus (HIV). Genital ulcers make HIV transmission between sexual partners more likely. Unfortunately, if the patient is treating himself, he may alter the lesions, making differential diagnosis especially difficult.

History and physical examination

Begin by asking the patient when he first noticed the lesion. Did it erupt after he began taking a new drug or after a trip out of the country? Has he had similar lesions before? If so, did he get medical treatment for them? Find out if he has been treating the lesion himself. If so, how? Does the lesion itch? If so, is the itching constant or does it bother him only at night? Note whether the lesion is painful. Ask for a description of any drainage from the lesion. Next, take a complete sexual history, noting the frequency of relations, number of sexual partners, and pattern of condom use.

Before you examine the patient, observe his clothing. Do his pants fit properly? Tight pants or underwear, especially those made of nonabsorbent fabrics, can promote the growth of bacteria and fungi. Examine the entire skin surface, noting the location, size, color, and pattern of the lesions. Do genital lesions resemble lesions on other parts of the body? Palpate for nodules, masses, and tenderness. Also, look for bleeding, edema, or signs of infection, such as purulent drainage or erythema. Finally, take the patient's vital signs.

Medical causes

Balanitis and balanoposthitis. Typically, balanitis (glans infection) and posthitis (prepuce infection) occur together (balanoposthitis), causing painful ulceration on the glans, foreskin, or penile shaft. Ulceration is usually preceded by 2 to 3 days of prepuce irritation and soreness, followed by a foul discharge and edema. The patient may then develop features of acute infection, such as a fever with chills, malaise, and dysuria. Without treatment, the ulcers may deepen and multiply. Eventually, the entire penis and scrotum may become gan-grenous, resulting in life-threatening sepsis.

Bowen's disease. Bowen's disease is a painless, premalignant lesion that commonly occurs on the penis or scrotum, but may also appear elsewhere. It appears as a brownish red, raised, scaly, indurated plaque with well-defined borders, which may ulcerate at its center.

Chancroid. Chancroid is an STD that's characterized by the eruption of one or more lesions, usually on the groin, inner thigh, or penis. Within 24 hours, the lesion changes from a reddened area to a small papule. (A similar papule may erupt on the tongue, lip, breast, or umbilicus.) It then becomes an inflamed pustule that rapidly ulcerates. This painful—and usually deep—ulcer bleeds easily and commonly has a purulent gray or yellow exudate covering its base. Rarely more than 2 cm in diameter, it's typically irregular in shape. The inguinal lymph nodes also enlarge, become very tender, and may drain pus.

Folliculitis and furunculosis. Hair follicle infection may cause red, sharply pointed lesions that are tender and swollen with central pustules. If folliculitis progresses to furunculosis, these lesions become hard, painful nodules that may gradually enlarge and rupture, discharging pus and necrotic material. Rupture relieves the pain, but erythema and edema may persist for days or weeks.

Genital herpes. Caused by herpesvirus type 1 or 2, genital herpes is an STD that produces fluid-filled vesicles on the glans penis, foreskin, or penile shaft and, occasionally, on the mouth or anus. Usually painless at first, these vesicles may rupture and become extensive, shallow, painful ulcers accompanied by redness, marked edema, and tender, inguinal lymph nodes. Other findings may include a fever, malaise, and dysuria. If the vesicles recur in the same area, the patient usually feels localized numbness and tingling before they erupt. Associated inflammation is typically less marked.

Genital warts. Most common in sexually active males, genital warts initially develop on the subpreputial sac or urethral meatus, and less commonly on the penile shaft; they then spread to the perineum and perianal area. These painless warts start as tiny red or pink swellings that may grow to 10.2 cm and become pedunculated. Multiple swellings are common, giving the warts a cauliflower appearance. Infected warts are also malodorous.

Leukoplakia. Leukoplakia is a precancerous disorder that's characterized by white, scaly patches on the glans and prepuce accompanied by skin thickening and occasionally fissures.

Pediculosis pubis. Pediculosis pubis is a parasitic infestation that's characterized by erythematous, itching papules in the pubic area and around the anus, abdomen, and thigh. Inspection may detect grayish white specks (lice eggs) attached to hair shafts. Skin irritation from scratching in these areas is common.

Penile cancer. Penile cancer usually produces a painless, enlarging wartlike lesion on the glans or foreskin. However, if the foreskin becomes unretractable, the patient may experience localized pain. Examination may reveal a foul-smelling discharge from the prepuce, a firm lump in the glans, and enlarged lymph nodes. Late signs and symptoms may include dysuria, pain, bleeding from the lesion, and urine retention and bladder distention associated with urinary tract obstruction.

Scabies. Mites that burrow under the skin in scabies may cause crusted lesions or large papules on the glans and shaft of the penis and on the scrotum. Lesions may also occur on the wrists, elbows, axillae, and waist. They're usually raised, threadlike, and 1 to 10 cm long and have a swollen nodule or red papule that contains the mite. Nocturnal itching is typical and commonly causes excoriation.

Syphilis. Two to four weeks after exposure to the spirochete *Treponema pallidum,* one or more primary lesions, or chancres, may erupt on the genitalia; occasionally, they also erupt elsewhere on the body, typically on the mouth or perianal area. The chancre usually starts as a small, red, fluid-filled papule and then erodes to form a painless, firm, indurated, shallow ulcer with a clear base and a scant, yellow serous discharge or, less commonly, a hard papule. This lesion gradually involutes and disappears. Painless, unilateral regional lymphadenopathy is also typical.

Tinea cruris. Also called *jock itch,* tinea cruris is a superficial fungal infection that usually causes sharply defined, slightly raised, scaling patches on the inner thigh or groin (typically bilaterally) and, less commonly, on the scrotum and penis. Pruritus may be severe.

Urticaria. Urticaria is a common allergic reaction that's characterized by intensely pruritic hives, which may appear on the genitalia, especially on the foreskin or shaft of the penis. These distinct, raised, evanescent wheals are surrounded by an erythematous flare.

Other causes

Drugs. Barbiturates, and certain broad-spectrum antibiotics, such as tetracycline and sulfonamides, may cause a fixed drug eruption and a genital lesion.

Nursing considerations

■ Screen every patient with penile lesions for STDs, using the dark-field examination and the Venereal Disease Research Laboratory (VDRL) test.

■ Prepare the patient for a biopsy to confirm or rule out penile cancer if indicated.

■ Provide emotional support, especially if cancer is suspected.

■ To prevent cross-contamination, wash your hands before and after every patient contact.

■ Wear gloves when handling urine or performing catheter care.

■ Dispose of all needles carefully, and double-bag all material contaminated by secretions.

Patient teaching

■ Explain to the patient the use of creams and ointments.

■ Discuss methods to reduce crusting and itching.

■ Emphasize the lesion changes the patient should report.

■ Discuss and teach the proper use of condoms and safer sex practices.

Gum bleeding
[Gingival bleeding]

Bleeding gums usually result from dental disorders; less commonly, they may stem from a blood dyscrasia or the effects of certain drugs. Physiologic causes of this common sign include pregnancy, which can produce gum swelling in the first or second trimester (pregnancy epulis); atmospheric pressure changes, which usually affect divers and aviators; and oral trauma. Bleeding ranges from slight oozing to life-threatening hemorrhage. It may be spontaneous or may follow trauma. Occasionally, direct pressure can control it.

ACTION STAT!

 If you detect profuse, spontaneous bleeding in the oral cavity, quickly check the patient's airway and look for signs of cardiovascular collapse, such as tachycardia and hy-

potension. Suction the patient. Apply direct pressure to the bleeding site. Expect to insert an airway, administer I.V. fluids, and collect serum samples for diagnostic evaluation.

History and physical examination

If gum bleeding isn't an emergency, obtain a history. Find out when the bleeding began. Has it been continuous or intermittent? Does it occur spontaneously or when the patient brushes his teeth or flosses? Have the patient show you the site of the bleeding, if possible.

Find out if the patient or any family members have bleeding tendencies; for example, ask about easy bruising and frequent nosebleeds. How much does the patient bleed after a tooth extraction? Does he have a history of liver or spleen disease? Next, check the patient's dental history. Find out how often he brushes his teeth, flosses, and goes to the dentist and what kind of toothbrush and floss he uses. Has he seen a dentist recently? To evaluate nutritional status, have the patient describe his normal diet and alcohol intake. Finally, note the prescription and over-the-counter drugs he takes.

Next, perform a complete oral examination. If the patient wears dentures, have him remove them. Examine the gums to determine the site and amount of bleeding. Gums normally appear pink and rippled with their margins snugly against the teeth. Check for inflammation, pockets around the teeth, swelling, retraction, hypertrophy, discoloration, and gum hyperplasia. Note obvious decay, discoloration, foreign material such as food, and absence of teeth.

Medical causes

Agranulocytosis. Spontaneous gum bleeding and other systemic hemorrhages may occur in agranulocytosis, which typically causes progressive fatigue and weakness, followed by signs of infection, such as a fever and chills. Inspection may reveal oral and perianal lesions, which are usually rough edged with a gray or black membrane.

Aplastic anemia. In aplastic anemia, profuse or scant gum bleeding may follow trauma. Other signs of bleeding, such as epistaxis and ecchymoses, are also characteristic. The patient exhibits progressive weakness and fatigue, shortness of breath, a headache, pallor and, possibly, a fever. Eventually, tachycardia and signs of heart failure, such as jugular vein distention and dyspnea, also develop.

Ehlers-Danlos syndrome. In Ehlers-Danlos syndrome, gums bleed easily after toothbrushing. Easy bruising and other signs of abnormal bleeding are also typical. The skin is fragile and hyperelastic; joints are hyperextendible.

Gingivitis. Reddened and edematous gums are characteristic of gingivitis. The gingivae between the teeth become bulbous and bleed easily with slight trauma. However, with acute necrotizing ulcerative gingivitis, bleeding is spontaneous and the gums become so painful that the patient may be unable to eat. A characteristic grayish yellow pseudomembrane develops over punched-out gum erosions. Offensive halitosis is typical and may be accompanied by a headache, malaise, fever, and cervical adenopathy.

Hemophilia. Hemorrhage occurs from many sites in the oral cavity, especially the gums. *Mild hemophilia* causes easy bruising, hematomas, epistaxis, bleeding gums, and prolonged bleeding during even minor surgery and up to 8 days afterward. *Moderate hemophilia* produces more frequent episodes of abnormal bleeding and occasional bleeding into the joints, which may cause swelling and pain. *Severe hemophilia* causes spontaneous or severe bleeding after minor trauma, possibly resulting in large subcutaneous and intramuscular hematomas. Bleeding into joints and muscles causes pain, swelling, extreme tenderness and, possibly, permanent deformity. Bleeding near peripheral nerves causes peripheral neuropathies, pain, paresthesia, and muscle atrophy. Signs of anemia and a fever may follow bleeding. Severe blood loss may lead to shock and death.

Hereditary hemorrhagic telangiectasia. Hereditary hemorrhagic telangiectasia is characterized by red to violet spiderlike hemorrhagic areas on the gums, which blanch on pressure and bleed spontaneously. These telangiectases may also occur on the lips, buccal mucosa, and palate; on the face, ears, scalp, hands, arms, and feet; and under the nails. Epistaxis commonly occurs early and is difficult to control. Hemoptysis and signs of GI bleeding may develop.

Leukemia. Easy gum bleeding, which is an early sign of acute monocytic, lymphocytic, or myelocytic leukemia, is accompanied by gum swelling, necrosis, and petechiae. The soft, tender gums appear glossy and bluish. *Acute leukemia* causes severe prostration marked by a high fever and bleeding tendencies, such as epistaxis and prolonged menses. It may also cause dyspnea, tachycardia, palpitations, and abdominal or bone pain. Later effects may include confusion, headaches, vomiting, seizures, papilledema, and nuchal rigidity.

Chronic leukemia usually develops insidiously, producing less-severe bleeding tendencies. Other effects may include anorexia, weight loss, a low-grade fever, chills, skin eruptions, and an enlarged spleen, tonsils, and lymph nodes. Signs of anemia, such as fatigue and pallor, may occur.

Pemphigoid (benign mucosal).
Pemphigoid typically causes thick-walled gum lesions that rupture, desquamate, and then bleed easily. Extensive scars form with healing, and the gums remain red for months. Lesions may also develop on other parts of the oral mucosa, conjunctiva and, less commonly, the skin. Secondary fibrous bands may lead to dysphagia, hoarseness, or blindness.

Periodontal disease. With periodontal disease, gum bleeding typically occurs after chewing, toothbrushing, or gum probing, but may also occur spontaneously. As gingivae separate from the bone, pus-filled pockets develop around the teeth; occasionally, pus can be expressed. Other findings include an unpleasant taste with halitosis, facial pain, loose teeth, and dental calculi and plaque.

Polycythemia vera. In polycythemia vera, engorged gums ooze blood after even slight trauma. This disorder usually turns the oral mucosa—especially the gums and tongue—a deep red-violet. Among associated findings are a headache, dyspnea, dizziness, fatigue, paresthesia, tinnitus, double or blurred vision, aquagenic pruritus, epigastric distress, weight loss, increased blood pressure, ruddy cyanosis, ecchymosis, and hepatosplenomegaly.

Thrombocytopenia. With thrombocytopenia, blood usually oozes between the teeth and gums; however, severe bleeding may follow minor trauma. Associated signs of hemorrhage include large blood-filled bullae in the mouth, petechiae, ecchymosis, epistaxis, and hematuria. Malaise, fatigue, weakness, and lethargy eventually develop.

Thrombocytopenic purpura (idiopathic). Profuse gum bleeding occurs in idiopathic thrombocytopenic purpura. Its classic feature, however, is spontaneous hemorrhagic skin lesions that range from pinpoint petechiae to massive hemorrhages. The patient has a tendency to bruise easily, develops petechiae on the oral mucosa, and may exhibit melena, epistaxis, or hematuria.

Vitamin K deficiency. The first sign of vitamin K deficiency is usually gums that bleed when the teeth are brushed. Other signs of abnormal bleeding, such as ecchymosis, epistaxis, and hematuria, may also occur. GI bleeding may produce hematemesis and melena; intracranial bleeding may cause a decreased level of consciousness and focal neurologic deficits.

Other causes

Drugs. Warfarin and heparin interfere with blood clotting and may cause prolonged gum bleeding. Abuse of aspirin and nonsteroidal anti-inflammatory drugs may alter platelets, producing bleeding gums. Localized gum bleeding may also occur with mucosal "aspirin burn" caused by dissolving aspirin near an aching tooth.

Nursing considerations
- Prepare the patient for diagnostic tests, such as blood studies or facial X-rays.
- Prepare him for the possibility of a packed red blood cell blood product transfusion, if necessary (platelets or fresh frozen plasma).
- When providing mouth care, avoid using lemon-glycerin swabs, which may burn or dry the gums.

Patient teaching
- Instruct the patient in proper mouth and gum care.
- Discuss signs and symptoms that require medical attention.
- Emphasize the importance of seeking regular dental care.

Gynecomastia

Occurring only in males, gynecomastia refers to increased breast size due to excessive mammary gland development. This change in breast size may be barely palpable or immediately obvious. Usually bilateral, gynecomastia may be associated with breast tenderness and milk secretion.

Normally, several hormones regulate breast development. Estrogens, growth hormone, and corticosteroids stimulate ductal growth, whereas progesterone and prolactin stimulate growth of the alveolar lobules. Although the pathophysiology of gynecomastia isn't fully understood, a hormonal imbalance—particularly a change in the estrogen-androgen ratio and an increase in prolactin—is a likely contributing factor. This explains why gynecomastia commonly results from the effects of estrogens and other drugs. It may also result from hormone-secreting tumors and from endocrine, genetic, hepatic, or adrenal disorders. Physiologic gynecomastia may occur in neonatal, pubertal, and geriatric males because of normal fluctuations in hormone levels.

History and physical examination

Begin the history by asking the patient when he first noticed his breast enlargement. How old was he at the time? Since then, have his breasts gotten progressively larger, smaller, or stayed the same? Does he also have breast tenderness or discharge? Have him describe the discharge, if any. Ask him if he's ever had his nipples pierced. If so, were there any complications due to the piercings? Next, take a thorough drug history, including prescription, over-the-counter, herbal, and street drugs. Then explore associated signs and symptoms, such as testicular mass or pain, loss of libido,

decreased sexual potency, and loss of chest, axillary, or facial hair.

Focus the physical examination on the breasts, testicles, and penis. As you examine the breasts, note asymmetry, dimpling, abnormal pigmentation, or ulceration. Observe the testicles for size and symmetry. Then palpate them to detect nodules, tenderness, or unusual consistency. Look for normal penile development after puberty, and note hypospadias.

Medical causes

Adrenal carcinoma. Estrogen production by an adrenal tumor may produce a feminizing syndrome in males characterized by bilateral gynecomastia, loss of libido, impotence, testicular atrophy, and reduced facial hair growth. Cushingoid signs, such as moon face and purple striae, may also occur.

Breast cancer. Painful unilateral gynecomastia develops rapidly in males with breast cancer. Palpation may reveal a hard or stony breast lump suggesting a malignant tumor. Breast examination may also detect changes in breast symmetry; skin changes, such as thickening, dimpling, peau d'orange, or ulceration; a warm, reddened area; and nipple changes, such as itching, burning, erosion, deviation, flattening, retraction, and a watery, bloody, or purulent discharge.

Hypothyroidism. Typically, hypothyroidism produces bilateral gynecomastia along with bradycardia, cold intolerance, weight gain despite anorexia, and mental dullness. The patient may display periorbital edema and puffiness in the face, hands, and feet. His hair appears brittle and sparse and his skin is dry, pale, cool, and doughy.

Klinefelter's syndrome. Painless bilateral gynecomastia first appears during adolescence in Klinefelter's syndrome, a genetic disorder. Before puberty, symptoms also include abnormally small testicles and a slight mental deficiency; after puberty, sparse facial hair, a small penis, decreased libido, and impotence.

Liver cancer. Liver cancer may produce bilateral gynecomastia and other characteristics of feminization, such as testicular atrophy, impotence, and reduced facial hair growth. The patient may complain of severe epigastric or right upper quadrant pain associated with a right upper quadrant mass. A large tumor may also produce a bruit on auscultation. Related findings may include anorexia, weight loss, dependent edema, fever, cachexia and, possibly, jaundice or ascites.

Pituitary tumor. A pituitary tumor is a hormone-secreting tumor that causes bilateral gynecomastia accompanied by galactorrhea, impotence, and decreased libido. Other hormonal effects may include enlarged hands and feet, coarse facial features with prognathism, voice deepening, weight gain, increased blood pressure, diaphoresis, heat intolerance, hyperpigmentation, and thickened, oily skin. Paresthesia or sensory loss and muscle weakness commonly affect the limbs. If the tumor expands, it may cause blurred vision, diplopia, a headache, or partial bitemporal hemianopia that may progress to blindness.

Reifenstein's syndrome. Reifenstein's syndrome is a genetic disorder that produces painless bilateral gynecomastia at puberty. Associated signs may include hypospadias, testicular atrophy, and an underdeveloped penis.

Other causes

Drugs. When gynecomastia is an effect of drugs, it's typically painful and unilateral. Estrogens used to treat prostate cancer, including diethylstilbestrol, estramustine, and chlorotrianisene, directly affect the estrogen-androgen ratio. Drugs that have an estrogen-like effect,

such as cardiac glycosides and human chorionic gonadotropin, may do the same. Regular use of alcohol, marijuana, or heroin reduces plasma testosterone levels, causing gynecomastia. Other drugs—such as flutamide, cyproterone, spironolactone, cimetidine, and ketoconazole—produce this sign by interfering with androgen production or action. Some common drugs, including phenothiazines, tricyclic antidepressants, and antihypertensives, produce gynecomastia in an unknown way.

Treatments. Gynecomastia may develop within weeks of starting hemodialysis for chronic renal failure. It may also follow major surgery or testicular irradiation.

Nursing considerations

- Apply cold compresses to the breasts and administer analgesics as needed for pain and discomfort.
- Prepare the patient for diagnostic tests, including chest and skull X-rays and blood hormone levels.
- Because gynecomastia may alter the patient's body image, provide emotional support.
- Administer tamoxifen, an antiestrogen, or testolactone, an inhibitor of testosterone-to-estrogen conversion, as ordered.
- Prepare the patient for surgical removal of breast tissue, as indicated, if drug treatment fails.

Patient teaching

- Reassure the patient that treatment can reduce gynecomastia.
- Explain all treatments and procedures to the patient.

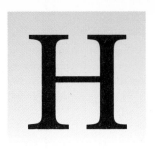

Halo vision

Halo vision refers to seeing rainbowlike, colored rings around lights or bright objects. This effect can be explained by the physical principle that as light passes through water (in the eye, through tears or the cells of various anteretinal media), it breaks up into spectral colors.

Halo vision usually develops suddenly; its duration depends on the causative disorder. It may occur with disorders associated with excessive tearing and corneal epithelial edema. Among these causes, the most common and significant is acute angle-closure glaucoma, which can lead to blindness. With this disorder, increased intraocular pressure (IOP) forces fluid into corneal tissues anterior to Bowman's membrane, causing edema. Halo vision is also an early symptom of cataracts, resulting from dispersion of light by abnormal opacities on the lens.

Nonpathologic causes of excessive tearing associated with halo vision include poorly fitted or overworn contact lenses, emotional extremes, and exposure to intense light such as in snow blindness.

History and physical examination

First, ask the patient how long he has been seeing halos around lights and when he usually sees them. The patient with glaucoma usually sees halos in the morning, when IOP is most elevated. Ask the patient if light bothers his eyes. Does he have eye pain? If so, have him describe it. Remember that halos associated with excruciating eye pain or a severe headache may point to acute angle-closure glaucoma, an ocular emergency. Note a history of glaucoma or cataracts.

Next, examine the patient's eyes, noting conjunctival injection, excessive tearing, and lens changes. Examine pupil size, shape, and response to light. Then test visual acuity by performing an ophthalmoscopic examination.

Medical causes

Cataract. Halo vision may be an early symptom of painless, progressive cataract formation. The glare of headlights may blind the patient, making nighttime driving impossible. Other features include blurred vision, impaired visual acuity, and lens opacity, all of which develop gradually.

Corneal endothelial dystrophy. Typically, halo vision is a late symptom of corneal endothelial dystrophy. Impaired visual acuity may also occur.

Glaucoma. Halo vision characterizes all types of glaucoma. Acute angle-closure glaucoma—an ophthalmic emergency—also causes blurred vision, followed by a severe headache or excruciating pain in and around the affected eye. Examination reveals a moderately dilated fixed pupil that doesn't respond to light, conjunctival injection, a cloudy cornea, impaired visual acuity and, possibly, nausea and vomiting.

Chronic angle-closure glaucoma usually produces no symptoms until pain and blindness occur in advanced disease. Sometimes, halos and blurred vision develop slowly.

With chronic open-angle glaucoma, halo vision is a late symptom that's accompanied by a mild eye ache, peripheral vision loss, and impaired visual acuity.

Nursing considerations

- To help minimize halo vision, remind the patient not to look directly at bright lights.

Patient teaching

- Teach the patient how to instill eyedrops if prescribed.
- Discuss the importance of reporting eye discharge, eye watering, blurred or cloudy vision, halos, floaters, flashes of light, or eye pain.

Headache

The most common neurologic symptom, headaches may be localized or generalized, producing mild to severe pain. About 90% of headaches are benign and can be described as vascular, muscle-contraction, or a combination of both. (See *Clinical features of headache,* page 298.) Occasionally, however, headaches indicate a severe neurologic disorder associated with intracranial inflammation, increased intracranial pressure (ICP), or meningeal irritation. They may also result from an ocular or a sinus disorder, tests, drugs, or other treatments.

Other causes of headache include a fever, eyestrain, dehydration, systemic

febrile illnesses, and stress. Headaches may occur in certain metabolic disturbances—such as hypoxemia, hypercapnia, hyperglycemia, and hypoglycemia—but they aren't a diagnostic or prominent symptom. Some individuals get headaches after seizures or from coughing, sneezing, heavy lifting, or stooping.

History and physical examination

If the patient reports a headache, ask him to describe its characteristics and location. How often does he get a headache? How long does a typical headache last? Does he have a history of high blood pressure? Try to identify precipitating factors, such as certain foods or exposure to bright lights. Ask what helps to relieve the headache. Does he experience stress at work or at home? Has he had trouble sleeping?

Take a drug and alcohol history, and ask about head trauma within the past 4 weeks. Has the patient recently experienced nausea, vomiting, photophobia, or vision changes? Does he feel drowsy, confused, or dizzy? Has he recently developed seizures or does he have a history of seizures?

Begin the physical examination by evaluating the patient's level of consciousness (LOC). Then check his vital signs. Be alert for signs of increased ICP—a widened pulse pressure, bradycardia, an altered respiratory pattern, and increased blood pressure. Check pupil size and response to light, and note any neck stiffness.

Medical causes

Anthrax (cutaneous). Along with a macular papular lesion that develops into a vesicle and finally a painless ulcer with anthrax, headache, lymphadenopathy, fever, and malaise may also occur.

Clinical features of headache

The International Headache Society classifies migraines as occurring with or without an aura. The differentiating characteristics of each type are listed here.

Migraines without an aura

Previously called *common migraines* or *hemicrania simplex*, migraine headaches without an aura are diagnosed when the patient has five attacks that include these symptoms:

- untreated or unsuccessfully treated headache lasting 4 to 72 hours
- two of the following: pain that's unilateral, pulsating, moderate or severe in intensity, or aggravated by activity
- nausea, vomiting, photophobia, or phonophobia.

Migraines with an aura

Previously called *classic, classical, ophthalmic, hemiplegic,* or *aphasic* migraines, migraine headaches with an aura are diagnosed when the patient has at least two attacks with three of these characteristics:

- one or more reversible aura symptoms (indicates focal cerebral cortical or brain stem dysfunction)
- one or more aura symptoms that develop over more than 4 minutes or two or more symptoms that occur in succession
- an aura symptom that lasts less than 60 minutes (per symptom)
- a headache that begins before, occurs with, or follows an aura with a free interval of less than 60 minutes.

Migraines with an aura must also have one of these characteristics to be classified as a typical aura:

- homonymous vision disturbance
- unilateral paresthesia, numbness, or both
- unilateral weakness
- aphasia or other speech difficulty.

Migraines also have one of these characteristics:

- the history and physical and neurologic examinations are negative for a disorder

- examinations suggest a disorder that's ruled out by appropriate investigation
- a disorder is present, but migraines don't occur for the first time in relation to the disorder.

Tension-type headaches

In contrast to migraines, episodic tension-type headaches are diagnosed when the headache occurs on fewer than 180 days per year or the patient has fewer than 15 headaches per month and these characteristics are present:

- a headache lasting from 30 minutes to 7 days
- pain that's pressing or tightening in quality, mild to moderate, bilateral, and not aggravated by activity
- photophobia or phonophobia occurring sometimes, but usually not nausea or vomiting.

Cluster headaches

Cluster headaches are a treatable type of vascular headache syndrome. Characteristics include:

- episodic type (more common)—one to three short-lived attacks of periorbital pain per day over a 4- to 8-week period followed by a pain-free interval averaging 1 year
- chronic type—occurring after an episodic pattern is established
- unilateral pain occurring without warning, reaching a crescendo within 5 minutes, and described as excruciating and deep
- attacks lasting from 30 minutes to 2 hours
- associated symptoms—may include tearing, reddening of the eye, nasal stuffiness, lid ptosis, and nausea.

Arteriovenous malformations. Less common than cerebral aneurysms, vascular malformations usually result from developmental defects of the cerebral veins and arteries. Although many are present from birth, they manifest in adulthood with a triad of symptoms: headache, hemorrhage, and seizures.

Brain abscess. With brain abscess, the headache is localized to the abscess site. Usually, it intensifies over a few days and is aggravated by straining. Accompanying the headache may be nausea, vomiting, and focal or generalized seizures. The patient's LOC varies from drowsiness to deep stupor. Depending on the abscess site, associated signs and symptoms may include aphasia, impaired visual acuity, hemiparesis, ataxia, tremors, and personality changes. Signs of infection, such as fever and pallor, usually develop late; however, if the abscess remains encapsulated, these signs may not appear.

Brain tumor. Initially, a tumor causes a localized headache near the tumor site; as the tumor grows, the headache becomes generalized. The pain is usually intermittent, deep seated, dull, and most intense in the morning. It's aggravated by coughing, stooping, Valsalva's maneuver, and changes in head position and relieved by sitting and rest. Associated signs and symptoms include personality changes, an altered LOC, motor and sensory dysfunction and, eventually, signs of increased ICP, such as vomiting, increased systolic blood pressure, and a widened pulse pressure.

Cerebral aneurysm (ruptured). Ruptured cerebral aneurysm is a life-threatening disorder that's characterized by a sudden, excruciating headache, which may be unilateral and usually peaks within minutes of the rupture. The patient may lose consciousness immediately or display a variably altered LOC. Depending on the severity and lo-cation of the bleeding, he may also exhibit nausea and vomiting; signs and symptoms of meningeal irritation, such as nuchal rigidity and blurred vision; hemiparesis; seizure activity; and other features.

Ebola virus. With ebola virus, headache is usually abrupt in onset, commonly occurring on the fifth day of illness. Additionally, the patient has a history of malaise, myalgia, a high fever, diarrhea, abdominal pain, dehydration, and lethargy. A maculopapular skin rash develops between the fifth and seventh days of the illness. Other possible findings include pleuritic chest pain; a dry, hacking cough; pronounced pharyngitis; hematemesis; melena; and bleeding from the nose, gums, and vagina. Death usually occurs in the second week of the illness, preceded by severe blood loss and shock.

Encephalitis. A severe, generalized headache is characteristic with encephalitis. Within 48 hours, the patient's LOC typically deteriorates—perhaps from lethargy to coma. Associated signs and symptoms include a fever, nuchal rigidity, irritability, seizures, nausea and vomiting, photophobia, cranial nerve palsies such as ptosis, and focal neurologic deficits, such as hemiparesis and hemiplegia.

Epidural hemorrhage (acute). Head trauma and a sudden, brief loss of consciousness usually precede acute epidural hemorrhage, which causes a progressively severe headache that's accompanied by nausea and vomiting, bladder distention, confusion, and then a rapid decrease in the patient's LOC. Other signs and symptoms include unilateral seizures, hemiparesis, hemiplegia, a high fever, a decreased pulse rate and bounding pulse, a widened pulse pressure, increased blood pressure, a positive Babinski's reflex, and decerebrate posture.

If the patient slips into a coma, his respirations deepen and become stertorous, then shallow and irregular, and eventually they cease. Pupil dilation may occur on the same side as the hemorrhage.

Glaucoma (acute angle-closure). Glaucoma is an ophthalmic emergency that may cause an excruciating headache as well as acute eye pain, blurred vision, halo vision, nausea, and vomiting. Assessment reveals conjunctival injection, a cloudy cornea, and a moderately dilated, fixed pupil.

Hantavirus pulmonary syndrome. Noncardiogenic pulmonary edema distinguishes hantavirus pulmonary syndrome. Common reasons for seeking treatment include flulike signs and symptoms—headache, myalgia, fever, nausea, vomiting, and a cough—followed by respiratory distress. Fever, hypoxia, and (in some patients) serious hypotension typify the hospital course. Other signs and symptoms include a rising respiratory rate (28 breaths/minute or more) and an increased heart rate (120 beats/minute or more).

Hypertension. Hypertension may cause a slightly throbbing occipital headache on awakening that decreases in severity during the day. However, if the patient's diastolic blood pressure exceeds 120 mm Hg, the headache remains constant. Associated signs and symptoms include an atrial gallop, restlessness, confusion, nausea and vomiting, blurred vision, seizures, and an altered LOC.

Influenza. A severe generalized or frontal headache usually begins suddenly with the flu. Accompanying signs and symptoms may last for 3 to 5 days and include stabbing retro-orbital pain, weakness, diffuse myalgia, fever, chills, coughing, rhinorrhea and, occasionally, hoarseness.

Listeriosis. Signs and symptoms of listeriosis include fever, myalgia, abdominal pain, nausea, vomiting, and diarrhea. If the infection spreads to the nervous system, meningitis may develop. These signs and symptoms include headache, nuchal rigidity, fever, and a change in the patient's LOC.

Meningitis. Meningitis is marked by the sudden onset of a severe, constant, generalized headache that worsens with movement. Associated signs include nuchal rigidity, positive Kernig's and Brudzinski's signs, hyperreflexia and, possibly, opisthotonos. A fever occurs early with meningitis and may be accompanied by chills. As ICP increases, vomiting and, occasionally, papilledema develop. Other features include an altered LOC, seizures, ocular palsies, facial weakness, and hearing loss.

Plague (Yersinia pestis). The pneumonic form of the plague causes a sudden onset of a headache, chills, fever, myalgia, a productive cough, chest pain, tachypnea, dyspnea, hemoptysis, respiratory distress, and cardiopulmonary insufficiency.

Postconcussional syndrome. A generalized or localized headache may develop 1 to 30 days after head trauma and last for 2 to 3 weeks. This characteristic symptom may be described as an aching, pounding, pressing, stabbing, or throbbing pain. The patient's neurologic examination is normal, but he may experience giddiness or dizziness, blurred vision, fatigue, insomnia, an inability to concentrate, and noise and alcohol intolerance.

Q Fever. Signs and symptoms of Q fever include severe headaches, fever, chills, malaise, chest pain, nausea, vomiting, and diarrhea. Fever may last for up to 2 weeks, and in severe cases, the patient may develop hepatitis or pneumonia.

Severe acute respiratory syndrome (SARS). SARS generally begins with a fever (usually greater than 100.4° F [38° C]). Other symptoms include headache; malaise; a dry, nonproductive cough; and dyspnea. The severity of the illness is highly variable, ranging from mild illness to pneumonia and, in some cases, progressing to respiratory failure and death.

Smallpox (variola major). Initial signs and symptoms of smallpox include a severe headache, backache, abdominal pain, a high fever, malaise, prostration, and a maculopapular rash on the mucosa of the mouth, pharynx, face, and forearms, and then the trunk and legs. The rash becomes vesicular, then pustular, and finally crusts and scabs, leaving a pitted scar. In fatal cases, death results from encephalitis, extensive bleeding, or secondary infection.

Subarachnoid hemorrhage. Subarachnoid hemorrhage commonly produces a sudden, severe headache along with nuchal rigidity, nausea and vomiting, seizures, dizziness, ipsilateral pupil dilation, and an altered LOC that may rapidly progress to coma. The patient also exhibits positive Kernig's and Brudzinski's signs, photophobia, blurred vision and, possibly, a fever. Focal signs and symptoms (such as hemiparesis, hemiplegia, sensory or vision disturbances, and aphasia) and signs of elevated ICP (such as bradycardia and increased blood pressure) may also occur.

Subdural hematoma. Typically associated with head trauma, acute and chronic subdural hematomas may cause a headache and decreased LOC. With *acute subdural hematoma,* head trauma also produces drowsiness, confusion, and agitation that may progress to coma. Later findings include signs of increased ICP and focal neurologic deficits such as hemiparesis.

Chronic subdural hematoma produces a dull, pounding headache that fluctuates in severity and is located over the hematoma. Weeks or months after the initial head trauma, the patient may experience giddiness, personality changes, confusion, seizures, and a progressively worsening LOC. Late signs may include unilateral pupil dilation, sluggish pupil reaction to light, and ptosis.

Tularemia. Signs and symptoms following inhalation of the bacterium *Francisella tularensis* include an abrupt onset of a headache, a fever, chills, generalized myalgia, a nonproductive cough, dyspnea, pleuritic chest pain, and empyema.

Typhus. Initial symptoms of typhus include a headache, myalgia, arthralgia, and malaise followed by an abrupt onset of chills, a fever, nausea, and vomiting. A maculopapular rash may be present in some cases.

West Nile encephalitis. Signs and symptoms of West Nile encephalitis include a fever, a headache, and body aches, commonly with a skin rash and swollen lymph glands. More severe infection is marked by a high fever, a headache, neck stiffness, stupor, disorientation, coma, tremors, occasional seizures, paralysis and, rarely, death.

Other causes

Diagnostic tests. A lumbar puncture, myelogram, or epidural or spinal procedure may produce a throbbing frontal headache that worsens on standing.

Drugs. Many drugs can cause headaches. For example, indomethacin produces headaches—usually in the morning—in many patients. Vasodilators and drugs with a vasodilating effect, such as nitrates, typically cause a throbbing headache. Headaches may also follow withdrawal from vasopressors, such as caffeine, ergotamine, and sympathomimetics.

Traction. Cervical traction with pins commonly causes a headache, which may be generalized or localized to pin insertion sites.

Nursing considerations
- Monitor the patient's vital signs and LOC.
- Watch for a change in the headache's severity or location.
- To help ease the headache, administer an analgesic, darken the patient's room, and minimize other stimuli.
- Prepare the patient for diagnostic tests, such as skull X-rays, a computed tomography scan, lumbar puncture, or cerebral arteriography.

Patient teaching
- Explain all procedures and treatments to the patient.
- Discuss the signs of reduced LOC and seizures that the patient or his caregivers should report.
- Explain ways to maintain a safe, quiet environment and reduce environmental stress.
- Discuss the proper use of analgesics.

Hearing loss

Affecting nearly 16 million Americans, hearing loss may be temporary or permanent and partial or complete. This common symptom may involve reception of low-, middle-, or high-frequency tones. If the hearing loss doesn't affect speech frequencies, the patient may be unaware of it.

Normally, sound waves enter the external auditory canal, and then travel to the middle ear's tympanic membrane and ossicles (incus, malleus, and stapes) and into the inner ear's cochlea. The cochlear division of cranial nerve (CN) VIII (auditory nerve) carries the sound impulse to the brain. This type of sound transmission, called *air conduction,* is normally better than bone conduction—sound transmission through bone to the inner ear.

Hearing loss can be classified as conductive, sensorineural, mixed, or functional. Conductive hearing loss results from external- or middle-ear disorders that block sound transmission. This type of hearing loss usually responds to medical or surgical intervention (or in some cases, both). Sensorineural hearing loss results from disorders of the inner ear or of CN VIII. Mixed hearing loss combines aspects of conductive and sensorineural hearing loss. Functional hearing loss results from psychological factors rather than identifiable organic damage.

Hearing loss may also result from trauma, infection, allergy, tumors, certain systemic and hereditary disorders, and the effects of ototoxic drugs and treatments. In most cases, however, it results from presbycusis, a type of sensorineural hearing loss that usually affects people older than age 50. Other physiologic causes of hearing loss include cerumen (earwax) impaction; barotitis media (unequal pressure on the eardrum) associated with descent in an airplane or elevator, diving, or close proximity to an explosion; and chronic exposure to noise over 90 decibels, which can occur on the job, with certain hobbies, or from listening to live or recorded music.

History and physical examination

If the patient reports hearing loss, ask him to describe it. Is it unilateral or bilateral? Continuous or intermittent? Ask about a family history of hearing loss. Then obtain the patient's medical history, noting chronic ear infections, ear surgery, and ear or head trauma. Has the patient recently had an upper respiratory tract infection? After taking a drug history, have the patient describe his occupation and work environment.

Next, explore associated signs and symptoms. Does the patient have ear pain? If so, is it unilateral or bilateral, or continuous or intermittent? Ask the patient if he has noticed discharge from one or both ears. If so, have him describe its color and consistency, and note when it began. Does he hear ringing, buzzing, hissing, or other noises in one or both ears? If so, are the noises constant or intermittent? Does he experience dizziness? If so, when did he first notice it?

Begin the physical examination by inspecting the external ear for inflammation, boils, foreign bodies, and discharge. Then apply pressure to the tragus and mastoid to elicit tenderness. If you detect tenderness or external ear abnormalities, notify the physician to discuss whether an otoscopic examination should be done. (See *Using an otoscope correctly*, page 223.) During the otoscopic examination, note color change, perforation, bulging, or retraction of the tympanic membrane, which normally looks like a shiny, pearl gray cone.

Next, evaluate the patient's hearing acuity, using the ticking watch and whispered voice tests. Then perform Weber's and the Rinne tests to obtain a preliminary evaluation of the type and degree of hearing loss. (See *Differentiating conductive from sensorineural hearing loss,* page 304.)

Medical causes

Acoustic neuroma. Acoustic neuroma, which is a CN VIII tumor, causes unilateral, progressive, sensorineural hearing loss. The patient may also develop tinnitus, vertigo, and—with cranial nerve compression—facial paralysis.

Adenoid hypertrophy. Eustachian tube dysfunction causes gradual conductive hearing loss accompanied by in-

termittent ear discharge. The patient also tends to breathe through his mouth and may complain of a sensation of ear fullness.

Aural polyps. If a polyp occludes the external auditory canal, partial hearing loss may occur. The polyp typically bleeds easily and is covered by a purulent discharge.

Cholesteatoma. Gradual hearing loss is characteristic of cholesteatoma. It can be accompanied by vertigo and, at times, facial paralysis. Examination reveals eardrum perforation, pearly white balls in the ear canal, and possible discharge.

Cyst. Ear canal obstruction by a sebaceous or dermoid cyst causes progressive conductive hearing loss. On inspection, the cyst looks like a soft mass.

External ear canal tumor (malignant). Progressive conductive hearing loss is characteristic of an external ear canal tumor and is accompanied by deep, boring ear pain, purulent discharge and, eventually, facial paralysis. The patient may develop a rash in the external canal or pinna of the ear. Examination may detect the granular, bleeding tumor.

Glomus jugulare tumor. Initially, this benign tumor causes mild, unilateral conductive hearing loss that becomes progressively more severe. The patient may report tinnitus that sounds like his heartbeat. Associated signs and symptoms include gradual congestion in the affected ear, throbbing or pulsating discomfort, bloody otorrhea, facial nerve paralysis, and vertigo. Although the tympanic membrane is normal, a reddened mass appears behind it.

Head trauma. Sudden conductive or sensorineural hearing loss may result from ossicle disruption, ear canal fracture, tympanic membrane perforation, or cochlear fracture associated with head trauma. Typically, the patient reports a

Differentiating conductive from sensorineural hearing loss

Weber's and the Rinne tests can help determine whether the patient's hearing loss is conductive or sensorineural. Weber's test evaluates bone conduction; the Rinne test, bone and air conduction. Using a 512-Hz tuning fork, perform these preliminary tests as described here.perform these preliminary tests as described here.

Weber's test

Place the base of a vibrating tuning fork firmly against the midline of the patient's skull at the forehead. Ask her if she hears the tone equally well in both ears. If she does, Weber's test is graded *midline*—a normal finding. In an abnormal Weber's test (graded *right* or *left*), sound is louder in one ear, suggesting a conductive hearing loss in that ear, or a sensorineural loss in the opposite ear.

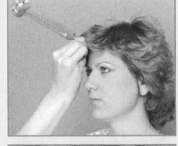

Rinne test

Hold the base of a vibrating tuning fork against the patient's mastoid process to test bone conduction. Then quickly move the vibrating fork in front of her ear canal to test air conduction. Ask her to tell you which location has the louder or longer sound. Repeat the procedure for the other ear. In a positive Rinne test, air conduction lasts longer or sounds louder than bone conduction—a normal finding. In a negative test, the opposite is true: Bone conduction lasts longer or sounds louder than air conduction.

After performing both tests, correlate the results with other assessment data.

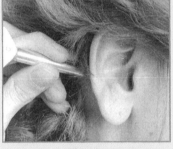

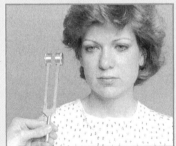

Implications of results

Conductive hearing loss produces:
- abnormal Weber's test result
- negative Rinne test result
- improved hearing in noisy areas
- normal ability to discriminate sounds
- difficulty hearing when chewing
- a quiet speaking voice.

Sensorineural hearing loss produces:
- positive Rinne test
- poor hearing in noisy areas
- difficulty hearing high-frequency sounds
- complaints that others mumble or shout
- tinnitus.

headache and exhibits bleeding from his ear. Neurologic features vary and may include impaired vision and an altered level of consciousness.

Ménière's disease. Initially, Ménière's disease, an inner ear disorder, produces intermittent, unilateral sensorineural hearing loss that involves only low tones. Later, hearing loss becomes constant and affects other tones. Associated signs and symptoms include intermittent severe vertigo, nausea and vomiting, a feeling of fullness in the ear, a roaring or hollow-seashell tinnitus, diaphoresis, and nystagmus.

Nasopharyngeal cancer. Nasopharyngeal cancer causes mild unilateral conductive hearing loss when it compresses the eustachian tube. Bone conduction is normal, and inspection reveals a retracted tympanic membrane backed by fluid. When this tumor obstructs the nasal airway, the patient may exhibit nasal speech and a bloody nasal and postnasal discharge. Cranial nerve involvement produces other findings, such as diplopia and rectus muscle paralysis.

Otitis externa. Conductive hearing loss resulting from debris in the ear canal characterizes acute and malignant otitis externa. With acute otitis externa, ear canal inflammation produces pain, itching, and a foul-smelling, sticky yellow discharge. Severe tenderness is typically elicited by chewing, opening the mouth, and pressing on the tragus or mastoid. The patient may also develop a low-grade fever, regional lymphadenopathy, a headache on the affected side, and mild to moderate pain around the ear that may later intensify. Examination may reveal greenish white debris or edema in the canal.

With malignant otitis externa, debris is also visible in the canal. This life-threatening disorder, which most commonly occurs in the patient with dia-betes, causes sensorineural hearing loss, pruritus, tinnitus, and severe ear pain.

Otitis media. *Otitis media* is a middle ear inflammation that typically produces unilateral conductive hearing loss. In patients with acute suppurative otitis media, the hearing loss develops gradually over a few hours and is usually accompanied by an upper respiratory tract infection with a sore throat, cough, nasal discharge, and headache. Related signs and symptoms include dizziness, a sensation of fullness in the ear, intermittent or constant ear pain, a fever, nausea, and vomiting. Rupture of the bulging, swollen tympanic membrane relieves the pain and produces a brief, bloody, purulent discharge. Hearing returns after the infection subsides.

Hearing loss also develops gradually in patients with *chronic otitis media*. Assessment may reveal a perforated tympanic membrane, purulent ear drainage, an earache, nausea, and vertigo.

Commonly associated with an upper respiratory tract infection or nasopharyngeal cancer, *serous otitis media* commonly produces a stuffy feeling in the ear and pain that worsens at night. Examination reveals a retracted—and perhaps discolored—tympanic membrane and possibly air bubbles behind the membrane.

Otosclerosis. Otosclerosis is a hereditary disorder in which unilateral conductive hearing loss usually begins when the patient is in his early twenties and may gradually progress to bilateral mixed loss. The patient may report tinnitus and an ability to hear better in a noisy environment. The deafness is usually noticed between ages 11 and 30.

Skull fracture. With a skull fracture, auditory nerve injury causes sudden unilateral sensorineural hearing loss. Accompanying signs and symptoms include ringing tinnitus, blood behind the tympanic membrane, scalp wounds, and other findings.

Temporal bone fracture. Temporal bone fracture can cause sudden unilateral sensorineural hearing loss accompanied by hissing tinnitus. The tympanic membrane may be perforated, depending on the fracture's location. Loss of consciousness, Battle's sign, and facial paralysis may also occur.

Tympanic membrane perforation. Commonly caused by trauma from sharp objects or rapid pressure changes, perforation of the tympanic membrane causes abrupt hearing loss along with ear pain, tinnitus, vertigo, and a sensation of fullness in the ear.

Other causes

Drugs. Ototoxic drugs typically produce ringing or buzzing tinnitus and a feeling of fullness in the ear. Chloroquine, cisplatin, vancomycin, and aminoglycosides (especially neomycin, kanamycin, and amikacin) may cause irreversible hearing loss. Loop diuretics, such as furosemide, ethacrynic acid, and bumetanide, usually produce a brief, reversible hearing loss. Quinine, quinidine, and high doses of erythromycin or salicylates (such as aspirin) may also cause reversible hearing loss.

Radiation therapy. Irradiation of the middle ear, thyroid, face, skull, or nasopharynx may cause eustachian tube dysfunction, resulting in hearing loss.

Surgery. Myringotomy, myringoplasty, simple or radical mastoidectomy, or fenestrations may cause scarring that interferes with hearing.

Nursing considerations

- When talking with the patient, remember to face him and speak slowly.
- Don't shout, smoke, eat, or chew gum when talking.
- Prepare the patient for audiometry and auditory evoked-response testing.

- Provide an alternate means of communication, if necessary.

Patient teaching

- Explain interventions to the patient, such as a hearing aid or cochlear implant to improve his hearing.
- Discuss the importance of ear protection and avoidance of loud noise.
- Stress the importance of following instructions for taking prescribed antibiotics.
- Explain the underlying cause of the hearing loss and its treatment.

Heat intolerance

Heat intolerance refers to the inability to withstand high temperatures or to maintain a comfortable body temperature. This symptom produces a continuous feeling of being overheated and, at times, profuse diaphoresis. It usually develops gradually and is chronic.

Most cases of heat intolerance result from thyrotoxicosis. With this disorder, excess thyroid hormone stimulates peripheral tissues, increasing basal metabolism and producing excess heat. Although rare, hypothalamic disease may also cause intolerance to heat and cold.

History and physical examination

Ask the patient when he first noticed his heat intolerance. Did he gradually use fewer blankets at night? Does he have to turn up the air conditioning to keep cool? Is it hard for him to adjust to warm weather? Does he sweat in a hot environment? Find out if his appetite or weight has changed. Also, ask about unusual nervousness or other personality changes. Then take a drug history, especially noting the use of amphetamines or amphetamine-like drugs. Ask the patient if he takes a thyroid drug. If so, what's the daily dose? When did he last take it?

As you begin the examination, notice how much clothing the patient is wearing. After taking his vital signs, inspect his skin for flushing and diaphoresis. Also, note tremors and lid lag.

Medical causes

Hypothalamic disease. With hypothalamic disease, body temperature fluctuates dramatically, causing alternating heat and cold intolerance. Related features include amenorrhea, disturbed sleep patterns, increased thirst and urination, increased appetite with weight gain, impaired visual acuity, a headache, and personality changes, such as bursts of rage or laughter. Common causes of hypothalamic disease are pituitary adenoma and hypothalamic and pineal tumors.

Thyrotoxicosis. A classic symptom of thyrotoxicosis, heat intolerance may be accompanied by an enlarged thyroid, nervousness, weight loss despite increased appetite, diaphoresis, diarrhea, tremor, and palpitations. Although exophthalmos is characteristic, many patients don't display this sign. Associated findings may affect virtually every body system. Some common findings include irritability, difficulty concentrating, mood swings, insomnia, muscle weakness, fatigue, lid lag, tachycardia, full and bounding pulse, a widened pulse pressure, dyspnea, amenorrhea, and gynecomastia. Typically, the patient's skin is warm and flushed; premature graying and alopecia occur in both sexes.

Other causes

Drugs. Amphetamines, amphetamine-like appetite suppressants, and excessive doses of thyroid hormone may cause heat intolerance. Anticholinergics may interfere with sweating, resulting in heat intolerance.

Nursing considerations

- Adjust the room temperature to make the patient comfortable.
- If the patient is diaphoretic, change his clothing and bed linens as necessary, and encourage him to drink lots of fluids.

Patient teaching

- Teach the patient about the disease process and its treatments.
- Discuss the importance of proper hygiene and drinking plenty of fluids.

Heberden's nodes

Heberden's nodes are painless, irregular, cartilaginous or bony enlargements of the distal interphalangeal joints of the fingers. They reflect degeneration of articular cartilage, which irritates the bone and stimulates osteoblasts, causing bony enlargement. Approximately 2 to 3 mm in diameter, Heberden's nodes develop on one or both sides of the dorsal midline. The dominant hand usually has larger nodes, which affect one or more fingers but not the thumb. (See *Recognizing Heberden's nodes,* page 308.)

Osteoarthritis is the most common cause of Heberden's nodes; in fact, more than one-half of all osteoarthritic patients have these nodes. Less commonly, repeated fingertip trauma may lead to node formation in only one joint ("baseball finger"). Because Heberden's nodes aren't associated with joint pain or loss of function, they aren't a primary indicator of osteoarthritis; however, they're a helpful adjunct to diagnosis.

History and physical examination

Begin by asking the patient if anyone else in his family has had Heberden's nodes or osteoarthritis. Are the patient's joints stiff? Does stiffness disappear with movement? Ask him which hand is

Recognizing Heberden's nodes

These painless bony enlargements of the distal interphalangeal finger joints appear in more than one-half of all patients with osteoarthritis.

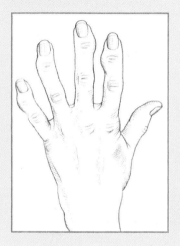

dominant. Also ask about repeated fingertip trauma associated with his job or sports.

Carefully palpate the nodes, noting any signs of inflammation, such as redness and tenderness. Then determine range of motion (ROM) in the fingers of each hand. As you do so, listen and feel for crepitation.

Medical causes

Osteoarthritis. This disorder commonly causes Heberden's nodes and may also cause nodes in the proximal interphalangeal joints (Bouchard's nodes). Its chief symptom, though, is joint pain that's aggravated by movement or weight bearing. Joints may also be tender and display restricted ROM. Typically, joint stiffness is triggered by disuse and relieved by brief exercise. Stiffness may be accompanied by bony enlargement and crepitus.

Nursing considerations
- Administer anti-inflammatories, as prescribed.
- For affected hand joints, use hot soaks and paraffin dips.

Patient teaching
- Remind the patient to exercise regularly.
- Teach the patient about his prescribed drugs and adverse effects that should be reported.
- Encourage the patient to avoid joint strain, for example, by maintaining a healthy body weight.

Hematemesis

Hematemesis, the vomiting of blood, usually indicates GI bleeding above the ligament of Treitz, which suspends the duodenum at its junction with the jejunum. Bright red or blood-streaked vomitus indicates fresh or recent bleeding. Dark red, brown, or black vomitus (the color and consistency of coffee grounds) indicates that blood has been retained in the stomach and partially digested.

Although hematemesis usually results from a GI disorder, it may stem from a coagulation disorder or a treatment that irritates the GI tract. Esophageal varices may also cause hematemesis. Swallowed blood from epistaxis or oropharyngeal erosion may also cause bloody vomitus. Hematemesis may be precipitated by straining, emotional stress, and the use of an anti-inflammatory, anticoagulant, or alcohol. In a patient with esophageal varices, hematemesis may be a result of trauma from swallowing hard or partially chewed food.

Hematemesis is always an important sign, but its severity depends on the amount, source, and rapidity of the bleeding. Massive hematemesis (vomiting 500 to 1,000 ml of blood) may be life-threatening.

ACTION STAT!

 If the patient has massive hematemesis, check his vital signs. If you detect signs of shock—such as tachypnea, hypotension, and tachycardia—place the patient in a supine position, and elevate his feet 20 to 30 degrees. Insert a large-bore I.V. catheter for emergency fluid replacement. Also, send a blood sample for typing and crossmatching, hemoglobin level, and hematocrit and administer oxygen. Emergency endoscopy may be necessary to locate, and possibly treat, the source of bleeding. Prepare to insert a nasogastric (NG) tube for suction or iced lavage. A Sengstaken-Blakemore tube may be used to compress esophageal varices. (See *Managing hematemesis with intubation,* page 310.)

History and physical examination

If the patient's hematemesis isn't immediately life-threatening, begin with a thorough history. First, have the patient describe the amount, color, and consistency of the vomitus. When did he first notice this sign? Has he ever had hematemesis before? Find out if he also has bloody or black, tarry stools. Note whether hematemesis is usually preceded by nausea, flatulence, diarrhea, or weakness. Has he recently had bouts of retching with or without vomiting?

Next, ask about a history of ulcers or of liver or coagulation disorders. Find out how much alcohol the patient drinks, if any. Does he regularly take aspirin or other nonsteroidal anti-inflam-

matory drug (NSAID), such as phenylbutazone or indomethacin? These drugs may cause erosive gastritis or ulcers. Does he take warfarin or other drugs with anticoagulant properties? These drugs increase the patient's risk of bleeding.

Begin the physical examination by checking for orthostatic hypotension, an early warning sign of hypovolemia. Take blood pressure and pulse with the patient in the supine, sitting, and standing positions. A decrease of 10 mm Hg or more in systolic pressure or an increase of 10 beats/minute or more in pulse rate indicates volume depletion. After obtaining other vital signs, inspect the mucous membranes, nasopharynx, and skin for signs of bleeding or other abnormalities. Finally, palpate the abdomen for tenderness, pain, or masses. Note lymphadenopathy.

Medical causes

Anthrax (GI). Initial signs and symptoms after eating contaminated meat from an animal infected with the gram-positive, spore-forming bacterium *Bacillus anthracis* include a loss of appetite, nausea, vomiting, and a fever. Signs and symptoms may progress to hematemesis, abdominal pain, and severe bloody diarrhea.

Coagulation disorders. Any disorder that disrupts normal clotting may result in GI bleeding and moderate to severe hematemesis. Bleeding may occur in other body systems as well, resulting in such signs as epistaxis and ecchymosis. Other associated effects vary, depending on the specific coagulation disorder, such as thrombocytopenia or hemophilia.

Esophageal cancer. A late sign of esophageal cancer, hematemesis may be accompanied by steady chest pain that radiates to the back. Other features include substantial fullness, severe dyspha-

Managing hematemesis with intubation

A patient with hematemesis needs to have a GI tube inserted to allow blood drainage, aspirate gastric contents, or facilitate gastric lavage, if necessary. Here are the most common tubes and their uses.

Nasogastric tubes

The Salem-Sump tube (at right), a double-lumen nasogastric (NG) tube, is used to remove stomach fluid and gas or to aspirate gastric contents. It may also be used for gastric lavage, drug administration, or feeding. Its main advantage over the Levin tube—a single-lumen NG tube—is that it allows atmospheric air to enter the patient's stomach so the tube can float freely instead of risking adhesion and damage to the gastric mucosa.

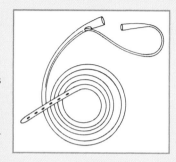

Wide-bore gastric tubes

The Edlich tube (at right) has one wide-bore lumen with four openings near the closed distal tip. A funnel or syringe can be connected at the proximal end. Like the other tubes, the Edlich tube can aspirate a large volume of gastric contents quickly.

The Ewald tube, a wide-bore tube that allows quick passage of a large amount of fluid and clots, is especially useful for gastric lavage in patients with profuse GI bleeding and in those who have ingested poison. Another wide-bore tube, the double-lumen Levacuator, has a large lumen for evacuation of gastric contents and a small one for lavage.

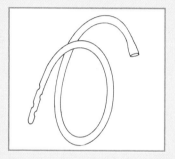

Esophageal tubes

The Sengstaken-Blakemore tube (at right), a triple-lumen double-balloon esophageal tube, provides a gastric aspiration port that allows drainage from below the gastric balloon. It can also be used to instill medication. A similar tube, the Linton shunt, can aspirate esophageal and gastric contents without risking necrosis because it has no esophageal balloon. The Minnesota esophagogastric tamponade tube, which has four lumina and two balloons, provides pressure-monitoring ports for both balloons without the need for Y-connectors.

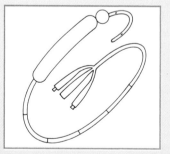

gia, nausea, vomiting with nocturnal regurgitation and aspiration, hemoptysis, a fever, hiccups, a sore throat, melena, and halitosis.

Esophageal rupture. The severity of hematemesis depends on the cause of the esophageal rupture. When an instrument damages the esophagus, hematemesis is usually slight. However, rupture due to Boerhaave's syndrome (increased esophageal pressure from vomiting or retching) or other esophageal disorders typically causes more severe hematemesis. This life-threatening disorder may also produce severe retrosternal, epigastric, neck, or scapular pain accompanied by chest and neck edema. Examination reveals subcutaneous crepitation in the chest wall, supraclavicular fossa, and neck. The patient may also show signs of respiratory distress, such as dyspnea and cyanosis.

Esophageal varices (ruptured). Life-threatening rupture of esophageal varices may produce coffee-ground or massive, bright red vomitus. Signs of shock, such as hypotension or tachycardia, may follow or even precede hematemesis if the stomach fills with blood before vomiting occurs. Other symptoms may include abdominal distention and melena or painless hematochezia, ranging from slight oozing to massive rectal hemorrhage.

Gastric cancer. Painless bright red or dark brown vomitus is a late sign of gastric cancer, which usually begins insidiously with upper abdominal discomfort. The patient then develops anorexia, mild nausea, and chronic dyspepsia unrelieved by antacids and exacerbated by food. Later symptoms may include fatigue, weakness, weight loss, feelings of fullness, melena, altered bowel habits, and signs of malnutrition, such as muscle wasting and dry skin.

Gastritis (acute). Hematemesis and melena are the most common signs of acute gastritis. They may even be the only signs, although mild epigastric discomfort, nausea, a fever, and malaise may also occur. Massive blood loss precipitates signs of shock. Typically, the patient has a history of alcohol abuse or has used aspirin or some other NSAID. Gastritis may also occur secondary to *Helicobacter pylori* infection.

Mallory-Weiss syndrome. Characterized by a mucosal tear of the mucous membrane at the junction of the esophagus and stomach, this syndrome may produce hematemesis and melena. It's commonly triggered by severe vomiting, retching, or straining (as from coughing), most commonly in alcoholics or in people whose pylorus is obstructed. Severe bleeding may precipitate signs of shock, such as tachycardia, hypotension, dyspnea, and cool, clammy skin.

Peptic ulcer. Hematemesis may occur when a peptic ulcer penetrates an artery, vein, or highly vascular tissue. Massive—and possibly life-threatening—hematemesis is typical when an artery is penetrated. Other features include melena or hematochezia, chills, a fever, and signs and symptoms of shock and dehydration, such as tachycardia, hypotension, poor skin turgor, and thirst. The patient may have a history of nausea, vomiting, epigastric tenderness, and epigastric pain that's relieved by foods or antacids. He may also have a history of habitually using tobacco, alcohol, or NSAIDs.

Other causes

Treatments. Traumatic NG or endotracheal intubation may cause hematemesis associated with swallowed blood. Nose or throat surgery may also cause this sign in the same way.

Nursing considerations

- Closely monitor the patient's vital signs, and watch for signs of shock.

- Check the patient's stools regularly for occult blood.
- Keep accurate intake and output records.
- Monitor NG drainage for blood.
- Place the patient on bed rest in low or semi-Fowler's position to prevent aspiration of vomitus.
- Keep suctioning equipment nearby, and use it as needed.
- Provide frequent oral hygiene and emotional support.
- Administer a histamine-2 receptor antagonist I.V.; vasopressin may be required for variceal hemorrhage.

Patient teaching

- Explain any food or fluid restrictions.
- Stress the importance of avoiding the use of alcohol.
- Teach the patient about prescribed medications and what drugs to avoid.

Hematochezia
[Rectal bleeding]

The passage of bloody stools, also known as *hematochezia,* usually indicates—and may be the first sign of—GI bleeding below the ligament of Treitz. However, this sign—usually preceded by hematemesis—may also accompany rapid hemorrhage of 1 L or more from the upper GI tract.

Hematochezia ranges from formed, blood-streaked stools to liquid, bloody stools that may be bright red, dark mahogany, or maroon. This sign usually develops abruptly and is heralded by abdominal pain.

Although hematochezia is commonly associated with GI disorders, it may also result from a coagulation disorder, exposure to toxins, or certain diagnostic tests. Always a significant sign, hematochezia may precipitate life-threatening hypovolemia.

ACTION STAT!

 If the patient has severe hematochezia, check his vital signs. If you detect signs of shock, such as hypotension and tachycardia, place the patient in a supine position and elevate his feet 20 to 30 degrees. Prepare to administer oxygen, and insert a large-bore I.V. catheter for emergency fluid replacement. Next, obtain a blood sample for typing and crossmatching, hemoglobin level, and hematocrit. Insert a nasogastric tube. Iced lavage may be indicated to control bleeding. Endoscopy may be necessary to detect the source of bleeding.

History and physical examination

If hematochezia isn't immediately life-threatening, ask the patient to fully describe the amount, color, and consistency of his bloody stools. (If possible, also inspect and characterize the stools yourself.) How long have the stools been bloody? Do they always look the same, or does the amount of blood seem to vary? Ask about associated signs and symptoms.

Next, explore the patient's medical history, focusing on GI and coagulation disorders. Ask about the use of GI irritants, such as alcohol, aspirin, and other nonsteroidal anti-inflammatory drugs (NSAIDs).

Begin the physical examination by checking for orthostatic hypotension, an early sign of shock. Take the patient's blood pressure and pulse while he's lying down, sitting, and standing. If systolic pressure decreases by 10 mm Hg or more or if the pulse rate increases by 10 beats/minute or more when he changes position, suspect volume depletion and impending shock.

Examine the skin for petechiae or spider angiomas. Palpate the abdomen for tenderness, pain, or masses. Also note lymphadenopathy. Finally, a digital rectal examination must be done to rule out rectal masses or hemorrhoids.

Medical causes

Anal fissure. Slight hematochezia characterizes anal fissure; blood may streak the stools or appear on toilet tissue. Accompanying hematochezia is severe rectal pain that may make the patient reluctant to defecate, thereby causing constipation.

Angiodysplastic lesions. Most common in elderly patients, these arteriovenous lesions of the ascending colon typically cause chronic, bright red rectal bleeding. Occasionally, this painless hematochezia may result in life-threatening blood loss and signs of shock, such as tachycardia and hypotension.

Coagulation disorders. Patients with a coagulation disorder (such as thrombocytopenia and disseminated intravascular coagulation) may experience GI bleeding marked by moderate to severe hematochezia. Bleeding may also occur in other body systems, producing such signs as epistaxis and purpura. Associated findings vary with the specific coagulation disorder.

Colitis. Ischemic colitis commonly causes bloody diarrhea, especially in elderly patients. Hematochezia may be slight or massive and is usually accompanied by severe, cramping lower abdominal pain and hypotension. Other effects include abdominal tenderness, distention, and absent bowel sounds. Severe colitis may cause life-threatening hypovolemic shock and peritonitis.

Ulcerative colitis typically causes bloody diarrhea that may also contain mucus. Hematochezia is preceded by mild to severe abdominal cramps and may cause slight to massive blood loss. Associated signs and symptoms include fever, tenesmus, anorexia, nausea, vomiting, hyperactive bowel sounds and, oc-

casionally, tachycardia. Weight loss and weakness occur late.

Colon cancer. Bright red rectal bleeding with or without pain is a telling sign of colon cancer especially in cancer of the left colon.

Usually, a left colon tumor causes early signs of obstruction, such as rectal pressure, bleeding, and intermittent fullness or cramping. As the disease progresses, the patient also develops obstipation, diarrhea or ribbon-shaped stools, and pain, which is typically relieved by the passage of stools or flatus. Stools are grossly bloody.

Early tumor growth in the right colon may cause melena, abdominal aching, pressure, and dull cramps. As the disease progresses, the patient develops weakness and fatigue. Later, he may also experience diarrhea, anorexia, weight loss, anemia, vomiting, an abdominal mass, and signs of obstruction, such as abdominal distention and abnormal bowel sounds.

Colorectal polyps. Colorectal polyps are the most common cause of intermittent hematochezia in adults younger than age 60; however, sometimes such polyps produce no symptoms. When located high in the colon, polyps may cause blood-streaked stools. The stools yield a positive response when tested with guaiac. If the polyps are located closer to the rectum, they may bleed freely.

Diverticulitis. Most common in the elderly patient, diverticulitis can suddenly cause mild to moderate rectal bleeding after the patient feels the urge to defecate. The bleeding may end abruptly or may progress to life-threatening blood loss with signs of shock. Associated signs and symptoms may include left lower quadrant pain that's relieved by defecation, alternating episodes of constipation and diarrhea, anorexia, nausea and vomiting, rebound tenderness, and a distended tympanic abdomen.

Dysentery. Bloody diarrhea is common in infection with *Shigella, Amoeba,* and *Campylobacter,* but rare with *Salmonella.* Abdominal pain or cramps, tenesmus, a fever, and nausea may also occur.

Esophageal varices (ruptured). In esophageal varices, a life-threatening disorder, hematochezia may range from slight rectal oozing to grossly bloody stools and may be accompanied by mild to severe hematemesis or melena. This painless but massive hemorrhage may precipitate signs of shock, such as tachycardia and hypotension. In fact, signs of shock occasionally precede overt signs of bleeding. Typically, the patient has a history of chronic liver disease.

Food poisoning (staphylococcal). The patient may have bloody diarrhea 1 to 6 hours after ingesting food toxins. Accompanying signs and symptoms include severe, cramping abdominal pain; nausea and vomiting; and prostration, all of which last a few hours.

Hemorrhoids. Hematochezia may accompany external hemorrhoids, which typically cause painful defecation, resulting in constipation. Less painful internal hemorrhoids usually produce more chronic bleeding with bowel movements, which may eventually lead to signs of anemia, such as weakness and fatigue.

Leptospirosis. The severe form of leptospirosis—*Weil's syndrome*—produces hematochezia or melena along with other signs of bleeding, such as epistaxis and hemoptysis. The bleeding is typically preceded by a sudden frontal headache and severe thigh and lumbar myalgia that may be accompanied by cutaneous hyperesthesia. Conjunctival suffusion is indicative. Bleeding is followed by chills, a rapidly rising fever and, perhaps, nausea and vomiting. A fever, a headache, and myalgia usually intensify and persist for weeks. Other findings may include right upper quadrant tenderness, hepatomegaly, and jaundice.

Peptic ulcer. Upper GI bleeding is a common complication in peptic ulcer. The patient may display hematochezia, hematemesis, or melena, depending on the rapidity and amount of bleeding. If the peptic ulcer penetrates an artery or vein, massive bleeding may precipitate signs of shock, such as hypotension and tachycardia. Other findings may include chills, a fever, nausea and vomiting, and signs of dehydration, such as dry mucous membranes, poor skin turgor, and thirst. The patient typically has a history of epigastric pain that's relieved by foods or antacids; he may also have a history of habitually using tobacco, alcohol, or NSAIDs.

Ulcerative proctitis. Ulcerative proctitis typically causes an intense urge to defecate, but the patient passes only bright red blood, pus, or mucus. Other common signs and symptoms include acute constipation and tenesmus.

Other causes
Diagnostic tests. Certain procedures, especially colonoscopy, polypectomy, hemorrhoidectomy, and proctosigmoidoscopy, may cause rectal bleeding. Bowel perforation is rare.

Nursing considerations
- Place the patient on bed rest.
- Check vital signs frequently, watching for signs of shock, such as hypotension, tachycardia, a weak pulse, and tachypnea.
- Monitor the patient's intake and output hourly.
- Monitor hemoglobin level and hematocrit.
- Administer blood products as ordered.
- Provide emotional support because hematochezia may frighten the patient.

- Prepare the patient for blood tests and GI procedures, such as endoscopy and GI X-rays.
- Visually examine the patient's stools and test them for occult blood.
- If necessary, send a stool specimen to the laboratory to check for parasites.

Patient teaching

- Explain signs and symptoms that require immediate medical attention.
- Teach the patient about ostomy self-care, as appropriate.
- Discuss proper bowel elimination habits.
- Explain dietary recommendations and restrictions.
- Teach the patient about prescribed medications.

Hematuria

A cardinal sign of renal and urinary tract disorders, hematuria is the abnormal presence of blood in urine. Strictly defined, it means three or more red blood cells (RBCs) per high-power microscopic field in urine. Microscopic hematuria is confirmed by an occult blood test, whereas macroscopic hematuria is immediately visible. However, macroscopic hematuria must be distinguished from pseudohematuria. (See *Confirming hematuria*.) Macroscopic hematuria may be continuous or intermittent, is commonly accompanied by pain, and may be aggravated by prolonged standing or walking.

Hematuria may be classified by the stage of urination it predominantly affects. Bleeding at the start of urination—initial hematuria—usually indicates urethral disease; bleeding at the end of urination—terminal hematuria—usually indicates disease of the bladder neck, posterior urethra, or prostate; bleeding throughout urination—total hema-

Confirming hematuria

If the patient's urine appears blood tinged, be sure to rule out pseudohematuria, red or pink urine caused by urinary pigments. First, carefully observe the urine specimen. If it contains red sediment, it's probably true hematuria.

Then check the patient's history for the use of drugs associated with pseudohematuria, including rifampin, chlorzoxazone, phenazopyridine, phenothiazines, doxorubicin, phensuximide, phenytoin, and daunomycin.

Ask about the patient's intake of beets, berries, or foods with red dyes that may color the urine red. Be aware that porphyrinuria and excess urate excretion can also cause pseudohematuria.

Finally, test the urine using a chemical reagent strip. This test can confirm even microscopic hematuria and can also estimate the amount of blood present.

turia—usually indicates disease above the bladder neck.

Hematuria may result from one of two mechanisms: rupture or perforation of vessels in the renal system or urinary tract, or impaired glomerular filtration, which allows RBCs to seep into the urine. The color of the bloody urine provides a clue to the source of the bleeding. Generally, dark or brownish blood indicates renal or upper urinary tract bleeding, whereas bright red blood indicates lower urinary tract bleeding.

Although hematuria usually results from renal and urinary tract disorders, it may also result from certain GI, prostate, vaginal, or coagulation disorders or from the effects of certain drugs. Invasive therapy and diagnostic tests that involve manipulative instrumentation of the renal and urologic systems may also cause hematuria. Nonpathologic hematuria may result from fever and hypercatabolic states. Transient hematuria may follow strenuous exercise.

History and physical examination

After detecting hematuria, take a pertinent health history. If hematuria is macroscopic, ask the patient when he first noticed blood in his urine. Does it vary in severity between voidings? Is it worse at the beginning, middle, or end of urination? Has it occurred before? Is the patient passing clots? To rule out artifactitious hematuria, ask about bleeding hemorrhoids or the onset of menses, if appropriate. Ask if there's pain or burning with hematuria episodes.

Ask about recent abdominal or flank trauma. Has the patient been exercising strenuously? Note a history of renal, urinary, prostatic, or coagulation disorders. Then obtain a drug history, noting anticoagulants or aspirin.

Begin the physical examination by palpating and percussing the abdomen and flanks. Next, percuss the costovertebral angle (CVA) to elicit tenderness. Check the urinary meatus for bleeding or other abnormalities. Using a chemical reagent strip, test a urine specimen for protein. A vaginal or digital rectal examination may be necessary.

Medical causes

Bladder cancer. A primary cause of gross hematuria in men, bladder cancer may also produce pain in the bladder, rectum, pelvis, flank, back, or leg. Other common features are nocturia, dysuria, urinary frequency and urgency, vomiting, diarrhea, and insomnia.

Bladder trauma. Gross hematuria is characteristic in traumatic rupture or perforation of the bladder. Typically, hematuria is accompanied by lower abdominal pain and, occasionally, anuria despite a strong urge to void. The patient may also develop swelling of the scrotum, buttocks, or perineum and signs of shock, such as tachycardia and hypotension.

Calculi. Bladder and *renal calculi* produce hematuria, which may be associated with signs of a urinary tract infection (UTI), such as dysuria and urinary frequency and urgency. Bladder calculi usually cause gross hematuria, referred pain to the lower back or penile or vulvar area and, in some patients, bladder distention.

Renal calculi may produce microscopic or gross hematuria. The cardinal symptom, however, is colicky pain that travels from the CVA to the flank, suprapubic region, and external genitalia when a calculus is passed. The pain may be excruciating at its peak. Other signs and symptoms may include nausea and vomiting, restlessness, a fever, chills, abdominal distention and, possibly, decreased bowel sounds.

Coagulation disorders. Macroscopic hematuria is usually the first sign of hemorrhage in coagulation disorders, such as thrombocytopenia or disseminated intravascular coagulation. Other features include epistaxis, purpura (petechiae and ecchymoses), and signs of GI bleeding.

Cortical necrosis (acute). Accompanying gross hematuria in acute cortical necrosis are intense flank pain, anuria, leukocytosis, and a fever.

Cystitis. Hematuria is a telling sign in all types of cystitis. *Bacterial cystitis* usually produces macroscopic hematuria with urinary urgency and frequency, dysuria, nocturia, and tenesmus. The patient complains of perineal and lumbar pain, suprapubic discomfort, and fatigue and occasionally has a low-grade fever.

More common in women, *chronic interstitial cystitis* occasionally causes grossly bloody hematuria. Associated features include urinary frequency, dysuria, nocturia, and tenesmus. Microscopic and macroscopic hematuria may occur with *tubercular cystitis,* which may also cause urinary urgency and frequency, dysuria, tenesmus, flank pain, fatigue, and anorexia. *Viral cystitis* usually produces hematuria, urinary urgency and frequency, dysuria, nocturia, tenesmus, and a fever.

Diverticulitis. When diverticulitis involves the bladder, it usually causes microscopic hematuria, urinary frequency and urgency, dysuria, and nocturia. Characteristic findings include left lower quadrant pain, abdominal tenderness, constipation or diarrhea and, at times, a palpable, firm, fixed, and tender abdominal mass. The patient may also develop mild nausea, flatulence, and a low-grade fever.

Glomerulonephritis. Acute glomerulonephritis usually begins with gross hematuria that tapers off to microscopic hematuria and red cell casts, which may persist for months. It may also produce oliguria or anuria, proteinuria, a mild fever, fatigue, flank and abdominal pain, generalized edema, increased blood pressure, nausea, vomiting, and signs of lung congestion, such as crackles and a productive cough.

Chronic glomerulonephritis usually causes microscopic hematuria accompanied by proteinuria, generalized edema, and increased blood pressure. Signs and symptoms of uremia may also occur in advanced disease.

Nephritis (interstitial). Typically, nephritis causes microscopic hematuria. However, the patient with acute interstitial nephritis may develop gross hematuria. Other findings are a fever, a maculopapular rash, and oliguria or anuria. In chronic interstitial nephritis, the patient has dilute—almost colorless—urine that may be accompanied by polyuria and increased blood pressure.

Nephropathy (obstructive). Obstructive nephropathy may cause microscopic or macroscopic hematuria, but urine is rarely grossly bloody. The patient may report colicky flank and abdominal pain, CVA tenderness, and anuria or oliguria that alternates with polyuria.

Polycystic kidney disease. Polycystic kidney disease is a hereditary disorder that may cause recurrent microscopic or gross hematuria. Although it commonly produces no symptoms before age 40, it may cause increased blood pressure, polyuria, dull flank pain, and signs of a UTI, such as dysuria and urinary frequency and urgency. Later, the patient develops a swollen, tender abdomen and lumbar pain that's aggravated by exertion and relieved by lying down. He may also have proteinuria and colicky abdominal pain from the ureteral passage of clots or calculi.

Prostatitis. Whether acute or chronic, prostatitis may cause macroscopic hematuria, usually at the end of urination. It may also produce urinary frequency and urgency and dysuria followed by visible bladder distention.

Acute prostatitis also produces fatigue, malaise, myalgia, polyarthralgia, a fever with chills, nausea, vomiting, perineal and low back pain, and a decreased libido. Rectal palpation reveals a tender, swollen, boggy, firm prostate.

Chronic prostatitis commonly follows an acute attack. It may cause persistent urethral discharge, dull perineal pain, ejaculatory pain, and a decreased libido.

Pyelonephritis (acute). Acute pyelonephritis typically produces microscopic or macroscopic hematuria that progresses to grossly bloody hematuria. After the infection resolves, microscopic hematuria may persist for a few months. Related signs and symptoms include a persistent high fever, unilateral or bilateral flank pain, CVA tenderness, shaking chills, weakness, fatigue, dysuria, urinary frequency and urgency, nocturia, and tenesmus. The patient may also exhibit nausea, anorexia, vomiting, and signs of paralytic ileus, such as hypoactive or absent bowel sounds and abdominal distention.

Renal cancer. The classic triad of signs and symptoms of renal cancer includes grossly bloody hematuria; dull, aching flank pain; and a smooth, firm, palpable flank mass. Colicky pain may accompany the passage of clots. Other findings include a fever, CVA tenderness, and increased blood pressure. In advanced disease, the patient may develop weight loss, nausea and vomiting, and leg edema with varicoceles.

Renal infarction. Typically, renal infarction produces gross hematuria. The patient may complain of constant, severe flank and upper abdominal pain accompanied by CVA tenderness, anorexia, and nausea and vomiting. Other findings include oliguria or anuria, proteinuria, hypoactive bowel sounds and, a day or two after infarction, a fever and increased blood pressure.

Renal papillary necrosis (acute). Acute renal papillary necrosis usually produces grossly bloody hematuria, which may be accompanied by intense flank pain, CVA tenderness, abdominal rigidity and colicky pain, oliguria or anuria, pyuria, fever, chills, vomiting, and hypoactive bowel sounds. Arthralgia and hypertension are common.

Renal trauma. About 80% of patients with renal trauma have microscopic or gross hematuria. Accompanying signs and symptoms may include flank pain, a palpable flank mass, oliguria, hematoma or ecchymoses over the upper abdomen or flank, nausea and vomiting, and hypoactive bowel sounds. Severe trauma may precipitate signs of shock, such as tachycardia and hypotension.

Renal tuberculosis. Gross hematuria is commonly the first sign of renal tuberculosis. It may be accompanied by urinary frequency, dysuria, pyuria, tenesmus, colicky abdominal pain, lumbar pain, and proteinuria.

Renal vein thrombosis. Grossly bloody hematuria usually occurs in renal vein thrombosis. In abrupt venous obstruction, the patient experiences severe flank and lumbar pain as well as epigastric and CVA tenderness. Other features include a fever, pallor, proteinuria, peripheral edema and, when the obstruction is bilateral, oliguria or anuria and other uremic signs. The kidneys are easily palpable. Gradual venous obstruction causes signs of nephrotic syndrome, proteinuria and, occasionally, peripheral edema.

Schistosomiasis. Schistosomiasis usually causes intermittent hematuria at the end of urination. It may be accompanied by dysuria, colicky renal and bladder pain, and palpable lower abdominal masses.

Sickle cell anemia. Sickle cell anemia is a hereditary disorder in which gross hematuria may result from congestion of the renal papillae. Associated signs and symptoms may include pallor, dehydration, chronic fatigue, polyarthralgia, leg ulcers, dyspnea, chest pain, impaired growth and development, hepatomegaly and, possibly, jaundice. Auscultation reveals tachycardia and systolic and diastolic murmurs.

Systemic lupus erythematosus (SLE). Gross hematuria and proteinuria may occur when SLE involves the kidneys. Cardinal associated features include nondeforming joint pain and stiffness, a butterfly rash, photosensitivity, Raynaud's phenomenon, seizures or psychoses, a recurrent fever, lymphadenopathy, oral or nasopharyngeal ulcers, anorexia, and weight loss.

Urethral trauma. Initial hematuria may occur, possibly with blood at the urinary meatus, local pain, and penile or vulvar ecchymoses.

Vasculitis. Hematuria is usually microscopic in vasculitis. Associated signs and symptoms include malaise, myalgia, polyarthralgia, a fever, increased blood pressure, pallor and, occasionally, anuria. Other features, such as urticaria and purpura, may reflect the etiology of vasculitis.

Other causes
Diagnostic tests. Renal biopsy is the diagnostic test most commonly associated with hematuria. This sign may also result from biopsy or manipulative instrumentation of the urinary tract such as in cystoscopy.

Drugs. Drugs that commonly cause hematuria are anticoagulants, aspirin (toxicity), analgesics, cyclophosphamide, metyrosine, phenylbutazone, oxyphenbutazone, penicillin, rifampin, and thiabendazole.

Treatments. Any therapy that involves manipulative instrumentation of the urinary tract, such as transurethral prostatectomy, may cause microscopic or macroscopic hematuria. Following a kidney transplant, a patient may experience hematuria with or without clots, which may require indwelling urinary catheter irrigation.

Nursing considerations
- Check vital signs frequently.
- Monitor intake and output, including the amount and pattern of hematuria.
- If the patient has an indwelling urinary catheter in place, ensure its patency and irrigate it if necessary to remove clots and tissue that may impede urine drainage.
- Administer prescribed analgesics, and enforce bed rest as indicated.

- Prepare the patient for diagnostic tests, such as blood and urine studies, cystoscopy, and renal X-rays or biopsy.
- Monitor hemoglobin level and hematocrit; administer blood products as ordered.

Patient teaching
- Show the patient how to collect urine specimens.
- Emphasize the need to increase fluid intake.
- Explain the underlying cause of hematuria and its treatment.

Hemianopsia

Hemianopsia is a loss of vision in one-half of the normal visual field (usually the right or left half) of one or both eyes. However, if the visual field defects are identical in both eyes but affect less than one-half of the field of vision in each eye (incomplete homonymous hemianopsia), the lesion may be in the occipital lobe; otherwise, it probably involves the parietal or temporal lobe. (See *Recognizing types of hemianopsia,* page 320.)

Hemianopsia is caused by a lesion affecting the optic chiasm, tract, or radiation. Defects in visual perception due to cerebral lesions are usually associated with impaired color vision.

History and physical examination
Suspect a visual field defect if the patient seems startled when you approach him from one side or if he fails to see objects placed directly in front of him. To help determine the type of defect, compare the patient's visual fields with your own—assuming that yours are normal. First, ask the patient to cover his right eye while you cover your left eye. Then move a pen or similarly shaped object from the periphery of his

Recognizing types of hemianopsia

Lesions of the optic pathways cause visual field defects. The lesion's site determines the type of defect. For example, a lesion of the optic chiasm involving only those fibers that cross over to the opposite side causes bitemporal hemianopsia—vision loss in the temporal half of each field. However, a lesion of the optic tract or a complete lesion of the optic radiation produces vision loss in the same half of each field—either left or right homonymous hemianopsia.

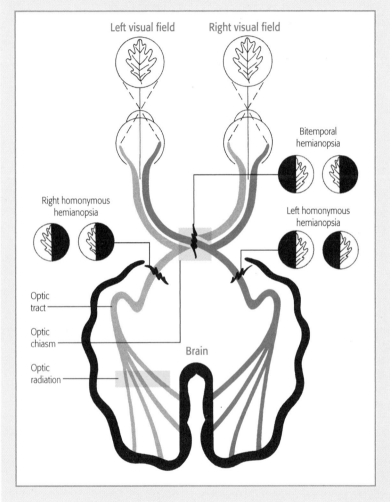

(and your) uncovered eye into his field of vision. Ask the patient to indicate when he first sees the object. Does he see it at the same time you do? After you do? Repeat this test in each quadrant of both eyes. Then, for each eye, plot the defect by shading the area of a circle that corresponds to the area of vision loss.

Next, evaluate the patient's level of consciousness (LOC), take his vital signs, and check his pupillary reaction and motor response. Ask if he has recently experienced a headache, dysarthria, or seizures. Does he have ptosis or facial or extremity weakness? Hallucinations or loss of color vision? When did neurologic symptoms start? Obtain a medical history, noting especially eye disorders, hypertension, diabetes mellitus, and recent head trauma.

Medical causes

Carotid artery aneurysm. An aneurysm in the internal carotid artery can cause contralateral or bilateral defects in the visual fields. It can also cause hemiplegia, a decreased LOC, a headache, aphasia, behavior disturbances, and unilateral hypoesthesia.

Occipital lobe lesion. The most common symptoms arising from a lesion of one occipital lobe are incomplete homonymous hemianopsia, scotomas, and impaired color vision. The patient may also experience visual hallucinations—flashes of light or color or visions of objects, people, animals, or geometric forms. These may appear in the defective field or may move toward it from the intact field.

Parietal lobe lesion. Parietal lobe lesion produces homonymous hemianopsia and sensory deficits, such as an inability to perceive body position or passive movement or to localize tactile, thermal, or vibratory stimuli. It may also cause apraxia and visual or tactile agnosia.

Pituitary tumor. A tumor that compresses nerve fibers supplying the nasal half of both retinas causes complete or partial bitemporal hemianopsia that first occurs in the upper visual fields but later can progress to blindness. Related findings include blurred vision, diplopia, a headache and, rarely, somnolence, hypothermia, and seizures.

Stroke. Hemianopsia can result when a hemorrhagic, thrombotic, or embolic stroke affects part of the optic pathway. Associated signs and symptoms vary according to the location and size of the stroke, but may include a decreased LOC; intellectual deficits, such as memory loss and poor judgment; personality changes; emotional lability; a headache; and seizures. The patient may also develop contralateral hemiplegia, dysarthria, dysphagia, ataxia, a unilateral sensory loss, apraxia, agnosia, aphasia, blurred vision, decreased visual acuity, and diplopia. He may also experience urine retention or incontinence, constipation, and vomiting.

Nursing considerations
- If the patient's visual field defect is significant, prepare him for further testing, such as perimetry or a tangent screen examination.
- To avoid startling the patient, approach him from the unaffected side and position his bed so that his unaffected side faces the door.
- If he's ambulatory, remove objects that could cause falls and alert him to other possible hazards.
- Place his clock and other personal objects within his field of vision, and avoid putting dangerous objects (such as hot dishes) where he can't see them.

Patient teaching
- Explain the extent of the defect to the patient so that he can learn to compensate for it.
- Advise him to scan his surroundings frequently, turning his head in the direction of the defective visual field.
- Discuss safety measures that may be needed.

Identifying hemoptysis

These guidelines will help you distinguish hemoptysis from epistaxis, hematemesis, and brown, red, or pink sputum.

Hemoptysis
Typically frothy because it's mixed with air, hemoptysis is commonly bright red with an alkaline pH (tested with nitrazine paper). It's strongly suggested by the presence of respiratory signs and symptoms, including a cough, a tickling sensation in the throat, and blood produced from repeated coughing episodes. (You can rule out epistaxis because the patient's nasal passages and posterior pharynx are usually clear.)

Hematemesis
The usual site of hematemesis is the GI tract; the patient vomits or regurgitates coffee-ground material that contains food particles, tests positive for occult blood, and has an acid pH. However, he may vomit bright red blood or swallowed blood from the oral cavity and nasopharynx. After an episode of hematemesis, the patient may have stools with traces of blood and may also complain of dyspepsia.

Brown, red, or pink sputum
Brown, red, or pink sputum can result from oxidation of inhaled bronchodilators. Sputum that looks like old blood may result from rupture of an amebic abscess into the bronchus. Red or brown sputum may occur in a patient with pneumonia caused by the enterobacterium *Serratia marcescens*.

Hemoptysis

Frightening to the patient and commonly ominous, hemoptysis is the expectoration of blood or bloody sputum from the lungs or tracheobronchial tree. It's sometimes confused with bleeding from the mouth, throat, nasopharynx, or GI tract. (See *Identifying hemoptysis*.) Expectoration of 200 ml of blood in a single episode suggests severe bleeding, whereas expectoration of 400 ml in 3 hours or more than 600 ml in 16 hours signals a life-threatening crisis.

Hemoptysis usually results from chronic bronchitis, lung cancer, or bronchiectasis. However, it may also result from inflammatory, infectious, cardiovascular, or coagulation disorders and, rarely, from a ruptured aortic aneurysm. In up to 15% of patients, the cause is unknown. The most common causes of *massive hemoptysis* are lung cancer, bronchiectasis, active tuberculosis (TB), and cavitary pulmonary disease from necrotic infections or TB.

Several pathophysiologic processes can cause hemoptysis. (See *What happens in hemoptysis.*)

ACTION STAT!

If the patient coughs up copious amounts of blood, endotracheal intubation may be required. Suction frequently to remove blood. Lavage may be necessary to loosen tenacious secretions or clots. Massive hemoptysis can cause airway obstruction and asphyxiation. Insert an I.V. catheter to allow fluid replacement, drug administration, and blood transfusions, if needed. An emergency bronchoscopy should be performed to identify the bleeding site. Monitor the patient's blood pressure and pulse to detect hypotension and tachycardia, and draw an arterial blood sample for laboratory analysis to monitor respiratory status.

History and physical examination

If hemoptysis is mild, ask the patient when it began. Has he ever coughed up blood before? About how much blood is he coughing up now and about how often? Ask about a history of cardiac, pulmonary, or bleeding disorders. If he's receiving anticoagulant therapy, find out the drug, its dosage and schedule, and the duration of therapy. Is he taking other prescription drugs? Does he smoke? Ask the patient if he has had a recent infection. Has he been exposed to TB? When was his last tine test and what were the results?

Take the patient's vital signs and examine his nose, mouth, and pharynx for sources of bleeding. Inspect the configuration of his chest and look for abnormal movement during breathing, the use of accessory muscles, and retractions. Observe his respiratory rate, depth, and rhythm. Finally, examine his skin for lesions.

Next, palpate the patient's chest for diaphragm level and for tenderness, respiratory excursion, fremitus, and abnormal pulsations; then percuss for flatness, dullness, resonance, hyperresonance, and tympany. Finally, auscultate the lungs, noting especially the quality and intensity of breath sounds. Also auscultate for heart murmurs, bruits, and pleural friction rubs.

Obtain a sputum specimen and examine it for overall quantity, for the amount of blood it contains, and for its color, odor, and consistency.

Medical causes

Blast lung injury. Although individuals with blast lung injury may not have obvious external chest injuries, they sometimes show other indications of internal damage, such as hemoptysis. Health care providers should evaluate survivors of explosive detonations for

What happens in hemoptysis

Hemoptysis results from bleeding into the respiratory tract by bronchial or pulmonary vessels. Bleeding reflects alterations in the vascular walls and in blood-clotting mechanisms. It can result from any of these pathophysiologic processes:

■ hemorrhage and diapedesis of red blood cells from the pulmonary microvasculature into the alveoli
■ necrosis of lung tissue that causes inflammation and rupture of blood vessels or hemorrhage into the alveolar spaces
■ rupture of an aortic aneurysm into the tracheobronchial tree
■ rupture of distended endobronchial blood vessels from pulmonary hypertension due to mitral stenosis
■ rupture of a pulmonary arteriovenous fistula or of bronchial or pulmonary artery or pulmonary venous collateral channels
■ sloughing of a caseous lesion into the tracheobronchial tree
■ ulceration and erosion of the bronchial epithelium.

other classic signs and symptoms of a blast lung injury, such as chest pain, cyanosis, dyspnea, and wheezing. Treatment includes careful administration of fluids and oxygen to ensure tissue perfusion.

Bronchial adenoma. Bronchial adenoma is an insidious disorder that causes recurring hemoptysis in up to 30% of patients, along with a chronic cough and local wheezing.

Bronchiectasis. Inflamed bronchial surfaces and eroded bronchial blood vessels cause hemoptysis, which can vary from blood-tinged sputum to blood (in about 20% of cases). The patient's sputum may also be copious, foul-smelling, and purulent. He may exhibit a chronic cough, coarse crackles, clubbing (a late sign), a fever, weight loss, fatigue, weakness, malaise, and dyspnea on exertion.

Bronchitis (chronic). The first sign of chronic bronchitis is typically a productive cough that lasts at least 3 months. Eventually this leads to the production of blood-streaked sputum; massive hemorrhage is unusual. Other respiratory effects include dyspnea, prolonged expirations, wheezing, scattered rhonchi, accessory muscle use, barrel chest, tachypnea, and clubbing (a late sign).

Coagulation disorders. Such disorders as thrombocytopenia and disseminated intravascular coagulation can cause hemoptysis. Besides their specific related findings, these disorders may share such general signs as multisystem hemorrhaging (for example, GI bleeding or epistaxis) and purpuric lesions.

Lung abscess. In about 50% of patients, lung abscess produces blood-streaked sputum resulting from bronchial ulceration, necrosis, and granulation tissue. Common associated findings include a cough with large amounts of purulent, foul-smelling sputum; a fever with chills; diaphoresis; anorexia; weight loss; a headache; weakness; dyspnea; pleuritic or dull chest pain; and clubbing. Auscultation reveals tubular or cavernous breath sounds and crackles. Percussion reveals dullness on the affected side.

Lung cancer. Ulceration of the bronchus commonly causes recurring hemoptysis (an early sign), which can vary from blood-streaked sputum to blood. Related findings include a productive cough, dyspnea, a fever, anorexia, weight loss, wheezing, and chest pain (a late symptom).

Plague (Yersinia pestis). The pneumonic form of this acute bacterial infection can produce hemoptysis, a productive cough, chest pain, tachypnea, dyspnea, increasing respiratory distress, and cardiopulmonary insufficiency, along with the sudden onset of chills, a fever, a headache, and myalgia.

Pneumonia. In up to 50% of cases, *Klebsiella* pneumonia produces dark brown or red (currant jelly) sputum, which is so tenacious that the patient has difficulty expelling it from his mouth. This type of pneumonia begins abruptly with chills, a fever, dyspnea, a productive cough, and severe pleuritic chest pain. Associated findings may include cyanosis, prostration, tachycardia, decreased breath sounds, and crackles.

Pneumococcal pneumonia causes pinkish or rusty mucoid sputum. It begins with sudden, shaking chills; a rapidly rising temperature; and, in over 80% of cases, tachycardia and tachypnea. Within a few hours, the patient typically experiences a productive cough along with severe, stabbing, pleuritic pain. The agonizing chest pain leads to rapid, shallow, grunting respirations with splinting. Examination reveals respiratory distress with dyspnea and accessory muscle use, crackles, and dullness on percussion over the affected lung. Malaise, weakness, myalgia, and prostration accompany a high fever.

Pulmonary edema. Severe cardiogenic or noncardiogenic pulmonary edema commonly causes frothy, blood-tinged pink sputum, which accompanies severe dyspnea, orthopnea, gasping, anxiety, cyanosis, diffuse crackles, a ventricular gallop, and cold, clammy skin. This life-threatening condition may also cause tachycardia, lethargy, cardiac arrhythmias, tachypnea, hypotension, and a thready pulse.

Pulmonary embolism with infarction. Hemoptysis is a common finding in pulmonary embolism with infarction, a life-threatening disorder, although massive hemoptysis is infrequent. Typical initial symptoms are dyspnea and anginal or pleuritic chest pain. Other common clinical features include tachycardia, tachypnea, a low-grade fever, and diaphoresis. Less commonly, splinting of the chest, leg edema, and—with a large embolus—cyanosis, syncope, and jugular vein distention may occur. Examination reveals decreased breath sounds, a pleural friction rub, crackles, diffuse wheezing, dullness on percussion, and signs of circulatory collapse (a weak, rapid pulse; hypotension), cerebral ischemia (transient loss of consciousness, seizures), and hypoxemia (restlessness and, particularly in elderly patients, hemiplegia and other focal neurologic deficits).

Pulmonary hypertension (primary). With pulmonary hyperension, features generally develop late. Hemoptysis, exertional dyspnea, and fatigue are common. Angina-like pain usually occurs with exertion and may radiate to the neck but not to the arms. Other findings include arrhythmias, syncope, a cough, and hoarseness.

Pulmonary TB. Blood-streaked or blood-tinged sputum commonly occurs in pulmonary TB; massive hemoptysis may occur in advanced cavitary TB. Accompanying respiratory findings include a chronic productive cough, fine crackles after coughing, dyspnea, dullness on percussion, increased tactile fremitus, and possible amphoric breath sounds. The patient may also develop night sweats, malaise, fatigue, a fever, anorexia, weight loss, and pleuritic chest pain.

Systemic lupus erythematosus (SLE). In 50% of patients with SLE, pleuritis and pneumonitis cause hemoptysis, a cough, dyspnea, pleuritic chest pain, and crackles. Related findings are a butterfly rash in the acute phase, nondeforming joint pain and stiffness, photosensitivity, Raynaud's phenomenon,

seizures or psychoses, anorexia with weight loss, and lymphadenopathy.

Tracheal trauma. Torn tracheal mucosa may cause hemoptysis, hoarseness, dysphagia, neck pain, airway occlusion, and respiratory distress.

Other causes

Diagnostic tests. Lung or airway injury from bronchoscopy, laryngoscopy, mediastinoscopy, or lung biopsy can cause bleeding and hemoptysis.

Nursing considerations

- If necessary, to protect the nonbleeding lung, place the patient in the lateral decubitus position, with the suspected bleeding lung facing down.
- Perform this maneuver with caution because hypoxemia may worsen with the healthy lung facing up.
- Prepare the patient for diagnostic tests to determine the cause of bleeding, such as a complete blood count, a sputum culture and smear, chest X-rays, coagulation studies, bronchoscopy, lung biopsy, pulmonary arteriography, and a lung scan.

Patient teaching

- Give the patient instructions for providing sputum specimens.
- Explain the underlying cause of hemoptysis and its treatment.
- Explain the importance of reporting recurrent episodes.

▌Hepatomegaly

Hepatomegaly, an enlarged liver, indicates potentially reversible primary or secondary liver disease. This sign may stem from diverse pathophysiologic mechanisms, including dilated hepatic sinusoids (in heart failure), persistently high venous pressure leading to liver congestion (in chronic constrictive pericarditis), dysfunction and engorgement

Percussing for liver size and position

With the patient in a supine position, begin at the right iliac crest to percuss up the right midclavicular line (MCL), as shown below. The percussion note becomes dull when you reach the liver's inferior border—usually at the costal margin, but sometimes at a lower point in the patient with liver disease. Mark this point and then percuss down from the right clavicle, again along the right MCL. The liver's superior border usually lies between the fifth and seventh intercostal spaces. Mark the superior border.

The distance between the two marked points represents the approximate span of the liver's right lobe, which normally ranges from 2¼″ to 4¾″ (6 to 12 cm).

Next, assess the liver's left lobe similarly, percussing along the sternal midline. Again, mark the points where you hear dull percussion notes. Also, measure the span of the left lobe, which normally ranges from 1½″ to 3⅛″ (4 to 8 cm). Record your findings for use as a baseline.

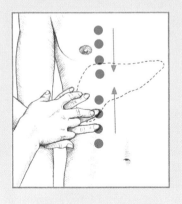

of hepatocytes (in hepatitis), fatty infiltration of parenchymal cells causing fibrous tissue (in cirrhosis), distention of liver cells with glycogen (in diabetes), and infiltration of amyloid (in amyloidosis).

Hepatomegaly may be confirmed by palpation, percussion, or radiologic tests. It may be mistaken for displacement of the liver by the diaphragm, in a respiratory disorder; by an abdominal tumor; by a spinal deformity, such as kyphosis; by the gallbladder; or by fecal material or a tumor in the colon.

History and physical examination

Hepatomegaly is seldom a patient's chief complaint. It usually comes to light during palpation and percussion of the abdomen.

If you suspect hepatomegaly, ask the patient about his use of alcohol and exposure to hepatitis. Also ask if he's currently ill or taking any prescribed drugs. If he complains of abdominal pain, ask him to locate and describe it.

Inspect the patient's skin and sclera for jaundice, dilated veins (suggesting generalized congestion), scars from previous surgery, and spider angiomas (commonly occurring in cirrhosis). Next, inspect the contour of his abdomen. Is it protuberant over the liver or distended (possibly from ascites)? Measure his abdominal girth.

Percuss the liver, but be careful to identify structures and conditions that can obscure dull percussion notes, such as the sternum, ribs, breast tissue, pleural effusions, and gas in the colon. (See *Percussing for liver size and position.*) Next, during deep inspiration, palpate the liver's edge; it's tender and rounded in hepatitis and cardiac decompensation, rocklike in carcinoma, and firm in cirrhosis.

Take the patient's baseline vital signs, and assess his nutritional status. An enlarged liver that's functioning poorly causes muscle wasting, exaggerated skeletal prominences, weight loss, thin hair, and edema.

Evaluate the patient's level of consciousness. When an enlarged liver loses its ability to detoxify waste products, the result is accumulation of metabolic substances toxic to brain cells. As a result, watch for personality changes, irritability, agitation, memory loss, an inability to concentrate and poor mentation, and—in a severely ill patient—decreased level of consciousness.

Medical causes

Amyloidosis. Amyloidosis is a rare disorder that may cause hepatomegaly and mild jaundice as well as renal, cardiac, and other GI effects.

Cirrhosis. Late in cirrhosis, the liver becomes enlarged, nodular, and hard. Other late signs and symptoms affect all body systems. Respiratory findings include limited thoracic expansion due to abdominal ascites, leading to hypoxia. Central nervous system findings include signs and symptoms of hepatic encephalopathy, such as lethargy, slurred speech, asterixis, peripheral neuritis, paranoia, hallucinations, extreme obtundation, and coma. Hematologic signs include epistaxis, easy bruising, and bleeding gums. Endocrine findings include testicular atrophy, gynecomastia, loss of chest and axillary hair, or menstrual irregularities. Integumentary effects include abnormal pigmentation, jaundice, severe pruritus, extreme dryness, poor tissue turgor, spider angiomas, and palmar erythema.

The patient may also develop fetor hepaticus, enlarged superficial abdominal veins, muscle atrophy, right upper quadrant pain that worsens when he sits up or leans forward, and a palpable spleen. Portal hypertension—elevated pressure in the portal vein—causes bleeding from esophageal varices.

Diabetes mellitus. Poorly controlled diabetes in overweight patients commonly produces fatty infiltration of the liver, hepatomegaly, and right upper quadrant tenderness along with polydipsia, polyphagia, and polyuria. These features are more common in type 2 than in type 1 diabetes. A chronically enlarged fatty liver typically produces no symptoms except for slight tenderness.

Granulomatous disorders. Sarcoidosis, histoplasmosis, and other such disorders commonly produce a slightly enlarged, firm liver.

Hepatic abscess. Hepatomegaly may accompany a fever (a primary sign), nausea, vomiting, chills, weakness, diarrhea, anorexia, an elevated right hemidiaphragm, and right upper quadrant pain and tenderness.

Hepatitis. In viral hepatitis, early signs and symptoms include nausea, anorexia, vomiting, fatigue, malaise, photophobia, a sore throat, a cough, and a headache. Hepatomegaly occurs in the icteric phase and continues during the recovery phase. Also, during the icteric phase, the early signs and symptoms diminish and others appear: liver tenderness, slight weight loss, dark urine, clay-colored stools, jaundice, pruritus, right upper quadrant pain, and splenomegaly.

Leukemia and lymphomas. Leukemia and lymphomas are proliferative blood cell disorders that typically cause moderate to massive hepatomegaly and splenomegaly as well as abdominal discomfort. General signs and symptoms include malaise, a low-grade fever, fatigue, weakness, tachycardia, weight loss, bleeding disorders, and anorexia.

Liver cancer. Primary liver tumors commonly cause irregular, nodular, firm hepatomegaly, with pain or tenderness in the right upper quadrant and a friction rub or bruit over the liver. Common related findings are weight loss, anorexia, cachexia, nausea, and vomiting. Peripheral edema, ascites, jaundice, and a palpable right upper quadrant mass may also develop. When metastatic liver tumors cause hepatomegaly, the patient's accompanying signs and symptoms reflect his primary cancer.

Mononucleosis (infectious). Occasionally, infectious mononucleosis causes hepatomegaly. Prodromal symptoms include a headache, malaise, and fatigue. After 3 to 5 days, the patient typically develops a sore throat, cervical lymphadenopathy, and temperature fluctuations. He may also develop stomatitis, palatal petechiae, periorbital edema, splenomegaly, exudative tonsillitis, pharyngitis and, possibly, a maculopapular rash.

Obesity. Hepatomegaly can result from fatty infiltration of the liver. Weight loss reduces the liver's size.

Pancreatic cancer. In pancreatic cancer, hepatomegaly accompanies such classic signs and symptoms as anorexia, weight loss, abdominal or back pain, and jaundice. Other findings include nausea, vomiting, a fever, fatigue, weakness, pruritus, and skin lesions (usually on the legs).

Pericarditis. In chronic constrictive pericarditis, an increase in systemic venous pressure produces marked congestive hepatomegaly. Distended jugular veins (more prominent on inspiration) are a common finding. The usual signs of cardiac disease typically are absent; other features include peripheral edema, ascites, fatigue, and decreased muscle mass.

Nursing considerations

- Prepare the patient for liver enzyme, alkaline phosphatase, bilirubin, albumin, and globulin studies to evaluate liver function and for X-rays, a liver scan, celiac arteriography, a computed tomography scan, and ultrasonography to confirm hepatomegaly.
- Provide bed rest, relief from stress, and adequate nutrition to help protect liver cells from further damage and to allow the liver to regenerate functioning cells.
- Monitor and restrict dietary protein as needed.
- Give hepatotoxic drugs or drugs metabolized by the liver in very small doses, if at all.

Patient teaching

- Explain the underlying disorder and its treatments.
- Stress the importance of avoiding alcohol and people with infections.
- Discuss the importance of pacing activities and rest periods.

Hoarseness

Hoarseness—a rough or harsh sound to the voice—can result from infections, inflammatory lesions, or exudates of the larynx; laryngeal edema; and compression or disruption of the vocal cords or recurrent laryngeal nerve. This common sign can also result from a thoracic aortic aneurysm, vocal cord paralysis, and systemic disorders such as rheumatoid arthritis. It's characteristically worsened by excessive alcohol intake, smoking, inhaling noxious fumes, excessive talking, and shouting.

Hoarseness can be acute or chronic. For example, chronic hoarseness and laryngitis result when irritating polyps or nodules develop on the vocal cords. Gastroesophageal reflux into the larynx should also be considered as a possible cause of chronic hoarseness. Hoarseness may also result from progressive atrophy of the laryngeal muscles and mucosa due to aging, which leads to diminished control of the vocal cords.

History and physical examination

Obtain a patient history. First, consider his age and sex; laryngeal cancer is most common in men between ages 50 and 70. Be sure to ask about the onset of hoarseness. Has the patient been overusing his voice? Has he experienced shortness of breath, a sore throat, a dry mouth, a cough, or difficulty swallowing dry food? In addition, ask if he has been in or near a fire within the past 48 hours. Be aware that an inhalation injury can cause sudden airway obstruction.

Next, explore associated symptoms. Does the patient have a history of cancer, rheumatoid arthritis, or aortic aneurysm? Does he regularly drink alcohol or smoke?

Inspect the oral cavity and pharynx for redness or exudate, possibly indicating an upper respiratory infection. Palpate the neck for masses and the cervical lymph nodes and thyroid for enlargement. Palpate the trachea—is it midline? Ask the patient to stick out his tongue; if he can't, he may have paralysis from cranial nerve involvement. Examine the eyes for corneal ulcers and enlarged lacrimal ducts (signs of Sjögren's syndrome). Dilated jugular and chest veins may indicate compression by an aortic aneurysm.

Take the patient's vital signs, noting especially a fever and bradycardia. Inspect for asymmetrical chest expansion or signs of respiratory distress—nasal flaring, stridor, and intercostal retractions. Then auscultate for crackles, rhonchi, wheezing, and tubular sounds, and percuss for dullness.

Medical causes

Gastroesophageal reflux. With gastroesophageal reflux, retrograde flow of gastric juices into the esophagus may then spill into the hypopharynx. This, in turn, irritates the larynx, resulting in hoarseness as well as a sore throat, a cough, throat clearing, and a sensation of a lump in the throat. The arytenoids and the vocal cords may appear red and swollen.

Hypothyroidism. With hypothyroidism, hoarseness may be an early sign. Others include fatigue, cold intolerance, weight gain despite anorexia, and menorrhagia.

Laryngeal cancer. Hoarseness is an early sign of vocal cord cancer, but may not occur until later in cancer of other laryngeal areas. The patient usually has a long history of smoking. Other common findings include a mild, dry cough; minor throat discomfort; otalgia; and, sometimes, hemoptysis.

Laryngeal leukoplakia. Leukoplakia is a common cause of hoarseness, especially in smokers. Histologic examination from direct laryngoscopy usually reveals mild, moderate, or severe dysphagia.

Laryngitis. Persistent hoarseness may be the only sign of chronic laryngitis. With acute laryngitis, hoarseness or a complete loss of voice develops suddenly. Related findings include pain (especially during swallowing or speaking), a cough, a fever, profuse diaphoresis, a sore throat, and rhinorrhea.

Rheumatoid arthritis. Hoarseness may signal laryngeal involvement in reumatoid arthritis. Other findings include pain, dysphagia, a sensation of fullness or tension in the throat, dyspnea on exertion, and stridor.

Thoracic aortic aneurysm. Thoracic aortic aneurysm typically produces no symptoms, but may cause hoarseness. Its most common symptom is penetrating pain that's especially severe when the patient is supine. Other clinical features include a brassy cough; dyspnea; wheezing; a substernal aching in the shoulders, lower back, or abdomen; a tracheal tug; facial and neck edema; jugular vein distention; dysphagia; prominent chest veins; stridor; and, possibly, paresthesia or neuralgia.

Tracheal trauma. Torn tracheal mucosa may cause hoarseness, hemoptysis, dysphagia, neck pain, airway occlusion, and respiratory distress.

Vocal cord paralysis. Unilateral vocal cord paralysis causes hoarseness and vocal weakness. Paralysis may accompany signs of trauma, such as pain and swelling of the head and neck.

Vocal cord polyps or nodules. Raspy hoarseness, the chief complaint, accompanies a chronic cough and a crackling voice.

Other causes

Inhalation injury. Inhalation injury from a fire or explosion produces hoarseness and coughing, singed nasal hairs, orofacial burns, and soot-stained sputum. Subsequent signs and symptoms include crackles, rhonchi, and wheezing, which rapidly deteriorate to respiratory distress.

Treatments. Occasionally, surgical trauma to the recurrent laryngeal nerve results in temporary or permanent unilateral vocal cord paralysis, leading to hoarseness. Prolonged intubation may cause temporary hoarseness.

Nursing considerations

■ Observe the patient for stridor, which may indicate bilateral vocal cord paralysis.
■ When hoarseness lasts for longer than 2 weeks, indirect or fiber-optic laryngoscopy is indicated to observe the larynx at rest and during phonation.

Patient teaching

■ Explain the importance of resting the voice.
■ Teach the patient alternative ways to communicate.

■ Stress the importance of avoiding alcohol, smoking, and second-hand smoke.

Homans' sign

Homans' sign is deep calf pain resulting from strong and abrupt dorsiflexion of the ankle. This pain results from venous thrombosis or inflammation of the calf muscles. However, because Homans' sign appears in only 35% of patients with these conditions, it's an unreliable indicator. (See *Eliciting Homans' sign.*) Even when accurate, Homans' sign doesn't indicate the extent of the venous disorder.

This elicited sign may be confused with continuous calf pain, which can result from strains, contusions, cellulitis, or arterial occlusion or with pain in the posterior ankle or Achilles tendon (for example, in a woman with Achilles tendons shortened from wearing high heels).

History and physical examination

When you detect Homans' sign, focus the patient history on signs and symptoms that can accompany deep vein thrombosis (DVT) or thrombophlebitis. These include throbbing, aching, heavy, or tight sensations in the calf as well as leg pain during or after exercise or routine activity. Also, ask about shortness of breath or chest pain, which may indicate pulmonary embolism. Be sure to ask about predisposing events, such as a leg injury, recent surgery, childbirth, use of hormonal contraceptives, associated diseases (cancer, nephrosis, hypercoagulable states), and prolonged inactivity or bed rest.

Next, inspect and palpate the patient's calf for warmth, tenderness, redness, swelling, and the presence of a palpable vein. If you strongly suspect DVT, elicit Homans' sign very carefully to

Eliciting Homans' sign

To elicit Homans' sign, first support the patient's thigh with one hand and his foot with the other. Bend his leg slightly at the knee, and then firmly and abruptly dorsiflex the ankle. Resulting deep calf pain indicates Homans' sign. (The patient may also resist ankle dorsiflexion or flex the knee involuntarily if Homans' sign is positive.)

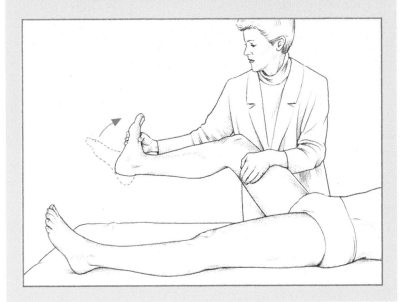

avoid dislodging the clot, which could cause pulmonary embolism, a life-threatening condition.

In addition, measure the circumferences of both the patient's calves. The calf with the positive Homans' sign may be larger because of edema and swelling.

Medical causes

Cellulitis (superficial). Superficial cellulitis typically affects the legs, but can also affect the arms, producing pain, redness, tenderness, and edema. Some patients also experience a fever, chills, tachycardia, a headache, and hypotension.

Deep vein thrombophlebitis. Homans' sign and calf tenderness may be the only clinical features of deep vein thrombophlebitis. However, the patient may also have severe pain, heaviness, warmth, and swelling of the affected leg; visible, engorged superficial veins or palpable, cordlike veins; and a fever, chills, and malaise.

DVT. DVT causes Homans' sign along with tenderness over the deep calf veins, slight edema of the calves and thighs, a low-grade fever, and tachycardia. If DVT affects the femoral and iliac veins, you'll notice marked local swelling and tenderness. If DVT causes venous obstruction, you'll notice cyanosis and possibly cool skin in the affected leg.

Popliteal cyst (ruptured). Rupture of this synovial cyst may produce Homans' sign as well as a sudden onset of calf tenderness, swelling, and redness.

DO'S & DON'TS

 Managing the patient with DVT

Deep vein thrombosis (DVT) occurs when a blood clot, or thrombus, occludes a vein and blocks blood flow. Most thrombi develop in the deep veins of the legs, but they can also develop in the veins of the pelvis, kidneys, liver, right side of the heart, and arms. DVT can lead to severe venous obstruction and injury, depending on thrombus size and collateral circulation.

Do's
- Administer anticoagulants as ordered.
- Place warm soaks over the affected area.
- Assess the patient's circulatory status, noting the quality of pulses in the affected limb.
- Monitor coagulation times if the patient is receiving anticoagulants.
- Watch for signs and symptoms of bleeding.
- Apply antiembolism stockings, as ordered.
- Be alert for signs and symptoms of pulmonary emboli.

Don'ts
- Depending on the severity of the thrombosis, the health care provider may restrict activity to bed rest.
- Avoid placing the affected arm or leg in a dependent position; keep it elevated on pillows above the level of the heart.
- Don't rub or massage the affected extremity.
- Avoid I.M. injections in the patient receiving an anticoagulant and tell him to avoid contact sports.
- Tell the patient not to take any new drugs without checking with his health care provider.

Nursing considerations
- Prepare the patient for a Doppler study of the lower extremities to assess blood flow and identify occlusions.
- Administer mild oral analgesics. (See *Managing the patient with DVT*.)
- Prepare the patient for further diagnostic tests, such as Doppler studies and venograms.
- Evaluate and monitor the affected leg for temperature and pulses.

Patient teaching
- Explain the use of elastic support stockings.
- Instruct the patient to keep the affected leg elevated while sitting and to avoid crossing his legs at the knees to prevent impairing circulation to the popliteal area.

- Explain the signs and symptoms of prolonged clotting times the patient should report.
- Stress the importance of follow-up appointments.
- Emphasize the importance of avoiding alcohol.
- Explain necessary dietary restrictions.
- Explain the drugs the patient needs to take.

Hyperpnea

Hyperpnea indicates increased respiratory effort for a sustained period—a normal rate (at least 12 breaths/minute) with increased depth (a tidal volume greater than 7.5 ml/kg), an increased rate (more than 20 breaths/minute) with normal depth, or increased rate and depth. This sign differs from sighing (intermittent deep inspirations) and may be associated with tachypnea (increased respiratory frequency).

The typical patient with hyperpnea breathes at a normal or increased rate and inhales deeply, displaying marked chest expansion. He may complain of shortness of breath if a respiratory disorder is causing hypoxemia, or he may not be aware of his breathing if a metabolic, psychiatric, or neurologic disorder is causing involuntary hyperpnea. Other causes of hyperpnea include profuse diarrhea or dehydration, loss of pancreatic juice or bile from GI drainage, and ureterosigmoidostomy. All these conditions and procedures cause a loss of bicarbonate ions, resulting in metabolic acidosis. Of course, hyperpnea may also accompany strenuous exercise, and voluntary hyperpnea can promote relaxation in the patient experiencing stress or pain—for example, a woman in labor.

Hyperventilation, a consequence of hyperpnea, is characterized by alkalosis (arterial pH above 7.45 and partial pressure of arterial carbon dioxide below 35 mm Hg). In central neurogenic hyperventilation, brain stem dysfunction (such as results from a severe cranial injury) increases the rate and depth of respirations. In acute intermittent hyperventilation, the respiratory pattern may be a response to hypoxemia, anxiety, fear, pain, or excitement. Hyperpnea may also be a compensatory mechanism to metabolic acidosis. Under these conditions, it's known as *Kussmaul's respirations*. (See *Kussmaul's respirations: A compensatory mechanism*.)

History and physical examination

If you observe hyperpnea in a patient whose other signs and symptoms signal a life-threatening emergency, you must intervene quickly and effectively. (See *Managing hyperpnea,* page 334.) Howev-

Kussmaul's respirations: A compensatory mechanism

Kussmaul's respirations—fast, deep breathing without pauses—characteristically sound labored, with deep breaths that resemble sighs. This breathing pattern develops when respiratory centers in the medulla detect decreased blood pH, thereby triggering compensatory fast and deep breathing to remove excess carbon dioxide and restore pH balance.

> Disorders (such as diabetes mellitus and renal failure), drug effects, and other conditions cause metabolic acidosis (loss of bicarbonate ions and retention of acid).

▼

> Blood pH decreases.

▼

> Kussmaul's respirations develop to blow off excess carbon dioxide.

▼

> Blood pH rises.

▼

> Respiratory rate and depth decrease (corrected pH) in effective compensation.

er, if the patient's condition isn't grave, first determine his level of consciousness (LOC). If he's alert (and if his hyperpnea isn't interfering with speaking), ask about recent illnesses or infections, ingestion of aspirin, and ingestion or inhalation of other drugs or chemicals. Find out if the patient has diabetes mellitus, renal disease, or pulmonary condition. Is he excessively thirsty or hungry? Has he recently had severe diarrhea or an upper respiratory tract infection?

ACTION STAT!

 # Managing hyperpnea

Carefully examine the patient with hyperpnea for related signs of life-threatening conditions, such as increased intracranial pressure (ICP), metabolic acidosis, diabetic ketoacidosis, and uremia.

Increased ICP

If you observe hyperpnea in a patient who has signs of head trauma (soft-tissue injury, edema, or ecchymoses on the face or head) from a recent accident and has lost consciousness, act quickly to prevent further brain stem injury and irreversible deterioration. Take the patient's vital signs, noting bradycardia, increased systolic blood pressure, and a widening pulse pressure (signs of increased ICP).

Examine the patient's pupillary reaction. Elevate the head of the bed 30 degrees (unless you suspect spinal cord injury), and insert an artificial airway. Connect the patient to a cardiac monitor, and continuously observe his respiratory pattern. Insert an I.V. catheter and begin fluids at a slow infusion rate and prepare to administer an osmotic diuretic, such as mannitol, to decrease cerebral edema. Catheterize the patient to measure urine output, administer supplemental oxygen, and keep emergency resuscitation equipment close by. Obtain an arterial blood gas analysis to help guide treatments.

Metabolic acidosis

If the patient with hyperpnea doesn't have a head injury, his increased respiratory rate probably indicates metabolic acidosis. If the patient's level of consciousness is decreased, check his chart for history data to help you determine the cause of his metabolic acidosis, and intervene appropriately. Suspect shock if the patient has cold, clammy skin. Palpate for a rapid, thready pulse and take his blood pressure, noting hypotension. Elevate the patient's legs 30 degrees,

apply pressure dressings to any obvious hemorrhage, insert several large-bore I.V. catheters, and prepare to administer fluids, vasopressors, and blood products.

A patient with hyperpnea who has a history of alcohol abuse, is vomiting profusely, has diarrhea or profuse abdominal drainage, has ingested an overdose of aspirin, or is cachectic and has a history of starvation may also have metabolic acidosis. Inspect his skin for dryness and poor turgor, indicating dehydration. Take his vital signs, looking for a low-grade fever and hypotension. Insert an I.V. catheter for fluid administration. Obtain blood specimens for electrolyte studies, and prepare to administer sodium bicarbonate, as ordered.

Diabetic ketoacidosis

If the patient has a history of diabetes mellitus, is vomiting, and has a fruity breath odor (acetone breath), suspect diabetic ketoacidosis. Catheterize him to monitor urine output. Infuse an I.V. saline solution. Perform a fingerstick to estimate blood glucose level with a reagent strip. Obtain a urine specimen to test for glucose and acetone, and obtain a blood specimen for glucose and ketone tests. Also administer fluids, insulin, potassium, and sodium bicarbonate I.V, as ordered.

Uremia

If the patient has a history of renal disease, an ammonia breath odor (uremic fetor), and a fine, white powder on his skin (uremic frost), suspect uremia. Insert an I.V. catheter and infuse fluids at a slow rate, and prepare to administer sodium bicarbonate if ordered. Monitor his cardiac rhythm for arrhythmias due to hyperkalemia. Monitor his serum electrolyte, blood urea nitrogen, and creatinine levels as well until hemodialysis or peritoneal dialysis begins.

Next, observe the patient for clues to his abnormal breathing pattern. Can he speak, or does he speak only in brief, choppy phrases? Is his breathing abnormally rapid? Examine the patient for cyanosis (especially of the mouth, lips, mucous membranes, and earlobes), restlessness, and anxiety—all signs of decreased tissue oxygenation, as occurs in shock. In addition, observe the patient for intercostal and abdominal retractions, use of accessory muscles, and diaphoresis, all of which may indicate deep breathing related to an insufficient oxygen supply. Next, inspect for draining wounds or signs of infection, and ask about nausea and vomiting. Take the patient's vital signs, including oxygen saturation, noting a fever, and examine his skin and mucous membranes for turgor, possibly indicating dehydration. Auscultate the patient's heart and lungs.

Medical causes

Head injury. Hyperpnea that results from a severe head injury is called *central neurogenic hyperventilation.* Whether its onset is acute or gradual, this type of hyperpnea indicates damage to the lower midbrain or upper pons. Accompanying signs reflect the site and extent of injury and can include loss of consciousness; soft-tissue injury or bony deformity of the face, head, or neck; facial edema; clear or bloody drainage from the mouth, nose, or ears; raccoon eyes; Battle's sign; an absent doll's eye sign; and motor and sensory disturbances.

Signs of increased intracranial pressure include decreased response to painful stimulation, loss of pupillary reaction, bradycardia, increased systolic pressure, and a widening pulse pressure.

Hyperventilation syndrome. Acute anxiety triggers episodic hyperpnea, resulting in respiratory alkalosis. Other findings may include agitation, vertigo, syncope, pallor, circumoral and peripheral paresthesia, muscle twitching, carpopedal spasm, weakness, and arrhythmias.

Hypoxemia. Many pulmonary disorders that cause hypoxemia—for example, pneumonia, pulmonary edema, chronic obstructive pulmonary disease, and pneumothorax—may cause hyperpnea and episodes of hyperventilation with chest pain, dizziness, and paresthesia. Other effects include dyspnea, a cough, crackles, rhonchi, wheezing, and decreased breath sounds.

Ketoacidosis. Alcoholic ketoacidosis (occurring most commonly in females with a history of alcohol abuse) typically follows cessation of drinking after a marked increase in alcohol consumption has caused severe vomiting. Kussmaul's respirations begin abruptly and are accompanied by vomiting for several days, a fruity breath odor, slight dehydration, abdominal pain and distention, and absent bowel sounds. The patient is alert and has a normal blood glucose level, unlike the patient with diabetic ketoacidosis.

Diabetic ketoacidosis is potentially life-threatening and typically produces Kussmaul's respirations. The patient usually experiences polydipsia, polyphagia, and polyuria before the onset of acidosis; he may have a history of diabetes mellitus. Other clinical features include a fruity breath odor; orthostatic hypotension; a rapid, thready pulse; generalized weakness; a decreased LOC (lethargy to coma); nausea; vomiting; anorexia; and abdominal pain.

Starvation ketoacidosis is also potentially life-threatening and can cause Kussmaul's respirations. Its onset is gradual; typical findings include signs of cachexia and dehydration, a decreased LOC, bradycardia, and a history of severely limited food intake.

Renal failure. Acute or chronic renal failure can cause life-threatening acidosis with Kussmaul's respirations. Signs and symptoms of severe renal failure include oliguria or anuria, uremic fetor, and yellow, dry, scaly skin. Other cutaneous signs include severe pruritus, uremic frost, purpura, and ecchymoses. The patient may complain of nausea and vomiting, weakness, burning pain in the legs and feet, and diarrhea or constipation.

As acidosis progresses, corresponding clinical features include frothy sputum, pleuritic chest pain, and signs of heart failure and pleural or pericardial effusion. Neurologic signs include an altered LOC (lethargy to coma), twitching, and seizures. Hyperkalemia and hypertension, if present, require rapid intervention to prevent cardiovascular collapse.

Sepsis. A severe infection may cause lactic acidosis, resulting in Kussmaul's respirations. Other findings include tachycardia, a fever or a low temperature, chills, a headache, lethargy, profuse diaphoresis, anorexia, a cough, wound drainage, burning on urination, confusion or a change in mental status, and other signs of local infection.

Shock. Potentially life-threatening metabolic acidosis produces Kussmaul's respirations, hypotension, tachycardia, narrowed pulse pressure, a weak pulse, dyspnea, oliguria, anxiety, restlessness, stupor that can progress to coma, and cool, clammy skin. Other clinical features may include external or internal bleeding (in hypovolemic shock); chest pain or arrhythmias and signs of heart failure (in cardiogenic shock); a high fever, chills and, rarely, hypothermia (in septic shock); or stridor due to laryngeal edema (in anaphylactic shock). The onset is usually acute in hypovolemic, cardiogenic, or anaphylactic shock, but it may be gradual in septic shock.

Other causes

Drugs. Toxic levels of salicylates, ammonium chloride, acetazolamide, and other carbonic anhydrase inhibitors can cause Kussmaul's respirations. So can ingestion of methanol and ethylene glycol, found in antifreeze solutions.

Nursing considerations

- Monitor vital signs, including oxygen saturation.
- Observe for increasing respiratory distress, an irregular respiratory pattern, or hypoxia—all of which signal deterioration.
- Start an I.V. line for administration of fluids, blood transfusions, and vasopressor drugs for hemodynamic stabilization, as ordered.
- Prepare to give ventilatory support.
- Obtain arterial blood gas analysis and blood chemistry studies, as ordered.

Patient teaching

- Teach the patient to monitor his blood glucose level, if appropriate.
- Stress the importance of compliance with diabetes therapy, if applicable.
- Explain any food and fluid restrictions.
- Teach the patient coughing and deep-breathing exercises.
- Discuss ways to avoid respiratory infection.

I

Impotence

Impotence is the inability to achieve and maintain penile erection sufficient to complete satisfactory sexual intercourse; ejaculation may be affected. Impotence varies from occasional and minimal to permanent and complete. Occasional impotence occurs in about one-half of adult American men, whereas chronic impotence affects about 10 million American men.

Impotence can be classified as primary or secondary. A man with primary impotence has never been potent with a sexual partner, but may achieve normal erections in other situations. This uncommon condition is difficult to treat. Secondary impotence carries a more favorable prognosis because, despite his present erectile dysfunction, the patient has completed satisfactory intercourse in the past.

Organic causes of impotence include vascular disease, diabetes mellitus, hypogonadism, a spinal cord lesion, alcohol and drug abuse, and surgical complications. Psychogenic causes range from performance anxiety and marital discord to moral or religious conflicts. Fatigue, poor health, age, and drugs can also disrupt normal sexual function.

History and physical examination

If the patient complains of impotence or of a condition that may be causing it, let him describe his problem without interruption. Then begin your examination with a psychosocial history. Is the patient married, single, or widowed? How long has he been married or had a sexual relationship? What's the age and health status of his sexual partner? Is he feeling stress or pressure from his partner to conceive a child? Find out about past marriages, if any, and ask him about his sexual experiences with former spouses. Ask about sexual activity outside marriage or his primary sexual relationship. Also ask about his job history, his typical daily activities, and his living situation. How well does he get along with others in his household?

Focus your medical history on the causes of erectile dysfunction. Does the patient have diabetes mellitus, hypertension, or heart disease? If so, ask about its onset and treatment. Also ask about neurologic diseases such as multiple sclerosis. Obtain a surgical history, emphasizing neurologic, vascular, and urologic surgery. If trauma may be causing the patient's impotence, find out the date of the injury as well as its severity, associated effects, and treatment. Ask about alcohol intake, drug use or abuse, smoking, diet, and exercise. Obtain a

Drugs that may cause impotence

Many commonly used drugs—especially antihypertensives—can cause impotence, which may be reversible if the drug is discontinued or the dosage reduced. Here are some examples.

- amitriptyline
- atenolol
- bicalutamide
- carbamazepine
- cimetidine
- clonidine
- desipramine
- digoxin
- escitalopram
- finasteride
- hydralazine
- imipramine
- methyldopa
- nortriptyline
- perphenazine
- prazosin
- propranolol
- thiazide diuretics
- thioridazine
- tranylcypromine

urologic history, including voiding problems and past injury.

Next, ask the patient when his impotence began. How did it progress? What's its current status? Make your questions specific, but remember that he may have difficulty discussing sexual problems or may not understand the physiology involved.

Other questions that can help yield helpful data include: When was the first time you remember not being able to initiate or maintain an erection? How often do you wake in the morning or at night with an erection? Do you have wet dreams? Has your sexual drive changed? How often do you try to have intercourse with your partner? How often

would you *like* to? Can you ejaculate with or without an erection? Do you experience orgasm with ejaculation?

Next, perform a brief physical examination. Inspect and palpate the genitalia and prostate for structural abnormalities. Assess the patient's sensory function, concentrating on the perineal area. Next, test motor strength and deep tendon reflexes in all extremities, and note other neurologic deficits. Take the patient's vital signs and palpate his pulses for quality. Note any signs of peripheral vascular disease, such as cyanosis and cool extremities. Auscultate for abdominal aortic, femoral, carotid, or iliac bruits, and palpate for thyroid gland enlargement.

Medical causes

Central nervous system disorders. Spinal cord lesions from trauma produce sudden impotence. A complete lesion above S2 (upper motor neuron lesion) disrupts descending motor tracts to the genital area, causing a loss of voluntary erectile control but not of reflex erection and reflex ejaculation. However, a complete lesion in the lumbosacral spinal cord (lower motor neuron lesion) causes a loss of reflex ejaculation and reflex erection. Spinal cord tumors and degenerative diseases of the brain and spinal cord (such as multiple sclerosis and amyotrophic lateral sclerosis) cause progressive impotence.

Endocrine disorders. Hypogonadism from testicular or pituitary dysfunction may lead to impotence from a deficient secretion of androgens (primarily testosterone). Adrenocortical and thyroid dysfunction and chronic hepatic disease may also cause impotence because these organs play a role (although minor) in sex hormone regulation.

Penile disorders. With Peyronie's disease, the penis is bent, making erection painful and penetration difficult and eventually impossible. Phimosis prevents erection until circumcision releases the constricted foreskin. Other inflammatory, infectious, or destructive diseases of the penis may also cause impotence.

Psychological distress. Impotence can result from diverse psychological causes, including depression, performance anxiety, memories of previous traumatic sexual experiences, moral or religious conflicts, and troubled emotional or sexual relationships.

Other causes

Alcohol and drugs. Alcoholism and drug abuse are associated with impotence, as are many prescription drugs, especially antihypertensives. (See *Drugs that may cause impotence.*)

Surgery. Surgical injury to the penis, bladder neck, urinary sphincter, rectum, or perineum can cause impotence, as can injury to local nerves or blood vessels.

Nursing considerations

- Ensure privacy, confirm confidentiality, and establish a rapport with the patient.
- Help the patient feel comfortable about discussing his sexuality.
- Adopt an accepting attitude about the sexual experiences and preferences of others.
- Prepare the patient for screening tests for hormonal irregularities, Doppler studies of penile blood pressure to rule out vascular insufficiency, voiding studies, nerve conduction tests, evaluation of nocturnal penile tumescence, and psychological screening.
- Discuss counseling for the patient and his sexual partner, if the patient has psychogenic impotence.
- Provide interventions to treat the cause, if the patient has organic impotence.

- Prepare the patient for other forms of treatment such as surgical revascularization, drug-induced erection, surgical repair of a venous leak, and penile prostheses.

Patient teaching

- Discuss the importance of maintaining follow-up appointments and therapy for underlying medical disorders.
- Encourage him to talk openly about his needs and desires, fears and anxieties, or misconceptions.
- Urge the patient to discuss his feelings with his partner as well as what role both of them want sexual activity to play in their lives.

Insomnia

Insomnia is the inability to fall asleep, remain asleep, or feel refreshed by sleep. Acute and transient during periods of stress, insomnia may become chronic, causing constant fatigue, extreme anxiety as bedtime approaches, and psychiatric disorders. This common complaint is experienced occasionally by about 25% of Americans and chronically by another 10%.

Physiologic causes of insomnia include jet lag, arguing, and lack of exercise. Pathophysiologic causes range from medical and psychiatric disorders to pain, adverse effects of a drug, and idiopathic factors. Complaints of insomnia are subjective and require close investigation; for example, the patient may mistakenly attribute his fatigue from an organic cause, such as anemia, to insomnia.

History and physical examination

Take a thorough sleep and health history. Find out when the patient's insomnia began and the circumstances surrounding it. Is the patient trying to stop using a sedative? Does he take a central nervous system (CNS) stimulant, such as an amphetamine, pseudoephedrine, a theophylline derivative, cocaine, or a drug that contains caffeine, or does he drink caffeinated beverages?

Find out if the patient has a chronic or acute condition, the effects of which may be disturbing his sleep, particularly cardiac or respiratory disease or painful or pruritic conditions. Ask if he has an endocrine or neurologic disorder, or a history of drug or alcohol abuse. Is he a frequent traveler who suffers from jet lag? Does he use his legs a lot during the day and then feel restless at night? Ask about daytime fatigue and regular exercise. Also ask if he commonly finds himself gasping for air, experiencing apnea, or frequently repositioning his body. If possible, consult the patient's spouse or sleep partner because the patient may be unaware of his own behavior. Ask how many pillows the patient uses to sleep.

Assess the patient's emotional status, and try to estimate his level of self-esteem. Ask about personal and professional problems and psychological stress. Also ask if he experiences hallucinations, and note behavior that may indicate alcohol or drug withdrawal. After reviewing complaints that suggest an undiagnosed disorder, perform a physical examination.

Medical causes
Alcohol withdrawal syndrome.
Abrupt cessation of alcohol intake after long-term use causes insomnia that may persist for up to 2 years. Other early effects of this acute syndrome include excessive diaphoresis, tachycardia, hypertension, tremors, restlessness, irritability, a headache, nausea, flushing, and nightmares. Progression to delirium tremens produces confusion, disorientation, paranoia, delusions, hallucinations, and seizures.

Generalized anxiety disorder. Anxiety can cause chronic insomnia as well as symptoms of tension, such as fatigue and restlessness; signs of autonomic hyperactivity, such as diaphoresis, dyspepsia, and high resting pulse and respiratory rates; and signs of apprehension.

Mood (affective) disorders. Depression commonly causes chronic insomnia with difficulty falling asleep, waking and being unable to fall back to sleep, or waking early in the morning. Related findings include dysphoria (a primary symptom), decreased appetite with weight loss or increased appetite with weight gain, and psychomotor agitation or retardation. The patient experiences loss of interest in his usual activities, feelings of worthlessness and guilt, fatigue, difficulty concentrating, indecisiveness, and recurrent thoughts of death.

Manic episodes produce a decreased need for sleep with an elevated mood and irritability. Related findings include increased energy and activity, fast speech, speeding thoughts, inflated self-esteem, easy distractibility, and involvement in high-risk activities such as reckless driving.

Nocturnal myoclonus (also known as periodic limb movement disorder*).* With nocturnal myoclonus, a seizure disorder, involuntary and fleeting muscle jerks of the legs occur every 20 to 40 seconds, disturbing sleep.

Restless leg syndrome. With restless leg syndrome, uncomfortable sensations in the legs cause uncontrollable urges to move the limbs. Although movement brings relief, sleep is usually disrupted, causing insomnia, which may be severe.

Sleep apnea syndrome. With sleep apnea syndrome, apneic periods begin with the onset of sleep, continue for 10 to 90 seconds, and end with a series of gasps and arousal. With central sleep apnea, respiratory movement ceases for

Tips for relieving insomnia

Common causes	Interventions
Acroparesthesia Improper positioning may compress superficial (ulnar, radial, and peroneal) nerves, disrupting circulation to the compressed nerve. This causes numbness, tingling, and stiffness in an arm or leg.	Teach the patient to assume a comfortable position in bed, with his limbs unrestricted. If he tends to awaken with a numb arm or leg, tell him to massage and move it until sensation returns completely and then to assume an unrestricted position.
Anxiety Physical and emotional stress produces anxiety, which causes autonomic stimulation.	Encourage the patient to discuss his fears and concerns, and teach him relaxation techniques, such as guided imagery and deep breathing. If ordered, administer a mild sedative, such as temazepam or another sedative hypnotic, before bedtime. Emphasize that these medications are to be used for the short term only.
Dyspnea With many cardiac and pulmonary disorders, a recumbent position and inactivity cause restricted chest expansion, secretion pooling, and pulmonary vascular congestion, leading to coughing and shortness of breath.	Elevate the head of the bed, or provide at least two pillows or a reclining chair to help the patient sleep. Suction him when he awakens, and encourage deep breathing and incentive spirometry every 2 to 4 hours. Also provide supplementary oxygen by nasal cannula. If the patient is pregnant, encourage her to sleep on her left side at a comfortable elevation to ease dyspnea.
Pain Chronic or acute pain from any cause can prevent or disrupt sleep.	Administer pain medication as ordered, 20 minutes before bedtime, and teach deep, even, slow breathing to promote relaxation. If the patient has back pain, help him lie on his side with his legs flexed. If he has epigastric pain, encourage him to take an antacid before bedtime and to sleep with the head of the bed elevated. If he has incisions, instruct him to splint during coughing or movement.
Pruritus A localized skin infection or a systemic disorder, such as liver failure, may produce intensely annoying itching, even during the night.	Wash the skin with a mild soap and water, and dry it thoroughly. Apply moisturizing lotion on dry, unbroken skin and an antipruritic, such as calamine lotion, on pruritic areas. Administer diphenhydramine or hydroxyzine to help minimize itching.

the apneic period; with obstructive sleep apnea, upper airway obstruction blocks incoming air, although breathing movements continue. Some patients display both types of apnea. Repeated possibly hundreds of times during the night, this cycle alternates with bradycardia and tachycardia. Associated findings include a morning headache, daytime fatigue, hypertension, ankle edema, and personality changes, such as hostility, paranoia, and agitated depression.

Other causes

Drugs. Use of, abuse of, or withdrawal from sedatives or hypnotics may produce insomnia. CNS stimulants—including amphetamines, theophylline derivatives, pseudoephedrine, cocaine, and caffeinated beverages—may also produce insomnia.

Nursing considerations

- Prepare the patient for tests to evaluate his insomnia, such as blood and urine studies for 17-hydroxycorticosteroids and catecholamines, polysomnography (including an EEG, electro-oculography, and electrocardiography), and sleep studies.
- Institute measures to help relieve insomnia. (See *Tips for relieving insomnia,* page 341.)

Patient teaching

- Teach the patient comfort and relaxation techniques to promote natural sleep.
- Advise him to awaken and retire at the same time each day and to exercise regularly, but not close to bedtime.
- Encourage the patient to avoid caffeinated beverages at least 3 hours before bedtime.
- Refer the patient to counseling or a sleep disorder clinic as needed.

Intermittent claudication

Most common in the legs, intermittent claudication is cramping limb pain brought on by exercise and relieved by 1 to 2 minutes of rest. This pain may be acute or chronic; when acute, it may signal acute arterial occlusion that requires immediate intervention. Intermittent claudication is most common in men ages 50 to 60 with a history of diabetes mellitus, hyperlipidemia, hypertension, or tobacco use. Without treatment, it may progress to pain at rest. With chronic arterial occlusion, limb loss is uncommon because collateral circulation usually develops.

With occlusive artery disease, intermittent claudication results from an inadequate blood supply. Pain in the calf (the most common area) or foot indicates disease of the femoral or popliteal arteries; pain in the buttocks and upper thigh, disease of the aortoiliac arteries. During exercise, the pain typically results from the release of lactic acid due to anaerobic metabolism in the ischemic segment, secondary to obstruction. When exercise stops, the lactic acid clears and the pain subsides.

Intermittent claudication may also have a neurologic cause: narrowing of the vertebral column at the level of the cauda equina. This condition creates pressure on the nerve roots to the lower extremities. Walking stimulates circulation to the cauda equina, causing increased pressure on those nerves and resultant pain.

Physical findings include pallor on elevation, rubor on dependency (especially the toes and soles), loss of hair on the toes, and diminished arterial pulses.

If the patient has sudden intermittent claudication with severe or aching leg pain at rest, check the leg's temperature and color and palpate femoral, popliteal, posterior tibial, and dorsalis pedis pulses. Ask about numbness and tingling. Suspect acute arterial occlusion if pulses are absent; if the leg feels cold and looks pale, cyanotic, or mottled; and if paresthesia and pain are present. Mark the area of pallor, cyanosis, or mottling, and reassess it frequently, noting an increase in the area.

Don't elevate the leg. Protect it, allowing nothing to press on it. Prepare the patient for preoperative blood tests, urinalysis, electrocardiography, chest Xrays, lower-extremity Doppler studies, and angiography. Insert an I.V. catheter, and administer an anticoagulant and analgesics as ordered.

History and physical examination

If the patient has chronic intermittent claudication, gather history data first. Ask how far he can walk before pain occurs and how long he must rest before it subsides. Can he walk less far now than before, or does he need to rest longer? Does the pain-rest pattern vary? Has this symptom affected his lifestyle?

Obtain a history of risk factors for atherosclerosis, such as smoking, diabetes, hypertension, and hyperlipidemia. Next, ask about associated signs and symptoms, such as paresthesia in the affected limb and visible changes in the color of the fingers (white to blue to pink) when he's smoking, exposed to cold, or under stress. If the patient is male, does he experience impotence?

Focus the physical examination on the cardiovascular system. Palpate for femoral, popliteal, dorsalis pedis, and posterior tibial pulses. Note character,

amplitude, and bilateral equality. Diminished or absent popliteal and pedal pulses with the femoral pulse present may indicate atherosclerotic disease of the femoral artery. Diminished femoral and distal pulses may indicate disease of the terminal aorta or iliac branches. Absent pedal pulses with normal femoral and popliteal pulses may indicate Buerger's disease.

Listen for bruits over the major arteries. Note color and temperature differences between his legs or compared with his arms; also note where on his leg the changes in temperature and color occur. Elevate the affected leg for 2 minutes; if it becomes pale or white, blood flow is severely decreased. When the leg dangles, how long does it take for color to return? (Thirty seconds or longer indicates severe disease.) If possible, check the patient's deep tendon reflexes (DTRs) after exercise; note if they're diminished in his lower extremities.

Examine the patient's feet, toes, and fingers for ulceration, and inspect his hands and lower legs for small, tender nodules and erythema along blood vessels. Note the quality of his nails and the amount of hair on his fingers and toes.

If the patient has arm pain, inspect his arms for a change in color (to white) on elevation. Next, palpate for changes in temperature, muscle wasting, and a pulsating mass in the subclavian area. Palpate and compare the radial, ulnar, brachial, axillary, and subclavian pulses to identify obstructed areas.

Medical causes

Arterial occlusion (acute). Acute arterial occlusion produces intense intermittent claudication. A saddle embolus may affect both legs. Associated findings include paresthesia, paresis, and a sensation of cold in the affected limb. The limb is cool, pale, and cyanotic (mottled) with absent pulses below the occlusion. Capillary refill time is increased.

Arteriosclerosis obliterans. Arteriosclerosis obliterans usually affects the femoral and popliteal arteries, causing intermittent claudication (the most common symptom) in the calf. Typical associated findings include diminished or absent popliteal and pedal pulses, coolness in the affected limb, pallor on elevation, and profound limb weakness with continuing exercise. Other possible findings include numbness, paresthesia and, in severe disease, pain in the toes or foot while at rest, ulceration, and gangrene.

Buerger's disease. Buerger's disease typically produces intermittent claudication of the instep. Early signs include migratory superficial nodules and erythema along extremity blood vessels (nodular phlebitis) as well as migratory venous phlebitis. With exposure to cold, the feet initially become cold, cyanotic, and numb; later, they redden, become hot, and tingle. Occasionally, Buerger's disease also affects the hands and can cause painful ulcerations on the fingertips. Other characteristic findings include impaired peripheral pulses, paresthesia of the hands and feet, and migratory superficial thrombophlebitis.

Neurogenic claudication. Neurospinal disease causes pain from neurogenic intermittent claudication that requires a longer rest time than the 2 to 3 minutes needed in vascular claudication. Associated findings include paresthesia, weakness and clumsiness when walking, and hypoactive DTRs after walking. Pulses are unaffected.

Nursing considerations

- Prepare the patient for diagnostic tests (Doppler flow studies, arteriography, and digital subtraction angiography) to determine the location and degree of occlusion.

Patient teaching

- Encourage the patient to exercise to improve collateral circulation and increase venous return.
- Advise the patient to avoid prolonged sitting or standing as well as crossing his legs at the knees.
- Discuss risk factors for intermittent claudication.
- Stress the importance of inspecting the legs and feet for ulcers.
- Teach signs and symptoms to report to the health care provider.

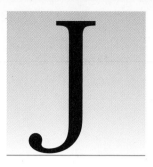

Jaundice
[Icterus]

A yellow discoloration of the skin, mucous membranes, or sclera of the eyes, jaundice indicates excessive levels of conjugated or unconjugated bilirubin in the blood. In fair-skinned patients, it's most noticeable on the face, trunk, and sclera; in dark-skinned patients, on the hard palate, sclera, and conjunctiva.

Jaundice is most apparent in natural sunlight. In fact, it may be undetectable in artificial or poor light. It's commonly accompanied by pruritus (because bile pigment damages sensory nerves), dark urine, and clay-colored stools.

Jaundice may result from any of three pathophysiologic processes. (See *Impaired bilirubin metabolism in jaundice,* page 346.) It may be the only warning sign of certain disorders such as pancreatic cancer.

History and physical examination

Documenting a history of the patient's jaundice is critical in determining its cause. Begin by asking the patient when he first noticed the jaundice. Does he also have pruritus, clay-colored stools, or dark urine? Ask about past episodes or a family history of jaundice. Does he have nonspecific signs or symptoms, such as fatigue, a fever, or chills; GI signs or symptoms, such as anorexia, abdominal pain, nausea, weight loss, or vomiting; or cardiopulmonary symptoms, such as shortness of breath or palpitations? Ask about alcohol use and a history of cancer or liver or gallbladder disease. Has the patient lost weight recently? Also, obtain a drug history. Ask about a history of hepatitis, gallstones, or liver or pancreatic disease.

Perform the physical examination in a room with natural light. Make sure that the orange-yellow hue is jaundice and not due to hypercarotenemia, which is more prominent on the palms and soles and doesn't affect the sclera. Inspect the patient's skin for texture and dryness and for hyperpigmentation and xanthomas. Look for spider angiomas or petechiae, clubbed fingers, and gynecomastia. If the patient has heart failure, auscultate for arrhythmias, murmurs, and gallops as well as crackles and abnormal bowel sounds. Palpate the lymph nodes for swelling and the abdomen for tenderness, pain, and swelling. Palpate and percuss the liver and spleen for enlargement, and test for ascites with the shifting dullness and fluid wave techniques. Obtain baseline data on the patient's mental status: Slight changes in sensorium may be an early sign of deteriorating hepatic function.

Impaired bilirubin metabolism in jaundice

Jaundice occurs in three forms: prehepatic, hepatic, and posthepatic. In all three, bilirubin levels in the blood increase due to impaired metabolism.

Prehepatic jaundice
With *prehepatic jaundice,* certain conditions and disorders, such as transfusion reactions and sickle cell anemia, cause massive hemolysis. Red blood cells rupture faster than the liver can conjugate bilirubin, so large amounts of unconjugated bilirubin pass into the blood, causing increased intestinal conversion of this bilirubin to water-soluble urobilinogen for excretion in urine and stools. (Unconjugated bilirubin is insoluble in water, so it can't be directly excreted in urine.)

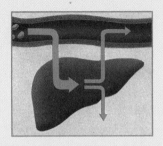

Hepatic jaundice
Hepatic jaundice results from the liver's inability to conjugate or excrete bilirubin, leading to increased blood levels of conjugated and unconjugated bilirubin. This occurs with such disorders as hepatitis, cirrhosis, and metastatic cancer and during the prolonged use of drugs metabolized by the liver.

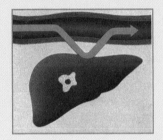

Posthepatic jaundice
With *posthepatic jaundice,* which occurs in patients with a biliary or pancreatic disorder, bilirubin forms at its normal rate, but inflammation, scar tissue, a tumor, or gallstones block the flow of bile into the intestine. This causes an accumulation of conjugated bilirubin in the blood. Water-soluble, conjugated bilirubin is excreted in urine.

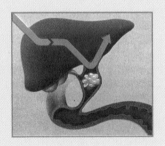

Medical causes
Carcinoma. *Cancer of the ampulla of Vater* initially produces fluctuating jaundice, mild abdominal pain, a recurrent fever, and chills. Occult bleeding may be its first sign. Other findings include weight loss, pruritus, and back pain.

Hepatic cancer (primary liver cancer or another cancer that has metastasized to the liver) may cause jaundice by causing obstruction of the bile duct. Even advanced cancer causes nonspecific signs and symptoms, such as right upper quadrant discomfort and tenderness, nausea, weight loss, and a slight fever. Examination may reveal irregular, nodular, firm hepatomegaly; ascites; peripheral edema; a bruit heard over the liver; and a right upper quadrant mass.

With *pancreatic cancer,* progressive jaundice—possibly with pruritus—may be the only sign. Related early findings are nonspecific, such as weight loss and back or abdominal pain. Other signs and symptoms include anorexia, nausea and vomiting, a fever, steatorrhea, fatigue, weakness, diarrhea, pruritus, and skin lesions (usually on the legs).

Cholangitis. Obstruction and infection in the common bile duct cause Charcot's triad: jaundice, right upper quadrant pain, and a high fever with chills.

Cholecystitis. Cholecystitis produces nonobstructive jaundice in about 25% of patients. Biliary colic typically peaks abruptly, persisting for 2 to 4 hours. The pain then localizes to the right upper quadrant and becomes constant. Local inflammation or passage of stones to the common bile duct causes jaundice. Other findings include nausea, vomiting (usually indicating the presence of a stone), a fever, profuse diaphoresis, chills, tenderness on palpation, a positive Murphy's sign and, possibly, abdominal distention and rigidity.

Cholelithiasis. Cholelithiasis commonly causes jaundice and biliary colic. It's characterized by severe, steady pain in the right upper quadrant or epigastrium that radiates to the right scapula or shoulder and intensifies over several hours. Accompanying signs and symptoms include nausea and vomiting, tachycardia, and restlessness. Occlusion of the common bile duct causes a fever, chills, jaundice, clay-colored stools, and abdominal tenderness. After consuming a fatty meal, the patient may experience vague epigastric fullness and dyspepsia.

Cirrhosis. With *Laënnec's cirrhosis,* mild to moderate jaundice with pruritus usually signals hepatocellular necrosis or progressive hepatic insufficiency. Common early findings include ascites, weakness, leg edema, nausea and vomiting, diarrhea or constipation, anorexia, weight loss, and right upper quadrant pain. Massive hematemesis and other bleeding tendencies may also occur.

Other findings include an enlarged liver and parotid gland, clubbed fingers, Dupuytren's contracture, mental changes, asterixis, fetor hepaticus, spider angiomas, and palmar erythema. Males may exhibit gynecomastia, scanty chest and axillary hair, and testicular atrophy; females may experience menstrual irregularities.

With *primary biliary cirrhosis,* fluctuating jaundice may appear years after the onset of other signs and symptoms, such as pruritus that worsens at bedtime (commonly the first sign), weakness, fatigue, weight loss, and vague abdominal pain. Itching may lead to skin excoriation. Associated findings include hyperpigmentation; indications of malabsorption, such as nocturnal diarrhea, steatorrhea, purpura, and osteomalacia; hematemesis from esophageal varices; ascites; edema; xanthelasmas; xanthomas on the palms, soles, and elbows; and hepatomegaly.

Dubin-Johnson syndrome. With Dubin-Johnson syndrome, which is a rare, chronic inherited syndrome, fluctuating jaundice that increases with stress is the major sign, appearing as late as age 40. Related findings include slight hepatic enlargement and tenderness, upper abdominal pain, nausea, and vomiting.

Heart failure. Jaundice due to liver dysfunction occurs in patients with severe right-sided heart failure. Other effects include jugular vein distention, cyanosis, dependent edema of the legs and sacrum, steady weight gain, confusion, hepatomegaly, nausea and vomiting, abdominal discomfort, and anorexia due to visceral edema. Ascites is a late sign. Oliguria, marked weakness, and anxiety may also occur. If left-sided heart failure develops first, other findings may include fatigue, dyspnea, orthopnea, paroxysmal nocturnal dyspnea, tachypnea, arrhythmias, and tachycardia.

Hepatic abscess. Multiple liver abscesses may cause jaundice, but the primary effects are a persistent fever with chills and sweating. Other findings include steady, severe pain in the right upper quadrant or midepigastrium that may be referred to the shoulder; nausea and vomiting; anorexia; hepatomegaly; an elevated right hemidiaphragm; and ascites.

Hepatitis. Dark urine and clay-colored stools usually develop before jaundice in the late stages of acute viral hepatitis. Early systemic signs and symptoms vary and include fatigue, nausea, vomiting, malaise, arthralgia, myalgia, a headache, anorexia, photophobia, pharyngitis, a cough, diarrhea or constipation, and a low-grade fever associated with liver and lymph node enlargement. During the *icteric phase* (which subsides within 2 to 3 weeks unless complications occur), systemic signs subside, but an enlarged, palpable liver may be present along with weight loss, anorexia, and right upper quadrant pain and tenderness.

Pancreatitis (acute). Edema of the head of the pancreas and obstruction of the common bile duct can cause jaundice; however, the primary symptom of acute pancreatitis is severe epigastric pain that commonly radiates to the back. Lying with the knees flexed on the chest or sitting up and leaning forward brings relief. Early associated signs and symptoms include nausea, persistent vomiting, abdominal distention, and Turner's or Cullen's sign. Other findings include a fever, tachycardia, abdominal rigidity and tenderness, hypoactive bowel sounds, and crackles.

Severe pancreatitis produces extreme restlessness; mottled skin; cold, diaphoretic extremities; paresthesia; and tetany—the last two being symptoms of hypocalcemia. Fulminant pancreatitis causes massive hemorrhage.

Sickle cell anemia. Hemolysis produces jaundice in the patient with sickle cell anemia. Other findings include impaired growth and development, increased susceptibility to infection, life-threatening thrombotic complications and, commonly, leg ulcers, swollen (painful) joints, a fever, and chills. Bone aches and chest pain may also occur. Severe hemolysis may cause hematuria and pallor, chronic fatigue, weakness, dyspnea (or dyspnea on exertion), and tachycardia. The patient may also have splenomegaly. During a sickle cell crisis, the patient may have severe bone, abdominal, thoracic, and muscular pain; a low-grade fever; and increased weakness, jaundice, and dyspnea.

Other causes

Drugs. Many drugs may cause hepatic injury and resultant jaundice. Examples include acetaminophen, phenylbutazone, I.V. tetracycline, isoniazid, hormonal contraceptives, sulfonamides, mercaptopurine, erythromycin estolate, niacin, troleandomycin, androgenic steroids, 3-hydroxy-3-methylglutaryl coenzyme A reductase inhibitors, phenothiazines, ethanol, methyldopa, rifampin, and dilantin.

Treatments. Upper abdominal surgery may cause postoperative jaundice, which occurs secondary to hepatocellular damage from the manipulation of organs, leading to edema and obstructed bile flow; from the administration of halothane; or from prolonged surgery resulting in shock, blood loss, or blood transfusion.

A surgical shunt used to reduce portal hypertension (such as a portacaval shunt) may also produce jaundice.

Nursing considerations

■ To decrease pruritus, frequently bathe the patient; apply an antipruritic lotion, such as calamine; and administer diphenhydramine or hydroxyzine.

▪ Prepare the patient for diagnostic tests to evaluate biliary and hepatic function, including laboratory studies (such as urine and fecal urobilinogen, serum bilirubin, liver enzyme, and cholesterol levels; prothrombin time; and a complete blood count), computed tomography, ultrasonography, cholangiography, liver biopsy, and exploratory laparotomy.

Patient teaching

▪ Teach the patient appropriate dietary changes.
▪ Discuss ways to reduce pruritis.
▪ Review with the patient prescribed medications and their possible adverse effects.

Jaw pain

Jaw pain may arise from either of the two bones that hold the teeth in the jaw—the maxilla (upper jaw) and the mandible (lower jaw). Jaw pain also includes pain in the temporomandibular joint (TMJ), where the mandible meets the temporal bone.

Jaw pain may develop gradually or abruptly and may range from barely noticeable to excruciating, depending on its cause. It usually results from disorders of the teeth, soft tissue, or glands of the mouth or throat or from local trauma or infection. Systemic causes include musculoskeletal, neurologic, cardiovascular, endocrine, immunologic, metabolic, and infectious disorders. Life-threatening disorders, such as a myocardial infarction (MI) and tetany, also produce jaw pain as well as certain drugs (especially phenothiazines) and dental or surgical procedures.

Jaw pain is seldom a primary indicator of any one disorder; however, some causes are medical emergencies.

ACTION STAT!

 Ask the patient when the jaw pain began. Did it arise suddenly or gradually? Is it more severe or frequent now than when it first occurred? Sudden severe jaw pain, especially when associated with chest pain, shortness of breath, or arm pain, requires prompt evaluation because it may herald a life-threatening MI. Perform an electrocardiogram and obtain blood samples for cardiac enzyme levels. Administer oxygen, morphine sulfate, and a vasodilator as indicated.

History and physical examination

Begin the patient history by asking him to describe the pain's character, intensity, and frequency. When did he first notice the jaw pain? Where on the jaw does he feel pain? Does the pain radiate to other areas? Sharp or burning pain arises from the skin or subcutaneous tissues. Causalgia, an intense burning sensation, usually results from damage to the fifth cranial, or trigeminal, nerve. This type of superficial pain is easily localized, unlike dull, aching, boring, or throbbing pain, which originates in muscle, bone, or joints. Also ask about aggravating or alleviating factors.

Ask about recent trauma, surgery, or procedures, especially dental work. Ask about associated signs and symptoms, such as joint or chest pain, dyspnea, palpitations, fatigue, a headache, malaise, anorexia, weight loss, intermittent claudication, diplopia, and hearing loss. (Keep in mind that jaw pain may accompany more characteristic signs and symptoms of life-threatening disorders such as chest pain in a patient with an MI.)

Focus your physical examination on the jaw. Inspect the painful area for redness, and palpate for edema or warmth.

Facing the patient directly, look for facial asymmetry indicating swelling. Check the TMJs by placing your fingertips just anterior to the external auditory meatus and asking the patient to open and close, and to thrust out and retract his jaw. Note the presence of crepitus, an abnormal scraping or grinding sensation in the joint. (Clicks heard when the jaw is widely spread apart are normal.) How wide can the patient open his mouth? Less than $1\frac{1}{8}''$ (3 cm) or more than $2\frac{3}{8}''$ (6 cm) between the upper and lower teeth is abnormal. Next, palpate the parotid area for pain and swelling, and inspect and palpate the oral cavity for lesions, elevation of the tongue, or masses.

Medical causes

Angina pectoris. Angina may produce jaw pain (usually radiating from the substernal area) and left arm pain. Angina is less severe than the pain of an MI. It's commonly triggered by exertion, emotional stress, or ingestion of a heavy meal and usually subsides with rest and the administration of nitroglycerin. Other signs and symptoms include shortness of breath, nausea and vomiting, tachycardia, dizziness, diaphoresis, belching, and palpitations.

Arthritis. With *osteoarthritis,* which usually affects the small joints of the hand, aching jaw pain increases with activity (talking, eating) and subsides with rest. Other features are crepitus heard and felt over the TMJ, enlarged joints with a restricted range of motion (ROM), and stiffness on awakening that improves with a few minutes of activity. Redness and warmth are usually absent.

Rheumatoid arthritis causes symmetrical pain in all joints (commonly affecting proximal finger joints first), including the jaw. The joints display limited ROM and are tender, warm, swollen, and stiff after inactivity, especially in the morning. Myalgia is common. Systemic signs and symptoms include fatigue, weight loss, malaise, anorexia, lymphadenopathy, and a mild fever. Painless, movable rheumatoid nodules may appear on the elbows, knees, and knuckles. Progressive disease causes deformities, crepitation with joint rotation, muscle weakness and atrophy around the involved joint, and multiple systemic complications.

Head and neck cancer. Many types of head and neck cancer, especially of the oral cavity and nasopharynx, produce aching jaw pain of insidious onset. Other findings include a history of leukoplakia; ulcers of the mucous membranes; palpable masses in the jaw, mouth, and neck; dysphagia; bloody discharge; drooling; lymphadenopathy; and trismus.

Hypocalcemic tetany. Besides painful muscle contractions of the jaw and mouth, hypocalcemic tetany—a life-threatening disorder—produces paresthesia and carpopedal spasms. The patient may complain of weakness, fatigue, and palpitations. Examination reveals hyperreflexia and positive Chvostek's and Trousseau's signs. Muscle twitching, choreiform movements, and muscle cramps may also occur. With severe hypocalcemia, laryngeal spasm may occur with stridor, cyanosis, seizures, and cardiac arrhythmias.

Ludwig's angina. Ludwig's angina is an acute streptococcal infection of the sublingual and submandibular spaces that produces severe jaw pain in the mandibular area with tongue elevation, sublingual edema, and drooling. A fever is a common sign. Progressive disease produces dysphagia, dysphonia, and stridor and dyspnea due to laryngeal edema and obstruction by an elevated tongue.

MI. Initially, MI causes intense, crushing substernal pain that's unrelieved by rest or nitroglycerin. The pain may radiate to the lower jaw, left arm, neck, back, or shoulder blades. (Rarely, jaw pain occurs without chest pain.) Other findings include pallor, clammy skin, dyspnea, excessive diaphoresis, nausea and vomiting, anxiety, restlessness, a feeling of impending doom, a low-grade fever, decreased or increased blood pressure, arrhythmias, an atrial gallop, new murmurs (in many cases from mitral insufficiency), and crackles.

Sinusitis. Maxillary sinusitis produces intense boring pain in the maxilla and cheek that may radiate to the eye. This type of sinusitis also causes a feeling of fullness, increased pain on percussion of the first and second molars and, in those with nasal obstruction, the loss of the sense of smell. Sphenoid sinusitis causes scanty nasal discharge and chronic pain at the mandibular ramus and vertex of the head and in the temporal area. Other signs and symptoms of both types of sinusitis include a fever, halitosis, a headache, malaise, a cough, and a sore throat.

Suppurative parotitis. Bacterial infection of the parotid gland by *Staphylococcus aureus* tends to develop in debilitated patients with dry mouth or poor oral hygiene. Besides the abrupt onset of jaw pain, a high fever, and chills, findings include erythema and edema of the overlying skin; a tender, swollen gland; and pus at the second top molar (Stensen's ducts). Infection may lead to disorientation; shock and death are common.

Temporal arteritis. Most common in women older than age 60, temporal arteritis produces sharp jaw pain after chewing or talking. Nonspecific signs and symptoms include a low-grade fever, generalized muscle pain, malaise, fatigue, anorexia, and weight loss. Vascular lesions produce jaw pain; a throbbing, unilateral headache in the fron-

totemporal region; swollen, nodular, tender and, possibly, pulseless temporal arteries; and, at times, erythema of the overlying skin.

TMJ syndrome. TMJ syndrome is a common syndrome that produces jaw pain at the TMJ; spasm and pain of the masticating muscle; clicking, popping, or crepitus of the TMJ; and restricted jaw movement. Unilateral, localized pain may radiate to other head and neck areas. The patient typically reports teeth clenching, bruxism, and emotional stress. He may also experience ear pain, a headache, deviation of the jaw to the affected side upon opening the mouth, and jaw subluxation or dislocation, especially after yawning.

Tetanus. A rare life-threatening disorder caused by a bacterial toxin, tetanus produces stiffness and pain in the jaw and difficulty opening the mouth. Early nonspecific signs and symptoms (commonly unnoticed or mistaken for influenza) include a headache, irritability, restlessness, a low-grade fever, and chills. Examination reveals tachycardia, profuse diaphoresis, and hyperreflexia. Progressive disease leads to painful, involuntary muscle spasms that spread to the abdomen, back, or face. The slightest stimulus may produce reflex spasms of any muscle group. Ultimately, laryngospasm, respiratory distress, and seizures may occur.

Trigeminal neuralgia. Trigeminal neuralgia is marked by paroxysmal attacks of intense unilateral jaw pain (stopping at the facial midline) or rapid-fire shooting sensations in one division of the trigeminal nerve (usually the mandibular or maxillary division). This superficial pain, felt mainly over the lips and chin and in the teeth, lasts from 1 to 15 minutes. Mouth and nose areas may be hypersensitive. Involvement of the ophthalmic branch of the trigeminal nerve causes a diminished or absent corneal reflex on the same side. Attacks can be triggered by mild stimulation of the nerve (for example, lightly touching the cheeks), exposure to heat or cold, or consumption of hot or cold foods or beverages.

Other causes
Drugs. Some drugs, such as phenothiazines, affect the extrapyramidal tract, causing dyskinesias; others cause tetany of the jaw secondary to hypocalcemia.

Nursing considerations
■ If the patient is in severe pain, withhold food, liquids, and oral medications until the diagnosis is confirmed.
■ Administer an analgesic as ordered, and monitor effect.
■ Prepare the patient for diagnostic tests such as jaw X-rays.
■ Apply an ice pack if the jaw is swollen, and discourage the patient from talking or moving his jaw.

Patient teaching
■ Explain the disorder and the treatments to the patient.
■ Teach the patient the proper way to insert mouth splints.
■ Discuss ways to reduce stress.
■ Explain the identification and avoidance of triggers.

Jugular vein distention

Jugular vein distention is the abnormal fullness and height of the pulse waves in the internal or external jugular veins. For a patient in a supine position with his head elevated 45 degrees, a pulse wave height greater than $1\frac{1}{4}''$ to $1\frac{1}{2}''$ (3 to 4 cm) above the angle of Louis indicates distention. Engorged, distended veins reflect increased venous pressure in the right side of the heart, which, in turn, indicates an increased central venous pressure. This common sign characteristically occurs in heart failure and other cardiovascular disorders, such as constrictive pericarditis, tricuspid stenosis, and obstruction of the superior vena cava.

ACTION STAT!

Evaluating jugular vein distention involves visualizing and assessing venous pulsations. (See *Evaluating jugular vein distention.*) If you detect jugular vein distention in the patient with pale, clammy skin who suddenly appears anxious and dyspneic, take his blood pressure. If you note hypotension and a paradoxical pulse, suspect cardiac tamponade. Elevate the foot of the bed 20 to 30 degrees, give supplemental oxygen, and monitor cardiac status and rhythm, oxygen saturation, and mental status. Insert an I.V. catheter for medication administration, and keep cardiopulmonary resuscitation equipment close by. Assemble the needed equipment for emergency pericardiocentesis (to relieve pressure on the heart). Throughout the procedure, monitor the patient's blood pressure, heart rhythm, respirations, and pulse oximetry.

History and physical examination
If the patient isn't in severe distress, obtain a history. Has he recently gained weight? Does he have difficulty putting on shoes? Are his ankles swollen? Ask about chest pain, shortness of breath, paroxysmal nocturnal dyspnea, anorexia, nausea or vomiting, and a history of cancer or cardiac, pulmonary, hepatic, or renal disease. Obtain a drug history, noting diuretic use and dosage. Is the patient taking drugs as prescribed? Ask the patient about his regular diet patterns, noting a high sodium intake.

Evaluating jugular vein distention

With the patient in a supine position, position him so that you can visualize jugular vein pulsations reflected from the right atrium. Elevate the head of the bed 45 to 90 degrees. (In the normal patient, veins distend only when the patient lies flat.)

Next, locate the angle of Louis (sternal notch)—the reference point for measuring venous pressure. To do so, palpate the clavicles where they join the sternum (the suprasternal notch). Place your first two fingers on the suprasternal notch. Then, without lifting them from the skin, slide them down the sternum until you feel a bony protuberance—this is the angle of Louis.

Find the internal jugular vein (which indicates venous pressure more reliably than the external jugular vein). Shine a flashlight across the patient's neck to create shadows that highlight his venous pulse. Be sure to distinguish jugular vein pulsations from carotid artery pulsations. One way to do this is to palpate the vessel: Arterial pulsations continue, whereas venous pulsations disappear with light finger pressure. Also, venous pulsations increase or decrease with changes in body position; arterial pulsations remain constant.

Next, locate the highest point along the vein where you can see pulsations. Using a centimeter ruler, measure the distance between that high point and the sternal notch. Record this finding as well as the angle at which the patient was lying. A finding greater than 1 1/4" to 1 1/2" (3 to 4 cm) above the sternal notch, with the head of the bed at a 45-degree angle, indicates jugular vein distention.

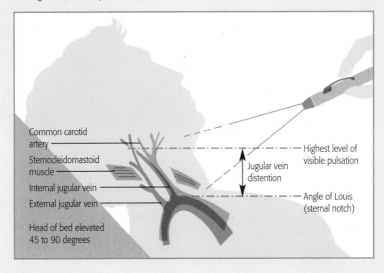

Common carotid artery

Sternocleidomastoid muscle

Internal jugular vein

External jugular vein

Head of bed elevated 45 to 90 degrees

Highest level of visible pulsation

Jugular vein distention

Angle of Louis (sternal notch)

Next, perform a physical examination, beginning with the patient's vital signs. Tachycardia, tachypnea, and increased blood pressure indicate fluid overload that's stressing the heart. Inspect and palpate the patient's extremities and face for edema. Then weigh the patient and compare that weight with his baseline.

Auscultate his lungs for crackles and his heart for gallops, a pericardial friction rub, and muffled heart sounds. Inspect his abdomen for distention, and palpate and percuss for an enlarged liver. Finally, monitor urine output and compare to fluid intake.

Medical causes

Cardiac tamponade. Cardiac tamponade is a life-threatening condition that produces jugular vein distention along with anxiety, restlessness, cyanosis, chest pain, dyspnea, hypotension, and clammy skin. It also causes tachycardia, tachypnea, muffled heart sounds, a pericardial friction rub, weak or absent peripheral pulses or pulses that decrease during inspiration (pulsus paradoxus), and hepatomegaly. The patient may sit upright or lean forward to ease breathing.

Heart failure. Sudden or gradual development of right-sided heart failure commonly causes jugular vein distention, along with weakness and anxiety, cyanosis, dependent edema of the legs and sacrum, steady weight gain, confusion, and hepatomegaly. Other findings include nausea and vomiting, abdominal discomfort, and anorexia due to visceral edema. Ascites is a late sign. Massive right-sided heart failure may produce anasarca and oliguria.

If left-sided heart failure precedes right-sided heart failure, jugular vein distention is a late sign. Other signs and symptoms include fatigue, dyspnea, orthopnea, paroxysmal nocturnal dyspnea, tachypnea, tachycardia, and arrhythmias. Auscultation reveals crackles and a ventricular gallop.

Hypervolemia. Markedly increased intravascular fluid volume causes jugular vein distention, along with rapid weight gain, elevated blood pressure, bounding pulse, peripheral edema, dyspnea, and crackles.

Pericarditis (chronic constrictive). Progressive signs and symptoms of restricted heart filling include jugular vein distention that's more prominent on inspiration (Kussmaul's sign). The patient usually complains of chest pain. Other signs and symptoms include fluid retention with dependent edema, hepatomegaly, ascites, and a pericardial friction rub.

Superior vena cava obstruction. A tumor or, rarely, thrombosis of the superior vena cava may gradually lead to jugular vein distention when the veins of the head, neck, and arms fail to empty effectively, causing facial, neck, and upper arm edema. Metastasis of a malignant tumor to the mediastinum may cause dyspnea, a cough, substernal chest pain, and hoarseness.

Nursing considerations

- If the patient has cardiac tamponade, prepare him for pericardiocentesis.
- Restrict fluids and monitor intake and output.
- Insert an indwelling urinary catheter if necessary.
- If the patient has heart failure, administer a diuretic.
- Routinely change his position to avoid skin breakdown from peripheral edema.
- Prepare the patient for central venous or pulmonary artery catheter insertion to measure right- and left-sided heart pressure and to monitor fluid status.

Patient teaching

- Explain food and fluid restrictions.
- Teach the patient to perform daily weight monitoring.
- Explain signs and symptoms that require immediate medical attention.
- Explain the importance of scheduled rest periods.

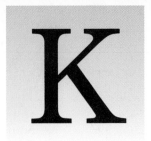

Kehr's sign

A cardinal sign of hemorrhage within the peritoneal cavity, Kehr's sign is referred left shoulder pain due to diaphragmatic irritation by intraperitoneal blood. The pain usually arises when the patient assumes the supine position or lowers his head. Such positioning increases the contact of free blood or clots with the left diaphragm, involving the phrenic nerve.

Kehr's sign usually develops right after the hemorrhage; however, its onset is sometimes delayed up to 48 hours. A classic symptom of a ruptured spleen, Kehr's sign also occurs in ruptured ectopic pregnancy.

ACTION STAT!

 After you detect Kehr's sign, quickly take the patient's vital signs. If the patient shows signs of hypovolemia, elevate his feet 30 degrees. In addition, insert a large-bore I.V. catheter for fluid and blood replacement and an indwelling urinary catheter. Begin monitoring intake and output. Draw blood to determine hematocrit, and provide supplemental oxygen.

History and physical examination

Ask the patient about recent abdominal injury. Take the patient's vital signs. Assess laboratory values of hemoglobin and hematocrit for evidence of blood loss. If Kehr's sign is detected, inspect the patient's abdomen for bruises and distention, and palpate for tenderness. Note any pain or abdominal guarding or rigidity. Percuss for Ballance's sign—an indicator of massive perisplenic clotting and free blood in the peritoneal cavity from a ruptured spleen.

Medical causes
Intra-abdominal hemorrhage.
Kehr's sign usually accompanies intense abdominal pain, abdominal rigidity, and muscle spasm that occurs with intra-abdominal hemorrhage. Other findings vary with the cause of bleeding. Many patients have a history of blunt or penetrating abdominal injuries.

Nursing considerations
- In anticipation of surgery, withhold oral intake.
- Prepare the patient for abdominal X-rays, a computed tomography scan, an ultrasound and, possibly, paracentesis, peritoneal lavage, and culdocentesis.
- Give an analgesic as ordered.

Patient teaching
- Explain all treatments to the patient.
- Discuss any food or fluid restrictions.

Kernig's sign

A reliable early indicator and tool used to diagnose meningeal irritation, Kernig's sign is hamstring stiffness and muscle pain when the examiner attempts to extend the knee while the hip and knee are flexed 90 degrees. This pain causes resistance to movement. However, when the patient's thigh isn't flexed to the abdomen, he can usually completely extend his leg. (See *Eliciting Kernig's sign*.) This sign is commonly elicited in meningitis or subarachnoid hemorrhage. With these potentially life-threatening disorders, hamstring muscle resistance results from stretching the blood- or exudate-irritated meninges surrounding spinal nerve roots.

Kernig's sign can also indicate a herniated disk or spinal tumor. With these disorders, sciatic pain results from disk or tumor pressure on spinal nerve roots.

History and physical examination
If you elicit Kernig's sign and suspect life-threatening meningitis or subarachnoid hemorrhage, immediately prepare for emergency intervention. (See *When Kernig's sign signals CNS crisis*.)

If you don't suspect meningeal irritation, ask the patient if he feels back pain that radiates down one or both legs. Does he also feel leg numbness, tingling, or weakness? Ask about other signs and symptoms, and find out if he has a history of cancer or back injury. Then perform a physical examination, concentrating on motor and sensory function.

ASSESSMENT TIP

 Eliciting Kernig's sign

To elicit Kernig's sign, place the patient in a supine position. Flex her leg at the hip and knee, as shown here. Then try to extend the leg while you keep the hip flexed. If the patient experiences pain and possibly spasm in the hamstring muscle and resists further extension, you can assume that meningeal irritation has occurred.

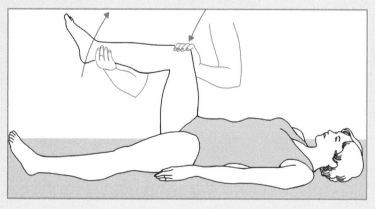

When Kernig's sign signals CNS crisis

Because Kernig's sign may signal meningitis or subarachnoid hemorrhage—life-threatening central nervous system (CNS) disorders—take the patient's vital signs at once to obtain baseline information. Then test for Brudzinski's sign to obtain further evidence of meningeal irritation. (See *Testing for Brudzinski's sign,* page 111.) Next, ask the patient or his family to describe the onset of illness. Typically, the progressive onset of a headache, a fever, nuchal rigidity, and confusion suggests meningitis. Conversely, the sudden onset of a severe headache, nuchal rigidity, photophobia and, possibly, loss of consciousness usually indicates subarachnoid hemorrhage.

Meningitis
If a diagnosis of meningitis is suspected, ask about recent infections, especially tooth abscesses. Ask about exposure to infected persons or places where meningitis is endemic. Meningitis is usually a complication of another bacterial infection, so draw blood for culture studies to determine the causative organism. Prepare the patient for a lumbar puncture (if a tumor or abscess can be ruled out). Also, find out if the patient has a history of I.V. drug abuse, an open head injury, or endocarditis. Insert an I.V. catheter, and immediately begin administering an antibiotic.

Subarachnoid hemorrhage
If subarachnoid hemorrhage is the suspected diagnosis, ask about a history of hypertension, cerebral aneurysm, head trauma, or arteriovenous malformation. Also ask about sudden withdrawal of an antihypertensive.

Check the patient's pupils for dilation, and assess him for signs of increasing intracranial pressure, such as bradycardia, increased systolic blood pressure, and a widened pulse pressure. Insert an I.V. catheter, and administer supplemental oxygen.

Medical causes
Lumbosacral herniated disk. Kernig's sign may be elicited in patients with lumbosacral herniated disk, but the cardinal and earliest feature is sciatic pain on the affected side or on both sides. Associated findings include postural deformity (lumbar lordosis or scoliosis), paresthesia, hypoactive deep tendon reflexes in the involved leg, and dorsiflexor muscle weakness.

Meningitis. Kernig's sign usually occurs early with meningitis, along with a fever and, possibly, chills. Other signs and symptoms of meningeal irritation include nuchal rigidity, hyperreflexia, Brudzinski's sign, and opisthotonos. As intracranial pressure (ICP) increases, headache and vomiting may occur. In severe meningitis, the patient may experience stupor, coma, and seizures. Cranial nerve involvement may produce ocular palsies, facial weakness, deafness, and photophobia. An erythematous maculopapular rash may occur in viral meningitis; a purpuric rash may be seen in those with meningococcal meningitis.

Spinal cord tumor. Kernig's sign can be elicited occasionally, but the earliest symptom is typically pain felt locally or along the spinal nerve, commonly in the leg. Associated findings include weakness or paralysis distal to the tumor, paresthesia, urine retention, urinary or fecal incontinence, and sexual dysfunction.

Subarachnoid hemorrhage. Kernig's and Brudzinski's signs can be elicited within minutes after the initial bleed in subarachnoid hemorrhage. The patient experiences a sudden onset of a severe headache that begins in a localized area and then spreads, pupillary inequality, nuchal rigidity, and a decreased level of consciousness. Photophobia, a fever, nausea and vomiting, dizziness, and seizures are possible. Focal signs include hemiparesis or hemiplegia, aphasia, and sensory or vision disturbances. Increasing ICP may produce bradycardia, increased blood pressure, respiratory pattern change, and rapid progression to coma.

Nursing considerations
■ Prepare the patient for diagnostic tests, such as a computed tomography scan, magnetic resonance imaging, spinal X-ray, myelography, and lumbar puncture.
■ Closely monitor the patient's vital signs, ICP, and cardiopulmonary and neurologic status.
■ Ensure bed rest, quiet environment, and minimal stress.
■ If the patient has a subarachnoid hemorrhage, darken the room and elevate the head of the bed at least 30 degrees to reduce ICP.
■ If he has a herniated disk or spinal tumor, he may require pelvic traction.

Patient teaching
■ Teach the patient and his family signs and symptoms of meningitis and treatment.
■ Discuss ways to prevent meningitis.
■ Explain activities that the patient with a herniated disk should avoid.
■ Teach the patient how to apply a back brace or cervical collar as ordered.

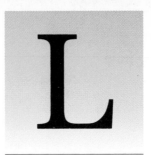

Leg pain

Although leg pain commonly signifies a musculoskeletal disorder, it can also result from a more serious vascular or neurologic disorder. The pain may arise suddenly or gradually and may be localized or affect the entire leg. Constant or intermittent, it may feel dull, burning, sharp, shooting, or tingling. Leg pain may affect locomotion, limiting weight bearing. Severe leg pain that follows cast application for a fracture may signal limb-threatening compartment syndrome. The sudden onset of severe leg pain in the patient with underlying vascular insufficiency may signal acute deterioration, possibly requiring an arterial graft or amputation. (See *Causes of local leg pain,* page 360.)

(See *Causes of local leg pain,* page 360.)

A C T I O N   S T A T !

 If the patient has acute leg pain and a history of trauma, quickly take his vital signs and determine the leg's neurovascular status. Observe the patient's leg position and check for swelling, gross deformities, or abnormal rotation. Also, be sure to check distal pulses and note skin color and temperature. A pale, cool, and pulseless leg may indicate impaired circulation, which may require emergency surgery.

History and physical examination

If the patient's condition permits, ask him when the pain began and have him describe its intensity, character, and pattern. Is the pain worse in the morning, at night, or with movement? If it doesn't prevent him from walking, must he rely on a crutch or other assistive device? Also ask him about the presence of other signs and symptoms.

Find out if the patient has a history of leg injury or surgery and if he or a family member has a history of joint, vascular, or back problems. Also ask which medications he's taking and whether they've helped to relieve his leg pain.

Begin the physical examination by watching the patient walk, if his condition permits. Observe how he holds his leg while standing and sitting. Palpate the legs, buttocks, and lower back to determine the extent of pain and tenderness. If a fracture has been ruled out, test the patient's range of motion (ROM) in the hip and knee. Also, check reflexes with the patient's leg straightened and raised, noting action that causes pain. Then compare both legs for symmetry, movement, and active ROM. Additionally, assess sensation and strength. If the patient wears a leg cast, splint, or restrictive dressing, carefully check distal

Causes of local leg pain

Various disorders cause hip, knee, ankle, or foot pain, which may radiate to surrounding tissues and be reported as leg pain. Local pain is commonly accompanied by tenderness, swelling, and deformity in the affected area.

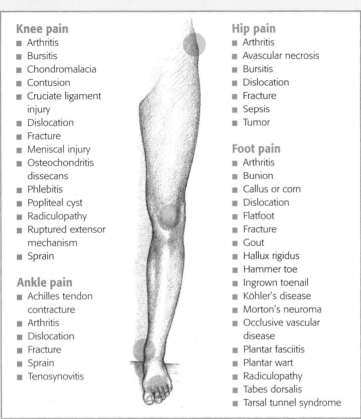

Knee pain
- Arthritis
- Bursitis
- Chondromalacia
- Contusion
- Cruciate ligament injury
- Dislocation
- Fracture
- Meniscal injury
- Osteochondritis dissecans
- Phlebitis
- Popliteal cyst
- Radiculopathy
- Ruptured extensor mechanism
- Sprain

Ankle pain
- Achilles tendon contracture
- Arthritis
- Dislocation
- Fracture
- Sprain
- Tenosynovitis

Hip pain
- Arthritis
- Avascular necrosis
- Bursitis
- Dislocation
- Fracture
- Sepsis
- Tumor

Foot pain
- Arthritis
- Bunion
- Callus or corn
- Dislocation
- Flatfoot
- Fracture
- Gout
- Hallux rigidus
- Hammer toe
- Ingrown toenail
- Köhler's disease
- Morton's neuroma
- Occlusive vascular disease
- Plantar fasciitis
- Plantar wart
- Radiculopathy
- Tabes dorsalis
- Tarsal tunnel syndrome

circulation, sensation, and mobility, and stretch his toes to elicit associated pain.

Medical causes

Bone cancer. Continuous deep or boring pain, commonly worse at night, may be the first symptom of bone cancer. Later, skin breakdown and impaired circulation may occur, along with cachexia, a fever, and impaired mobility.

Compartment syndrome. Progressive, intense lower leg pain that increases with passive muscle stretching is a cardinal sign of compartment syndrome, a limb-threatening disorder. Restrictive dressings or traction may aggravate the pain, which typically worsens despite analgesic administration. Other findings include muscle weakness and paresthesia, but apparently normal distal circulation. With irreversible muscle ischemia, paralysis and an absent pulse also occur.

Fracture. A fracture causes severe, acute pain accompanies swelling and ecchymosis in the affected leg. Movement produces extreme pain, and the leg may be unable to bear weight. Neurovascular status distal to the fracture may be impaired, causing paresthesia, an absent pulse, mottled cyanosis, and cool skin. Deformity, muscle spasms, and bony crepitation may also occur.

Infection. Local leg pain, erythema, swelling, streaking, and warmth characterize soft-tissue and bone infections. A fever and tachycardia may be present with other systemic signs.

Occlusive vascular disease. Occlusive vascular disease causes continuous cramping pain in the legs and feet that may worsen with walking, inducing claudication. The patient may report increased pain at night, cold feet, cold intolerance, numbness, and tingling. Examination may reveal ankle and lower leg edema, decreased or absent pulses, and increased capillary refill time.

Sciatica. With sciatica, pain is described as shooting, aching, or tingling and radiates down the back of the leg along the sciatic nerve. Typically, activity exacerbates the pain and rest relieves it. The patient may limp to avoid exacerbating the pain and may have difficulty moving from a sitting to a standing position.

Strain or sprain. Acute strain causes sharp, transient pain and rapid swelling, followed by leg tenderness and ecchymosis. Chronic strain produces stiffness, soreness, and generalized leg tenderness several hours after the injury; active and passive motion may be painful or impossible. A sprain causes local pain, especially during joint movement; ecchymosis and, possibly, local swelling and loss of mobility develop.

Thrombophlebitis. Thrombophebitis causes discomfort that may range from calf tenderness to severe pain and be accompanied by swelling, warmth, and a feeling of heaviness in the affected leg. The patient may also develop a fever, chills, malaise, muscle cramps, and a positive Homans' sign. Assessment may reveal superficial veins that are visibly engorged; palpable, hard, thready, and cordlike; and sensitive to pressure.

Varicose veins. With varicose veins, mild to severe leg symptoms may develop, including nocturnal cramping; a feeling of heaviness; diffuse, dull aching after prolonged standing or walking; and aching during menses. Assessment may reveal palpable nodules, orthostatic edema, and stasis pigmentation of the calves and ankles.

Venous stasis ulcer. Localized pain and bleeding arise from infected ulcerations on the lower extremities. Mottled, bluish pigmentation is characteristic, and local edema may occur.

Nursing considerations

- If the patient has acute leg pain, closely monitor his neurovascular status by frequently checking distal pulses and evaluating the legs for temperature, color, and sensation.
- Monitor thigh and calf circumference to evaluate bleeding into tissues from a possible fracture site.
- Prepare the patient for X-rays.
- Use sandbags to immobilize his leg; apply ice and, if needed, skeletal traction.
- If a fracture isn't suspected, prepare the patient for laboratory tests to detect an infectious agent or for venography, Doppler ultrasonography, plethysmography, or angiography to determine vascular competency.
- Withhold food and fluids until the need for surgery has been ruled out.
- Administer an anticoagulant and antibiotic as needed.

Patient teaching

- Explain the use of anti-inflammatory drugs, ROM exercises, and assistive devices.
- Discuss lifestyle changes that should be made.
- Teach appropriate positioning to enhance blood flow and venous return.
- Discuss the need for physical therapy.

Level of consciousness, decreased

A decrease in the level of consciousness (LOC), from lethargy to stupor to coma, usually results from a neurologic disorder and may signal a life-threatening complication, such as hemorrhage, trauma, or cerebral edema. However, this sign can also result from a metabolic, GI, musculoskeletal, urologic, or cardiopulmonary disorder; severe nutritional deficiency; the effects of toxins; or drug use. LOC can deteriorate suddenly or gradually and can remain altered temporarily or permanently.

Consciousness is affected by the reticular activating system (RAS), an intricate network of neurons with axons extending from the brain stem, thalamus, and hypothalamus to the cerebral cortex. A disturbance in any part of this integrated system prevents the intercommunication that makes consciousness possible. Loss of consciousness can result from a bilateral cerebral disturbance, an RAS disturbance, or both. Cerebral dysfunction characteristically produces the least dramatic decrease in a patient's LOC. In contrast, dysfunction of the RAS produces the most dramatic decrease in LOC—coma.

The most sensitive indicator of a decreased LOC is a change in the patient's mental status. The Glasgow Coma Scale, which measures a patient's ability to respond to verbal, sensory, and motor stimulation, can be used to quickly evaluate a patient's LOC.

 After evaluating the patient's airway, breathing, and circulation, use the Glasgow Coma Scale to quickly determine his LOC and to obtain baseline data. (See *Glasgow Coma Scale*.) Insert an artificial airway, elevate the head of the bed 30 degrees and, if spinal cord injury has been ruled out, turn the patient's head to the side. Prepare to suction the patient if necessary. You may need to hyperventilate him to reduce carbon dioxide levels and decrease intracranial pressure (ICP). Then determine the rate, rhythm, and depth of spontaneous respirations. Support his breathing with a handheld resuscitation bag, if necessary. If the patient's Glasgow Coma Scale score is less than 9, endotracheal intubation and resuscitation may be necessary.

Continue to monitor the patient's vital signs, being alert for signs of increasing ICP, such as bradycardia and a widening pulse pressure. When his airway, breathing, and circulation are stabilized, perform a neurologic examination.

History and physical examination

Try to obtain history information from the patient, if he's alert, and from his family. Did the patient complain of a headache, dizziness, nausea, vision or hearing disturbances, weakness, fatigue, or other problems before his LOC decreased? Has his family noticed changes in the patient's behavior, personality, memory, or temperament? Also ask about a history of neurologic disease, cancer, or recent trauma or infections; drug and alcohol use; and the development of other signs and symptoms.

Glasgow Coma Scale

You've probably heard such terms as *lethargic, obtunded,* and *stuporous* used to describe a progressive decrease in a patient's level of consciousness (LOC). However, the Glasgow Coma Scale provides a more accurate, less subjective method of recording such changes, grading consciousness in relation to eye opening and motor and verbal responses.

To use the Glasgow Coma Scale, test the patient's ability to respond to verbal, motor, and sensory stimulation. The scoring system doesn't determine the exact LOC, but it does provide an easy way to describe the patient's basic status and helps to detect and interpret changes from baseline findings. A decreased reaction score in one or more categories may signal an impending neurologic crisis. A total score of less than 9 indicates severe brain damage.

Test	Reaction	Score
Eye opening response	Open spontaneously	4
	Open to verbal command	3
	Open to pain	2
	No response	1
Best motor response	Obeys verbal command	6
	Localizes painful stimulus	5
	Flexion—withdrawal	4
	Flexion—abnormal (decorticate rigidity)	3
	Extension (decerebrate rigidity)	2
	No response	1
Best verbal response	Oriented and converses	5
	Disoriented and converses	4
	Inappropriate words	3
	Incomprehensible sounds	2
	No response	1
Total		3 to 15

Because a decreased LOC can result from a disorder affecting any body system, tailor the remainder of your evaluation according to the patient's associated symptoms.

Medical causes

Adrenal crisis. A decreased LOC, ranging from lethargy to coma, may develop within 8 to 12 hours of the onset of adrenal crisis. Early associated findings include progressive weakness, irritability, anorexia, a headache, nausea and vomiting, diarrhea, abdominal pain, and a fever. Later signs and symptoms include hypotension; a rapid, thready pulse; oliguria; cool, clammy skin; and flaccid extremities. The patient with chronic adrenocortical hypofunction may have hyperpigmented skin and mucous membranes.

Brain abscess. With a brain abscess, decreased LOC varies from drowsiness to deep stupor, depending on the abscess size and site. Early signs and symptoms—a constant intractable headache, nausea, vomiting, and seizures—reflect increasing ICP. Typical later features include ocular disturbances (nystagmus, vision loss, and pupillary inequality) and signs of infection such as a fever. Other findings may include personality changes, confusion, abnormal behavior, dizziness, facial weakness, aphasia, ataxia, tremor, and hemiparesis.

Brain tumor. With a brain tumor, the patient's LOC decreases slowly, from lethargy to coma. He may also experience apathy, behavior changes, memory loss, a decreased attention span, a morning headache, dizziness, vision loss, ataxia, and sensorimotor disturbances. Aphasia and seizures are possible, along with signs of hormonal imbalance, such as fluid retention or amenorrhea. Signs and symptoms vary according to the location and size of the tumor. In later stages, papilledema, vomiting, bradycardia, and a widening pulse pressure also appear. In the final stages, the patient may exhibit decorticate or decerebrate posture.

Cerebral aneurysm (ruptured). Somnolence, confusion and, at times, stupor characterize a moderate cerebral bleed; deep coma occurs with severe bleeding, which can be fatal. The onset is usually abrupt, with a sudden, severe headache and nausea and vomiting. Nuchal rigidity, back and leg pain, a fever, restlessness, irritability, occasional seizures, and blurred vision point to meningeal irritation. The type and severity of other findings vary with the site and severity of the hemorrhage and may include hemiparesis, hemisensory defects, dysphagia, and visual defects.

Diabetic ketoacidosis. Diabetic ketoacidosis produces a rapid decrease in the patient's LOC, ranging from lethargy to coma, commonly preceded by polydipsia, polyphagia, and polyuria. The patient may complain of weakness, anorexia, abdominal pain, nausea, and vomiting. He may also exhibit orthostatic hypotension; a fruity breath odor; Kussmaul's respirations; warm, dry skin; and a rapid, thready pulse. Untreated, this condition invariably leads to coma and death.

Encephalitis. Within 24 to 48 hours after onset of encephalitis, the patient may develop changes in his LOC ranging from lethargy to coma. Other possible findings include an abrupt onset of a fever, a headache, nuchal rigidity, nausea, vomiting, irritability, personality changes, seizures, aphasia, ataxia, hemiparesis, nystagmus, photophobia, myoclonus, and cranial nerve palsies.

Encephalomyelitis (postvaccinal). Postvaccinal encephalomyelitis is a life-threatening disorder that produces rapid deterioration in the patient's LOC, from drowsiness to coma. He also experiences a rapid onset of a fever, a headache, nuchal rigidity, back pain, vomiting, and seizures.

Encephalopathy. With *hepatic encephalopathy,* signs and symptoms develop in four stages: in the prodromal stage, slight personality changes (disorientation, forgetfulness, slurred speech) and slight tremor; in the impending stage, tremor progressing to asterixis (the hallmark of hepatic encephalopathy), lethargy, aberrant behavior, and apraxia; in the stuporous stage, stupor and hyperventilation, with the patient noisy and abusive when aroused; in the comatose stage, coma with decerebrate posture, hyperactive reflexes, a positive Babinski's reflex, and fetor hepaticus.

With *life-threatening hypertensive encephalopathy,* the LOC progressively decreases from lethargy to stupor to coma. Besides markedly elevated blood pressure, the patient may experience a severe headache, vomiting, seizures, vision disturbances, transient paralysis and, eventually, Cheyne-Stokes respirations.

With *hypoglycemic encephalopathy,* the patient's LOC rapidly deteriorates from lethargy to coma. Early signs and symptoms include nervousness, restlessness, agitation, and confusion; hunger; alternate flushing and cold sweats; and a headache, trembling, and palpitations. Blurred vision progresses to motor weakness, hemiplegia, dilated pupils, pallor, a decreased pulse rate, shallow respirations, and seizures. Flaccidity and decerebrate posture appear late.

Depending on its severity, *hypoxic encephalopathy* produces a sudden or gradual decrease in the LOC, leading to coma and brain death. Initially, the patient appears confused and restless, with cyanosis and increased heart and respiratory rates and blood pressure. Later, his respiratory pattern becomes abnormal, and assessment reveals a decreased pulse, blood pressure, and deep tendon reflexes (DTRs); a positive Babinski's reflex; an absent doll's eye sign; and fixed pupils.

With *uremic encephalopathy,* the LOC decreases gradually from lethargy to coma. Initially, the patient may appear apathetic, inattentive, confused, and irritable and may complain of a headache, nausea, fatigue, and anorexia. Other findings include vomiting, tremors, edema, papilledema, hypertension, cardiac arrhythmias, dyspnea, crackles, oliguria, and Kussmaul's and Cheyne-Stokes respirations.

Heatstroke. With heatstroke, as body temperature increases, the patient's LOC gradually decreases from lethargy to coma. Early signs and symptoms include malaise, tachycardia, tachypnea, orthostatic hypotension, muscle cramps, rigidity, and syncope. The patient may be irritable, anxious, and dizzy and may report a severe headache. At the onset of heatstroke, the patient's skin is hot,

flushed, and diaphoretic with blotchy cyanosis; later, when his fever exceeds 105° F (40.5° C), his skin becomes hot, flushed, and anhidrotic. Pulse and respiratory rate increase markedly, and blood pressure drops precipitously. Other findings include vomiting, diarrhea, dilated pupils, and Cheyne-Stokes respirations.

Hypernatremia. Hypernatremia, life-threatening if acute, causes the patient's LOC to deteriorate from lethargy to coma. He's irritable and exhibits twitches progressing to seizures. Other associated signs and symptoms include a weak, thready pulse; nausea; malaise; a fever; thirst; flushed skin; and dry mucous membranes.

Hyperosmolar hyperglycemic nonketotic syndrome (HHNS). LOC decreases rapidly from lethargy to coma with HHNS. Early findings include polyuria, polydipsia, weight loss, and weakness. Later, the patient may develop hypotension, poor skin turgor, dry skin and mucous membranes, tachycardia, tachypnea, oliguria, and seizures.

Hypokalemia. LOC gradually decreases to lethargy with hypokalemia; coma is rare. Other findings include confusion, nausea, vomiting, diarrhea, and polyuria; weakness, decreased reflexes, and malaise; and dizziness, hypotension, arrhythmias, and abnormal electrocardiogram results.

Hyponatremia. Hyponatremia, life-threatening if acute, produces a decreased LOC in late stages. Early nausea and malaise may progress to behavior changes, confusion, lethargy, incoordination and, eventually, seizures and coma.

Hypothermia. With severe hypothermia (temperature below 90° F [32.2° C]), the patient's LOC decreases from lethargy to coma. DTRs disappear, and ventricular fibrillation occurs, possibly followed by cardiopulmonary arrest. With mild to moderate hypothermia, the patient may experience memory loss and slurred speech as well as shivering, weakness, fatigue, and apathy. Other early signs and symptoms include ataxia, muscle stiffness, and hyperactive DTRs; diuresis; tachycardia and decreased respiratory rate and blood pressure; and cold, pale skin. Later, muscle rigidity and decreased reflexes may develop, along with peripheral cyanosis, bradycardia, arrhythmias, severe hypotension, a decreased respiratory rate with shallow respirations, and oliguria.

Intracerebral hemorrhage. Intracerebral hemorrhage is a life-threatening disorder that produces a rapid, steady loss of consciousness within hours, commonly accompanied by a severe headache, dizziness, nausea, and vomiting. Associated signs and symptoms vary and may include increased blood pressure, irregular respirations, a positive Babinski's reflex, seizures, aphasia, decreased sensations, hemiplegia, decorticate or decerebrate posture, and dilated pupils.

Listeriosis. If listeriosis spreads to the nervous system and causes meningitis, signs and symptoms include a decreased LOC, a fever, a headache, and nuchal rigidity. Early signs and symptoms of listeriosis include a fever, myalgia, abdominal pain, nausea, vomiting, and diarrhea.

Meningitis. Confusion and irritability are expected; however, stupor, coma, and seizures may occur in the patient with severe meningitis. A fever develops early, possibly accompanied by chills. Associated findings include a severe headache, nuchal rigidity, hyperreflexia and, possibly, opisthotonos. The patient exhibits Kernig's and Brudzinski's signs and, possibly, ocular palsies, photophobia, facial weakness, and hearing loss.

Pontine hemorrhage. A sudden, rapid decrease in the patient's LOC to the point of coma occurs within minutes and death within hours of pontine hemorrhage. The patient may also exhibit total paralysis, decerebrate posture, a positive Babinski's reflex, an absent doll's eye sign, and bilateral miosis (however, the pupils remain reactive to light).

Seizure disorders. A *complex partial seizure* produces a decreased LOC, manifested as a blank stare, purposeless behavior (picking at clothing, wandering, lip smacking or chewing motions), and unintelligible speech. The seizure may be heralded by an aura and followed by several minutes of mental confusion.

An *absence seizure* usually involves a brief change in the patient's LOC, indicated by blinking or eye rolling, a blank stare, and slight mouth movements.

A *generalized tonic-clonic seizure* typically begins with a loud cry and sudden loss of consciousness. Muscle spasm alternates with relaxation. Tongue biting, incontinence, labored breathing, apnea, and cyanosis may also occur. Consciousness returns after the seizure, but the patient remains confused and may have difficulty talking. He may complain of drowsiness, fatigue, a headache, muscle aching, and weakness and may fall into a deep sleep.

An *atonic seizure* produces sudden unconsciousness for a few seconds.

Status epilepticus, rapidly recurring seizures without intervening periods of physiologic recovery and return of consciousness, can be life-threatening.

Shock. A decreased LOC—lethargy progressing to stupor and coma—occurs late in shock. Associated findings include confusion, anxiety, and restlessness; hypotension; tachycardia; a weak pulse with narrowing pulse pressure; dyspnea; oliguria; and cool, clammy skin.

Hypovolemic shock is generally the result of massive or insidious bleeding, either internally or externally. Cardiogenic shock may produce chest pain or arrhythmias and signs of heart failure, such as dyspnea, a cough, edema, jugular vein distention, and weight gain. Septic shock may be accompanied by a high fever and chills. Anaphylactic shock usually involves stridor in response to an allergen.

Stroke. When a stroke occurs, changes in the patient's LOC vary in degree and onset, depending on the lesion's size and location and the presence of edema. A thrombotic stroke usually follows multiple transient ischemic attacks (TIAs) or an episode of atrial fibrillation. Changes in the LOC may be abrupt or take several minutes, hours, or days. An embolic stroke occurs suddenly, and deficits reach their peak almost at once. Deficits associated with a hemorrhagic stroke usually develop over minutes or hours.

Associated findings vary with the stroke type and severity and may include disorientation; intellectual deficits, such as memory loss and poor judgment; personality changes; and emotional lability. Other possible findings include dysarthria, dysphagia, ataxia, aphasia, apraxia, agnosia, unilateral sensorimotor loss, and vision disturbances. In addition, urine retention, incontinence, constipation, a headache, vomiting, and seizures may occur.

Subdural hemorrhage (acute). Acute subdural hemorrhage is a potentially life-threatening disorder in which agitation and confusion are followed by a progressively decreasing LOC from somnolence to coma. The patient may also experience a headache, a fever, unilateral pupil dilation, decreased pulse and respiratory rates, a widening pulse pressure, seizures, hemiparesis, and a positive Babinski's reflex.

Thyroid storm. The patient's LOC decreases suddenly with thyroid storm and can progress to coma. Irritability, restlessness, confusion, and psychotic behavior precede the deterioration. Associated signs and symptoms include tremors and weakness; vision disturbances; tachycardia, arrhythmias, angina, and acute respiratory distress; warm, moist, flushed skin; and vomiting, diarrhea, and a fever of up to 105° F (40.5° C).

TIA. When a TIA occurs, the patient's LOC decreases abruptly (with varying severity) and gradually returns to normal within 24 hours. Site-specific findings may include vision loss, nystagmus, aphasia, dizziness, dysarthria, unilateral hemiparesis or hemiplegia, tinnitus, paresthesia, dysphagia, or staggering or incoordinated gait.

West Nile encephalitis. Signs and symptoms of West Nile encephalitis include fever, headache, and body aches, commonly with a skin rash and swollen lymph glands. More severe infection is marked by high fever, headache, neck stiffness, stupor, disorientation, coma, tremors, occasional seizures, paralysis and, rarely, death.

Other causes

Alcohol. Alcohol use causes varying degrees of sedation, irritability, and incoordination; intoxication commonly causes stupor.

Drugs. Sedation and other degrees of a decreased LOC can result from an overdose of a barbiturate, another central nervous system depressant, or aspirin.

Nursing considerations
- Reassess the patient's LOC and neurologic status at least hourly.
- Carefully monitor ICP and intake and output.
- Ensure airway patency and proper nutrition.
- Keep the patient on bed rest and maintain seizure precautions.

■ Keep emergency resuscitation equipment at the patient's bedside.

■ Prepare the patient for a computed tomography scan of the head, magnetic resonance imaging of the brain, EEG, and lumbar puncture.

■ Elevate the head of the bed to at least 30 degrees.

■ Don't administer an opioid or sedative because either may further decrease the patient's LOC and hinder an accurate, meaningful neurologic examination.

■ Talk to the patient even if he appears comatose; your voice may help reorient him to reality.

Patient teaching

■ Explain the underlying cause of decreased LOC and its treatments and procedures to the patient and his family.

■ Teach them about safety and seizure precautions.

■ Provide referrals to sources of support.

■ Discuss quality of life issues, if appropriate.

Light flashes
[Photopsias]

A cardinal symptom of vision-threatening retinal detachment, light flashes can occur locally or throughout the visual field. The patient usually reports seeing spots, stars, or lightning-type streaks. Flashes can occur suddenly or gradually and can indicate temporary or permanent vision impairment.

In most cases, light flashes signal the splitting of the posterior vitreous membrane into two layers; the inner layer detaches from the retina, and the outer layer remains fixed to it. The sensation of light flashes may result from vitreous traction on the retina, hemorrhage caused by a tear in the retinal capillary, or strands of solid vitreous floating in a local pool of liquid vitreous.

ACTION STAT!

If light flashes occur suddenly, restrict the patient's eye and body movement until retinal detachment is ruled out.

History and physical examination

Ask the patient when the light flashes began. Can he pinpoint their location, or do they occur throughout the visual field? If the patient is experiencing eye pain or a headache, have him describe it. Ask if the patient wears or has ever worn corrective lenses and if he or a family member has a history of eye or vision problems. Also ask if the patient has other medical problems—especially hypertension or diabetes mellitus, which can cause retinopathy and, possibly, retinal detachment. Obtain an occupational history because light flashes may be related to job stress or eye strain.

Next, perform a complete eye and vision examination, especially if trauma is apparent or suspected. Begin by inspecting the external eye, lids, lashes, and tear puncta for abnormalities and the iris and sclera for signs of bleeding. Observe pupillary size and shape; check for reaction to light, accommodation, and consensual light response. Then test visual acuity in each eye. Also test visual fields; document any light flashes that the patient reports during this test.

Medical causes

Head trauma. A patient who has sustained minor head trauma may report "seeing stars" when the injury occurs. He may also complain of localized pain at the injury site, a generalized headache, and dizziness. Later, he may develop nausea, vomiting, and a decreased level of consciousness.

Migraine headache. Light flashes—possibly accompanied by an aura—may herald a classic migraine headache. As these symptoms subside, the patient typically experiences a severe, throbbing, unilateral headache that usually lasts 1 to 12 hours and may be accompanied by paresthesia of the lips, face, or hands; slight confusion; dizziness; photophobia; nausea; and vomiting.

Retinal detachment. Light flashes described as floaters or spots are localized in the portion of the visual field where the retina is detaching. With macular involvement, the patient may experience painless vision impairment resembling a curtain covering the visual field.

Vitreous detachment. Visual floaters may accompany a sudden onset of light flashes. Usually, just one eye is affected.

Nursing considerations

■ If the patient has retinal detachment, prepare him for reattachment surgery.
■ If the patient doesn't have retinal detachment, reassure him that the light flashes are temporary and don't indicate eye damage.
■ For the patient with a migraine headache, maintain a quiet, darkened environment; encourage sleep; and administer an analgesic as ordered.

Patient teaching

■ Explain that after surgery the patient may need to wear bilateral eye patches.
■ Explain any activity and position restrictions that may be required.

Low birth weight

Two groups of neonates are born weighing less than the normal minimum birth weight of 5½ lb (2,500 g)—those who are born prematurely (before 37 weeks' gestation) and those who are small for gestational age (SGA). Premature neonates weigh an appropriate amount for their gestational age and probably would have matured normally if carried to term. Conversely, SGA neonates weigh less than normal for their age; however, their organs are mature. Differentiating between the two groups helps direct the search for a cause.

In the premature neonate, low birth weight usually results from a disorder that prevents the uterus from retaining the fetus, interferes with the normal course of pregnancy, causes premature separation of the placenta, or stimulates uterine contractions before term. In the SGA neonate, intrauterine growth may be retarded by a disorder that interferes with placental circulation, fetal development, or maternal health. (See *Maternal causes of low birth weight.*)

Regardless of cause, low birth weight is associated with higher neonate mor-

---

Maternal causes of low birth weight

If the neonate is small for his gestational age, consider these possible maternal causes:
■ acquired immunodeficiency syndrome
■ alcohol or opioid abuse
■ chronic maternal illness
■ cigarette smoking
■ hypertension
■ hypoxemia
■ malnutrition
■ toxemia.
If the neonate is born prematurely, consider these common maternal causes:
■ abruptio placentae
■ amnionitis
■ cocaine or crack use
■ incompetent cervix
■ placenta previa
■ polyhydramnios
■ preeclampsia
■ premature rupture of membranes
■ severe maternal illness
■ urinary tract infection.

Ballard Scale for calculating gestational age

NEUROMUSCULAR MATURITY

NEUROMUSCULAR MATURITY SIGN	SCORE							RECORD SCORE HERE
	– 1	0	1	2	3	4	5	
POSTURE	–						–	
SQUARE WINDOW (Wrist)	>90°	90°	60°	45°	30°	0°	–	
ARM RECOIL	–	180°	140° to 180°	110° to 140°	90° to 100°	<90°	–	
POPLITEAL ANGLE	180°	160°	140°	120°	100°	90°	<90°	
SCARF SIGN							–	
HEEL TO EAR							–	

TOTAL NEUROMUSCULAR MATURITY SCORE

PHYSICAL MATURITY

PHYSICAL MATURITY SIGN	SCORE							RECORD SCORE HERE
	–1	0	1	2	3	4	5	
SKIN	Sticky, friable, transparent	Gelatinous, red, translucent	Smooth, pink; visible vessels	Superficial peeling or rash; few visible vessels	Cracking; pale areas; rare visible vessels	Parchment-like; deep cracking; no visible vessels	Leathery, cracked, wrinkled	
LANUGO	None	Sparse	Abundant	Thinning	Bald areas	Mostly bald		
PLANTAR SURFACE	Heel-toe 40 to 50 mm: –1; <40 mm: –2	>50 mm; no crease	Faint red marks	Anterior transverse crease only	Creases over anterior two-thirds	Creases over entire sole	–	
BREAST	Imperceptible	Barely perceptible	Flat areola, no bud	Stippled areola; 1- to 2-mm bud	Raised areola; 3- to 4-mm bud	Full areola; 5- to 10-mm bud	–	
EYE AND EAR	Lids fused, loosely: –1; tightly: –2	Lids open; pinna flat, stays folded	Slightly curved pinna; soft, slow recoil	Well-curved pinna; soft but ready recoil	Formed and firm; instant recoil	Thick cartilage; ear stiff	–	
GENITALIA, (Male)	Scrotum flat, smooth	Scrotum empty; faint rugae	Testes in upper canal; rare rugae	Testes descending; few rugae	Testes down; good rugae	Testes pendulous; deep rugae	–	
GENITALIA, (Female)	Clitoris prominent; labia flat	Prominent clitoris; small labia minora	Prominent clitoris; enlarging minora	Majora and minora equally prominent	Majora large; minora small	Majora cover clitoris and minora	–	

TOTAL PHYSICAL MATURITY SCORE

SCORE

Neuromuscular _____

Physical _____

Total _____

MATURITY RATING

TOTAL MATURITY SCORE	GESTATIONAL AGE (WEEKS)
–10	20
–5	22
0	24
5	26
10	28
15	30
20	32
25	34
30	36
35	38
40	40
45	42
50	44

GESTATIONAL AGE (Weeks)

By dates _____

By ultrasound _____

By score _____

Adapted with permission from Ballard, J.L. "New Ballard Score Expanded to Include Extremely Premature Infants," *Journal of Pediatrics* 119(3):417-23, 1991.

bidity and mortality; in fact, these neonates are 20 times more likely to die within the first month of life. Low birth weight can also signal a life-threatening emergency.

SGA neonates who will demonstrate catch-up growth do so by 8 to 12 months. Some SGA neonates will remain below the 10th percentile. Weight of the premature neonate should be corrected for gestational age by approximately 24 months.

ACTION STAT!

 Because low birth weight may be associated with poorly developed body systems, particularly the respiratory system, monitor the neonate's respiratory status. Be alert for signs of distress, such as apnea, grunting respirations, intercostal or xiphoid retractions, or a respiratory rate exceeding 60 breaths/minute after the first hour of life. If you detect any of these signs, prepare to provide respiratory support. Endotracheal intubation or supplemental oxygen with an oxygen hood may be needed.

Monitor the neonate's axillary temperature. Decreased fat reserves may keep him from maintaining normal body temperature, and a drop below 97.8° F (36.5° C) exacerbates respiratory distress by increasing oxygen consumption. To maintain normal body temperature, use an overbed warmer or an Isolette. (If these are unavailable, use a wrapped rubber bottle filled with warm water, but be careful to avoid hyperthermia.) Cover the neonate's head to prevent heat loss.

History and physical examination

As soon as possible, evaluate the neonate's neuromuscular and physical maturity to determine gestational age. (See *Ballard Scale for calculating gestational age.*) Follow with a routine neonatal examination.

Medical causes

This section lists some fetal and placental causes of low birth weight as well as the associated signs and symptoms present in the neonate at birth.

Chromosomal aberrations. Abnormalities in the number, size, or configuration of chromosomes can cause low birth weight and possibly multiple congenital anomalies in a premature or SGA neonate. For example, a neonate with trisomy 21 (Down syndrome) may be SGA and have prominent epicanthal folds, a flat-bridged nose, a protruding tongue, palmar simian creases, muscular hypotonia, and an umbilical hernia.

Cytomegalovirus infection. Although low birth weight in cytomegalovirus infection is usually associated with premature birth, the neonate may be SGA. Assessment at birth may reveal these classic signs: petechiae and ecchymoses, jaundice, and hepatosplenomegaly, which increases for several days. The neonate may also have a high fever, lymphadenopathy, tachypnea, and dyspnea, along with prolonged bleeding at puncture sites.

Placental dysfunction. With placental dysfunction, low birth weight and a wasted appearance occur in an SGA neonate. He may be symmetrically short or may appear relatively long for his low weight. Additional findings reflect the underlying cause. For example, if maternal hyperparathyroidism caused placental dysfunction, the neonate may exhibit muscle jerking and twitching, carpopedal spasm, ankle clonus, vomiting, tachycardia, and tachypnea.

Rubella (congenital). Usually, the low-birth-weight neonate with congenital rubella is born at term but is SGA. A characteristic "blueberry muffin" rash accompanies cataracts, purpuric lesions, hepatosplenomegaly, and a large anterior fontanel. Abnormal heart sounds, if present, vary with the type of associated congenital heart defect.

Varicella (congenital). With congenital varicella, low birth weight is accompanied by cataracts and skin vesicles.

Nursing considerations

- Initiate feedings as soon as possible and continue to feed the neonate every 2 to 3 hours.
- Provide gavage or I.V. nutrition for the sick or very premature neonate.
- Check abdominal girth daily or more frequently if indicated, and check stools for blood to detect necrotizing enterocolitis.
- Prepare for a sepsis workup if signs of infection are associated with low birth weight.
- Check the neonate's vital signs every 15 minutes for the first hour and at least once every hour thereafter until his condition stabilizes.
- Be alert for changes in temperature or behavior, feeding problems, respiratory distress, or periods of apnea—possible indications of infection.
- Monitor blood glucose levels and watch for signs and symptoms of hypoglycemia, such as irritability, jitteriness, tremors, seizures, irregular respirations, lethargy, and a high-pitched or weak cry.
- If the neonate is receiving supplemental oxygen, carefully monitor arterial blood gas values and the oxygen concentration of inspired air to prevent retinopathy.
- Monitor the neonate's urine output by weighing diapers before and after voiding.
- Check urine color, measure specific gravity, and test for the presence of glucose, blood, or protein.
- Watch for changes in the neonate's skin color because increasing jaundice may indicate hyperbilirubinemia.

Patient teaching

- Explain disorder and all procedures and treatments to the parents.
- Encourage the parents to participate in their neonate's care to strengthen bonding.

Lymphadenopathy

Lymphadenopathy—enlargement of one or more lymph nodes—may result from increased production of lymphocytes or reticuloendothelial cells or from infiltration of cells that aren't normally present. This sign may be generalized (involving three or more node groups) or localized. Generalized lymphadenopathy may be caused by an inflammatory process, such as bacterial or viral infection, connective tissue disease, an endocrine disorder, or neoplasm. Localized lymphadenopathy most commonly results from infection or trauma affecting a specific area. (See *Areas of localized lymphadenopathy,* page 374, and *Causes of localized lymphadenopathy,* page 375.)

Normally, lymph nodes are discrete, mobile, soft, nontender and, except in children, nonpalpable. (However, palpable nodes may be normal in adults.) Nodes that are more than ⅜″ (1 cm) in diameter are cause for concern. They may be tender, and the skin overlying the lymph node may be erythematous, suggesting a draining lesion. Alternatively, they may be hard and fixed, tender or nontender, suggesting a malignant tumor.

History and physical examination

Ask the patient when he first noticed the swelling and whether it's located on one side of his body or both. Are the swollen areas sore, hard, or red? Ask the patient if he has recently had an infection or other health problem. Also ask if a biopsy has ever been done on any node because this may indicate a previously diagnosed cancer. Find out if the patient has a family history of cancer.

Palpate the entire lymph node system to determine the extent of lymphadenopathy and to detect other areas of local enlargement. Use the pads of your index and middle fingers to move the skin over underlying tissues at the nodal area. If you detect enlarged nodes, note their size in centimeters and whether they're fixed or mobile, tender or nontender, and erythematous or not. Note their texture: Is the node discrete, or does the area feel matted? If you detect tender, erythematous lymph nodes, check the area drained by that part of the lymph system for signs of infection, such as erythema and swelling. Also, palpate for and percuss the spleen.

Medical causes

Acquired immunodeficiency syndrome (AIDS). Besides lymphadenopathy, findings with AIDS include a history of fatigue, night sweats, afternoon fevers, diarrhea, weight loss, and a cough with several concurrent infections appearing soon afterward.

Anthrax (cutaneous). Lymphadenopathy, malaise, headache, and fever may develop with cutaneous anthrax, along with a lesion that progresses into a painless, necrotic-centered ulcer.

Brucellosis. With brucellosis, generalized lymphadenopathy usually affects cervical and axillary lymph nodes, making them tender. It usually begins insidiously with easy fatigability, malaise, a headache, backache, anorexia, weight loss, and arthralgia; it may also begin abruptly with chills, a fever that usually rises in the morning and subsides during the day, and diaphoresis.

Cytomegalovirus infection (CMV). CMV causes generalized lymphadenopathy occurs in the immunocompromised

Areas of localized lymphadenopathy

When you detect an enlarged lymph node, palpate the entire lymph node system to determine the extent of lymphadenopathy. Include the lymph nodes indicated here in your assessment.

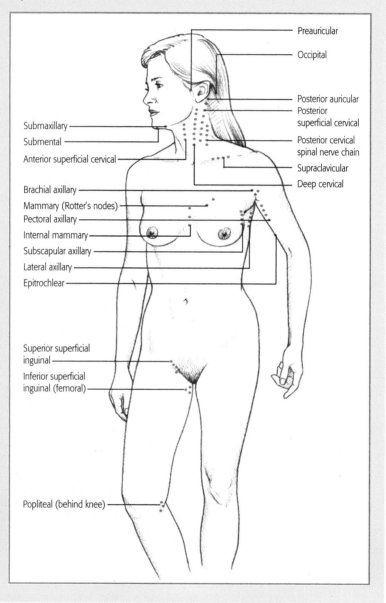

Causes of localized lymphadenopathy

Various disorders can cause localized lymphadenopathy, but this sign usually results from infection or trauma affecting the specific area. Here you'll find some common causes of lymphadenopathy listed according to the areas affected.

Auricular

- Erysipelas
- Herpes zoster ophthalmicus
- Infection
- Rubella
- Squamous cell carcinoma
- Styes or chalazion
- Tularemia

Axillary

- Breast cancer
- Infection
- Lymphoma
- Mastitis

Cervical

- Cat-scratch fever
- Facial or oral cancer
- Infection
- Mononucleosis
- Mucocutaneous lymph node syndrome
- Rubella
- Rubeola
- Thyrotoxicosis
- Tonsillitis
- Tuberculosis
- Varicella

Inguinal and femoral

- Carcinoma
- Chancroid
- Infection
- Lymphogranuloma venereum
- Syphilis

Occipital

- Infection
- Roseola
- Scalp infection
- Seborrheic dermatitis
- Tick bite
- Tinea capitis

Popliteal

- Infection

Submaxillary and submental

- Cystic fibrosis
- Dental infection
- Gingivitis
- Glossitis
- Infection

Supraclavicular

- Infection
- Neoplastic disease

patient and is accompanied by fever, malaise, rash, and hepatosplenomegaly.

Hodgkin's disease. The extent of lymphadenopathy with Hodgkin's disease reflects the stage of malignancy—from stage I involvement of a single lymph node region to stage IV generalized lymphadenopathy. Common early signs and symptoms include pruritus and, in older patients, fatigue, weakness, night sweats, malaise, weight loss, and an unexplained fever (usually up to 101° F [38.3° C]). Also, if mediastinal lymph nodes enlarge, tracheal and esophageal pressure produces dyspnea and dysphagia.

Kawasaki syndrome. Cervical lymphadenopathy is a characteristic sign of Kawasaki syndrome, a potentially life-threatening illness. Affected individuals present with a high, spiking fever, along with other diagnostic signs including erythema, bilateral conjunctival injection, and swelling in the peripheral extremities. Kawasaki syndrome isn't contagious, however the cause remains unknown and the disease typically affects children under age 5. Prompt detection and treatment with I.V. gamma globulin is essential in preventing serious complications, such as coronary artery dilations and aneurysms.

Leptospirosis. Lymphadenopathy is uncommon in leptospirosis, a rare disease. More common findings include a sudden onset of a fever and chills, malaise, myalgia, a headache, nausea and vomiting, and abdominal pain.

Leukemia (acute lymphocytic). With acute lymphocytic leukemia, generalized lymphadenopathy is accompanied by fatigue, malaise, pallor, and a low-grade fever. The patient also experiences prolonged bleeding time, swollen gums, weight loss, bone or joint pain, and hepatosplenomegaly.

Leukemia (chronic lymphocytic). With chronic lymphocytic leukemia, generalized lymphadenopathy appears early, along with fatigue, malaise, and a fever. As the disease progresses, hepatosplenomegaly, severe fatigue, and weight loss occur. Other late findings include bone tenderness, edema, pallor, dyspnea, tachycardia, palpitations, bleeding, anemia, and macular or nodular lesions.

Lyme disease. Spread by the bite of certain ticks, Lyme disease begins with a skin lesion called *erythema chronicum migrans*. As the disease progresses, the patient may suffer from lymphadenopathy, constant malaise and fatigue, an intermittent headache, a fever, chills, and aches. He may go on to develop arthralgia and, eventually, neurologic and cardiac abnormalities.

Monkeypox. Lymphadenopathy is the one symptom that clearly distinguishes monkeypox from smallpox. Humans infected with monkeypox usually develop cervical or inguinal lymphadenopathy, along with other characteristic symptoms such as fever, chills, throat pain, muscle aches, and rash. This rare viral disease acquired its name after being discovered in laboratory monkeys; however, many other animals can carry this disease. Although the monkeypox virus is similar to smallpox, the smallpox vaccine is only used in limited circumstances to protect certain at-risk individuals against the disease.

Mononucleosis (infectious). With infectious mononucleosis, characteristic, painful lymphadenopathy involves cervical, axillary, and inguinal nodes. Posterior cervical adenopathy is also common. Typically, prodromal symptoms—such as a headache, malaise, and fatigue—occur 3 to 5 days before the appearance of the classic triad of lymphadenopathy, a sore throat, and temperature fluctuations with an evening peak of about 102° F (38.9° C). Hepatosplenomegaly may develop, along with findings of stomatitis, exudative tonsillitis, or pharyngitis.

Mycosis fungoides. Lymphadenopathy occurs in stage III of mycosis fungoides, a rare, chronic malignant lymphoma. It's accompanied by ulcerated brownish red tumors that are painful and itchy.

Non-Hodgkin's lymphoma. Painless enlargement of one or more peripheral lymph nodes is the most common sign of non-Hodgkin's lymphoma, with generalized lymphadenopathy characterizing stage IV. Dyspnea, a cough, and hepatosplenomegaly occur, along with systemic complaints of a fever of up to 101° F (38.3° C), night sweats, fatigue, malaise, and weight loss.

Plague (Yersinia pestis). Signs and symptoms of the bubonic form of plague, a bacterial infection, include lymphadenopathy, a fever, and chills.

Rheumatoid arthritis. Lymphadenopathy is an early, nonspecific finding in rheumatoid arthritis and is associated with fatigue, malaise, a continuous low-grade fever, weight loss, and vague arthralgia and myalgia. Later, the patient develops joint tenderness, swelling, and warmth; joint stiffness after inactivity (especially in the morning); and subcutaneous nodules on the elbows. Eventually joint deformity, muscle weakness, and atrophy may occur.

Sarcoidosis. With sarcoidosis, generalized, bilateral hilar and right paratracheal forms of lymphadenopathy (seen on chest X-ray) with splenomegaly are common. Initial findings are arthralgia, fatigue, malaise, weight loss, and pulmonary symptoms. Other findings vary with the site and extent of fibrosis. Typical cardiopulmonary findings include breathlessness, a cough, substernal chest pain, and arrhythmias. About 90% of patients have an abnormal chest X-ray at some time during their illness. Musculoskeletal and cutaneous features may include muscle weakness and pain, phalangeal and nasal mucosal lesions, and subcutaneous skin nodules. Common ophthalmic findings include eye pain, photophobia, and nonreactive pupils. Central nervous system involvement may produce cranial or peripheral nerve palsies and seizures.

Sjögren's syndrome. Lymphadenopathy of the parotid and submaxillary nodes may occur in Sjögren's syndrome, a rare disorder. Assessment reveals cardinal signs of dry mouth, eyes, and mucous membranes, which may be accompanied by photosensitivity, poor vision, eye fatigue, nasal crusting, and epistaxis.

Syphilis (secondary). Generalized lymphadenopathy occurs in the second stage of syphilis and may be accompanied by a macular, papular, pustular, or nodular rash on the arms, trunk, palms, soles, face, and scalp. A palmar rash is a significant diagnostic sign. Headache, malaise, anorexia, weight loss, nausea, vomiting, sore throat, and low-grade fever may occur.

Systemic lupus erythematosus (SLE). With SLE, generalized lymph-adenopathy typically accompanies the hallmark butterfly rash, photosensitivity, Raynaud's phenomenon, and joint pain and stiffness. Pleuritic chest pain and a cough may appear with systemic findings, such as a fever, anorexia, and weight loss.

Tuberculous lymphadenitis. Lymphadenopathy that occurs with tuberculous lymphadenitis may be generalized or restricted to superficial lymph nodes. Affected lymph nodes may become fluctuant and drain to surrounding tissue. They may be accompanied by a fever, chills, weakness, and fatigue.

Waldenström's macroglobulinemia. Lymphadenopathy may appear along with hepatosplenomegaly in Waldenström's macroglobulinemia. Associated findings include retinal hemorrhage, pallor, and signs of heart failure, such as jugular vein distention and crackles. The patient shows a decreased level of consciousness, abnormal reflexes, and signs of peripheral neuritis. Weakness, fatigue, weight loss, epistaxis, and GI bleeding may also occur. Circulatory impairment occurs because of increased blood viscosity.

Other causes

Drugs. Phenytoin may cause generalized lymphadenopathy.

Immunizations. Typhoid vaccination may cause generalized lymphadenopathy.

Nursing considerations

- If the patient is uncomfortable, provide an antipyretic, tepid sponge bath, or a hypothermia blanket.
- Expect to obtain blood for routine blood work, platelet and white blood cell counts, liver and renal function studies, erythrocyte sedimentation rate, and blood cultures.
- Prepare the patient for other diagnostic tests, such as chest X-ray, computed to-

mography, liver and spleen scan, lymph node biopsy, or lymphography, to visualize the lymphatic system.

■ If tests reveal infection, check your facility's policy regarding infection control and isolation precautions.

Patient teaching

■ Explain to the patient all diagnostic tests or procedures.

■ Teach the patient ways to prevent infection.

■ Explain the signs and symptoms of infection the patient should report.

■ Explain the reasons for any isolation precautions.

■ Stress the importance of a healthy diet and rest.

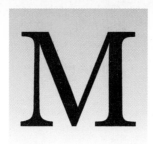

McBurney's sign

A telltale indicator of localized peritoneal inflammation in acute appendicitis, McBurney's sign is tenderness elicited by palpating the right lower quadrant over McBurney's point. McBurney's point is about 2″ (5 cm) above the anterior superior spine of the ilium, on the line between the spine and the umbilicus where pressure produces pain and tenderness in acute appendicitis. Before McBurney's sign is elicited, the abdomen is inspected for distention, auscultated for hypoactive or absent bowel sounds, and tested for tympany.

History and physical examination

Ask the patient to describe the abdominal pain. When did it begin? Does coughing, movement, eating, or elimination worsen or help relieve it? Ask about the development of other signs and symptoms, such as vomiting and a low-grade fever. Ask the patient to point to the spot where the pain is worst.

Continue light palpation of the patient's abdomen to detect additional tenderness, rigidity, guarding, or pain. Observe the patient's facial expression for signs of pain, such as grimacing or wincing. (See *Eliciting McBurney's sign*.)

Eliciting McBurney's sign

To elicit McBurney's sign, help the patient into a supine position, with his knees slightly flexed and his abdominal muscles relaxed. Then, palpate deeply and slowly in the right lower quadrant over McBurney's point—located about 2″ (5 cm) from the ilium's right anterior superior spine, on a line between the spine and the umbilicus. Point pain and tenderness, a positive McBurney's sign, indicates appendicitis.

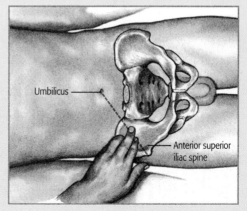

Umbilicus

Anterior superior iliac spine

 Managing the patient with appendicitis

The most common abdominal surgical disease, appendicitis, is inflammation of the vermiform appendix because of an obstruction. Although appendicitis may occur at any age and affects both sexes equally, it's most common between puberty and age 30. Since the advent of antibiotics, the incidence and the death rate of appendicitis have declined. If left untreated, gangrene and perforation develop within 36 hours.

Do's

■ Administer I.V. fluids to prevent dehydration.
■ Administer a systemic antibiotic to reduce the risk of postoperative infection.
■ Place the patient in Fowler's position to minimize pain.
■ Monitor vital signs frequently.
■ Assess for signs and symptoms of perforation, such as fever, a change in pain characteristics, generalized right lower quadrant pain or abdominal tenderness, and a rigid abdomen.

Don'ts

■ Never administer a cathartic or enema; these risk rupturing the appendix.
■ Don't give the patient anything by mouth because the patient may require surgery.
■ Don't apply heat to the right lower quadrant of the patient's abdomen; heat increases the risk of rupture.

Auscultate the abdomen, noting decreased bowel sounds.

Medical causes

Appendicitis. McBurney's sign appears within the first 2 to 12 hours after the onset of appendicitis, after initial pain in the epigastric and periumbilical area shifts to the right lower quadrant (McBurney's point). This persistent pain increases with walking or coughing. Nausea and vomiting may occur from the start. Boardlike abdominal rigidity and rebound tenderness that worsen as the condition progresses accompany cutaneous hyperalgia, fever, constipation or diarrhea, tachycardia, retractive respirations, anorexia, and moderate malaise.

Rupture of the appendix causes sudden cessation of pain. Then signs and symptoms of peritonitis develop, such as severe abdominal pain, pallor, hypoactive or absent bowel sounds, diaphoresis, and a high fever.

Nursing considerations

■ Draw blood for laboratory tests such as a complete blood count, including a white blood cell count, erythrocyte sedimentation rate, and blood cultures. (See *Managing the patient with appendicitis.*)
■ Prepare the patient for abdominal X-rays or computed tomography to confirm appendicitis.
■ Prepare the patient for an appendectomy.

Patient teaching

■ Explain the disease process and what to expect following surgery.
■ Instruct the patient on wound care.
■ Discuss any activity restrictions.

McMurray's sign

McMurray's sign is a palpable, audible click or pop that occurs when the tibia is rotated on the femur. It results when gentle manipulation of the leg traps torn cartilage and then lets it snap free. This indicates medial meniscal injury. Because eliciting this sign forces the surface of the tibial plateau against the femoral condyles, such manipulation is contraindicated in patients with suspected fractures of the tibial plateau or femoral condyles. (See *Eliciting McMurray's sign.*)

A positive McMurray's sign augments other findings commonly associated with meniscal injury, such as severe joint line tenderness, locking or clicking of the joint, and a decreased range of motion (ROM).

History and physical examination

After McMurray's sign has been elicited, find out if the patient is experiencing acute knee pain. Then ask him to describe a recent knee injury. For example, did his injury place twisting external or internal force on the knee, or did he experience blunt knee trauma from a fall? Also, ask about previous knee injury, surgery, prosthetic replacement, or other joint problems, such as arthritis, that could have weakened the knee. Ask if anything aggravates or relieves the pain and if he needs assistance to walk.

ASSESSMENT TIP

 Eliciting McMurray's sign

Eliciting McMurray's sign requires special training and gentle manipulation of the patient's leg to avoid extending a meniscal tear or locking the knee. To elicit McMurray's sign, place the patient in a supine position and flex his affected knee until his heel nearly touches his buttock. Place your thumb and index finger on either side of the knee joint space and grasp his heel with your other hand. Then rotate the foot and lower leg laterally to test the posterior aspect of the medial meniscus.

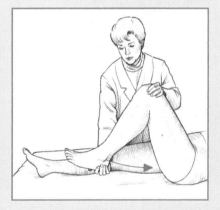

Keeping the patient's foot in a lateral position, extend the knee to a 90-degree angle to test the anterior aspect of the medial meniscus. A palpable or audible click indicates injury to meniscal structures.

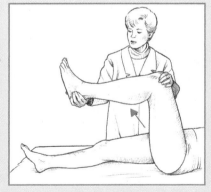

Have the patient point to the exact area of pain. Assess the leg's ROM, both passive and with resistance. Next, check for cruciate ligament stability by noting anterior or posterior movement of the tibia on the femur (drawer sign). Finally, measure the quadriceps muscles in both legs for symmetry.

Medical causes

Meniscal tear. McMurray's sign can usually be elicited with a meniscal tear injury. Associated signs and symptoms include acute knee pain at the medial or lateral joint line (depending on injury site) and decreased ROM or locking of the knee joint. Quadriceps weakening and atrophy may also occur.

Nursing considerations

- Prepare the patient for knee X-rays, arthroscopy, and arthrography, and obtain any previous X-rays for comparison.
- If trauma precipitated the knee pain and McMurray's sign, prepare the patient for aspiration of the joint.
- Immobilize and apply ice to the knee.
- Apply a knee immobilizer and prepare the patient for a cast, if appropriate.

Patient teaching

- Explain the purpose of elevating the affected leg.
- Review activity restrictions, as appropriate.
- Demonstrate the proper use of assistive devices.
- Explain how to use analgesics and anti-inflammatory drugs correctly.
- Discuss lifestyle modifications, if needed.

 Melena

A common sign of upper GI bleeding, melena is the passage of black, tarry stools containing digested blood. The characteristic color results from bacterial degradation and hydrochloric acid acting on the blood as it travels through the GI tract. At least 60 ml of blood in the GI tract is needed to produce this sign. (See *Comparing melena with hematochezia.*)

Severe melena can signal acute bleeding and life-threatening hypovolemic shock. Usually, melena indicates bleeding from the esophagus, stomach, or duodenum, although it can also indicate bleeding from the jejunum, ileum, or ascending colon. This sign can also result from swallowing blood, as in epistaxis; from taking certain drugs; or from ingesting alcohol. Because false melena may be caused by ingestion of lead, iron, bismuth, or licorice (which produces black stools without the presence of blood), all black stools should be tested for occult blood.

ACTION STAT!

 If the patient is experiencing severe melena, quickly take his orthostatic vital signs to detect hypovolemic shock. A decline of 10 mm Hg or more in systolic pressure or an increase of 10 beats/minute or more in the pulse rate indicates volume depletion. Quickly examine the patient for other signs of shock, such as tachycardia, tachypnea, and cool, clammy skin. Insert a large-bore I.V. catheter to administer replacement fluids and allow for blood transfusion. Obtain hematocrit, prothrombin time, International Normalized Ratio levels, and partial thromboplastin time. Place the patient flat with his feet elevated. Administer supplemental oxygen as needed.

History and physical examination

If the patient's condition permits, ask when he discovered that his stools were black and tarry. Ask about the frequency

Comparing melena with hematochezia

With GI bleeding, the site, amount, and rate of blood flow through the GI tract determine if a patient will develop melena (black, tarry stools) or hematochezia (bright red, blood stools). Usually, melena indicates *upper* GI bleeding, and hematochezia indicates *lower* GI bleeding. However, with some disorders, melena may alternate with hematochezia. This chart helps differentiate these two commonly related signs.

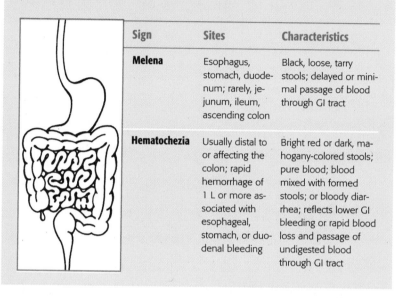

	Sign	Sites	Characteristics
	Melena	Esophagus, stomach, duodenum; rarely, jejunum, ileum, ascending colon	Black, loose, tarry stools; delayed or minimal passage of blood through GI tract
	Hematochezia	Usually distal to or affecting the colon; rapid hemorrhage of 1 L or more associated with esophageal, stomach, or duodenal bleeding	Bright red or dark, mahogany-colored stools; pure blood; blood mixed with formed stools; or bloody diarrhea; reflects lower GI bleeding or rapid blood loss and passage of undigested blood through GI tract

and quantity of bowel movements. Has he had melena before? Ask about other signs and symptoms, notably hematemesis or hematochezia, and about use of anti-inflammatories, alcohol, or other GI irritants. Also, find out if he has a history of GI lesions. Ask if the patient takes iron supplements, which may also cause black stools. Obtain a drug history, noting the use of warfarin or other anticoagulants.

Next, inspect the patient's mouth and nasopharynx for evidence of bleeding. Perform an abdominal examination that includes inspection, auscultation, palpation, and percussion. Then perform a rectal examination.

Medical causes

Colon cancer. On the right side of the colon, early tumor growth may cause melena accompanied by abdominal aching, pressure, or cramps. As the disease progresses, the patient develops weakness, fatigue, and anemia. Eventually, he also experiences diarrhea or obstipation, anorexia, weight loss, vomiting, and other signs and symptoms of intestinal obstruction.

With a tumor on the left side of the colon, melena is a rare sign until late in the disease. Early tumor growth commonly causes rectal bleeding with intermittent abdominal fullness or cramping and rectal pressure. As the disease progresses, the patient may develop obstipation, diarrhea, or pencil-shaped stools. At this stage, bleeding from the colon is signaled by melena or bloody stools.

Ebola virus. Melena, hematemesis, and bleeding from the nose, gums, and vagina may occur later with Ebola virus. Patients usually report an abrupt onset of headache, malaise, myalgia, high fever, diarrhea, abdominal pain, dehydration, and lethargy on the fifth day of illness. Pleuritic chest pain, a dry hacking cough, and pharyngitis have also been noted. A maculopapular rash develops between days 5 and 7 of the illness.

Esophageal cancer. Melena is a late sign of esophageal cancer. Increasing obstruction first produces painless dysphagia, then rapid weight loss. The patient may experience steady chest pain with substernal fullness, nausea, vomiting, and hematemesis. Other findings include hoarseness, a persistent cough (possibly hemoptysis), hiccups, a sore throat, and halitosis. In the later stages, signs and symptoms include painful dysphagia, anorexia, and regurgitation.

Esophageal varices (ruptured). Ruptured esophageal varices is a life-threatening disorder that can produce melena, hematochezia, and hematemesis. Melena is preceded by signs of shock, such as tachycardia, tachypnea, hypotension, and cool, clammy skin. Agitation or confusion signals developing hepatic encephalopathy.

Gastritis. Melena and hematemesis are common with gastritis. The patient may also experience mild epigastric or abdominal discomfort that's exacerbated by eating, belching, nausea, vomiting, and malaise.

Mallory-Weiss syndrome. Mallory-Weiss syndrome is characterized by massive bleeding from the upper GI tract due to a tear in the mucous membrane of the esophagus or the junction of the esophagus and the stomach. Melena and hematemesis follow vomit-

ing. Severe upper abdominal bleeding leads to signs and symptoms of shock, such as tachycardia, tachypnea, hypotension, and cool, clammy skin. The patient may also report epigastric or back pain.

Mesenteric vascular occlusion. Mesenteric vascular occlusion is a life-threatening disorder that produces slight melena with 2 or 3 days of persistent, mild abdominal pain. Later, abdominal pain becomes severe and may be accompanied by tenderness, distention, guarding, and rigidity. The patient may also experience anorexia, vomiting, fever, and profound shock.

Peptic ulcer. With a peptic ulcer, melena may signal life-threatening hemorrhage from vascular penetration. The patient may also develop decreased appetite, nausea, vomiting, hematemesis, hematochezia, and left epigastric pain that's gnawing, burning, or sharp and may be described as heartburn or indigestion. With hypovolemic shock come tachycardia, tachypnea, hypotension, dizziness, syncope, and cool, clammy skin.

Small-bowel tumors. Small-bowel tumors may bleed and produce melena. Other signs and symptoms include abdominal pain, distention, and an increasing frequency and pitch of bowel sounds.

Thrombocytopenia. Melena or hematochezia may accompany other manifestations of bleeding tendency that occurs with thrombocytoenia: hematemesis, epistaxis, petechiae, ecchymoses, hematuria, vaginal bleeding, and characteristic blood-filled oral bullae. Typically, the patient displays malaise, fatigue, weakness, and lethargy.

Typhoid fever. Melena or hematochezia occurs late in typhoid fever and may occur with hypotension and hypothermia. Other late findings include mental dullness or delirium, marked abdominal distention and diarrhea, marked weight loss, and profound fatigue.

Yellow fever. Melena, hematochezia, and hematemesis are ominous signs of hemorrhage, a classic feature of yellow fever, which occurs along with jaundice. Other findings include fever, headache, nausea, vomiting, epistaxis, albuminuria, petechiae and mucosal hemorrhage, and dizziness.

Other causes

Drugs and alcohol. Aspirin, other nonsteroidal anti-inflammatory drugs, or alcohol can cause melena as a result of gastric irritation.

Nursing considerations

■ Monitor the patient's vital signs, and look closely for signs of hypovolemic shock.
■ Encourage bed rest, if the patient is unstable.
■ Provide good skin care and monitor skin integrity.
■ Insert a nasogastric tube, if indicated, to assist with drainage of gastric contents and decompression.
■ Prepare the patient for diagnostic tests, including blood studies, gastroscopy or other endoscopic studies, barium swallow, and upper GI series, and for blood transfusions as indicated by his hematocrit.

Patient teaching

■ Explain the underlying cause of melena and its treatment.
■ Explain bowel elimination changes that the patient needs to report.
■ Stress the importance of colorectal cancer screening.
■ Reinforce the need to avoid aspirin, other nonsteroidal anti-inflammatory drugs, and alcohol.

Menorrhagia

Abnormally heavy or long menstrual bleeding, menorrhagia may occur as a single episode or a chronic sign. In menorrhagia, bleeding is heavier than the patient's normal menstrual flow; menstrual blood loss is 80 ml or more per monthly period. A form of dysfunctional uterine bleeding, menorrhagia can result from endocrine and hematologic disorders, stress, and certain drugs and procedures.

ACTION STAT!

 Evaluate the patient's hemodynamic status by taking orthostatic vital signs. Insert a large-gauge I.V. catheter to begin fluid replacement if the patient shows an increase of 10 beats/minute in pulse rate, a decrease of 10 mm Hg in systolic blood pressure, or other signs of hypovolemic shock, such as pallor, tachycardia, tachypnea, and cool, clammy skin. Place the patient in a supine position with her feet elevated, and administer supplemental oxygen as needed.

Monitor menstrual pads to obtain information related to the quality and quantity of bleeding. Prepare the patient for a pelvic examination to help determine the cause of bleeding.

History and physical examination

When the patient's condition permits, obtain a history. Determine her age at menarche, the duration of menses, and the interval between them. Establish the date of the patient's last menses, and ask about recent changes in her normal menstrual pattern. Have the patient describe the character and amount of bleeding. For example, how many pads or tampons does the patient use per period? Has she noted clots or tissue in the blood? Also ask about the development of other signs and symptoms before and during her menses.

Next, ask if the patient is sexually active. Does she use a method of birth control? If so, what kind? Could the patient be pregnant? Be sure to note the number of pregnancies, the outcome of each, and any pregnancy-related complications. Find out the dates of her most recent pelvic examination and Papanicolaou smear and the details of any previous gynecologic infections or neoplasms. Also, be sure to ask about previous episodes of abnormal bleeding and the outcome of any treatment. If possible, obtain a pregnancy history of the patient's mother, and determine if the patient was exposed in utero to diethylstilbestrol. (This drug has been linked to vaginal adenosis.)

Be sure to ask the patient about her general health and medical history. Note particularly if the patient or her family has a history of thyroid, adrenal, or hepatic disease; blood dyscrasias; or tuberculosis because these may predispose the patient to menorrhagia. Also, ask about the patient's past surgical procedures and recent emotional stress. Find out if the patient has undergone X-ray or other radiation therapy, because this may indicate prior treatment for menorrhagia. Obtain a thorough drug and alcohol history, noting the use of anticoagulants or aspirin. Prepare the patient for a pelvic examination, and obtain blood samples and urine specimens for pregnancy testing.

Medical causes

Blood dyscrasias. Menorrhagia is one of several possible signs of a bleeding disorder. Other possible associated findings include epistaxis, bleeding gums, purpura, hematemesis, hematuria, and melena.

Hypothyroidism. Menorrhagia is a common early sign of hypothyroidism and is accompanied by such nonspecific findings as fatigue, cold intolerance, constipation, and weight gain despite anorexia. As hypothyroidism progresses, intellectual and motor activity decrease; the skin becomes dry, pale, cool, and doughy; the hair becomes dry and sparse; and the nails become thick and brittle. Myalgia, hoarseness, a decreased libido, and infertility commonly occur. Eventually, the patient develops a characteristic dull, expressionless face and edema of the face, hands, and feet.

Also, deep tendon reflexes are delayed, and bradycardia and abdominal distention may occur.

Uterine fibroids. Menorrhagia is the most common sign of uterine fibroids, but other forms of abnormal uterine bleeding as well as dysmenorrhea or leukorrhea can also occur. Possible related findings include abdominal pain, a feeling of abdominal heaviness, a backache, constipation, urinary urgency or frequency, and an enlarged uterus, which is usually nontender.

Other causes

Drugs. The use of a hormonal contraceptive may cause a sudden onset of profuse, prolonged menorrhagia. Anticoagulants have also been associated with excessive menstrual flow. Injectable or implanted contraceptives may cause menorrhagia in some women.

Intrauterine devices. Menorrhagia can result from the use of intrauterine contraceptive devices.

Nursing considerations
■ Monitor the patient's vital signs and observe closely for signs of hypovolemia.
■ Encourage the patient to maintain an adequate fluid intake, insert an I.V.

catheter for fluid or blood administration.

■ Monitor intake and output, and estimate uterine blood loss by recording the number of sanitary napkins or tampons used during an abnormal menses and comparing this with usage during a normal menses.

■ Obtain blood samples for hematocrit, prothrombin time, partial thromboplastin time, and International Normalized Ratio levels.

Patient teaching

■ Explain all procedures and treatments to the patient.

■ Discuss the need to rest and to avoid strenuous activities until bleeding subsides.

■ Teach signs and symptoms that require immediate medical attention.

▌Metrorrhagia

Metrorrhagia—uterine bleeding that occurs irregularly between menses—is usually light, although it can range from staining to hemorrhage. Usually, this common sign reflects slight physiologic bleeding from the endometrium during ovulation. However, metrorrhagia may be the only indication of an underlying gynecologic disorder and can also result from stress, drugs, treatments, and intrauterine devices.

History and physical examination

Begin your evaluation by obtaining a thorough menstrual history. Ask the patient when she began menstruating, the duration of menses, the interval between them, and the average number of tampons or pads she uses each month. Establish when metrorrhagia occurs in relation to her menses. Does she experience other signs or symptoms? Find out the date of her last menses, and ask

about other changes in her normal menstrual pattern. Ask for details of previous gynecologic problems. If applicable, obtain a contraceptive and obstetric history. Record the dates of her last Papanicolaou (Pap) smear and pelvic examination. Ask the patient if she is sexually active. Next, ask about her general health and any recent changes. Is she under emotional stress? If possible, obtain a pregnancy history of the patient's mother. Was the patient exposed in utero to diethylstilbestrol? (This drug has been linked to vaginal adenosis.)

Prepare the patient for a pelvic examination if indicated, and obtain blood samples and a urine specimen for pregnancy testing.

Medical causes

Cervicitis. Cervicitis may cause spontaneous bleeding, spotting, or posttraumatic bleeding. Assessment reveals red, granular, irregular lesions on the external cervix. Purulent vaginal discharge (with or without odor), lower abdominal pain, and fever may occur.

Dysfunctional uterine bleeding. Abnormal uterine bleeding not caused by pregnancy or major gynecologic disorders usually occurs as metrorrhagia, although menorrhagia is possible. Bleeding may be profuse or scant, intermittent or constant.

Endometrial polyps. In most patients, endometrial polyps cause abnormal bleeding, usually intermenstrual or postmenopausal; however, some patients do remain asymptomatic.

Endometriosis. Metrorrhagia (usually premenstrual) may be the only indication of endometriosis or it may accompany cyclical pelvic discomfort, infertility, and dyspareunia. A tender, fixed adnexal mass may be palpable on bimanual examination.

Endometritis. Endometritis causes metrorrhagia, purulent vaginal discharge, and enlargement of the uterus. It also produces fever, lower abdominal pain, and abdominal muscle spasm.

Gynecologic cancer. Metrorrhagia is commonly an early sign of cervical or uterine cancer. Later, the patient may experience weight loss, pelvic pain, fatigue and, possibly, an abdominal mass.

Uterine leiomyomas. Besides metrorrhagia, uterine leiomyomas may cause increasing abdominal girth and heaviness in the abdomen, constipation, and urinary frequency or urgency. The patient may report pain if the uterus attempts to expel the tumor through contractions and if the tumors twist or necrose after circulatory occlusion or infection, but the patient with leiomyomas is usually asymptomatic.

Vaginal adenosis. Vaginal adenosis commonly produces metrorrhagia. Palpation reveals roughening or nodules in affected vaginal areas.

Other causes

Drugs. Anticoagulants and oral, injectable, or implanted contraceptives may cause metrorrhagia.

Surgery and procedures. Cervical conization and cauterization may cause metrorrhagia.

Nursing considerations

- Encourage bed rest to reduce bleeding.
- Give an analgesic for discomfort.

Patient teaching

- Explain signs and symptoms that require immediate attention.
- Explain all procedures and treatments.
- Discuss the importance of regular gynecologic examinations and Pap smears.

Miosis

Miosis—pupillary constriction caused by contraction of the sphincter muscle in the iris—occurs normally as a re-sponse to fatigue, increased light, or administration of a miotic; as part of the eye's accommodation reflex; and as part of the aging process (pupil size steadily decreases from adolescence to about age 60). However, it can also stem from an ocular or neurologic disorder, trauma, use of a systemic drug, or contact lens overuse. A rare form of miosis—Argyll Robertson pupils—can stem from tabes dorsalis and diverse neurologic disorders. Occurring bilaterally, these miotic (commonly pinpoint), unequal, and irregularly shaped pupils don't dilate properly with mydriatic use and fail to react to light, although they do constrict on accommodation.

History and physical examination

Begin by asking the patient if he has experienced other ocular symptoms, and have him describe their onset, duration, and intensity. Does he wear contact lenses? During your history, be sure to ask about trauma, serious systemic disease, and the use of topical and systemic drugs.

Next, perform a thorough eye examination. Test visual acuity in each eye, with and without correction, paying particular attention to blurred or decreased vision in the miotic eye. Examine and compare the pupils for size (many people have a normal discrepancy), color, shape, reaction to light, accommodation, and consensual light response. Examine the eyes for additional signs, and then evaluate extraocular muscle function by assessing the six cardinal fields of gaze.

Medical causes

Cerebrovascular arteriosclerosis. Miosis is usually unilateral with cerebrovascular arteriosclerosis, depending on the site and extent of vascular damage. Other findings include blurred vision, slurred speech or possibly aphasia, loss of muscle tone, memory loss, vertigo, and headache.

Cluster headache. Ipsilateral miosis, tearing, conjunctival injection, and ptosis commonly accompany a severe cluster headache, along with facial flushing and sweating, bradycardia, restlessness, and nasal stuffiness or rhinorrhea.

Corneal foreign body. With a corneal foreign body, miosis in the affected eye occurs with pain, a foreign-body sensation, slight vision loss, conjunctival injection, photophobia, and profuse tearing.

Corneal ulcer. With a corneal ulcer, miosis in the affected eye appears with moderate pain, blurred vision and possibly some vision loss, and diffuse conjunctival injection.

Horner syndrome. Moderate miosis is common in Horner syndrome and occurs ipsilaterally to the spinal cord lesion. Related ipsilateral findings include a sluggish pupillary reflex, slight enophthalmos, moderate ptosis, facial anhidrosis, transient conjunctival injection, and a vascular headache. When the syndrome is congenital, the iris on the affected side may appear lighter.

Hyphema. Usually the result of blunt trauma, hyphema can cause miosis with moderate pain, blurred vision, diffuse conjunctival injection, and slight eyelid swelling. The eyeball may feel harder than normal.

Iritis (acute). With iritis, miosis typically occurs in the affected eye along with decreased pupillary reflex, severe eye pain, photophobia, blurred vision, conjunctival injection and, possibly, pus accumulation in the anterior chamber. The eye appears cloudy, the iris bulges, and the pupil is constricted on ophthalmic examination.

Neuropathy. Two forms of neuropathy occasionally produce Argyll Robertson pupils. With diabetic neuropathy, related effects include paresthesia and other sensory disturbances, extremity pain, orthostatic hypotension, impotence, incontinence, and leg muscle weakness and atrophy.

With alcoholic neuropathy, related effects include progressive, variable muscle weakness and wasting; various sensory disturbances; and hypoactive deep tendon reflexes.

Parry-Romberg syndrome. Parry-Romberg syndrome typically produces miosis, sluggish pupillary reflexes, enophthalmos, nystagmus, ptosis, and different-colored irises.

Pontine hemorrhage. Bilateral miosis is characteristic of a pontine hemorrhage, along with a rapid onset of coma, total paralysis, decerebrate posture, an absent doll's eye sign, and a positive Babinski's sign.

Uveitis. Anterior uveitis commonly produces miosis in the affected eye, moderate to severe eye pain, severe conjunctival injection, photophobia, and pus in the anterior chamber.

With posterior uveitis, miosis is accompanied by a gradual onset of eye pain, photophobia, visual floaters, blurred vision, conjunctival injection and, commonly, a distorted pupil shape.

Other causes

Chemical burns. An opaque cornea may make miosis hard to detect. However, chemical burns may also cause moderate to severe pain, diffuse conjunctival injection, an inability to keep the eye open, blurred vision, and blistering.

Drugs. Such topical drugs as acetylcholine, carbachol, demecarium bromide, echothiophate iodide, and pilocarpine are used to treat eye disorders specifically for their miotic effect. Such systemic drugs as barbiturates, cholinergics, anticholinesterases, clonidine (overdose), guanethidine monosulfate, opiates, and reserpine also cause miosis, as does general anesthesia.

Nursing considerations

- Reassure and support the patient.
- Prepare the patient for diagnostic tests, which may include a complete ophthalmologic examination or a neurologic workup.

Patient teaching

- Demonstrate how to correctly instill eyedrops.
- Explain measures to relieve eye pain or discomfort.

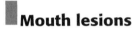

Mouth lesions

Mouth lesions include ulcers (the most common type), cysts, firm nodules, hemorrhagic lesions, papules, vesicles, bullae, and erythematous lesions. They may occur anywhere on the lips, cheeks, hard and soft palate, salivary glands, tongue, gingivae, or mucous membranes. Many are painful and can be readily detected. Some, however, produce no symptoms; when they occur deep in the mouth, they may be discovered only through a complete oral examination. (See *Common mouth lesions*.)

Mouth lesions can result from trauma, infection, systemic disease, drug use, or radiation therapy.

History and physical examination

Begin your evaluation with a thorough history. Ask the patient when the lesions appeared and whether he has noticed odor or drainage or experienced pain. Also ask about associated complaints, particularly skin lesions. Obtain a complete drug history, including drug allergies and antibiotic use, and a complete medical history. Note especially malignancy, sexually transmitted disease, I.V. drug use, recent infection, or trauma.

Ask about his dental history, including oral hygiene habits, the frequency of dental examinations, and the date of his most recent dental visit.

Next, perform a complete oral examination, noting lesion sites and character. Examine the patient's lips for color and texture. Inspect and palpate the buccal mucosa and tongue for color, texture, and contour; note especially painless ulcers on the sides or base of the tongue. Hold the tongue with a piece of gauze, lift it, and examine its underside and the floor of the mouth. Depress the tongue with a tongue blade, and examine the oropharynx. Inspect the teeth and gums, noting missing, broken, or discolored teeth; dental caries; excessive debris; and bleeding, inflamed, swollen, or discolored gums. Note any odor.

Palpate the neck for adenopathy, especially in patients who use tobacco or ingest alcohol excessively.

Medical causes

Acquired immunodeficiency syndrome (AIDS). Oral lesions may be an early indication of the immunosuppression that's characteristic of AIDS. Fungal infections can occur, with oral candidiasis being the most common. Bacterial or viral infections of the oral mucosa, tongue, gingivae, and periodontal tissue may also occur.

The primary oral neoplasm associated with AIDS is Kaposi's sarcoma. The tumor is usually found on the hard palate and may appear initially as a flat or raised lesion that produces no symptoms and ranges from red to blue to purple. As these tumors grow, they may ulcerate and become painful.

Actinomycosis (cervicofacial). Actinomycosis is a chronic fungal infection that typically produces small, firm, flat, and usually painless swellings on the oral mucosa and under the skin of the

Common mouth lesions

Squamous cell carcinoma

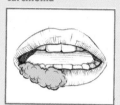

Ulceration from tongue biting

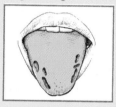

Recurrent aphthous stomatitis

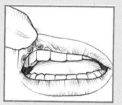

Lichen planus

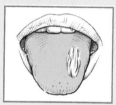

Gingival hyperplasia

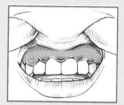

Syphilitic chancre (rare)

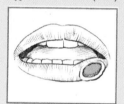

jaw and neck. Swellings may indurate and abscess, producing fistulas and sinus tracts with a characteristic purulent yellow discharge.

Behçet's syndrome. Behçet's syndrome produces small, painful ulcers on the lips, gums, buccal mucosa, and tongue. In severe cases, the ulcers also develop on the palate, pharynx, and esophagus. The ulcers typically have a reddened border and are covered with a gray or yellow exudate. Similar lesions appear on the scrotum and penis or labia majora; small pustules or papules on the trunk and limbs; and painful erythematous nodules on the shins. Ocular lesions may also develop.

Candidiasis. Candidiasis characteristically produces soft, elevated plaques on the buccal mucosa, tongue, and sometimes the palate, gingivae, and floor of the mouth; the plaques may be wiped away. The lesions of acute atrophic candidiasis are red and painful. The lesions of chronic hyperplastic candidiasis are white and firm. Localized areas of redness, pruritus, and a foul odor may be present.

Discoid lupus erythematosus. Oral lesions are common with discoid lupus erythematosus, typically appearing on the tongue, buccal mucosa, and palate as erythematous areas with white spots and radiating white striae. Associated findings include skin lesions on the face, possibly extending to the neck, ears, and scalp; if the scalp is involved, alopecia may result. Hair follicles are enlarged and filled with scales.

Erythema multiforme. Erythema multiforme produces a sudden onset of vesicles and bullae on the lips and buccal mucosa. Also, erythematous macules and papules form symmetrically on the hands, arms, feet, legs, face, and neck and, possibly, in the eyes and on the genitalia. Lymphadenopathy may also occur. With visceral involvement, other findings include fever, malaise, cough, throat and chest pain, vomiting, diarrhea, myalgia, arthralgia, fingernail loss, blindness, hematuria, and signs of renal failure.

Gingivitis (acute necrotizing ulcerative). Gingivitis causes a sudden onset of gingival ulcers covered with a grayish white pseudomembrane. Other findings include tender or painful gingivae, intermittent gingival bleeding, halitosis, enlarged lymph nodes in the neck, and fever.

Herpes simplex I. With primary herpes simplex I infection, a brief period of prodromal tingling and itching, which is accompanied by fever and pharyngitis, is followed by eruption of small and irritating vesicles on part of the oral mucosa, especially the tongue, gums, and cheeks. Vesicles form on an erythematous base and then rupture, leaving a painful ulcer, followed by a yellowish crust. Other findings include submaxillary lymphadenopathy, increased salivation, halitosis, anorexia, and keratoconjunctivitis.

Herpes zoster. Herpes zoster may produce painful vesicles on the buccal mucosa, tongue, uvula, pharynx, and larynx. Small red nodules typically erupt unilaterally around the thorax or vertically on the arms and legs, and rapidly become vesicles filled with clear fluid or pus; vesicles dry and form scabs about 10 days after eruption. Fever and general malaise accompany pruritus, paresthesia or hyperesthesia, and tenderness along the course of the involved sensory nerve.

Inflammatory fibrous hyperplasia. Inflammatory fibrous hyperplasia is a painless nodular swelling of the buccal mucosa characterized by pink, smooth, pedunculated areas of soft tissue.

Leukoplakia, erythroplakia. Leukoplakia is a white lesion that can't be removed simply by rubbing the mucosal surface—unlike candidiasis. It may occur in response to chronic irritation from dentures or from tobacco use or pipe smoking, or it may represent dysplasia or early squamous cell carcinoma. Erythroplakia is red and edematous and has a velvety surface. About 90% of all cases of erythroplakia are either dysplasia or cancer.

Pemphigoid (benign mucosal). Pemphigoid is characterized by thick-walled vesicles on the oral mucous membranes, the conjunctiva and, less commonly, the skin. Mouth lesions typically develop months or even years before other manifestations and may occur as desquamative patchy gingivitis or as a vesicobullous eruption. Secondary fibrous bands may lead to dysphagia, hoarseness, and blindness. Recurrent skin lesions include vesicobullous eruptions, usually on the inguinal area and extremities, and an erythematous, vesicobullous plaque on the scalp and face near the affected mucous membranes.

Pemphigus. Pemphigus is characterized by thin-walled vesicles and bullae that appear in cycles on skin or mucous membranes that otherwise appear normal. On the oral mucosa, bullae rupture, leaving painful lesions and raw patches that bleed easily. Associated findings include bullae anywhere on the body, denudation of the skin, and pruritus.

Pyogenic granuloma. Pyogenic granuloma is a soft, tender nodule, papule, or polypoid mass of excessive granulated tissue that usually appears on the gingivae, but can also erupt on the lips, tongue, or buccal mucosa. The lesions bleed easily because they contain many capillaries. The affected area may be smooth or have a warty surface; erythema develops in the surrounding mucosa. The lesions may ulcerate, producing a purulent exudate.

Squamous cell carcinoma. Squamous cell carcinoma is typically a painless ulcer with an elevated, indurated border. It may erupt in areas of leuko-plakia and is most common on the lower lip, but it may also occur on the edge of the tongue or floor of the mouth. High risk factors include chronic tobacco use and alcohol intake.

Stomatitis (aphthous). Stomatitis is characterized by painful ulcerations of the oral mucosa, usually on the dorsum of the tongue, gingivae, and hard palate.

With recurrent aphthous stomatitis minor, the ulcer begins as one or more erosions covered by a gray membrane and surrounded by a red halo. It's commonly found on the buccal and lip mucosa and junction, tongue, soft palate, pharynx, gingivae, and all places not bound to the periosteum.

With recurrent aphthous stomatitis major, large, painful ulcers commonly occur on the lips, cheek, tongue, and soft palate; they may last up to 6 weeks and leave a scar.

Syphilis. Primary syphilis typically produces a solitary painless, red ulcer (chancre) on the lip, tongue, palate, tonsil, or gingivae. The ulcer appears as a crater with undulated, raised edges and a shiny center; lip chancres may develop a crust. Similar lesions may appear on the fingers, breasts, or genitals, and regional lymph nodes may become enlarged and tender.

During the secondary stage, multiple painless ulcers covered by a grayish white plaque may erupt on the tongue, gingivae, or buccal mucosa. A macular, papular, pustular, or nodular rash appears, usually on the arms, trunk, palms, soles, face, and scalp; genital lesions usually subside. Other findings include generalized lymphadenopathy, headache, malaise, anorexia, weight loss, nausea, vomiting, a sore throat, low-grade fever, metrorrhagia, and post-coital bleeding.

At the tertiary stage, lesions (usually gummas—chronic, painless, superficial nodules or deep granulomatous lesions) develop on the skin and mucous membranes, especially the tongue and palate.

Systemic lupus erythematosus (SLE). Oral lesions are common with SLE and appear as erythematous areas associated with edema, petechiae, and superficial ulcers with a red halo and a tendency to bleed. Primary effects include nondeforming arthritis, a butterfly rash across the nose and cheeks, and photosensitivity.

Other causes
Drugs. Various chemotherapeutic agents can directly produce stomatitis. Also, allergic reactions to penicillin, sulfonamides, gold, quinine, streptomycin, phenytoin, aspirin, and barbiturates commonly cause lesions to develop and erupt. Inhaled steroids used for pulmonary disorders can also cause oral lesions.

Radiation therapy. Radiation therapy may cause oral lesions.

Nursing considerations
- If the patient's mouth ulcers are painful, provide a topical anesthetic such as lidocaine.
- Encourage or provide regular oral hygiene.

Patient teaching
- Tell the patient which irritants he should avoid.
- Teach proper mouth care and oral hygiene.
- Review any prescribed medications.

▌Murmurs

Murmurs are auscultatory sounds heard within the heart chambers or major arteries. They're classified by their timing and duration in the cardiac cycle, auscultatory location, loudness, configuration, pitch, and quality.

Timing can be characterized as systolic (between S_1 and S_2), holosystolic (continuous throughout systole), diastolic (between S_2 and S_1), or continuous throughout systole and diastole; systolic and diastolic murmurs can be further characterized as early, middle, or late.

Location refers to the area of maximum loudness, such as the apex, the lower left sternal border, or an intercostal space. *Loudness* is graded on a scale of 1 to 6. A grade 1 murmur is very faint, only detected after careful auscultation. A grade 2 murmur is a soft, evident murmur. Murmurs considered to be grade 3 are moderately loud. A grade 4 murmur is a loud murmur with a possible intermittent thrill. Grade 5 murmurs are loud and associated with a palpable precordial thrill. Grade 6 murmurs are loud and, like grade 5 murmurs, are associated with a thrill. A grade 6 murmur is audible even when the stethoscope is lifted from the thoracic wall.

Configuration, or shape, refers to the nature of loudness—crescendo (grows louder), decrescendo (grows softer), crescendo-decrescendo (first rises, then falls), decrescendo-crescendo (first falls, then rises), plateau (even intensity), or variable (uneven intensity). The murmur's *pitch* may be high or low. Its *quality* may be described as harsh, rumbling, blowing, scratching, buzzing, musical, or squeaking.

Murmurs can reflect accelerated blood flow through normal or abnormal valves; forward blood flow through a narrowed or irregular valve or into a dilated vessel; blood backflow through an incompetent valve, septal defect, or patent ductus arteriosus; or decreased blood viscosity. Commonly the result of organic heart disease, murmurs occasionally may signal an emergency situation—for example, a loud holosystolic murmur after an acute myocardial infarction (MI) may signal papillary muscle rupture or a ventricular septal defect. Murmurs may also result from surgical implantation of a prosthetic valve. (See *When murmurs mean emergency.*)

Some murmurs are innocent, or functional. An *innocent systolic murmur* is generally soft, medium-pitched, and loudest along the left sternal border at the second or third intercostal space. It's exacerbated by physical activity, excitement, fever, pregnancy, anemia, or thyrotoxicosis. Examples include Still's murmur in children and mammary souffle, commonly heard over either breast during late pregnancy and early postpartum. (See *Detecting congenital murmurs,* pages 396 and 397.)

History and physical examination

If you discover a murmur, try to determine its type through careful auscultation. (See *Identifying common murmurs,* page 398.) Use the bell of your stethoscope for low-pitched murmurs and the diaphragm for high-pitched murmurs.

Next, obtain a patient history. Ask if the murmur is a new discovery or if it has been known since birth or childhood. Find out if the patient has experienced associated symptoms, particularly palpitations, dizziness, syncope, chest pain, dyspnea, and fatigue. Explore the patient's medical history, noting especially an incidence of rheumatic fever, recent dental work, heart disease, or heart surgery, particularly prosthetic valve replacement.

Perform a systematic physical examination. Note especially the presence of cardiac arrhythmias, jugular vein distention, and such pulmonary signs and symptoms as dyspnea, orthopnea, and crackles. Is the patient's liver tender or palpable? Does he have peripheral edema?

When murmurs mean emergency

Although not usually a sign of an emergency, murmurs—especially newly developed ones—may signal a serious complication in patients with bacterial endocarditis or a recent acute myocardial infarction (MI).

When caring for a patient with known or suspected bacterial endocarditis, carefully auscultate for new murmurs. Their development, along with crackles, jugular vein distention, orthopnea, and dyspnea, may signal heart failure.

Regular auscultation is also important in a patient who has experienced an acute MI. A loud decrescendo holosystolic murmur at the apex that radiates to the axilla and left sternal border or throughout the chest is significant, particularly in association with a widely split S_2 and an atrial gallop (S_4). This murmur, when accompanied by signs of acute pulmonary edema, usually indicates the development of acute mitral insufficiency due to rupture of the chordae tendineae—a medical emergency.

Medical causes

Aortic insufficiency. Acute aortic insufficiency typically produces a soft, short diastolic murmur over the left sternal border that's best heard when the patient sits and leans forward and at the end of a forced held expiration. S_2 may be soft or absent. Sometimes, a soft, short midsystolic murmur may also be heard over the second right intercostal space. Associated findings include tachycardia, dyspnea, jugular vein distention, crackles, increased fatigue, and pale, cool extremities.

Chronic aortic insufficiency causes a high-pitched, blowing, decrescendo diastolic murmur that's best heard over the second or third right intercostal space or the left sternal border with the patient sitting, leaning forward, and holding his breath after deep expiration. An Austin Flint murmur—a rumbling, mid-to-late diastolic murmur best heard at the apex—may also occur. Complications may not develop until the patient is between ages 40 and 50; then, typical findings include palpitations, tachycardia, angina, increased fatigue, dyspnea, orthopnea, and crackles.

Aortic stenosis. With aortic stenosis, the murmur is systolic, beginning after S_1 and ending at or before aortic valve closure. It's harsh and grating, medium-pitched, and crescendo-decrescendo. Loudest over the second right intercostal space when the patient is sitting and leaning forward, this murmur may also be heard at the apex, at the suprasternal notch (Erb's point), and over the carotid arteries.

If the patient has advanced disease, S_2 may be heard as a single sound, with inaudible aortic closure. An early systolic ejection click at the apex is typical, but is absent when the valve is severely calcified. Associated signs and symptoms usually don't appear until age 30 in congenital aortic stenosis, ages 30 to 65 in stenosis due to rheumatic disease, and after age 65 in calcific aortic stenosis. They may include dizziness, syncope, dyspnea on exertion, paroxysmal nocturnal dyspnea, fatigue, and angina.

Cardiomyopathy (hypertrophic). Hypertrophic cardiomyopathy generates a harsh late-systolic murmur, ending at S_2. Best heard over the left sternal bor-

(Text continues on page 398.)

Detecting congenital murmurs

Heart defect	Type of murmur
Aortopulmonary septal defect	*Small defect:* a continuous rough or crackling murmur best heard at the upper left sternal border and below the left clavicle, possibly accompanied by a systolic ejection click. *Large defect:* a harsh systolic murmur heard at the left sternal border.
Atrial septal defect	A midsystolic, spindle-shaped murmur of grade 2 or 3 intensity heard at the upper left sternal border, with a fixed splitting of S_2. Large shunts may also produce a low- to medium-pitched early diastolic murmur over the lower left sternal border.
Bicuspid aortic valve	An early systolic, loud, high-pitched ejection sound or click that's best heard at the apex and is commonly accompanied by a soft, early or midsystolic murmur at the upper right sternal border. The aortic component of S_2 is usually accentuated at the apex. This murmur may not be recognized until early childhood.
Coarctation of the aorta	Usually a systolic ejection click at the base of the heart, at the apex, and occasionally over the carotid arteries, usually accompanied by a systolic ejection murmur at the base. This disorder may also produce a blowing diastolic murmur of aortic insufficiency or an apical pansystolic murmur of unknown origin.
Common atrioventricular canal defects (endocardial cushion defect)	*With a competent mitral valve:* a midsystolic, spindle-shaped murmur of grade 2 or 3 intensity heard at the upper left sternal border, with a fixed splitting of S_2; may be accompanied by a low- to medium-pitched early diastolic murmur over the lower left sternal border. *With an incompetent mitral valve:* an early systolic or holosystolic decrescendo murmur at the apex, along with a widely split S_2 and commonly an S_4.
Ebstein's anomaly	A soft, high-pitched holosystolic blowing murmur that increases with inspiration (Carvallo's sign); best heard over the lower left sternal border and the xiphoid area; possibly accompanied by a low-pitched diastolic rumbling murmur at the apex. Fixed splitting of S_2 and a loud split S_4 also occur.
Left ventricular–right atrial communication	A holosystolic, decrescendo murmur of grades 2 to 4 intensity heard along the lower left sternal border, accompanied by a normal S_2; large shunts also produce a diastolic rumbling murmur over the apex.
Mitral atresia	A nonspecific systolic murmur and a diastolic flow rumble at the lower left sternal border, with one loud S_2.

Detecting congenital murmurs *(continued)*

Heart defect	Type of murmur
Partial anomalous pulmonary venous connection	A midsystolic, spindle-shaped grade 2 or 3 murmur at the upper left sternal border, possibly accompanied by a low- to medium-pitched early diastolic murmur over the lower left sternal border.
Patent ductus arteriosus	A continuous rough or crackling murmur best heard at the upper left sternal border and below the left clavicle. The murmur is accentuated late in systole.
Pulmonic insufficiency	An early to mid-diastolic, soft, medium-pitched crescendo-decrescendo murmur best heard at the second or third right intercostal space.
Pulmonic stenosis	An early systolic, harsh, crescendo-decrescendo murmur of grades 4 to 6 intensity heard at the second left intercostal space, possibly radiating along the left sternal border.
Single atrium	A holosystolic regurgitant murmur at the apex, accompanied by a fixed splitting of S_2.
Supravalvular aortic stenosis	A systolic ejection murmur best heard over the second right intercostal space or higher in the episternal notch or over the lower right side of the neck. The aortic closure sound is usually preserved, and no ejection clicks are heard.
Tetralogy of Fallot	A midsystolic murmur with a systolic thrill palpable at the left mid-sternal border; softer murmurs occurring earlier in systole generally indicate a more severe obstruction.
Tricuspid atresia	Variable, depending on associated defects.
Trilogy of Fallot	A systolic, harsh, crescendo-decrescendo murmur, best heard at the upper left sternal border with radiation toward the left clavicle. The pulmonic component of S_2 becomes progressively softer with increasing degrees of obstruction.
Ventricular septal defect	*Small defect:* usually a holosystolic (but may be limited to early or midsystole), grades 2 to 4 decrescendo murmur heard along the lower left sternal border, accompanied by a normal S_2. *Large defect:* a holosystolic murmur at the lower left sternal border and a midsystolic rumbling murmur at the apex, accompanied by an increased S_1 at the lower left sternal border and an increased pulmonic component of S_2.

Identifying common murmurs

The timing and configuration of a murmur can help you identify its underlying cause. Learn to recognize the characteristics of these common murmurs.

Aortic insufficiency (chronic)
Thickened valve leaflets fail to close correctly, permitting blood backflow into the left ventricle.

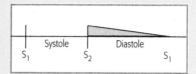

Aortic stenosis
Thickened, scarred, or calcified valve leaflets impede ventricular systolic ejection.

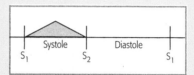

Mitral prolapse
An incompetent mitral valve bulges into the left atrium because of an enlarged posterior leaflet and elongated chordae tendineae.

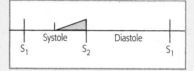

Mitral insufficiency (chronic)
Incomplete mitral valve closure permits backflow of blood into the left atrium.

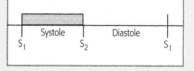

Mitral stenosis
Thickened or scarred valve leaflets cause valve stenosis and restrict blood flow.

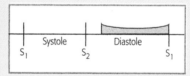

der and at the apex, the murmur is commonly accompanied by an audible S_3 or S_4. The murmur decreases with squatting and increases with sitting down. Major associated symptoms are dyspnea and chest pain; palpitations, dizziness, and syncope may also occur.

Mitral insufficiency. Acute mitral insufficiency is characterized by a medium-pitched blowing, early systolic or holosystolic decrescendo murmur at the apex, along with a widely split S_2 and commonly an S_4. This murmur doesn't

get louder on inspiration as with tricuspid insufficiency. Associated findings typically include tachycardia and signs of acute pulmonary edema.

Chronic mitral insufficiency produces a high-pitched, blowing, holosystolic plateau murmur that's loudest at the apex and usually radiates to the axilla or back. Fatigue, dyspnea, and palpitations may also occur.

Mitral prolapse. Mitral prolapse generates a midsystolic to late-systolic click with a high-pitched late-systolic crescendo murmur, best heard at the apex. Occasionally, multiple clicks may be heard, with or without a systolic murmur. Associated findings include cardiac awareness, migraine headaches, dizziness, weakness, syncope, palpitations, chest pain, dyspnea, severe episodic fatigue, mood swings, and anxiety.

Mitral stenosis. With mitral stenosis, the murmur is soft, low-pitched, rumbling, crescendo-decrescendo, and diastolic, accompanied by a loud S_1 or an opening snap—a cardinal sign. It's best heard at the apex with the patient in the left lateral position. Mild exercise helps make this murmur audible.

With severe stenosis, the murmur of mitral insufficiency may also be heard. Other findings include hemoptysis, exertional dyspnea and fatigue, and signs of acute pulmonary edema.

Myxomas. A left atrial myxoma (most common) usually produces a mid-diastolic murmur and a holosystolic murmur that's loudest at the apex, with an S_4, an early diastolic thudding sound (tumor plop), and a loud, widely split S_1. Related features include dyspnea, orthopnea, chest pain, fatigue, weight loss, and syncope.

A right atrial myxoma causes a late-diastolic rumbling murmur, a holosystolic crescendo murmur, and tumor plop, best heard at the lower left sternal border. Other findings include fatigue, peripheral edema, ascites, and hepatomegaly.

A left ventricular myxoma (rare) produces a systolic murmur, best heard at the lower left sternal border; arrhythmias; dyspnea; and syncope.

A right ventricular myxoma commonly generates a systolic ejection murmur with delayed S_2 and a tumor plop, best heard at the left sternal border. It's accompanied by peripheral edema, hepatomegaly, ascites, dyspnea, and syncope.

Papillary muscle rupture. With papillary muscle rupture—a life-threatening complication of an acute MI—a loud holosystolic murmur can be auscultated at the apex. Related findings include severe dyspnea, chest pain, syncope, hemoptysis, tachycardia, and hypotension.

Rheumatic fever with pericarditis. With rheumatic fever, a pericardial friction rub along with murmurs and gallops are heard best with the patient leaning forward on his hands and knees during forced expiration. The most common murmurs heard are the systolic murmur of mitral insufficiency, a midsystolic murmur due to swelling of the mitral valve leaflet, and the diastolic murmur of aortic insufficiency. Other signs and symptoms include fever, joint and sternal pain, edema, and tachypnea.

Tricuspid insufficiency. Tricuspid insufficiency is characterized by a soft, high-pitched, holosystolic blowing murmur that increases with inspiration (Carvallo's sign), decreases with exhalation and Valsalva's maneuver, and is best heard over the lower left sternal border and the xiphoid area. Following a lengthy period without symptoms, exertional dyspnea and orthopnea may develop, along with jugular vein distention, ascites, peripheral cyanosis and edema, muscle wasting, fatigue, weakness, and syncope.

Tricuspid stenosis. Tricuspid stenosis produces a diastolic murmur similar to that of mitral stenosis, but louder with inspiration and decreased with exhalation and Valsalva's maneuver. S_1 may also be louder. Associated signs and symptoms include fatigue, syncope, peripheral edema, jugular vein distention, ascites, hepatomegaly, and dyspnea.

Other causes

Treatments. Prosthetic valve replacement may cause variable murmurs, depending on the location, valve composition, and method of operation.

Nursing considerations

▪ Prepare the patient for diagnostic tests, such as electrocardiography, echocardiography, and angiography.
▪ Administer an antibiotic and an anticoagulant as appropriate.
▪ Because a cardiac abnormality is frightening to the patient, provide emotional support.
▪ Monitor the patient's heart rhythm and vital signs.

Patient teaching

▪ Explain the use of prophylactic antibiotics.
▪ Explain signs and symptoms that require prompt medical attention.

Muscle atrophy
[Muscle wasting]

Muscle atrophy results from denervation or prolonged muscle disuse. When deprived of regular exercise, muscle fibers lose bulk and length, producing a visible loss of muscle size and contour and apparent emaciation or deformity in the affected area. Even slight atrophy usually causes some loss of motion or power.

Atrophy usually results from neuromuscular disease or injury. However, it may also stem from certain metabolic and endocrine disorders and prolonged immobility. Some muscle atrophy also occurs with aging.

History and physical examination

Ask the patient when and where he first noticed the muscle wasting and how it has progressed. Also ask about associated signs and symptoms, such as weakness, pain, loss of sensation, and recent weight loss. Review the patient's medical history for chronic illnesses; musculoskeletal or neurologic disorders, including trauma; and endocrine and metabolic disorders. Ask about his use of alcohol and drugs, particularly steroids.

Begin the physical examination by determining the location and extent of atrophy. Visually evaluate small and large muscles. Check all major muscle groups for size, tonicity, and strength. (See *Testing muscle strength,* pages 410 and 411.) Measure the circumference of all limbs, comparing sides. (See *Measuring limb circumference.*) Check for muscle contractures in all limbs by fully extending joints and noting pain or resistance. Complete the examination by palpating peripheral pulses for quality and rate, assessing sensory function in and around the atrophied area, and testing deep tendon reflexes (DTRs).

Medical causes

Amyotrophic lateral sclerosis (ALS). Initial symptoms of ALS include muscle weakness and atrophy that typically begin in one hand, spread to the arm, and then develop in the other hand and arm. Eventually, weakness and atrophy spread to the trunk, neck, tongue, larynx, pharynx, and legs; progressive respiratory muscle weakness leads to respiratory insufficiency. Other findings include muscle flaccidity, fasciculations, hyperactive DTRs, slight leg muscle spasticity, dysphagia, impaired speech, excessive drooling, and depression.

Burns. Fibrous scar tissue formation, pain, and loss of serum proteins from severe burns can limit muscle movement, resulting in atrophy.

Hypothyroidism. Reversible weakness and atrophy of proximal limb muscles may occur in hypothyroidism. Associated findings commonly include muscle cramps and stiffness; cold intolerance; weight gain despite anorexia; mental dullness; dry, pale, cool, doughy skin; puffy face, hands, and feet; and bradycardia.

Meniscal tear. Quadriceps muscle atrophy, resulting from prolonged knee immobility and muscle weakness, is a classic sign of meniscal tear.

Multiple sclerosis. Multiple sclerosis may produce arm and leg atrophy as a result of chronic progressive weakness; spasticity and contractures may also develop. Associated signs and symptoms typically wax and wane and include diplopia and blurred vision, nystagmus, hyperactive DTRs, sensory loss or paresthesia, dysarthria, dysphagia, incoordination, an ataxic gait, intention tremors, emotional lability, impotence, and urinary dysfunction.

Osteoarthritis. Osteoarthritis eventually causes atrophy proximal to involved joints as a result of progressive weakness and disuse. Other late signs and symptoms include bony joint deformities, such as Heberden's nodes on the distal interphalangeal joints, Bouchard's nodes on the proximal interphalangeal joints, crepitus and fluid accumulation, and contractures.

Parkinson's disease. With Parkinson's disease, muscle rigidity, weakness, and disuse may produce muscle atrophy. The patient may exhibit insidious resting tremors that usually begin in the fingers (pill-rolling tremor), worsen with stress, and ease with purposeful movement and sleep. He may also develop bradykinesia; a characteristic propulsive gait; a high-pitched, monotone voice; masklike facies; drooling; dysphagia; dysarthria; and, occasionally, oculogyric crisis or blepharospasm.

Peripheral neuropathy. With peripheral neuropathy, muscle weakness progresses slowly to flaccid paralysis and eventually atrophy. Distal extremity

Measuring limb circumference

To ensure accurate and consistent limb circumference measurements, mark and use a consistent reference point each time and measure with the limb in full extension. The illustration below shows the correct reference points for arm and leg measurements.

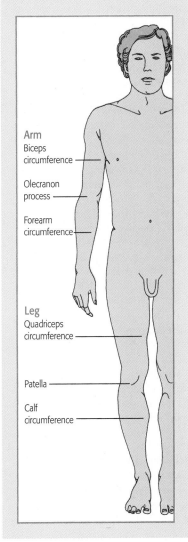

Arm
Biceps circumference

Olecranon process

Forearm circumference

Leg
Quadriceps circumference

Patella

Calf circumference

muscles are generally affected first. Associated findings include a loss of vibration sense; paresthesia, hyperesthesia, or anesthesia in the hands and feet; mild to sharp, burning pain; anhidrosis; glossy red skin; and diminished or absent DTRs.

Protein deficiency. If chronic, protein deficiency may lead to muscle weakness and atrophy. Other findings include chronic fatigue, apathy, anorexia, dry skin, peripheral edema, and dull, sparse, dry hair.

Rheumatoid arthritis. Muscle atrophy occurs in the late stages of rheumatoid arthritis as joint pain and stiffness decrease range of motion (ROM) and discourage muscle use.

Spinal cord injury. Trauma to the spinal cord can produce severe muscle weakness and flaccid, then spastic, paralysis, eventually leading to atrophy. Other signs and symptoms depend on the level of injury, but may include respiratory insufficiency or paralysis, sensory losses, bowel and bladder dysfunction, hyperactive DTRs, a positive Babinski's reflex, sexual dysfunction, priapism, hypotension, and anhidrosis (usually unilateral).

Other causes

Drugs. Prolonged steroid therapy interferes with muscle metabolism and leads to atrophy, most prominently in the limbs.

Immobility. Prolonged immobilization from bed rest, casts, splints, or traction may cause muscle weakness and atrophy.

Nursing considerations
▪ Help the patient maintain muscle length by encouraging him to perform frequent, active ROM exercises.
▪ If he can't actively move a joint, provide active assistive or passive exercises, and apply splints or braces to maintain muscle length.
▪ If you find resistance to full extension during exercise, consult the physical therapist.
▪ Use heat, pain medication, or relaxation techniques to relax resistant muscles.
▪ Prepare the patient for electromyography, nerve conduction studies, muscle biopsy, and X-rays or computed tomography scans.

Patient teaching
▪ Teach the patient to use necessary assistive devices properly to ensure his safety and prevent falls.
▪ Discuss safety measures that that patient should follow.
▪ Teach exercises that the patient can perform at home and increase in intensity as his muscle strength improves.

▎Muscle flaccidity
[Muscle hypotonicity]

Flaccid muscles are profoundly weak and soft, with decreased resistance to movement, increased mobility, and a greater than normal range of motion (ROM). The result of disrupted muscle innervation, flaccidity can be localized to a limb or muscle group or generalized over the entire body. Its onset may be acute, as in trauma, or chronic, as in neurologic disease.

ACTION STAT!

 If the patient's muscle flaccidity results from trauma, make sure his cervical spine has been stabilized. Quickly assess his respiratory status. If you note signs and symptoms of respiratory insufficiency—dyspnea, shallow respirations, nasal flaring, cyanosis, and decreased oxygen saturation—administer oxygen by nasal cannula or mask. Intubation and mechanical ventilation may be necessary.

History and physical examination

If the patient isn't in distress, ask about the onset and duration of muscle flaccidity and precipitating factors. Ask about associated symptoms, notably weakness, other muscle changes, and sensory loss or paresthesia.

Examine the affected muscles for atrophy, which indicates a chronic problem. Test muscle strength, and check deep tendon reflexes (DTRs) in all limbs. Then perform a complete neurologic examination.

Medical causes

Amyotrophic lateral sclerosis. Progressive muscle weakness and paralysis are accompanied by generalized flaccidity. Typically, these effects begin in one hand, spread to the arm, and then develop in the other hand and arm. Eventually, they spread to the trunk, neck, tongue, larynx, pharynx, and legs; progressive respiratory muscle weakness leads to respiratory insufficiency. Other findings include muscle cramps and coarse fasciculations, hyperactive DTRs, slight leg muscle spasticity, dysphagia, dysarthria, excessive drooling, and depression.

Brain lesions. Frontal and parietal lobe lesions may cause contralateral flaccidity, weakness or paralysis and, eventually, spasticity and possibly contractures. Other findings include hyperactive DTRs, a positive Babinski's sign, loss of proprioception, stereognosis, graphesthesia, anesthesia, and thermanesthesia.

Guillain-Barré syndrome. Guillain-Barré syndrome causes muscle flaccidity. Progression is typically symmetrical and ascending, moving from the feet to the arms and facial nerves within 24 to 72 hours of its onset. Associated findings include sensory loss or paresthesia, absent DTRs, tachycardia (or, less commonly, bradycardia), fluctuating hypertension and orthostatic hypotension, diaphoresis, incontinence, dysphagia, dysarthria, hypernasality, and facial diplegia. Weakness may progress to total motor paralysis and respiratory failure.

Huntington's disease. Besides flaccidity, progressive mental status changes up to and including dementia and choreiform movements are major symptoms of Huntington's disease. Others include poor balance, hesitant or explosive speech, dysphagia, impaired respirations, and incontinence.

Muscle disease. Muscle weakness and flaccidity are features of myopathies and muscular dystrophies.

Peripheral nerve trauma. Flaccidity, paralysis, and loss of sensation and reflexes in the traumatized innervated area can occur.

Peripheral neuropathy. With peripheral neuropathy, flaccidity usually occurs in the legs as a result of chronic progressive muscle weakness and paralysis. It may also cause mild to sharp burning pain, glossy red skin, anhidrosis, and a loss of vibration sensation. Paresthesia, hyperesthesia, or anesthesia may affect the hands and feet. DTRs may be hypoactive or absent.

Seizure disorder. Brief periods of syncope and generalized flaccidity commonly follow a generalized tonic-clonic seizure.

Spinal cord injury. Spinal shock can result in acute muscle flaccidity or spasticity below the level of injury. Associated signs and symptoms also occur below the level of injury and may include paralysis; absent DTRs; analgesia; thermanesthesia; loss of proprioception and vibration, touch, and pressure sensation; and anhidrosis (usually unilateral). Hypotension, bowel and bladder dysfunction, and impotence or priapism may also occur. Injury in the C1 to C5 region can produce respiratory paralysis and bradycardia.

Nursing considerations

- Provide regular, systematic, passive ROM exercises to preserve joint mobility and increase circulation.
- Reposition the patient every 2 hours to protect him from skin breakdown.
- Pad bony prominences and other pressure points.
- Treat isolated flaccidity by supporting the affected limb with a sling or splint.
- Consult a physical therapist and an occupational therapist to formulate a personalized therapy regimen and foster independence.
- Prepare the patient for diagnostic tests, such as cranial and spinal X-rays, computed tomography scans, and electromyography.

Patient teaching

- Teach the patient how to use assistive devices.
- Review the prescribed exercise regimen.

Muscle spasms
[Muscle cramps]

Muscle spasms are strong, painful contractions of the muscles. They can occur in virtually any muscle, but are most common in the calf and foot. Muscle spasms typically occur from simple muscle fatigue, after exercise, and during pregnancy. However, they may also occur with electrolyte imbalances and neuromuscular disorders or as the result of certain drugs. They're typically precipitated by movement, especially a quick or jerking movement, and can usually be relieved by slow stretching of the muscle.

ACTION STAT!

If the patient complains of frequent or unrelieved spasms in many muscles, accompanied by paresthesia in his hands and feet, quickly attempt to elicit Chvostek's and Trousseau's signs. If these signs are present, suspect hypocalcemia. Evaluate respiratory function, watching for the development of laryngospasm; provide supplemental oxygen as necessary, and prepare to intubate the patient and provide mechanical ventilation. Draw blood for calcium and electrolyte levels and arterial blood gas analysis, and insert an I.V. catheter for administration of a calcium supplement. Monitor the patient's cardiac status, and prepare to begin resuscitation if necessary.

History and physical examination

If the patient isn't in distress, ask when the muscle spasms began. Does a particular activity precipitate them? How long do they last? How painful are they? Did anything worsen or lessen the spasm? Ask about other symptoms, such as muscle weakness, sensory loss, or paresthesia.

Evaluate muscle strength and tone. Then, check all major muscle groups and note whether movement precipitate spasms. Test the presence and quality of all peripheral pulses, and examine the limbs for color and temperature changes. Test the capillary refill time (normal is less than 3 seconds), and inspect for edema, especially in the involved area. Observe for signs and symptoms of dehydration such as dry mucous membranes. Obtain a thorough drug and diet history. Ask the patient if he has had recent vomiting or diarrhea. Finally, test reflexes and sensory function in all extremities.

Medical causes

Amyotrophic lateral sclerosis (ALS).
With ALS, muscle spasms may accompany progressive muscle weakness and atrophy that typically begin in one hand, spread to the arm, and then spread to the other hand and arm. Eventually, muscle weakness and atrophy affect the trunk, neck, tongue, larynx, pharynx, and legs; progressive respiratory muscle weakness leads to respiratory insufficiency. Other findings include muscle flaccidity progressing to spasticity, coarse fasciculations, hyperactive deep tendon reflexes (DTRs), dysphagia, impaired speech, excessive drooling, and depression.

Arterial occlusive disease. Arterial occlusion typically produces muscle spasms and intermittent claudication in the leg, with residual pain. Associated findings are usually localized to the legs and feet and include loss of peripheral pulses, pallor or cyanosis, decreased sensation, hair loss, dry or scaling skin, edema, and ulcerations.

Cholera. With cholera, muscle spasms, severe water and electrolyte loss, thirst, weakness, decreased skin turgor, oliguria, tachycardia, and hypotension occur along with abrupt watery diarrhea and vomiting.

Dehydration. With dehydration, sodium loss may produce limb and abdominal cramps. Other findings include a slight fever, decreased skin turgor, dry mucous membranes, tachycardia, orthostatic hypotension, muscle twitching, seizures, nausea, vomiting, and oliguria.

Hypocalcemia. The classic feature of hypocalcemia is tetany—a syndrome of muscle cramps and twitching, carpopedal and facial muscle spasms, and seizures, possibly with stridor. Chvostek's and Trousseau's signs may be elicited. Related findings include paresthesia of the lips, fingers, and toes; choreiform

movements; hyperactive DTRs; fatigue; palpitations; and cardiac arrhythmias.

Muscle trauma. Excessive muscle strain may cause mild to severe spasms. The injured area may be painful, swollen, reddened, or warm.

Respiratory alkalosis. With respiratory alkalosis, an acute onset of muscle spasms may be accompanied by twitching and weakness, carpopedal spasms, circumoral and peripheral paresthesia, vertigo, syncope, pallor, and extreme anxiety. With severe alkalosis, cardiac arrhythmias may occur.

Spinal injury or disease. Muscle spasms can result from spinal injury, such as a cervical extension injury or spinous process fracture, or from spinal disease such as infection.

Other causes

Drugs. Common muscle spasm-producing drugs include diuretics, corticosteroids, and estrogens.

Nursing considerations
- Help alleviate muscle spasms by slowly stretching the affected muscle in the direction opposite the contraction.
- If necessary, administer a mild analgesic.
- Prepare the patient for diagnostic studies, such as serum calcium, sodium and carbon dioxide levels, thyroid function tests, and blood flow studies or arteriography.

Patient teaching
- Discuss measures for pain relief.
- Teach the patient how to use assistive devices, if appropriate.
- Teach about dietary changes that may help to decrease muscle spasms.

Muscle spasticity
[Muscle hypertonicity]

Spasticity is a state of excessive muscle tone manifested by increased resistance to stretching and heightened reflexes. It's commonly detected by evaluating a muscle's response to passive movement; a spastic muscle offers more resistance when the passive movement is performed quickly. Caused by an upper motor neuron lesion, spasticity usually occurs in the arm and leg muscles. Long-term spasticity results in muscle fibrosis and contractures. (See *How spasticity develops.*)

History and physical examination

When you detect muscle spasticity, ask the patient about its onset, duration, and progression. What, if any, events precipitate its onset? Has he experienced other muscular changes or related symptoms? Does his medical history reveal an incidence of trauma or a degenerative or vascular disease?

Take the patient's vital signs, and perform a complete neurologic and musculoskeletal examination. Test reflexes and evaluate motor and sensory function in all limbs. Evaluate muscles for wasting and contractures.

<small>ALERT</small>

 During your examination, keep in mind that generalized spasticity and trismus in a patient with a recent skin puncture or laceration indicates tetanus. If you suspect this rare disorder, look for signs of respiratory distress. Provide ventilatory support, if necessary, and monitor the patient closely.

Medical causes

Amyotrophic lateral sclerosis (ALS). ALS commonly produces spasticity, spasms, coarse fasciculations, hyperactive deep tendon reflexes (DTRs), and a positive Babinski's sign. Earlier effects include progressive muscle weakness and flaccidity that typically begin in the hands and arms and eventually spread to the trunk, neck, larynx, pharynx, and legs; progressive respiratory muscle weakness leads to respiratory insufficiency. Other findings include dysphagia, dysarthria, excessive drooling, and depression.

Epidural hemorrhage. With epidural hemorrhage, bilateral limb spasticity is a late and ominous sign. Other findings include a momentary loss of consciousness after head trauma, followed by a lucid interval and then a rapid deterioration in the level of consciousness (LOC). The patient may also develop unilateral hemiparesis or hemiplegia; seizures; fixed, dilated pupils; a high fever; a decreased and bounding pulse; a widened pulse pressure; elevated blood pressure; an irregular respiratory pattern; and decerebrate posture. A positive Babinski's sign can be elicited.

Spinal cord injury. Muscle spasticity commonly results from cervical and high thoracic spinal cord injury, especially from incomplete lesions. Spastic paralysis in the affected limbs follows initial flaccid paralysis; typically, spasticity and muscle atrophy increase for up to 1½ to 2 years after the injury, and then gradually regress to flaccidity. Associated signs and symptoms vary with the level of injury, but may include respiratory insufficiency or paralysis, sensory losses, bowel and bladder dysfunction, hyperactive DTRs, a positive Babinski's sign, sexual dysfunction, priapism, hypotension, anhidrosis, and bradycardia.

Stroke. Spastic paralysis may develop on the affected side following the acute stage of a stroke. Associated findings vary with the site and extent of vascular damage and may include dysarthria,

How spasticity develops

Motor activity is controlled by pyramidal and extrapyramidal tracts that originate in the motor cortex, basal ganglia, brain stem, and spinal cord. Nerve fibers from the various tracts converge and synapse at the anterior horn in the spinal cord. Together, they maintain segmental muscle tone by modulating the stretch reflex arc. This arc, shown in simplified form below, is basically a negative feedback loop in which muscle stretch (stimula-tion) causes reflexive contraction (inhibition), thus maintaining muscle length and tone.

Damage to certain tracts results in a loss of inhibition and a disruption of the stretch reflex arc. Uninhibited muscle stretch produces exaggerated, uncontrolled muscle activity, accentuating the reflex arc and eventually resulting in spasticity.

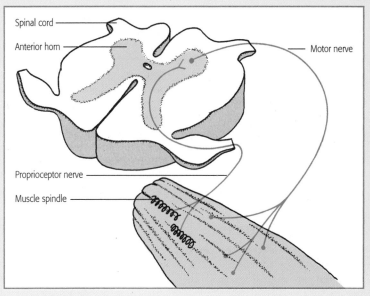

aphasia, ataxia, apraxia, agnosia, ipsilateral paresthesia or sensory loss, vision disturbances, altered LOC, amnesia and poor judgment, personality changes, emotional lability, bowel and bladder dysfunction, headache, vomiting, and seizures.

Tetanus. Tetanus is a rare, life-threatening disease that produces varying degrees of muscle spasticity. In generalized tetanus—the most common form—early signs and symptoms include painful jaw and neck stiffness, trismus, headache, irritability, restlessness, a low-grade fever with chills, tachycardia, diaphoresis, and hyperactive DTRs. As the disease progresses, painful involuntary spasms may spread and cause boardlike abdominal rigidity, opisthotonos, and a characteristic grotesque grin known as *risus sardonicus*. Reflex spasms may occur in any muscle group with the slightest stimulus. Glottal, pharyngeal, or respiratory muscle involvement can cause death by asphyxia or cardiac failure.

Nursing considerations

■ Prepare the patient for diagnostic tests, which may include electromyography, muscle biopsy, or intracranial or spinal magnetic resonance imaging or computed tomography.

■ Administer pain medication and an antispasmodic, as ordered.

■ Perform passive range-of-motion exercises, splinting, traction, and application of heat to help relieve spasms and prevent contractures.

■ Maintain a calm, quiet environment to help relieve muscle spasms and prevent recurrence, and encourage bed rest.

■ In cases of prolonged, uncontrollable muscle spasticity, as with spastic paralysis, prepare the patient for nerve blocks or surgical transection to provide permanent relief, as indicated.

Patient teaching

■ Teach the patient to use assistive devices as needed.

■ Help the patient to identify ways to maintain independence.

Muscle weakness

Muscle weakness is detected by observing and measuring the strength of an individual muscle or muscle group. It can result from a malfunction in the cerebral hemispheres, brain stem, spinal cord, nerve roots, peripheral nerves, or myoneural junctions and within the muscle itself. Muscle weakness occurs with certain neurologic, musculoskeletal, metabolic, endocrine, and cardiovascular disorders; as a response to certain drugs; and after prolonged immobilization.

History and physical examination

Begin by determining the location of the patient's muscle weakness. Ask if he has difficulty with specific movements such as rising from a chair. Find out when he first noticed the weakness; ask him whether it worsens with exercise or as the day progresses. Also ask about related symptoms, especially muscle or joint pain, altered sensory function, and fatigue.

Obtain a medical history, noting especially chronic disease, such as hyperthyroidism; musculoskeletal or neurologic problems, including recent trauma; a family history of chronic muscle weakness, especially in males; and alcohol and drug use.

Focus your physical examination on evaluating muscle strength. Test all major muscles bilaterally. (See *Testing muscle strength,* pages 410 and 411.) When testing, make sure that the patient's effort is constant; if it isn't, suspect pain or other reluctance to make the effort. If the patient complains of pain, ease or discontinue testing and have him try the movements again. Remember that the patient's dominant arm, hand, and leg are somewhat stronger than their nondominant counterparts. Besides testing individual muscle strength, test for range of motion (ROM) of all major joints (such as shoulder, elbow, wrist, hip, knee, and ankle). Also test sensory function in the involved areas, and test deep tendon reflexes (DTRs) bilaterally.

Medical causes

Amyotrophic lateral sclerosis (ALS). ALS typically begins with muscle weakness and atrophy in one hand that rapidly spread to the arm and then to the other hand and arm. Eventually, these effects spread to the trunk, neck, tongue, larynx, pharynx, and legs; progressive respiratory muscle weakness leads to respiratory insufficiency.

Anemia. With anemia, varying degrees of muscle weakness and fatigue are exacerbated by exertion and temporarily relieved by rest. Other signs and symptoms include pallor, tachycardia, paresthesia, and bleeding tendencies.

Brain tumor. Signs and symptoms of muscle weakness vary with a brain tumor's location and size. Associated findings include headache, vomiting, diplopia, decreased visual acuity, decreased level of consciousness (LOC), pupillary changes, decreased motor strength, hemiparesis, hemiplegia, diminished sensations, ataxia, seizures, and behavioral changes.

Guillain-Barré syndrome. Rapidly progressive, symmetrical weakness and pain ascends from the feet to the arms and facial nerves and may progress to total motor paralysis and respiratory failure. With Guillain-Barré syndrome, associated findings include sensory loss or paresthesia, muscle flaccidity, loss of DTRs, tachycardia or bradycardia, fluctuating hypertension and orthostatic hypotension, diaphoresis, bowel and bladder incontinence, facial diplegia, dysphagia, dysarthria, and hypernasality.

Herniated disk. Pressure on nerve roots of herniated disk leads to muscle weakness, disuse and, ultimately, atrophy. The primary symptom is severe low back pain, possibly radiating to the buttocks, legs, and feet—usually on one side. Diminished reflexes and sensory changes may also occur.

Hypercortisolism. Hypercortisolism may cause limb weakness and eventually atrophy. Related cushingoid features include buffalo hump, moon face, truncal obesity, purple striae, thin skin, acne, elevated blood pressure, fatigue, hyperpigmentation, easy bruising, poor wound healing, and diaphoresis. The male patient may be impotent; the female patient may exhibit hirsutism and menstrual irregularities.

Myasthenia gravis. Gradually progressive skeletal muscle weakness and fatigue are the cardinal symptoms of myasthenia gravis. Typically, weakness is mild upon awakening, but worsens during the day. Early signs include weak eye closure, ptosis, and diplopia; blank, masklike facies; difficulty chewing and swallowing; nasal regurgitation of fluid with hypernasality; and a hanging jaw and bobbing head. Respiratory muscle involvement may eventually lead to respiratory failure.

Osteoarthritis. Osteoarthritis is a chronic disorder that causes progressive muscle disuse and weakness that lead to atrophy.

Parkinson's disease. Muscle weakness accompanies rigidity in Parkinson's disease. Related findings include a unilateral pill-rolling tremor, a propulsive gait, dysarthria, bradykinesia, drooling, dysphagia, masklike facies, and a high-pitched, monotone voice.

Peripheral nerve trauma. Prolonged pressure on or injury to a peripheral nerve causes muscle weakness and atrophy. Other findings include paresthesia or sensory loss, pain, and loss of reflexes supplied by the damaged nerve.

Potassium imbalance. With hypokalemia, temporary generalized muscle weakness may be accompanied by nausea, vomiting, diarrhea, decreased mentation, leg cramps, diminished reflexes, malaise, polyuria, dizziness, hypotension, and arrhythmias.

With hyperkalemia, weakness may progress to flaccid paralysis accompanied by irritability and confusion, hyperreflexia, paresthesia or anesthesia, oliguria, anorexia, nausea, diarrhea, abdominal cramps, tachycardia or bradycardia, and arrhythmias.

Rhabdomyolysis. Signs and symptoms of rhabdomyolysis include muscle weakness or pain, fever, nausea, vomiting, malaise, and dark urine. Acute renal failure, due to renal structure obstruction and injury from the kidneys' attempt to filter myoglobin from the

(Text continues on page 412.)

Testing muscle strength

Obtain an overall picture of the patient's motor function by testing strength in 10 selected muscle groups. Ask him to attempt normal range-of-motion movements against your resistance. If the muscle group is weak, vary the amount of resistance as necessary to permit accurate assessment. If necessary, position the patient so his limbs don't have to resist gravity, and repeat the test.

Arm muscles

Biceps. With your hand on the patient's hand, have him flex his forearm against your resistance. Watch for biceps contraction.

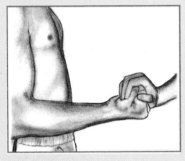

Deltoid. With the patient's arm fully extended, place one hand over his deltoid muscle and the other on his wrist. Ask him to abduct his arm to a horizontal position against your resistance; as he does so, palpate for deltoid contraction.

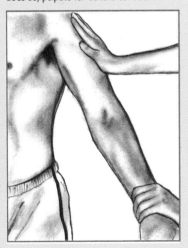

Triceps. Have the patient abduct and hold his arm midway between flexion and extension. Hold and support his arm at the wrist, and ask him to extend it against your resistance. Watch for triceps contraction.

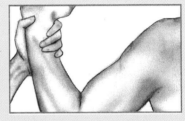

Dorsal interossei. Have the patient extend and spread his fingers, and tell him to try to resist your attempt to squeeze them together.

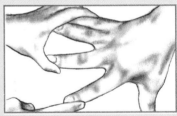

Forearm and hand (grip). Have the patient grasp your middle and index fingers and squeeze as hard as he can. To prevent pain or injury to the examiner, the examiner should cross his fingers.

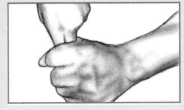

Rate muscle strength on a scale of 0 to 5:

0 = No evidence of muscle contraction
1 = Visible or palpable contraction but no movement
2 = Full muscle movement with force of gravity eliminated
3 = Full muscle movement against gravity but no movement against resistance
4 = Full muscle movement against gravity; partial movement against resistance
5 = Full muscle movement against both gravity and resistance—normal strength

Leg muscles

Anterior tibial. With the patient's leg extended, place your hand on his foot and ask him to dorsiflex his ankle against your resistance. Palpate for anterior tibial contraction.

Extensor hallucis longus. With your finger on the patient's great toe, have him dorsiflex the toe against your resistance. Palpate for extensor hallucis contraction.

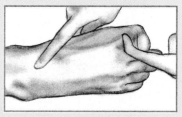

Quadriceps. Have the patient bend his knee slightly while you support his lower leg. Then ask him to extend the knee against your resistance; as he's doing so, palpate for quadriceps contraction.

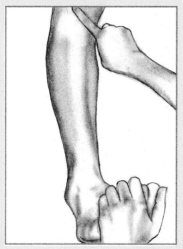

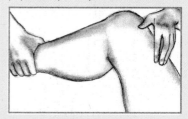

Psoas. While you support his leg, have the patient raise his knee and then flex his hip against your resistance. Watch for psoas contraction.

Gastrocnemius. With the patient on his side, support his foot and ask him to plantar flex his ankle against your resistance. Palpate for gastrocnemius contraction.

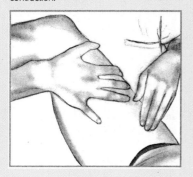

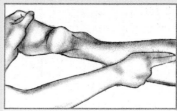

bloodstream, is a common complication.

Rheumatoid arthritis. With rheumatoid arthritis, symmetrical muscle weakness may accompany increased warmth, swelling, and tenderness in involved joints; pain; and stiffness, restricting motion.

Seizure disorder. Temporary generalized muscle weakness may occur after a generalized tonic-clonic seizure; other postictal findings include headache, muscle soreness, and profound fatigue.

Spinal trauma and disease. Trauma to the spine can cause severe muscle weakness, leading to flaccidity or spasticity and, eventually, paralysis. Infection, tumor, and cervical spondylosis or stenosis can also cause muscle weakness.

Stroke. Depending on the site and extent of damage, a stroke may produce contralateral or bilateral weakness of the arms, legs, face, and tongue, possibly progressing to hemiplegia and atrophy. Associated effects include dysarthria, aphasia, ataxia, apraxia, agnosia, ipsilateral paresthesia or sensory loss, vision disturbances, altered LOC, amnesia and poor judgment, personality changes, bowel and bladder dysfunction, headache, vomiting, and seizures.

Other causes

Drugs. Generalized muscle weakness can result from prolonged corticosteroid use, digoxin, and excessive doses of dantrolene. Aminoglycoside antibiotics may worsen muscle weakness in patients with myasthenia gravis.

Immobility. Immobilization in a cast, a splint, or traction can lead to muscle weakness in the involved extremity; prolonged bed rest or inactivity results in generalized muscle weakness.

Nursing considerations

- Provide assistive devices as necessary.

- Protect the patient from injury.
- If sensory loss occurs, guard against pressure ulcer formation and thermal injury.
- With chronic weakness, provide ROM exercises or splint limbs as necessary.
- Allow for adequate rest periods.
- Administer pain medications as needed.
- Prepare the patient for blood tests, muscle biopsy, electromyography, nerve conduction studies, and X-rays or computed tomography scans.

Patient teaching

- Teach the patient how to use assistive devices as necessary.
- Explain the importance of frequent position changes and rest periods.
- Explain the cause of muscle weakness and the treatment plan.

▌Mydriasis

Mydriasis—pupillary dilation caused by contraction of the dilator of the iris—is a normal response to decreased light, strong emotional stimuli, and topical administration of mydriatic and cycloplegic drugs. It can also result from ocular and neurologic disorders, eye trauma, and disorders that decrease the level of consciousness (LOC). Mydriasis may be an adverse effect of antihistamines or other drugs.

History and physical examination

Begin by asking the patient about eye problems, such as pain, blurring, diplopia, or visual field defects. Obtain a health history, focusing on eye or head trauma, glaucoma and other ocular problems, and neurologic and vascular disorders. In addition, obtain a complete drug history.

Grading pupil size

To accurately evaluate pupil size, compare the patient's pupils with the scale shown here. Keep in mind that the maximum constriction may be less than 1 mm and the maximum dilation greater than 9 mm.

1 mm	2 mm	3 mm
4 mm	5 mm	6 mm
7 mm	8 mm	9 mm

Next, perform a thorough eye examination. Inspect and compare the pupils' size, color, and shape—many people normally have unequal pupils. (See *Grading pupil size.*) Also, test each pupil for light reflex, consensual response, and accommodation. Perform a swinging flashlight test to evaluate a decreased response to direct light coupled with a normal consensual response (Marcus Gunn pupil). Be sure to check the eyes for ptosis, swelling, and ecchymosis. Test visual acuity in both eyes with and without correction. Evaluate extraocular muscle function by checking the six cardinal fields of gaze.

Keep in mind that mydriasis appears in two ocular emergencies: acute angle-closure glaucoma and traumatic iridoplegia.

Medical causes

Adie's syndrome. Adie's syndrome is characterized by abrupt unilateral my-driasis, poor or absent pupillary reflexes, visual blurring, and cramplike eye pain. Deep tendon reflexes (DTRs) may be hyperactive or absent, especially the ankle and knee jerk reflexes.

Aortic arch syndrome. Bilateral pupillary mydriasis commonly occurs late in aortic arch syndrome. Other ocular findings include visual blurring, transient vision loss, and diplopia. Related findings include dizziness and syncope; neck, shoulder, and chest pain; bruits; loss of radial and carotid pulses; paresthesia; and intermittent claudication. Blood pressure may be decreased in the arms.

Botulism. Botulism toxin causes bilateral mydriasis, usually 12 to 36 hours after ingestion. Other early findings are a loss of pupillary reflexes, visual blurring, diplopia, ptosis, strabismus and extraocular muscle palsies, anorexia, nausea, vomiting, diarrhea, and dry mouth. Vertigo, hearing loss, hoarseness, hypernasality, dysarthria, dysphagia, progressive muscle weakness, and a loss of DTRs soon follow.

Carotid artery aneurysm. With carotid artery aneurysm, unilateral mydriasis may be accompanied by bitemporal hemianopsia, decreased visual acuity, hemiplegia, decreased LOC, headache, aphasia, behavioral changes, and hypoesthesia.

Glaucoma (acute angle-closure). Acute angle-closure glaucoma is an ocular emergency that's characterized by moderate mydriasis and the loss of pupillary reflex in the affected eye, accompanied by an abrupt onset of excruciating pain, redness, decreased visual acuity, visual blurring, halo vision, conjunctival injection, and a cloudy cornea. Without treatment, permanent blindness occurs in 2 to 5 days.

Oculomotor nerve palsy. Unilateral mydriasis is commonly the first sign of oculomotor nerve palsy. It's soon followed by ptosis, diplopia, decreased pupillary reflexes, exotropia, and complete loss of accommodation. Focal neurologic signs may accompany signs of increased intracranial pressure.

Traumatic iridoplegia. Eye trauma can paralyze the sphincter of the iris, causing mydriasis and the loss of pupillary reflex; usually, this is transient. Associated findings include a quivering iris (iridodonesis), ecchymosis, pain, and swelling.

Other causes

Drugs. Mydriasis can be caused by anticholinergics, antihistamines, sympathomimetics, barbiturates (in overdose), estrogens, and tricyclic antidepressants; it also commonly occurs early in general anesthesia induction. Topical mydriatics and cycloplegics, such as phenylephrine, atropine, homatropine, scopolamine, cyclopentolate, and tropicamide, are ad-

ministered specifically for their mydriatic effects.

Surgery. Traumatic mydriasis commonly results from ocular surgery.

Nursing considerations
■ Prepare the patient for diagnostics tests, such as a complete ophthalmologic examination and a thorough neurologic workup.

Patient teaching
■ Explain diagnostic tests to the patient.
■ If the patient's mydriasis is the result of mydriatic drugs received during an eye examination, explain that he'll temporarily experience some photophobia and loss of accommodation.

Myoclonus

Myoclonus—sudden, shocklike contractions of a single muscle or muscle group—occurs with various neurologic disorders and may herald the onset of a seizure. These contractions may be isolated or repetitive, rhythmic or arrhythmic, symmetrical or asymmetrical, synchronous or asynchronous, and generalized or focal. They may be precipitated by bright flickering lights, a loud sound, or unexpected physical contact. One type, *intention myoclonus,* is evoked by intentional muscle movement.

Myoclonus occurs normally just before falling asleep and as a part of the natural startle reaction. It also occurs with some poisonings and, rarely, as a complication of hemodialysis.

ACTION STAT!

 If you observe myoclonus, check for seizure activity. Take the patient's vital signs to rule out arrhythmias or an occluded airway. Have resuscitation equipment on hand.

If the patient has a seizure, gently help him lie down. Place a pillow or a rolled-up towel under his head to prevent injury. Loosen constrictive clothing, especially around the neck, and turn his head (gently, if possible) to one side to prevent airway occlusion or aspiration of secretions or vomitus.

History and physical examination

If the patient is stable, evaluate his level of consciousness (LOC) and mental status. Ask about the frequency, severity, location, and circumstances of myoclonus. Has he ever had a seizure? If so, did myoclonus precede it? Is myoclonus ever precipitated by a sensory stimulus? During the physical examination, check for muscle rigidity and wasting, and test deep tendon reflexes. Then perform a neurologic examination.

Medical causes

Alzheimer's disease. Generalized myoclonus may occur in advanced stages of Alzheimer's disease, a slowly progressive dementia. Other late findings include mild choreoathetoid movements, muscle rigidity, bowel and bladder incontinence, delusions, and hallucinations.

Creutzfeldt-Jakob disease. Diffuse myoclonic jerks appear early in Creutzfeldt-Jakob disease. Initially random, they gradually become more rhythmic and symmetrical, usually occurring in response to sensory stimuli. Associated effects include ataxia, aphasia, hearing loss, muscle rigidity and wasting, fasciculations, hemiplegia, and vision disturbances, or possibly, blindness.

Encephalitis (viral). With viral encephalitis, myoclonus is usually intermittent and either localized or generalized. Associated findings vary, but may include rapidly decreasing LOC, fever, headache, irritability, nuchal rigidity,

vomiting, seizures, aphasia, ataxia, hemiparesis, facial muscle weakness, nystagmus, ocular palsies, and dysphagia.

Encephalopathy. Hepatic encephalopathy occasionally produces myoclonic jerks in association with asterixis and focal or generalized seizures.

Hypoxic encephalopathy may produce generalized myoclonus or seizures almost immediately after restoration of cardiopulmonary function. The patient may also have a residual intention myoclonus.

Uremic encephalopathy commonly produces myoclonic jerks and seizures. Other signs and symptoms include apathy, fatigue, irritability, headache, confusion, gradually decreasing LOC, nausea, vomiting, oliguria, edema, and papilledema. The patient may also exhibit elevated blood pressure, dyspnea, arrhythmias, and abnormal respirations.

Epilepsy. With idiopathic epilepsy, localized myoclonus is usually confined to an arm or leg and occurs singly or in short bursts, usually upon awakening. It's usually more frequent and severe during the prodromal stage of a major generalized seizure, after which it diminishes in frequency and intensity.

Myoclonic jerks are usually the first signs of myoclonic epilepsy, the most common cause of progressive myoclonus. At first, myoclonus is infrequent and localized, but over a period of months, it becomes more frequent and involves the entire body, disrupting voluntary movement (intention myoclonus). As the disease progresses, myoclonus is accompanied by generalized seizures and dementia.

Other causes

Drug withdrawal. Myoclonus may be seen in patients with alcohol, opioid, or sedative withdrawal or delirium tremens.

Poisoning. Acute intoxication with methyl bromide, bismuth, or strychnine may produce an acute onset of myoclonus and confusion.

Nursing considerations

- If the patient's myoclonus is progressive, institute seizure precautions.
- Keep an oral airway and suction equipment at his bedside, and pad the bed's side rails.
- Because myoclonus may cause falls, remove potentially harmful objects from the patient's environment, and remain with him while he walks.
- As needed, administer drugs that suppress myoclonus: ethosuximide, L-5-hydroxytryptophan, phenobarbital, clonazepam, or carbidopa.
- Prepare the patient for an electroencephalogram, as indicated, to evaluate myoclonus and related brain activity.

Patient teaching

- Instruct the patient and his family about the need for safety precautions.
- Talk with the patient and family about seizure precautions.
- Refer the patient to social service or community resources, as needed.
- Explain the cause of myoclonic movement and the treatment plan.

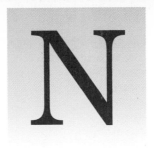

Nasal flaring

Nasal flaring is the abnormal dilation of the nostrils. Usually occurring during inspiration, nasal flaring may occasionally occur during expiration or throughout the respiratory cycle. It indicates respiratory dysfunction, ranging from mild difficulty to potentially life-threatening respiratory distress.

ACTION STAT!

 If you note nasal flaring in the patient, quickly evaluate his respiratory status. Absent breath sounds, cyanosis, diaphoresis, and tachycardia point to complete airway obstruction. As necessary, deliver back blows or abdominal thrusts (Heimlich maneuver) to relieve the obstruction. If these don't clear the airway, emergency intubation or tracheostomy and mechanical ventilation may be needed.

If the patient's airway isn't obstructed but he displays breathing difficulty, give oxygen by nasal cannula or face mask. Intubation and mechanical ventilation may be necessary. Insert an I.V. catheter for fluid and drug administration. Begin cardiac monitoring. Obtain a chest X-ray and samples for arterial blood gas (ABG) analysis and electrolyte studies.

History and physical examination

When the patient's condition is stabilized, obtain a pertinent history. Ask about cardiac and pulmonary disorders such as asthma. Does the patient have allergies? Has he experienced a recent illness, such as a respiratory tract infection, or trauma? Does the patient smoke or have a history of smoking? Obtain a drug history.

Medical causes

Acute respiratory distress syndrome (ARDS). ARDS causes increased respiratory difficulty and hypoxemia, with nasal flaring, dyspnea, tachypnea, diaphoresis, cyanosis, scattered crackles, and rhonchi. It also produces tachycardia, anxiety, and decreased level of consciousness (LOC).

Airway obstruction. Complete obstruction above the tracheal bifurcation causes sudden nasal flaring, absent breath sounds despite intercostal retractions and marked accessory muscle use, tachycardia, diaphoresis, cyanosis, decreasing LOC and, eventually, respiratory arrest.

Partial obstruction causes nasal flaring with inspiratory stridor, gagging, wheezing, a violent cough, marked accessory muscle use, agitation, cyanosis, and hoarseness.

Anaphylaxis. Severe anaphylactic reactions can produce respiratory distress with nasal flaring, stridor, wheezing, accessory muscle use, intercostal retractions, and dyspnea. Associated signs and symptoms include nasal congestion, sneezing, pruritus, urticaria, erythema, diaphoresis, angioedema, weakness, hoarseness, dysphagia and, rarely, vomiting, nausea, diarrhea, urinary urgency, and incontinence. Cardiac arrhythmias and signs of shock may occur late.

Asthma (acute). An asthma attack can cause nasal flaring, dyspnea, tachypnea, prolonged expiratory wheezing, accessory muscle use, cyanosis, and a dry or productive cough. Auscultation may reveal rhonchi, crackles, and decreased or absent breath sounds. Other findings include anxiety, tachycardia, and increased blood pressure.

Chronic obstructive pulmonary disease (COPD). COPD can lead to acute respiratory failure secondary to pulmonary infection or edema. Nasal flaring is accompanied by prolonged pursed-lip expiration; accessory muscle use; a loose, rattling, productive cough; cyanosis; reduced chest expansion; crackles; rhonchi; wheezing; and dyspnea.

Pneumothorax. Pneumothorax is an acute disorder that can result in respiratory distress with nasal flaring, dyspnea, tachypnea, shallow respirations, hyperresonance or tympany on percussion, agitation, jugular vein distention, tracheal deviation, and cyanosis. Other findings typically include sharp chest pain, tachycardia, hypotension, cold and clammy skin, diaphoresis, subcutaneous crepitation, and anxiety. Breath sounds may be decreased or absent on the affected side; similarly, chest wall motion may be decreased on the affected side.

Similar findings can occur with *hydrothorax, chylothorax,* or *hemothorax,*

depending on the amount of fluid accumulation.

Pulmonary edema. Pulmonary edema typically produces nasal flaring, severe dyspnea, wheezing, and a cough that produces frothy, pink sputum. Increased accessory muscle use may occur with tachycardia, cyanosis, hypotension, crackles, jugular vein distention, peripheral edema, and decreased LOC.

Pulmonary embolus. Signs of pulmonary embolus, a potentially life-threatening disorder, may include nasal flaring, dyspnea, tachypnea, wheezing, cyanosis, a pleural friction rub, and a productive cough (possibly hemoptysis). Its other effects include sudden chest tightness or pleuritic pain, tachycardia, atrial arrhythmias, hypotension, a low-grade fever, syncope, marked anxiety, and restlessness.

Other causes

Diagnostic tests. Pulmonary function tests, such as vital capacity testing, can produce nasal flaring with forced inspiration or expiration.

Treatments. Certain respiratory treatments, such as deep breathing, can cause nasal flaring.

Nursing considerations

- To help ease breathing, place the patient in high Fowler's position.
- If he's at risk for aspirating secretions, place him in a modified Trendelenburg or side-lying position.
- If necessary, suction frequently to remove oropharyngeal secretions.
- Administer humidified oxygen to thin secretions and decrease airway drying and irritation.
- Provide adequate hydration to liquefy secretions.
- Reposition the patient every hour, and encourage coughing and deep breathing.

■ Avoid administering sedatives or opiates, which can depress the cough reflex or respirations.
■ Continually assess the patient's respiratory status, and check his vital signs and oxygen saturation every 30 minutes, or as necessary.
■ Prepare the patient for diagnostic tests, such as chest X-rays, a lung scan, pulmonary arteriography, sputum culture, complete blood count, ABG analysis, and 12-lead electrocardiogram.

Patient teaching
■ Explain all procedures and treatments to the patient.
■ Review treatment of the underlying disorder.
■ Discuss the continued importance of not smoking.
■ Demonstrate how to use an inhaler correctly.

Nausea

Nausea is a sensation of profound revulsion to food or of impending vomiting. Typically accompanied by autonomic signs, such as hypersalivation, diaphoresis, tachycardia, pallor, and tachypnea, it's closely associated with anorexia and vomiting.

Nausea, a common symptom of GI disorders, also occurs with fluid and electrolyte imbalance; infection; metabolic, endocrine, labyrinthine, and cardiac disorders; and as a result of drug therapy, surgery, and radiation. Commonly present during the first trimester of pregnancy, nausea may also arise from severe pain, anxiety, alcohol intoxication, overeating, or ingestion of distasteful food or liquids.

History and physical examination
Begin by obtaining a complete medical history. Focus on GI, endocrine, and metabolic disorders; recent infections; and cancer and its treatment. Ask about drug use and alcohol consumption. If the patient is a female of childbearing age, ask if she is or could be pregnant. Have the patient describe the onset, duration, and intensity of the nausea as well as what causes or relieves it. Ask about related complaints, particularly vomiting (such as color and amount), abdominal pain, anorexia and weight loss, changes in bowel habits or stool character, excessive belching or flatus, and a sensation of bloating.

Inspect the skin for jaundice, bruises, and spider angiomas, and assess skin turgor. Next, inspect the abdomen for distention, auscultate for bowel sounds and bruits, palpate for rigidity and tenderness, and test for rebound tenderness. Palpate and percuss the liver for enlargement. Assess other body systems as appropriate.

Medical causes
Adrenal insufficiency. Common GI findings in adrenal insufficiency include nausea, vomiting, anorexia, and diarrhea. Other findings include weakness; fatigue; weight loss; bronze-colored skin; hypotension; a weak, irregular pulse; vitiligo; and depression.

Anthrax (GI). Initial signs and symptoms of GI anthrax include nausea, vomiting, loss of appetite, and fever. Signs and symptoms may progress to abdominal pain, severe bloody diarrhea, and hematemesis.

Appendicitis. With acute appendicitis, a brief period of nausea may accompany the onset of abdominal pain. Pain typically begins as vague epigastric or periumbilical discomfort and rapidly progresses to severe stabbing pain localized in the right lower quadrant (McBurney's sign). Associated findings usually include abdominal rigidity and tenderness, cutaneous hyperalgesia, fever, constipation or diarrhea, tachycardia, anorexia, moderate malaise, and positive psoas (increased abdominal pain occurs when the examiner places his hand above the patient's right knee and the patient flexes his right hip against resistance) and obturator signs (internal rotation of the right leg with the leg flexed to 90 degrees at the hip and knee with a resulting tightening of the internal obturator muscle that causes abdominal discomfort).

Cholecystitis (acute). With acute cholecystitis, nausea commonly follows severe right upper quadrant pain that may radiate to the back or shoulders, usually following meals. Associated findings include mild vomiting, flatulence, abdominal tenderness and, possibly, rigidity and distention, fever with chills, diaphoresis, and a positive Murphy's sign.

Cholelithiasis. With cholelithiasis, nausea accompanies attacks of severe right upper quadrant or epigastric pain after eating fatty foods. Other associated findings include vomiting, abdominal tenderness and guarding, flatulence, belching, epigastric burning, tachycardia, and restlessness. Occlusion of the common bile duct may cause jaundice, clay-colored stools, fever, and chills.

Cirrhosis. Insidious early signs and symptoms of cirrhosis typically include nausea and vomiting, anorexia, abdominal pain, and constipation or diarrhea. As the disease progresses, jaundice and hepatomegaly may occur with abdominal distention, spider angiomas, palmar erythema, severe pruritus, dry skin, fetor hepaticus, enlarged superficial abdominal veins, mental changes, and bilateral gynecomastia and testicular atrophy or menstrual irregularities.

Diverticulitis. Besides nausea, diverticulitis causes intermittent crampy abdominal pain, constipation or diarrhea, a low-grade fever, and commonly a palpable, tender, firm, fixed mass.

Escherichia coli *O157:H7*. Signs and symptoms of *E. coli* infection include nausea, watery or bloody diarrhea, vomiting, fever, and abdominal cramps. In children younger than age 5 and in the elderly, hemolytic uremic syndrome—in which red blood cells are destroyed—may develop. This may ultimately lead to acute renal failure.

Gastritis. Nausea is common with gastritis, especially after ingestion of alcohol, aspirin, spicy foods, or caffeine. Vomiting of mucus or blood, epigastric pain, belching, fever, and malaise may also occur.

Gastroenteritis. Usually viral, gastroenteritis causes nausea, vomiting, diarrhea, and abdominal cramping. Fever, malaise, hyperactive bowel sounds, abdominal pain and tenderness, and possible dehydration and electrolyte imbalances may also develop.

Heart failure. Heart failure may produce nausea and vomiting, particularly with right-sided heart failure. Associated findings include tachycardia, a ventricular gallop, profound fatigue, dyspnea, crackles, peripheral edema, jugular vein distention, ascites, nocturia, and diastolic hypertension.

Hepatitis. Nausea is an insidious early symptom of viral hepatitis. Vomiting, fatigue, myalgia and arthralgia, headache, anorexia, photophobia, pharyngitis, cough, and fever also occur early in the preicteric phase.

Hyperemesis gravidarum. Unremitting nausea and vomiting that persist beyond the first trimester are characteristic of hyperemesis gravidarum. Vomitus ranges from undigested food, mucus, and bile early in the disorder to a coffee-ground appearance in later stages. Associated findings include weight loss, signs of dehydration, headache, and delirium.

Intestinal obstruction. Nausea commonly occurs, especially with high small-intestinal obstruction. Vomiting may be bilious or fecal; abdominal pain is usually episodic and colicky, but can become severe and steady with strangulation. Constipation occurs early in large-intestinal obstruction and later in small-intestinal obstruction; obstipation may signal complete obstruction. Bowel sounds are typically hyperactive in partial obstruction and hypoactive or absent in complete obstruction. Abdominal distention and tenderness occur, possibly with visible peristaltic waves and a palpable abdominal mass.

Labyrinthitis. Nausea and vomiting commonly occur with labyrinthitis. More significant findings include severe vertigo, progressive hearing loss, nystagmus, tinnitus and, possibly, otorrhea.

Listeriosis. Signs and symptoms of listeriosis include nausea, vomiting, diarrhea, fever, myalgia, and abdominal pain. If listerosis spreads to the nervous system and causes meningitis, signs and symptoms include fever, headache, nuchal rigidity, and a change in the level of consciousness (LOC).

Ménière's disease. Ménière's disease causes sudden, brief, recurrent attacks of nausea, vomiting, vertigo, tinnitus, diaphoresis, and nystagmus. It also causes hearing loss and ear fullness.

Mesenteric venous thrombosis. An insidious or acute onset of nausea, vomiting, and abdominal pain occurs with mesenteric venous thrombosis, along with diarrhea or constipation, abdominal distention, hematemesis, and melena.

Metabolic acidosis. Metabolic acidosis may produce nausea and vomiting, anorexia, diarrhea, Kussmaul's respirations, and decreased LOC.

Migraine headache. Nausea and vomiting may occur in the prodromal stage of a migraine headache, along with photophobia, light flashes, increased sensitivity to noise, light-headedness and, possibly, partial vision loss and paresthesia of the lips, face, and hands.

Motion sickness. With motion sickness, nausea and vomiting are brought on by motion or rhythmic movement. Headache, dizziness, fatigue, diaphoresis, hypersalivation, and dyspnea may also occur.

Myocardial infarction (MI). Nausea and vomiting may occur with an MI, but the cardinal symptom is severe substernal chest pain that may radiate to the left arm, jaw, or neck. Dyspnea, pallor, clammy skin, diaphoresis, altered blood pressure, and arrhythmias also occur.

Norovirus infection. Acute gastroenteritis from noroviruses commonly causes infected individuals to experience nausea. Common accompanying symptoms include vomiting, diarrhea, and abdominal pain or cramping. Less commonly, individuals may develop low-grade fever, headache, chills, muscle aches, and generalized tiredness.

Pancreatitis (acute). Nausea, usually followed by vomiting, is an early symptom of pancreatitis. Other common findings include steady, severe pain in the epigastrium or left upper quadrant that may radiate to the back; abdominal tenderness and rigidity; anorexia; diminished bowel sounds; and fever. Tachycardia, restlessness, hypotension, skin mottling, and cold, sweaty extremities may occur in severe cases.

Peptic ulcer. With peptic ulcer, nausea and vomiting may follow attacks of sharp or gnawing, burning epigastric pain. Attacks typically occur when the stomach is empty or after the ingestion of alcohol, caffeine, or aspirin; they're relieved by eating food or taking an antacid or antisecretory. Hematemesis or melena may also occur.

Peritonitis. With peritonitis, nausea and vomiting usually accompany acute abdominal pain localized to the area of inflammation. Other findings include a high fever with chills; tachycardia; hypoactive or absent bowel sounds; abdominal distention, rigidity, and tenderness (including rebound tenderness); positive obturator sign and obturator weakness; pale, cold skin; diaphoresis; hypotension; shallow respirations; and hiccups.

Preeclampsia. Nausea and vomiting commonly occur with preeclampsia along with rapid weight gain, epigastric pain, oliguria, a severe frontal headache, hyperreflexia, and blurred or double vision. The classic diagnostic triad of signs include hypertension, proteinuria, and edema.

Q fever. Signs and symptoms of Q fever include nausea, vomiting, diarrhea, fever, chills, severe headache, malaise, and chest pain. In severe cases, the patient may develop hepatitis or pneumonia.

Rhabdomyolysis. Signs and symptoms of rhabdomyolysis include nausea, vomiting, muscle weakness or pain, fever, malaise, and dark urine. Acute renal failure is the most commonly reported complication of the disorder. It results from renal structure obstruction and injury during the kidneys' attempt to filter myoglobin from the bloodstream.

Typhus. With typhus, an abrupt onset of nausea, vomiting, fever, and chills follows the initial symptoms of headache, myalgia, arthralgia, and malaise.

Other causes

Drugs. Common nausea-producing drugs include antineoplastics, opiates, ferrous sulfate, levodopa, oral potassium chloride replacements, estrogens, sulfa-salazine, antibiotics, quinidine, anesthetics, cardiac glycosides, theophylline (overdose), and nonsteroidal antiinflammatory drugs.

Radiation and surgery. Radiation therapy can cause nausea and vomiting. Postoperative nausea and vomiting are common, especially after abdominal surgery.

Nursing considerations

- If the patient is experiencing severe nausea, prepare him for blood tests to determine fluid and electrolyte status and acid-base balance.
- To prevent aspiration, elevate the patient's head or position him on his side.
- Because pain can precipitate or intensify nausea, administer pain medications promptly, as needed.
- If possible, give medications by injection or suppository to prevent exacerbating nausea.
- Be alert for abdominal distention and hypoactive bowel sounds which may indicate gastric retention.
- Be prepared to insert a nasogastric tube, as needed.
- Prepare the patient for such procedures as a computed tomography scan, an ultrasound scan, endoscopy, and colonoscopy.
- Consult the nutritionist to determine the patient's need for parenteral nutrition.

Patient teaching

- Teach the patient to breathe deeply to ease his nausea.
- Discuss triggers for nausea and how to avoid them.
- Teach the patient the importance of aspiration precautions.

Neck pain

Neck pain may originate from any neck structure, ranging from the meninges and cervical vertebrae to its blood vessels, muscles, and lymphatic tissue. This symptom can also be referred from other areas of the body. Its location, onset, and pattern help determine the origin and underlying causes. Neck pain usually results from trauma and degenerative, congenital, inflammatory, metabolic, and neoplastic disorders.

ACTION STAT!

If the patient's neck pain is due to trauma, immediately ensure proper cervical spine immobilization, preferably with a long backboard and a Philadelphia collar. (See *Applying a Philadelphia collar*.) Then take his vital signs, and perform a quick neurologic examination. If he shows signs of respiratory distress, administer oxygen. Endotracheal intubation or tracheostomy and mechanical ventilation may be necessary. Ask the patient (or a family member, if the patient can't answer) how the injury occurred. Then examine the neck for abrasions, swelling, lacerations, erythema, and ecchymoses.

History and physical examination

If the patient hasn't sustained trauma, find out the severity and onset of his neck pain. Where specifically in the neck does he feel pain? Does anything relieve or worsen the pain? Does any particular event precipitate the pain? Also, ask about other symptoms, such as headaches or back pain. Next, focus on the patient's current and past illnesses and injuries, diet, drug history, and family health history.

Thoroughly inspect the patient's neck, shoulders, and cervical spine for swelling, masses, erythema, and ecchymoses. Assess active range of motion

Applying a Philadelphia collar

A lightweight molded polyethylene collar designed to hold the neck straight with the chin slightly elevated and tucked in, the Philadelphia cervical collar immobilizes the cervical spine, decreases muscle spasms, and relieves some pain. It also prevents further injury and promotes healing. When applying the collar, fit it snugly around the patient's neck and attach the Velcro fasteners or buckles at the back. Be sure to check the patient's airway and his neurovascular status to ensure that the collar isn't too tight. Also, make sure that the collar isn't placed too high in front, which can hyperextend the neck. In a patient with a neck sprain, hyperextension may cause the ligaments to heal in a shortened position; in a patient with a cervical spine fracture, it could cause serious neurologic damage.

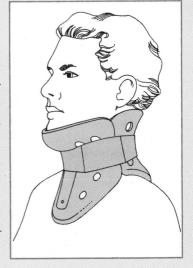

(ROM) in his neck by having him perform flexion, extension, rotation, and lateral side bending. Note the degree of pain produced by these movements. Examine his posture, and test and compare bilateral muscle strength. Check the sensation in his arms, and assess his hand grasp and arm reflexes. Attempt to elicit Brudzinski's and Kernig's signs if there isn't a history of neck trauma, and palpate the cervical lymph nodes for enlargement.

Medical causes

Ankylosing spondylitis. Intermittent, moderate to severe neck pain and stiffness with severely restricted ROM is characteristic of ankylosing spondylitis. Intermittent low back pain and stiffness and arm pain are generally worse in the morning or after periods of inactivity and are usually relieved after exercise. Related findings also include a low-grade fever, limited chest expansion, malaise, anorexia, fatigue and, occasionally, iritis.

Cervical extension injury. Anterior or posterior neck pain may develop within hours or days following a whiplash injury. Anterior pain usually diminishes within several days, but posterior pain persists and may even intensify. Associated findings include tenderness, swelling and nuchal rigidity, arm or back pain, an occipital headache, muscle spasms, visual blurring, and unilateral miosis on the affected side.

Cervical spine fracture. Fracture at C1 to C4 can cause sudden death; survivors may experience severe neck pain that restricts all movement, an intense occipital headache, quadriplegia, deformity, and respiratory paralysis.

Cervical spine tumor. Metastatic cervical spine tumors typically produce persistent neck pain that increases with movement and isn't relieved by rest; primary tumors cause mild to severe pain along a specific nerve root. Other findings depend on the lesions and may include paresthesia, arm and leg weakness that progresses to atrophy and paralysis, and bladder and bowel incontinence.

Cervical spondylosis. Cervical spondylosis produces posterior neck pain that restricts movement and is aggravated by it. Pain may radiate down either arm and may accompany paresthesia, weakness, and stiffness.

Esophageal trauma. An esophageal mucosal tear or a pulsion diverticulum may produce mild neck pain, chest pain, edema, hemoptysis, and dysphagia.

Herniated cervical disk. A herniated cervical disk characteristically causes variable neck pain that restricts movement and is aggravated by it. It also causes referred pain along a specific dermatome, paresthesia and other sensory disturbances, and arm weakness.

Laryngeal cancer. Neck pain that radiates to the ear develops late in laryngeal cancer. The patient may also develop dysphagia, dyspnea, hemoptysis, stridor, hoarseness, and cervical lymphadenopathy.

Lymphadenitis. With lymphadenitis, enlarged and inflamed cervical lymph nodes cause acute pain and tenderness. Fever, chills, and malaise may also occur.

Meningitis. With meningitis, neck pain may accompany characteristic nuchal rigidity. Related findings include fever, headache, photophobia, positive Brudzinski's and Kernig's signs, and decreased level of consciousness (LOC).

Neck sprain. Minor neck sprains typically produce pain, slight swelling, stiffness, and restricted ROM. Ligament rupture causes pain, marked swelling, ecchymosis, muscle spasms, and nuchal rigidity with head tilt.

Rheumatoid arthritis. Rheumatoid arthritis usually affects peripheral joints, but it can also involve the cervical vertebrae. Acute inflammation may cause moderate to severe pain that radiates along a specific nerve root; increased warmth, swelling, and tenderness in involved joints; stiffness, restricting ROM; paresthesia and muscle weakness; low-grade fever; anorexia; malaise; fatigue; and possible neck deformity. Some pain and stiffness remain after the acute *phase.*

Spinous process fracture. A fracture near the cervicothoracic junction produces acute pain radiating to the shoulders. Associated findings include swelling, exquisite tenderness, restricted ROM, muscle spasms, and deformity.

Subarachnoid hemorrhage. Subarachnoid hemorrhage is a life-threatening condition that may cause moderate to severe neck pain and rigidity, headache, and decreased LOC. Kernig's and Brudzinski's signs are present.

Thyroid trauma. Besides mild to moderate neck pain, thyroid trauma may cause local swelling and ecchymosis. If a hematoma forms, it can cause dyspnea.

Torticollis. Torticollis is a neck deformity in which severe neck pain accompanies recurrent unilateral stiffness and muscle spasms that produce a characteristic head tilt.

Tracheal trauma. A fracture of the tracheal cartilage, a life-threatening condition, produces moderate to severe neck pain and respiratory difficulty.

Torn tracheal mucosa produces mild to moderate pain and may result in airway occlusion, hemoptysis, hoarseness, and dysphagia.

Nursing considerations

■ Promote patient comfort by giving an anti-inflammatory and an analgesic, as needed.

■ Assist the patient to find positions that make him most comfortable.

■ Prepare him for diagnostic tests, such as X-rays, a computed tomography scan, blood tests, and cerebrospinal fluid analysis.

Patient teaching

■ Teach the patient how to apply a cervical collar, as appropriate.

■ Explain any activity restrictions.

■ Check that the patient knows how to perform any prescribed exercises correctly.

■ Teach about medications and their adverse effects.

Nipple discharge

Nipple discharge can occur spontaneously or can be elicited by nipple stimulation. It's characterized as intermittent or constant, unilateral or bilateral, and by color, consistency, and composition. Its incidence increases with age and parity. This sign rarely occurs (but is more likely to be pathologic) in men and in nulligravid, regularly menstruating women. It's relatively common and typically normal in parous women. A thick, grayish discharge—benign epithelial debris from inactive ducts—can usually be elicited in middle-aged parous women. Colostrum, a thin, yellowish or milky discharge, commonly occurs in the last weeks of pregnancy.

Nipple discharge can signal serious underlying disease, particularly when accompanied by other breast changes. Significant causes include endocrine disorders, cancer, certain drugs, and blocked lactiferous ducts.

History and physical examination

Ask the patient when she first noticed the discharge, and determine its duration, extent, quantity, color, consistency,

Eliciting nipple discharge

If the patient has a history or evidence of nipple discharge, you can attempt to elicit it during your examination. Help the patient into a supine position, and gently squeeze her nipple between your thumb and index finger; note any discharge through the nipple. Then place your fingers on the areola, as shown below, and palpate the entire areolar surface, watching for a discharge through areolar ducts.

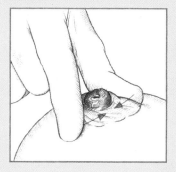

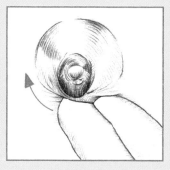

Obtain a complete gynecologic and obstetric history, and determine her normal menstrual cycle and the date of her last menses. Ask if she experiences breast swelling and tenderness, bloating, irritability, headaches, abdominal cramping, nausea, or diarrhea before or during menses. Note the number, date, and outcome of her pregnancies and, if she breast-fed, the approximate time of her last lactation. Also, check for risk factors of breast cancer—family history, previous or current malignancies, nulliparity or first pregnancy after age 30, early menarche, or late menopause.

Is the patient taking hormones (such as hormonal contraceptives or hormone replacement therapy), antihypertensives, or psychotropic drugs?

Start your physical examination by characterizing the discharge. If the discharge isn't frank, try to elicit it. (See *Eliciting nipple discharge.*) Then examine the nipples and breasts with the patient in four different positions: sitting with her arms at her sides; with her arms overhead; with her hands pressing on her hips; and leaning forward so her breasts are suspended. Check for nipple deviation, flattening, retraction, redness, asymmetry, thickening, excoriation, erosion, or cracking. Inspect her breasts for asymmetry, irregular contours, dimpling, erythema, and peau d'orange. With the patient in a supine position, palpate the breasts and axillae for lumps, giving special attention to the areolae. Note the size, location, delineation, consistency, and mobility of any lump you find.

Medical causes

Breast abscess. Breast abscess may produce a thick, purulent discharge from a cracked nipple or infected duct. Associated findings include an abrupt onset of a high fever with chills; breast pain, tenderness, and erythema; a palpa-

and smell, if any. Is the discharge spontaneous or does it have to be expressed? Has she had other nipple and breast changes, such as pain, tenderness, itching, warmth, changes in contour, and lumps? If she reports a lump, question her about its onset, location, size, and consistency. Ask about other symptoms, such as fever and malaise.

ble soft nodule or generalized induration; and possibly, nipple retraction.

Breast cancer. Breast cancer may cause bloody, watery, or purulent discharge from a normal-appearing nipple. Characteristic findings include a hard, irregular, fixed lump; erythema; dimpling; peau d'orange; changes in contour; nipple deviation, flattening, or retraction; axillary lymphadenopathy; and, possibly, breast pain.

Choriocarcinoma. Galactorrhea (a white or grayish milky discharge) may result from this highly malignant neoplasm, which can follow pregnancy. Other characteristics include persistent uterine bleeding and bogginess after delivery or curettage and vaginal masses.

Intraductal papilloma. Intraductal papilloma is the primary cause of nipple discharge in the nonpregnant, non–breast-feeding woman. Unilateral serous, serosanguineous, or bloody nipple discharge—usually from only one duct—is its predominant sign. Discharge may be intermittent or profuse and constant and can usually be stimulated by gentle pressure around the areola. Subareolar nodules, breast pain, and tenderness may occur.

Mammary duct ectasia. A thick, sticky, grayish discharge from multiple ducts may be the first sign of mammary duct ectasia. The discharge may be bilateral and is usually spontaneous. Other findings include a rubbery, poorly delineated lump beneath the areola, with a blue-green discoloration of the overlying skin; nipple retraction; and redness, swelling, tenderness, and burning pain in the areola and nipple.

Paget's disease. With Paget's disease, serous or bloody discharge emits from denuded skin on the nipple, which is red, intensely itchy and, possibly, eroded or excoriated. The discharge is usually unilateral.

Prolactin-secreting pituitary tumor. Bilateral galactorrhea may occur with prolactin-secreting pituitary tumor. Other findings include amenorrhea, infertility, decreased libido and vaginal secretions, headaches, and blindness.

Proliferative (fibrocystic) breast disease. Proliferative breast disease occasionally causes a bilateral clear, milky, or straw-colored discharge, which is rarely purulent or bloody. Multiple round, soft, tender nodules are usually palpable in both breasts, although they may occur singly. Usually, nodules are mobile and are located in the upper outer quadrant. Nodule size, tenderness, and discharge increase during the luteal phase of the menstrual cycle. Symptoms then regress after menses.

Other causes

Drugs. Galactorrhea can be caused by psychotropic agents, particularly phenothiazines and tricyclic antidepressants; some antihypertensives (such as reserpine and methyldopa); hormonal contraceptives; cimetidine; metoclopramide; and verapamil.

Surgery. Chest wall surgery may stimulate the thoracic nerves, causing intermittent bilateral galactorrhea.

Nursing considerations

▪ Apply a breast binder, which may reduce discharge by eliminating nipple stimulation.
▪ Prepare the patient for diagnostic tests such as tissue biopsy (if a breast lump is found), cytologic study of the discharge, mammography, ultrasonography, transillumination, and serum prolactin level.

Patient teaching

▪ Explain when to seek medical attention.
▪ Discuss the importance of breast self-examination, medical appointments, and mammograms.

■ Explain the nature and origin of the patient's nipple discharge and the treatment plan.

Nipple retraction

Nipple retraction, the inward displacement of the nipple below the level of surrounding breast tissue, may indicate an inflammatory breast lesion or cancer. It results from scar tissue formation within a lesion or large mammary duct. As the scar tissue shortens, it pulls adjacent tissue inward, causing nipple deviation, flattening and, finally, retraction.

History and physical examination

Ask the patient when she first noticed the nipple retraction. Has she experienced other nipple changes, such as itching, discoloration, discharge, or excoriation? Has she noticed breast pain, lumps, redness, swelling, or warmth? Has she had a fever? Obtain a history, noting risk factors of breast cancer, such as a family history or previous malignancy.

Carefully examine both nipples and breasts with the patient sitting upright with her arms at her sides; with her hands pressing on her hips; with her arms overhead; and leaning forward so her breasts hang. Look for redness, excoriation, and discharge; nipple flattening and deviation; and breast asymmetry, dimpling, or contour differences. (See *Differentiating nipple retraction from inversion*.)

Try to evert the nipple by gently squeezing the areola. With the patient in a supine position, palpate both breasts for lumps, especially beneath the areola. Mold breast skin over the lump or gently pull it up toward the clavicle, looking for accentuated nipple retraction. Also, palpate axillary lymph nodes.

Differentiating nipple retraction from inversion

Nipple retraction is sometimes confused with nipple inversion, a common abnormality that's congenital in many patients and doesn't usually signal underlying disease. A *retracted* nipple appears flat and broad, whereas an *inverted* nipple can be pulled out from the sulcus where it hides.

Nipple retraction

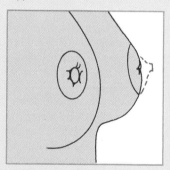

Nipple inversion

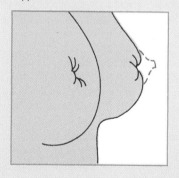

Medical causes

Breast abscess. Breast abscess occasionally produces unilateral nipple retraction. More common findings include a high fever with chills; breast pain, erythema, and tenderness; breast induration or a soft mass; and cracked, sore nipples, possibly with a purulent discharge.

Breast cancer. With breast cancer, unilateral nipple retraction is commonly accompanied by a hard, fixed, nontender nodule beneath the areola as well as other breast nodules. Other nipple changes include itching, burning, erosion, and watery or bloody discharge. Breast changes commonly include dimpling, altered contour, peau d'orange, ulceration, tenderness (possibly pain), redness, and warmth. Axillary lymph nodes may be enlarged.

Mammary duct ectasia. Nipple retraction commonly occurs along with a poorly defined, rubbery nodule beneath the areola, with a blue-green skin discoloration; areolar burning, itching, swelling, tenderness, and erythema; and nipple pain with a thick, sticky, grayish, multiductal discharge.

Mastitis. Nipple retraction, deviation, cracking, or flattening may occur in mastitis with a firm and indurated or tender, flocculent, discrete breast nodule; warmth; erythema; tenderness; and edema. Fatigue, high fevers, and chills may also be present.

Other causes
Surgery. Previous breast surgery may cause underlying scarring and retraction.

Nursing considerations
- Prepare the patient for diagnostic tests, including mammography, cytology of nipple discharge, and biopsy.

Patient teaching
- Teach the patient to perform monthly breast self-examination.
- Advise the patient to seek medical attention for breast changes.
- Explain the cause of the nipple retraction and the treatment plan.

▌Nocturia

Nocturia—excessive urination at night—may result from disruption of the normal diurnal pattern of urine concentration or from overstimulation of the nerves and muscles that control urination. Normally, more urine is concentrated during the night than during the day. As a result, most people excrete three to four times more urine during the day and can sleep for 6 to 8 hours during the night without being awakened. The patient with nocturia may awaken one or more times during the night to empty his bladder of 700 ml or more of urine.

Although nocturia usually results from renal and lower urinary tract disorders, it may result from certain cardiovascular, endocrine, and metabolic disorders. This common sign may also result from drugs that induce diuresis, particularly when they're taken at night, and from drinking large quantities of fluids, especially caffeinated beverages or alcohol, at bedtime.

History and physical examination
Begin by exploring the history of the patient's nocturia. When did it begin? How often does it occur? Can the patient identify a specific pattern or precipitating factors? Also, note the volume of urine voided. Ask the patient about changes in the color, odor, or consistency of his urine. Has the patient changed his usual pattern or volume of fluid intake? Next, explore associated symptoms. Ask about pain or burning on urination, difficulty initiating a urine stream, costovertebral angle (CVA) tenderness, and flank, upper abdominal, or suprapubic pain.

Determine if the patient or his family has a history of renal or urinary tract disorders or endocrine and metabolic diseases, particularly diabetes. Is the patient taking a drug that increases urine output, such as a diuretic, a cardiac glycoside, or an antihypertensive?

Focus your physical examination on palpating and percussing the kidneys, CVA, and bladder. Carefully inspect the urinary meatus. Inspect a urine specimen for color, odor, and the presence of sediment.

Medical causes

Benign prostatic hyperplasia (BPH). BPH produces nocturia when significant urethral obstruction develops. Typically, it causes frequency, hesitancy, incontinence, reduced force and caliber of the urine stream and, possibly, hematuria. Oliguria may also occur. Palpation reveals a distended bladder and an enlarged prostate. The patient may also complain of lower abdominal fullness, perineal pain, and constipation. Obstruction may lead to renal failure.

Cystitis. All three forms of cystitis may cause nocturia marked by frequent, small voidings and accompanied by dysuria and tenesmus.

Bacterial cystitis may also cause urinary urgency; hematuria; fatigue; suprapubic, perineal, flank, and lower back pain; and, occasionally, a low-grade fever. Most common in women between ages 25 and 60, chronic interstitial cystitis is characterized by Hunner's ulcers—small, punctate, bleeding lesions in the bladder; it also causes gross hematuria. Because symptoms resemble bladder cancer, this must be ruled out.

Viral cystitis also causes urinary urgency, hematuria, and fever.

Diabetes insipidus. The result of antidiuretic hormone deficiency, diabetes insipidus usually produces nocturia early in its course. It's characterized by periodic voiding of moderate to large amounts of urine. Diabetes insipidus can also produce polydipsia and dehydration.

Diabetes mellitus. An early sign of diabetes mellitus, nocturia involves voiding frequent, large amounts of urine. Associated features include daytime polyuria, polydipsia, polyphagia, frequent urinary tract infections, recurrent yeast infections, vaginitis, weakness, fatigue, weight loss and, possibly, signs of dehydration, such as dry mucous membranes and poor skin turgor.

Hypercalcemic nephropathy. With hypercalcemic nephropathy, nocturia involves the periodic voiding of moderate to large amounts of urine. Related findings include daytime polyuria, polydipsia and, occasionally, hematuria and pyuria.

Prostate cancer. Prostate cancer usually produces no symptoms in the early stages. Later, it produces nocturia characterized by difficulty voiding. Other characteristic effects include dysuria (most common symptom), difficulty initiating a urine stream, an interrupted urine stream, bladder distention, urinary frequency, weight loss, pallor, weakness, perineal pain, and constipation. Palpation reveals a hard, irregularly shaped, nodular prostate.

Pyelonephritis (acute). Nocturia is common with acute pyelonephritis and is usually characterized by voiding of moderate amounts of urine, which may appear cloudy. Associated signs and symptoms include a high, sustained fever with chills, fatigue, unilateral or bilateral flank pain, CVA tenderness, weakness, dysuria, hematuria, urinary frequency and urgency, and tenesmus. Occasionally, anorexia, nausea, vomiting, diarrhea, and hypoactive bowel sounds may also occur.

Renal failure (chronic). Nocturia occurs relatively early in chronic renal failure and is usually characterized by voiding of moderate amounts of urine. As the disorder progresses, oliguria or even anuria develops. Other widespread effects of chronic renal failure include fatigue, an ammonia breath odor, Kussmaul's respirations, peripheral edema, elevated blood pressure, a decreased level of consciousness, confusion, emotional lability, muscle twitching, anorexia, a metallic taste in the mouth, constipation or diarrhea, petechiae, ecchymoses, pruritus, yellow- or bronze-tinged skin, nausea, and vomiting.

Other causes
Drugs. Any drug that mobilizes edematous fluid or produces diuresis (for example, a diuretic or cardiac glycoside) may cause nocturia; obviously, this effect depends on when the drug is ingested.

Nursing considerations
▪ Monitor the patient's vital signs, intake and output, and daily weight.
▪ Document the frequency of nocturia, the amount, and specific gravity.
▪ Administer fluids to maintain fluid balance.
▪ Plan administration of a diuretic for daytime hours, if possible.
▪ Plan rest periods to compensate for sleep lost because of nocturia.
▪ Prepare the patient for diagnostic tests, which may include routine urinalysis; urine concentration and dilution studies; serum blood urea nitrogen, creatinine, and electrolyte levels; and cystoscopy.

Patient teaching
▪ Explain the importance of reducing fluid intake before bed.
▪ Reinforce the importance of voiding before bedtime.
▪ Explain the cause of the patient's nocturia and the treatment plan.

▌Nuchal rigidity

Commonly an early sign of meningeal irritation, nuchal rigidity refers to neck stiffness that prevents flexion. To elicit this sign, attempt to passively flex the patient's neck and touch his chin to his chest. If nuchal rigidity is present, this maneuver triggers pain and muscle spasms. (Make sure that there's no cervical spinal misalignment, such as a fracture or dislocation, before testing for nuchal rigidity. Severe spinal cord damage could result.) The patient may also notice nuchal rigidity when he attempts to flex his neck during daily activities. This sign isn't reliable in children and infants.

Nuchal rigidity may herald life-threatening subarachnoid hemorrhage or meningitis. It may also be a late sign of cervical arthritis, in which joint mobility is gradually lost.

ACTION STAT!

After eliciting nuchal rigidity, attempt to elicit Kernig's and Brudzinski's signs. Quickly evaluate the patient's level of consciousness (LOC). Take his vital signs. If you note signs of increased intracranial pressure (ICP), such as increased systolic pressure, bradycardia, and a widened pulse pressure, insert an I.V. catheter for drug and fluid administration. Administer oxygen as necessary. Draw a sample for routine blood studies such as a complete blood count with a white blood cell count and electrolyte levels.

History and physical examination
Obtain a patient history, relying on family members if an altered LOC prevents the patient from responding. Ask about the onset and duration of neck stiffness.

Were there precipitating factors? Also ask about associated signs and symptoms, such as headache, fever, nausea and vomiting, and motor and sensory changes. Check for a history of hypertension, head trauma, cerebral aneurysm or arteriovenous malformation, endocarditis, recent infection (such as sinusitis or pneumonia), or recent dental work. Then, obtain a complete drug history.

If the patient has no other signs of meningeal irritation, ask about a history of arthritis or neck trauma. Can the patient recall pulling a muscle in his neck? Inspect the patient's hands for swollen, tender joints, and palpate the neck for pain or tenderness.

Medical causes

Cervical arthritis. With cervical arthritis, nuchal rigidity develops gradually. Initially, the patient may complain of neck stiffness in the early morning or after a period of inactivity. Stiffness then becomes increasingly severe and frequent. Pain on movement, especially with lateral motion or head turning, is common. Typically, arthritis also affects other joints, especially those in the hands.

Encephalitis. Encephalitis is a viral infection that may cause nuchal rigidity accompanied by other signs of meningeal irritation, such as positive Kernig's and Brudzinski's signs. Usually, nuchal rigidity appears abruptly and is preceded by headache, vomiting, and fever. The patient may display rapidly decreasing LOC, progressing from lethargy to coma within 24 to 48 hours of onset. Associated features include seizures, ataxia, hemiparesis, nystagmus, and cranial nerve palsies, such as dysphagia and ptosis.

Listeriosis. If listeriosis spreads to the nervous system, meningitis may develop. Signs and symptoms include nuchal rigidity, fever, headache, change in LOC, myalgia, abdominal pain, nausea, vomiting, and diarrhea.

Meningitis. Nuchal rigidity is an early sign of meningitis and is accompanied by other signs of meningeal irritation— positive Kernig's and Brudzinski's signs, hyperreflexia and, possibly, opisthotonos. Other early features include fever with chills, headache, photophobia, and vomiting. Initially, the patient is confused and irritable; later, he may become stuporous and seizure-prone or may slip into a coma. Cranial nerve involvement may cause ocular palsies, facial weakness, and hearing loss. An erythematous papular rash occurs in some forms of viral meningitis; a purpuric rash may occur in meningococcal meningitis.

Subarachnoid hemorrhage. Nuchal rigidity develops immediately after bleeding into the subarachnoid space. Examination may detect positive Kernig's and Brudzinski's signs. The patient may experience an abrupt onset of a severe headache, photophobia, fever, nausea and vomiting, dizziness, cranial nerve palsies, and focal neurologic signs, such as hemiparesis or hemiplegia. His LOC deteriorates rapidly, possibly progressing to coma. Signs of increased ICP, such as bradycardia and altered respirations, may also occur.

Nursing considerations

- Prepare the patient for diagnostic tests, such as computed tomography scans, magnetic resonance imaging, and cervical spinal X-rays.
- Monitor the patient's vital signs, intake and output, and neurologic status closely.
- Avoid routine administration of opioid analgesics because these may mask signs of increasing ICP.

- Enforce strict bed rest; keep the head of the bed elevated at least 30 degrees to help minimize ICP.

Patient teaching
- Explain all procedures and diagnostic tests to the patient and his family.
- Orient the patient, as appropriate.
- Explain the cause of nuccal rigidity and the treatment plan.

Nystagmus

Nystagmus refers to the involuntary oscillations of one or, more commonly, both eyeballs. These oscillations are usually rhythmic and may be horizontal, vertical, rotary, or mixed. They may be transient or sustained and may occur spontaneously or on deviation or fixation of the eyes. Minor degrees of nystagmus at the extremes of gaze are normal. Nystagmus when the eyes are stationary and looking straight ahead is always abnormal. Although nystagmus is fairly easy to identify, the patient may be unaware of it unless it affects his vision.

Nystagmus may be classified as pendular or jerk. *Pendular nystagmus* consists of horizontal (pendular) or vertical (seesaw) oscillations that are equal in rate in both directions and resemble the movements of a clock's pendulum. *Jerk nystagmus* (convergence-retraction, downbeat, and vestibular), which is more common than pendular nystagmus, has a fast component and then a slow—perhaps unequal—corrective component in the opposite direction. (See *Classifying nystagmus,* page 434.)

Nystagmus is considered a *supranuclear* ocular palsy—that is, it results from disorders of the visual perceptual area, vestibular system, cerebellum, or brain stem rather than in the extraocular muscles or cranial nerves III, IV, and VI. Its causes are varied and include brain stem or cerebellar lesions, multiple sclerosis, encephalitis, labyrinthine disease, and drug toxicity. Occasionally, nystagmus is entirely normal; it's also considered a normal response in the unconscious patient during the doll's eye test (oculocephalic stimulation) or the cold caloric water test (oculovestibular stimulation).

History and physical examination
Begin by asking the patient how long he has had nystagmus. Does it occur intermittently? Does it affect his vision? Ask about recent infection, especially of the ear or respiratory tract, and about head trauma and cancer. Does the patient or anyone in his family have a history of stroke? Then explore associated signs and symptoms. Ask about vertigo, dizziness, tinnitus, nausea or vomiting, numbness, weakness, bladder dysfunction, and fever.

Begin the physical examination by assessing the patient's level of consciousness (LOC) and vital signs. Be alert for signs of increased intracranial pressure (ICP), such as pupillary changes, drowsiness, elevated systolic pressure, and an altered respiratory pattern. Next, assess nystagmus fully by testing extraocular muscle function: Ask the patient to focus straight ahead and then to follow your finger up, down, and in an "X" across his face. Note when nystagmus occurs as well as its velocity and direction. Finally, test reflexes, motor and sensory function, and the cranial nerves.

Medical causes
Brain tumor. An insidious onset of jerk nystagmus may occur with tumors of the brain stem and cerebellum. Associated characteristics include deafness, dysphagia, nausea and vomiting, vertigo, and ataxia. Brain stem compression by the tumor may cause signs of in-

Classifying nystagmus

Jerk nystagmus

Convergence-retraction nystagmus refers to the irregular jerking of the eyes back into the orbit during upward gaze. It can indicate midbrain tegmental damage.

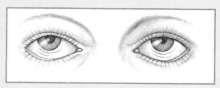

Downbeat nystagmus refers to the irregular downward jerking of the eyes during downward gaze. It can signal lower medullary damage.

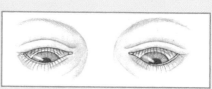

Vestibular nystagmus, the horizontal or rotary movement of the eyes, suggests vestibular disease or cochlear dysfunction.

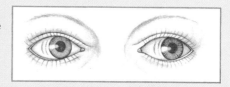

Pendular nystagmus

Horizontal, or *pendular, nystagmus* refers to oscillations of equal velocity around a center point. It can indicate congenital loss of visual acuity or multiple sclerosis.

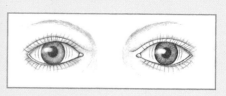

Vertical, or *seesaw, nystagmus* is the rapid, seesaw movement of the eyes: one eye appears to rise while the other appears to fall. It suggests an optic chiasm lesion.

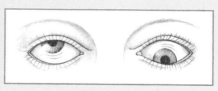

creased ICP, such as altered LOC, bradycardia, a widening pulse pressure, and an elevated systolic blood pressure.

Encephalitis. With encephalitis, jerk nystagmus is typically accompanied by altered LOC ranging from lethargy to coma. Usually, it's preceded by sudden onset of fever, headache, and vomiting. Among other features are nuchal rigidity, seizures, aphasia, ataxia, photophobia,

and cranial nerve palsies, such as dysphagia and ptosis.

Head trauma. Brain stem injury may cause jerk nystagmus, which is usually horizontal. The patient may also display pupillary changes, an altered respiratory pattern, altered LOC, and decerebrate posture.

Labyrinthitis (acute). Acute labyrinthitis causes a sudden onset of jerk nystagmus, accompanied by dizziness, vertigo, tinnitus, nausea, and vomiting. The fast component of the nystagmus is toward the unaffected ear. Gradual sensorineural hearing loss may also occur.

Ménière's disease. Ménière's disease is characterized by acute attacks of jerk nystagmus, severe nausea and vomiting, dizziness, vertigo, progressive hearing loss, tinnitus, and diaphoresis. Typically, the direction of jerk nystagmus varies from one attack to the next. Attacks may last from 10 minutes to several hours.

Stroke. A stroke involving the posterior inferior cerebellar artery may cause sudden horizontal or vertical jerk nystagmus that may be gaze dependent. Other findings include dysphagia, dysarthria, loss of pain and temperature sensation on the ipsilateral face and contralateral trunk and limbs, ipsilateral Horner's syndrome (unilateral ptosis, pupillary constriction, and facial anhidrosis), and cerebellar signs, such as ataxia and vertigo. Signs of increased ICP (such as altered LOC, bradycardia, a widening pulse pressure, and an elevated systolic pressure) may also occur.

Other causes

Drugs and alcohol. Jerk nystagmus may result from barbiturate, phenytoin, or carbamazepine toxicity or from alcohol intoxication.

Nursing considerations

- Prepare the patient for diagnostic tests, such as electronystagmography and a cerebral computed tomography scan.
- Provide for the patient's safety.

Patient teaching

- Instruct the patient about safety measures.
- Tell the patient to avoid sudden position changes.

- Explain the cause of the nystagmus and the treatment plan.

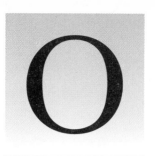

Ocular deviation

Ocular deviation refers to abnormal eye movement that may be conjugate (both eyes move together) or disconjugate (one eye moves separately from the other). This common sign may result from ocular, neurologic, endocrine, and systemic disorders that interfere with the muscles, nerves, or brain centers governing eye movement. Occasionally, it signals a life-threatening disorder such as a ruptured cerebral aneurysm. (See *Ocular deviation: Its characteristics and causes in cranial nerve damage.*)

Normally, eye movement is directly controlled by the extraocular muscles innervated by the oculomotor, trochlear, and abducens nerves (cranial nerves III, IV, and VI). Together, these muscles and nerves direct a visual stimulus to fall on corresponding parts of the retina. Disconjugate ocular deviation may result from unequal muscle tone (nonparalytic strabismus) or muscle paralysis associated with cranial nerve damage (paralytic strabismus). Conjugate ocular deviation may result from disorders that affect the centers in the cerebral cortex and brain stem responsible for conjugate eye movement. Typically, such disorders cause gaze palsy—difficulty moving the eyes in one or more directions.

History and physical examination

If the patient isn't in distress, find out how long he has had the ocular deviation. Is it accompanied by double vision, eye pain, or headache? Also, ask if he has noticed associated motor or sensory changes or fever.

Check for a history of hypertension, diabetes, allergies, and thyroid, neurologic, or muscular disorders. Then obtain a thorough ocular history. Has the patient ever had extraocular muscle imbalance, eye or head trauma, or eye surgery?

During the physical examination, observe the patient for partial or complete ptosis. Does he spontaneously tilt his head or turn his face to compensate for

Ocular deviation: Its characteristics and causes in cranial nerve damage

Characteristics	Cranial nerve and extraocular muscles involved	Probable causes
Inability to move the eye upward, downward, inward, and outward; drooping eyelid; and, except in diabetes, a dilated pupil in the affected eye	Oculomotor nerve (cranial nerve [CN] III); medial rectus, superior rectus, inferior rectus, and inferior oblique muscles	Cerebral aneurysm, diabetes, temporal lobe herniation from increased intracranial pressure, brain tumor
Loss of downward and outward movement in the affected eye	Trochlear nerve (CN IV); superior oblique muscle	Head trauma
Loss of outward movement in the affected eye	Abducens nerve (CN VI); lateral rectus muscle	Brain tumor

ocular deviation? Check for eye redness or periorbital edema. Assess the patient's visual acuity, and then evaluate extraocular muscle function by testing the six cardinal fields of gaze.

Medical causes

Brain tumor. The nature of ocular deviation depends on the site and extent of the brain tumor. Associated signs and symptoms include headaches that are most severe in the morning, behavioral changes, memory loss, dizziness, confusion, vision loss, motor and sensory dysfunction, aphasia and, possibly, signs of hormonal imbalance. The patient's LOC may slowly deteriorate from lethargy to coma. Late signs include papilledema, vomiting, increased systolic blood pressure, widening pulse pressure, and decorticate posture.

Cavernous sinus thrombosis. With cavernous sinus thrombosis, ocular deviation may be accompanied by diplopia, photophobia, exophthalmos, orbital and eyelid edema, corneal haziness, diminished or absent pupillary reflexes, and impaired visual acuity. Other fea-

tures include a high fever, headache, malaise, nausea and vomiting, seizures, and tachycardia. Retinal hemorrhage and papilledema are late signs.

Diabetes mellitus. A leading cause of isolated third cranial nerve palsy, especially in the middle-aged patient with long-standing mild diabetes, diabetes mellitus may cause ocular deviation and ptosis. Typically, the patient also complains of the sudden onset of diplopia and pain.

Encephalitis. Encephalitis causes ocular deviation and diplopia in some cases. Typically, it begins abruptly with fever, headache, and vomiting, followed by signs of meningeal irritation (for example, nuchal rigidity) and neuronal damage (for example, seizures, aphasia, ataxia, hemiparesis, cranial nerve palsies, and photophobia). The patient's LOC may rapidly deteriorate from lethargy to coma within 24 to 48 hours after onset.

Head trauma. The nature of ocular deviation depends on the site and extent of head trauma. The patient may have visible soft-tissue injury, bony deformity, facial edema, and clear or bloody otorrhea or rhinorrhea. Besides these obvious signs of trauma, he may also develop blurred vision, diplopia, nystagmus, behavioral changes, headache, motor and sensory dysfunction, and decreased LOC that may progress to coma. Signs of increased intracranial pressure—such as bradycardia, increased systolic pressure, and widening pulse pressure—may also occur.

Orbital blowout fracture. With an orbital blowout fracture, the inferior rectus muscle may become entrapped, resulting in limited extraocular movement and ocular deviation. Typically, the patient's upward gaze is absent; other directions of gaze may be affected if edema is dramatic. The globe may also be displaced downward and inward. Associated signs and symptoms include pain, diplopia, nausea, periorbital edema, and ecchymosis.

Orbital tumor. Ocular deviation occurs as the orbital tumor gradually enlarges. Associated findings include proptosis, diplopia and, possibly, blurred vision.

Stroke. Stroke, a life-threatening disorder, may cause ocular deviation, depending on the site and extent of the stroke. Accompanying features are also variable and include altered LOC, contralateral hemiplegia and sensory loss, dysarthria, dysphagia, homonymous hemianopsia, blurred vision, and diplopia. In addition, the patient may develop urine retention or incontinence or both, constipation, behavioral changes, headache, vomiting, and seizures.

Thyrotoxicosis. Thyrotoxicosis may produce exophthalmos—proptotic or protruding eyes—which, in turn, causes limited extraocular movement and ocular deviation. Usually, the patient's upward gaze weakens first, followed by diplopia. Other features are lid retrac-

tion, a wide-eyed staring gaze, excessive tearing, edematous eyelids and, sometimes, an inability to close the eyes. Cardinal features of thyrotoxicosis include tachycardia, palpitations, weight loss despite increased appetite, diarrhea, tremors, an enlarged thyroid, dyspnea, nervousness, diaphoresis, heat intolerance, and an atrial or a ventricular gallop.

Nursing considerations

■ Monitor the patient's vital signs and neurologic status if you suspect an acute neurologic disorder.
■ Take seizure precautions, if necessary.
■ Prepare the patient for diagnostic tests, such as blood studies, orbital and skull X-rays, and a CT scan.

Patient teaching

■ Explain the disorder and its treatment.
■ Discuss with the patient and his family changes in LOC that need to be reported.
■ Talk about how to maintain a safe environment.
■ Teach ways of reducing environmental stress.

Oligomenorrhea

In most women, menstrual bleeding occurs every 28 days, plus or minus 4 days. Although some variation is normal, menstrual bleeding at intervals of greater than 36 days may indicate oligomenorrhea—abnormally infrequent menstrual bleeding characterized by three to six menstrual cycles per year. When menstrual bleeding does occur, it's usually profuse, prolonged (up to 10 days), and laden with clots and tissue. Occasionally, scant bleeding or spotting occurs between these heavy menses.

Oligomenorrhea may develop suddenly or it may follow a period of gradually lengthening cycles. Although oligomenorrhea may alternate with normal menstrual bleeding, it can progress to secondary amenorrhea.

Because oligomenorrhea is commonly associated with anovulation, it's common in infertile, early postmenarchal, and perimenopausal women. This sign usually reflects abnormalities of the hormones that govern normal endometrial function. It may result from ovarian, hypothalamic, pituitary, thyroid, and other metabolic disorders and from the effects of certain drugs. It may also result from emotional or physical stress, such as sudden weight change, a debilitating illness, or rigorous physical training.

History and physical examination

After asking the patient's age, find out when menarche occurred. Has the patient ever experienced normal menstrual cycles? When did she begin having abnormal cycles? Ask her to describe the pattern of bleeding. How many days does the bleeding last, and how frequently does it occur? Are there clots and tissue fragments in her menstrual flow? Note when she last had menses.

Next, determine if she's having symptoms of ovulatory bleeding. Does she experience mild, cramping abdominal pain 14 days before she bleeds? Is the bleeding accompanied by premenstrual symptoms, such as breast tenderness, irritability, bloating, weight gain, nausea, and diarrhea? Does she have cramping or pain with bleeding? Also, check for a history of infertility. Does the patient have children? Is she trying to conceive? Ask if she's currently using hormonal contraceptives or if she has ever used them in the past. If she has, find out when she stopped taking them.

Then ask about previous gynecologic disorders such as ovarian cysts. If the patient is breast-feeding, has she experienced problems with milk production?

If she hasn't been breast-feeding recently, has she noticed milk leaking from her breasts? Ask about recent weight gain or loss. Is the patient less than 80% of her ideal weight? If so, does she claim that she's overweight? Ask if she's exercising more vigorously than usual.

Screen for metabolic disorders by asking about excessive thirst, frequent urination, or fatigue. Has the patient been jittery or had palpitations? Ask about headaches, dizziness, and impaired peripheral vision. Complete the history by finding out what drugs the patient is taking.

Begin the physical examination by taking the patient's vital signs and weighing her. Inspect for increased facial hair growth, sparse body hair, male distribution of fat and muscle, acne, and clitoral enlargement. Note if the skin is abnormally dry or moist, and check hair texture. Also, be alert for signs of psychological or physical stress. Rule out pregnancy by a blood or urine pregnancy test.

Medical causes

Adrenal hyperplasia. With adrenal hyperplasia, oligomenorrhea may occur with signs of androgen excess, such as clitoral enlargement and male distribution of hair, fat, and muscle mass.

Anorexia nervosa. Anorexia nervosa may cause sporadic oligomenorrhea or amenorrhea. Its cardinal symptom, however, is a morbid fear of being fat associated with weight loss of more than 20% of ideal body weight. Typically, the patient displays dramatic skeletal muscle atrophy and loss of fatty tissue; dry or sparse scalp hair; lanugo on the face and body; and blotchy or sallow, dry skin. Other symptoms include constipation, a decreased libido, and sleep disturbances.

Diabetes mellitus. Oligomenorrhea may be an early sign in diabetes mellitus. In type 1 diabetes, the patient may have never had normal menses. Associated findings include excessive hunger, polydipsia, polyuria, weakness, fatigue, dry mucous membranes, poor skin turgor, irritability and emotional lability, and weight loss.

Hypothyroidism. Besides oligomenorrhea, hypothyroidism may result in fatigue; forgetfulness; cold intolerance; unexplained weight gain; constipation; bradycardia; decreased mental acuity; dry, flaky, inelastic skin; puffy face, hands, and feet; hoarseness; periorbital edema; ptosis; dry, sparse hair; and thick, brittle nails.

Prolactin-secreting pituitary tumor. Oligomenorrhea or amenorrhea may be the first sign of a prolactin-secreting pituitary tumor. Accompanying findings include unilateral or bilateral galactorrhea, infertility, loss of libido, and sparse pubic hair. Headache and visual field disturbances—such as diminished peripheral vision, blurred vision, diplopia, and hemianopia—signal tumor expansion.

Thyrotoxicosis. Thyrotoxicosis may produce oligomenorrhea along with reduced fertility. Cardinal findings include irritability, weight loss despite increased appetite, dyspnea, tachycardia, palpitations, diarrhea, tremors, diaphoresis, heat intolerance, an enlarged thyroid and, possibly, exophthalmos.

Other causes

Drugs. Drugs that increase androgen levels—such as corticosteroids, corticotropin, anabolic steroids, danocrine, and injectable and implanted hormonal contraceptives—may cause oligomenorrhea. Hormonal contraceptives may be associated with delayed resumption of normal menses when their use is discontinued; however, 95% of women resume normal menses within 3 months. Other drugs that may cause oligomenor-

rhea include phenothiazine derivatives and amphetamines, and antihypertensive drugs, which increase prolactin levels.

Nursing considerations

- Prepare the patient for diagnostic tests, such as blood hormone levels, thyroid studies, or pelvic imaging studies.

Patient teaching

- Teach the patient techniques of recording basal body temperature.
- Explain the use of a home ovulation test.
- Provide information about the use of contraceptives.
- Teach about the cause of oligomenorrhea and the treatment plan.

▌Oliguria

A cardinal sign of renal and urinary tract disorders, oliguria is clinically defined as urine output of less than 400 ml/24 hours. Typically, this sign occurs abruptly and may herald serious—possibly life-threatening—hemodynamic instability. Its causes can be classified as prerenal (decreased renal blood flow), intrarenal (intrinsic renal damage), or postrenal (urinary tract obstruction); the pathophysiology differs for each classification. (See *How oliguria develops,* pages 442 and 443.) Oliguria associated with a prerenal or postrenal cause is usually promptly reversible with treatment, although it may lead to intrarenal damage if untreated. However, oliguria associated with an intrarenal cause is usually more persistent and may be irreversible.

History and physical examination

Begin by asking the patient about his usual daily voiding pattern, including frequency and amount. When did he first notice changes in this pattern and in the color, odor, or consistency of his urine? Ask about pain or burning on urination. Has the patient had a fever? Note his normal daily fluid intake. Has he recently been drinking more or less than usual? Has his intake of caffeine or alcohol changed drastically? Has he had recent episodes of diarrhea or vomiting that might cause fluid loss? Next, explore associated complaints, especially fatigue, loss of appetite, thirst, dyspnea, chest pain, or recent weight gain or loss (in dehydration).

Check for a history of renal, urinary tract, or cardiovascular disorders. Note recent traumatic injury or surgery associated with significant blood loss as well as recent blood transfusions. Was the patient exposed to nephrotoxic agents, such as heavy metals, organic solvents, anesthetics, or radiographic contrast media? Next, obtain a drug history.

Begin the physical examination by taking the patient's vital signs and weighing him. Assess his overall appearance for edema. Palpate both kidneys for tenderness and enlargement, and percuss for costovertebral angle (CVA) tenderness. Also, inspect the flank area for edema or erythema. Auscultate the heart and lungs for abnormal sounds and the flank area for renal artery bruits. Assess the patient for edema or signs of dehydration such as dry mucous membranes.

Obtain a urine specimen and inspect it for abnormal color, odor, or sediment. Use reagent strips to test for glucose, protein, and blood. Also, use a urinometer to measure specific gravity.

Medical causes

Acute tubular necrosis (ATN). An early sign of ATN, oliguria may occur abruptly (in shock) or gradually (in nephrotoxicity). Usually, it persists for about 2 weeks, followed by polyuria. Related features include signs of hyper-

kalemia (muscle weakness and cardiac arrhythmias), uremia (anorexia, confusion, lethargy, twitching, seizures, pruritus, and Kussmaul's respirations), and heart failure (edema, jugular vein distention, crackles, and dyspnea).

Calculi. Oliguria or anuria may result from calculi lodging in the kidneys, ureters, bladder outlet, or urethra. Associated signs and symptoms include urinary frequency and urgency, dysuria, and hematuria or pyuria. Usually, the patient experiences renal colic—excruciating pain that radiates from the CVA to the flank, the suprapubic region, and the external genitalia. This pain may be accompanied by nausea, vomiting, hypoactive bowel sounds, abdominal distention and, occasionally, fever and chills.

Cholera. With cholera, severe water and electrolyte loss lead to oliguria, thirst, weakness, muscle cramps, decreased skin turgor, tachycardia, hypotension, and abrupt watery diarrhea and vomiting. Death may occur in hours without treatment.

Glomerulonephritis (acute). Acute glomerulonephritis produces oliguria or anuria. Other features are a mild fever, fatigue, gross hematuria, proteinuria, generalized edema, elevated blood pressure, headache, nausea and vomiting, flank and abdominal pain, and signs of pulmonary congestion (dyspnea and a productive cough).

Heart failure. Oliguria may occur with left-sided heart failure as a result of low cardiac output and decreased renal perfusion. Accompanying signs and symptoms include dyspnea, fatigue, weakness, peripheral edema, jugular vein distention, tachycardia, tachypnea, crackles, and a dry or productive cough. With advanced or chronic heart failure, the patient may also develop orthopnea, cyanosis, clubbing, a ventricular gallop,

How oliguria develops

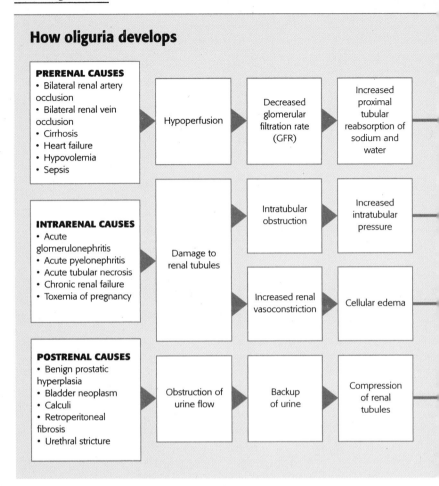

PRERENAL CAUSES
• Bilateral renal artery occlusion
• Bilateral renal vein occlusion
• Cirrhosis
• Heart failure
• Hypovolemia
• Sepsis

Hypoperfusion → Decreased glomerular filtration rate (GFR) → Increased proximal tubular reabsorption of sodium and water

INTRARENAL CAUSES
• Acute glomerulonephritis
• Acute pyelonephritis
• Acute tubular necrosis
• Chronic renal failure
• Toxemia of pregnancy

Damage to renal tubules → Intratubular obstruction → Increased intratubular pressure

Increased renal vasoconstriction → Cellular edema

POSTRENAL CAUSES
• Benign prostatic hyperplasia
• Bladder neoplasm
• Calculi
• Retroperitoneal fibrosis
• Urethral stricture

Obstruction of urine flow → Backup of urine → Compression of renal tubules

diastolic hypertension, cardiomegaly, and hemoptysis.

Hypovolemia. Any disorder that decreases circulating fluid volume can produce oliguria. Associated findings include orthostatic hypotension, apathy, lethargy, fatigue, gross muscle weakness, anorexia, nausea, profound thirst, dizziness, sunken eyeballs, poor skin turgor, and dry mucous membranes.

Pyelonephritis (acute). Accompanying the sudden onset of oliguria with acute pyelonephritis are a high fever with chills, fatigue, flank pain, CVA tenderness, weakness, nocturia, dysuria,

hematuria, urinary frequency and urgency, and tenesmus. The urine may appear cloudy. Occasionally, the patient also experiences anorexia, diarrhea, and nausea and vomiting.

Renal failure (chronic). Oliguria is a major sign of end-stage chronic renal failure. Associated findings reflect progressive uremia and include fatigue, weakness, irritability, uremic fetor, ecchymoses and petechiae, peripheral edema, elevated blood pressure, confusion, emotional lability, drowsiness, coarse muscle twitching, muscle cramps, peripheral neuropathies, anorexia, a metal-

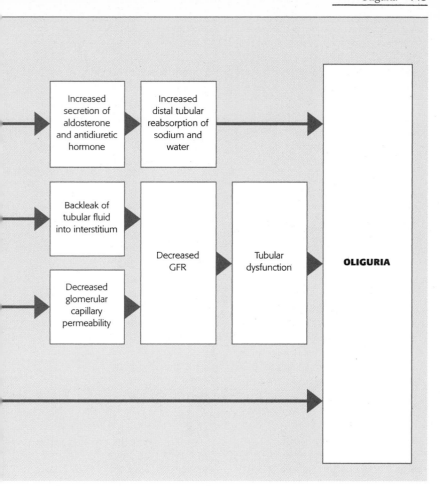

lic taste in the mouth, nausea and vomiting, constipation or diarrhea, stomatitis, pruritus, pallor, and yellow- or bronze-tinged skin. Eventually, seizures, coma, and uremic frost may develop.

Renal vein occlusion (bilateral). Bilateral renal vein occlusion occasionally causes oliguria accompanied by acute low back and flank pain, CVA tenderness, fever, pallor, hematuria, enlarged and palpable kidneys, edema and, possibly, signs of uremia.

Toxemia of pregnancy. With severe preeclampsia, oliguria may be accompanied by elevated blood pressure, dizzi-

ness, diplopia, blurred vision, epigastric pain, nausea and vomiting, irritability, and a severe frontal headache. Typically, oliguria is preceded by generalized edema and sudden weight gain of more than 3 lb (1.4 kg) per week during the second trimester, or more than 1 lb (0.45 kg) per week during the third trimester. If preeclampsia progresses to eclampsia, the patient develops seizures and may slip into coma.

Urethral stricture. Urethral stricture produces oliguria accompanied by chronic urethral discharge, urinary frequency and urgency, dysuria, pyuria, and a diminished urine stream. As the obstruction worsens, urine extravasation may lead to formation of urinomas and urosepsis.

Other causes

Diagnostic studies. Radiographic studies that use contrast media may cause nephrotoxicity and oliguria.

Drugs. Oliguria may result from drugs that cause decreased renal perfusion (diuretics), nephrotoxicity (most notably, aminoglycosides and chemotherapeutic drugs), urine retention (adrenergics and anticholinergics), or urinary obstruction associated with precipitation of urinary crystals (sulfonamides and acyclovir).

Nursing considerations

■ Monitor the patient's vital signs, intake and output, and daily weight.
■ Depending on the cause of oliguria, restrict fluids to between 0.6 and 1 L more than the patient's urine output for the previous day.
■ Provide a diet low in sodium, potassium, and protein.
■ Prepare the patient for diagnostic tests, such as laboratory tests (including serum blood urea nitrogen and creatinine levels, urea and creatinine clearance, urine sodium levels, and urine osmolality), abdominal X-rays, ultrasonography, a computed tomography scan, cystography, and a renal scan.
■ Prepare the patient for dialysis.

Patient teaching

■ Explain any fluid and dietary restrictions.
■ Explain the underlying disorder and the treatment plan.

Opisthotonos

A sign of severe meningeal irritation, opisthotonos is a severe, prolonged spasm characterized by a strongly arched, rigid back; a hyperextended neck; the heels bent back; and the arms and hands flexed at the joints. Usually, this posture occurs spontaneously and continuously; however, it may be aggravated by movement. Presumably, opisthotonos represents a protective reflex because it immobilizes the spine, alleviating the pain associated with meningeal irritation.

Usually caused by meningitis, opisthotonos may also result from subarachnoid hemorrhage, Arnold-Chiari syndrome, and tetanus. Occasionally, it occurs in achondroplastic dwarfism, although not necessarily as an indicator of meningeal irritation.

Opisthotonos is far more common in children—especially infants—than in adults. It's also more exaggerated in children because of nervous system immaturity. (See *Opisthotonos: Sign of meningeal irritation.*)

ACTION STAT!

 If the patient is stuporous or comatose and displays opisthotonos, immediately evaluate his vital signs. Employ resuscitative measures, as appropriate. Place the patient in bed, with side rails raised and padded, or in a crib.

History and physical examination

If the patient's condition permits, obtain a history. If the patient is a young child or an infant, consult with a relative. Ask about a history of cerebral aneurysm or arteriovenous malformation and about hypertension. Note a recent infection that may have spread to the nervous system. Explore associated findings, such as fever, headaches, chills, and vomiting.

Focus the physical examination on the patient's neurologic status. Evaluate

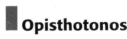

Opisthotonos: Sign of meningeal irritation

In the characteristic posture, the back is severely arched with the neck hyperextended. The heels bend back on the legs, and the arms and hands flex rigidly at the joints, as shown below.

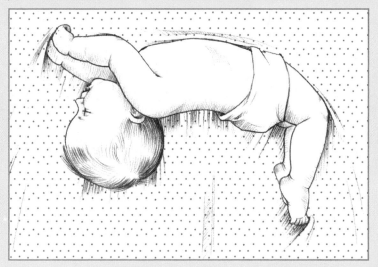

his level of consciousness (LOC) and test sensorimotor and cranial nerve function. Then check for Brudzinski's and Kernig's signs and for nuchal rigidity.

Medical causes

Arnold-Chiari syndrome. With Arnold-Chiari syndrome, opisthotonos typically occurs with hydrocephalus and its characteristic enlarged head; thin, shiny scalp with distended veins; and underdeveloped neck muscles. The infant usually also exhibits a high-pitched cry, abnormal leg muscle tone, anorexia, vomiting, nuchal rigidity, irritability, noisy respirations, and a weak sucking reflex.

Meningitis. With meningitis, opisthotonos accompanies other signs of meningeal irritation, including nuchal rigidity, positive Brudzinski's and Kernig's signs, and hyperreflexia. This disor-

der also causes cardinal signs of infection (moderate to high fever with chills and malaise) and of increased intracranial pressure (ICP) (headache, vomiting and, eventually, papilledema). Other features include irritability; photophobia; diplopia, deafness, and other cranial nerve palsies; and decreased LOC that may progress to seizures and coma.

Subarachnoid hemorrhage. Subarachnoid hemorrhage may produce opisthotonos along with other signs of meningeal irritation, such as nuchal rigidity and positive Kernig's and Brudzinski's signs. Focal signs of hemorrhage, such as a severe headache, hemiplegia or hemiparesis, aphasia, and photophobia, along with other vision problems, may also occur. With increasing ICP, the patient may develop bradycardia, elevated blood pressure, an altered respiratory pattern, seizures, and vomiting. His LOC may rapidly deteriorate, resulting in coma; then, decerebrate posture may alternate with opisthotonos.

Tetanus. Tetanus is a life-threatening infection that can cause opisthotonos. Initially, trismus occurs. Eventually, muscle spasms may affect the abdomen, producing boardlike rigidity; the back, resulting in opisthotonos; or the face, producing risus sardonicus. Spasms may affect the respiratory muscles, causing distress. Tachycardia, diaphoresis, hyperactive deep tendon reflexes, and seizures may also develop.

Other causes

Antipsychotics. Phenothiazines and other antipsychotic drugs may cause opisthotonos, usually as part of an acute dystonic reaction.

Nursing considerations

■ Assess the patient's neurologic status and check his vital signs frequently.
■ Make the patient as comfortable as possible; place him in a side-lying position with pillows for support.
■ If meningitis is suspected, institute respiratory isolation.
■ Prepare the patient for diagnostic tests, such as lumbar puncture, computed tomography scan, or magnetic resonance imaging.

Patient teaching

■ Teach the patient and his family about the patient's condition and its treatment.
■ Offer emotional support and refer the patient and his family to appropriate support groups and community resources.

Orthopnea

Orthopnea—difficulty breathing in the supine position—is a common symptom of cardiopulmonary disorders that produce dyspnea. It's usually a subtle symptom; the patient may complain that he can't catch his breath when lying down, or he may mention that he sleeps most comfortably in a reclining chair or propped up by pillows. Derived from this complaint is the common classification of two- or three-pillow orthopnea.

Orthopnea presumably results from increased hydrostatic pressure in the pulmonary vasculature related to gravitational effects in the supine position. It may be aggravated by obesity or pregnancy, which restricts diaphragmatic excursion. Sitting in an upright position relieves orthopnea by placing much of the pulmonary vasculature above the left atrium, which reduces mean hydrostatic pressure, and by enhancing diaphragmatic excursion, which increases inspiratory volume.

History and physical examination

Begin by asking about a history of cardiopulmonary disorders, such as myocardial infarction, rheumatic heart disease, valvular disease, asthma, emphysema, or chronic bronchitis. Does the patient smoke? If so, how much? Explore associated symptoms, noting especially complaints of coughing, nocturnal or exertional dyspnea, fatigue, weakness, loss of appetite, or chest pain. Does the patient use alcohol or have a history of heavy alcohol use?

When examining the patient, check for other signs of increased respiratory effort, such as accessory muscle use, shallow respirations, and tachypnea. Also note barrel chest. Inspect the patient's skin for pallor or cyanosis and the fingers for clubbing. Observe and palpate for edema, and check for jugular vein distention. Auscultate the lungs for crackles, rhonchi, or wheezing. Also auscultate the heart. Monitor the patient's oxygen saturation.

Medical causes

Chronic obstructive pulmonary disease (COPD). COPD typically produces orthopnea and other dyspneic complaints, accompanied by accessory muscle use, tachypnea, tachycardia, and paradoxical pulse. Auscultation may reveal diminished breath sounds, rhonchi, crackles, and wheezing. The patient may also exhibit a dry or productive cough with copious sputum. Other features include anorexia, weight loss, and edema. Barrel chest, cyanosis, and clubbing are usually late signs.

Left-sided heart failure. Orthopnea occurs late in left-sided heart failure. If heart failure is acute, orthopnea may begin suddenly; if chronic, it may become constant. The earliest symptom of this disorder is progressively severe dyspnea. Other common early symptoms include Cheyne-Stokes respirations, paroxysmal nocturnal dyspnea, fatigue, weakness, and cough that may occasionally produce clear or blood-tinged sputum. Tachycardia, tachypnea, and crackles may also occur.

Other late findings include cyanosis, clubbing, a ventricular gallop, and hemoptysis. Left-sided heart failure may also lead to signs of shock, such as hypotension, a thready pulse, and cold, clammy skin.

Mediastinal tumor. Orthopnea is an early sign of a mediastinal tumor, resulting from pressure of the tumor against the trachea, bronchus, or lung when the patient lies down. However, he may be asymptomatic until the tumor enlarges. Then it produces retrosternal chest pain, a dry cough, hoarseness, dysphagia, stertorous respirations, palpitations, and cyanosis. Examination reveals suprasternal retractions on inspiration, bulging of the chest wall, tracheal deviation, dilated jugular and superficial chest veins, and face, neck, and arm edema.

Nursing considerations

- To relieve orthopnea, place the patient in semi-Fowler's or high Fowler's position.
- Alternatively, have the patient lean over a bedside table with his chest forward.
- Administer oxygen via nasal cannula, if indicated.
- Administer a diuretic, if needed.
- For the patient with left-sided heart failure, give angiotensin-converting enzyme inhibitors, unless contraindicated.
- Monitor intake and output.
- Prepare the patient for diagnostic testing, such as an electrocardiogram, chest X-ray, pulmonary function tests, and arterial blood gas analysis.
- Assist with insertion of a central venous catheter or pulmonary artery catheter to measure central venous pressure and pulmonary artery wedge pressure and cardiac output, respectively.

Patient teaching

- Explains signs and symptoms that require prompt medical attention.
- Discuss any dietary and fluid restrictions.
- Reinforce the need to monitor weight daily.
- Explain diagnostic tests, diagnosis, and treatment plan.

Orthostatic hypotension
[Postural hypotension]

In orthostatic hypotension, the patient's blood pressure drops 15 to 20 mm Hg or more—with or without an increase in the heart rate of at least 20 beats/minute—when he rises from a supine to a sitting or standing position. (Blood pressure should be measured 5 minutes after the patient has changed his position.) This common sign indicates failure of compensatory vasomotor responses to adjust to position changes. It's typically associated with light-headedness, syncope, or blurred vision and may occur in a hypotensive, normotensive, or hypertensive patient. Although commonly a nonpathologic sign in an elderly person, orthostatic hypotension may result from prolonged bed rest, fluid and electrolyte imbalance, endocrine or systemic disorders, and the effects of drugs.

To detect orthostatic hypotension, take and compare blood pressure readings with the patient supine, sitting, and then standing.

ACTION STAT!

 If you detect orthostatic hypotension, quickly check for tachycardia, altered level of consciousness (LOC), and pale, clammy skin. If these signs are present, suspect hypovolemic shock. Insert a large-bore I.V. catheter for fluid or blood replacement. Take the patient's vital signs every 15 minutes, and monitor his intake and output. Encourage bed rest until condition is stable.

History and physical examination

If the patient is in no danger, obtain a history. Ask the patient if he frequently experiences dizziness, weakness, or fainting when he stands. Also ask about associated symptoms, particularly fatigue, orthopnea, impotence, nausea, headaches, abdominal or chest discomfort, and GI bleeding. Then obtain a complete drug history.

Begin the physical examination by checking the patient's skin turgor. Palpate peripheral pulses and auscultate the heart and lungs. Finally, test muscle strength and observe the patient's gait for unsteadiness.

Medical causes

Adrenal insufficiency. Adrenal insufficiency typically begins insidiously, with progressively severe signs and symptoms. Orthostatic hypotension may be accompanied by fatigue, muscle weakness, poor coordination, anorexia, nausea and vomiting, fasting hypoglycemia, weight loss, abdominal pain, irritability, and a weak, irregular pulse. Another common feature is hyperpigmentation—bronze coloring of the skin—which is especially prominent on the face, lips, gums, tongue, buccal mucosa, elbows, palms, knuckles, waist, and knees. Diarrhea, constipation, a decreased libido, amenorrhea, and syncope may also occur along with enhanced taste, smell, and hearing and cravings for salty food.

Alcoholism. Chronic alcoholism can lead to the development of peripheral neuropathy, which can present as orthostatic hypotension. Impotence is also a major issue in these patients. Other symptoms include numbness, tingling, nausea, vomiting, changes in bowel habits, and bizarre behavior.

Amyloidosis. Orthostatic hypotension is commonly associated with amyloid infiltration of the autonomic nerves. Associated signs and symptoms vary widely and include angina, tachycardia, dyspnea, orthopnea, fatigue, and cough.

Hyperaldosteronism. Hyperaldosteronism typically produces orthostatic hypotension with sustained elevated blood pressure. Most other clinical effects of hyperaldosteronism result from hypokalemia, which increases neuromuscular irritability and produces muscle weakness, intermittent flaccid paralysis, fatigue, headache, paresthesia and, possibly, tetany with positive Trousseau's and Chvostek's signs. The patient may also exhibit vision disturbances, nocturia, polydipsia, and personality changes. Diabetes mellitus is a common finding.

Hyponatremia. With hyponatremia, orthostatic hypotension is typically accompanied by headache, profound thirst, tachycardia, nausea and vomiting, abdominal cramps, muscle twitching and weakness, fatigue, oliguria or anuria, cold clammy skin, poor skin turgor, irritability, seizures, and decreased LOC. Cyanosis, a thready pulse and, eventually, vasomotor collapse may occur with a severe sodium deficit. Common causes include adrenal insufficiency, hypothyroidism, syndrome of inappropriate antidiuretic hormone secretion, and the use of thiazide diuretics.

Hypovolemia. Mild to moderate hypovolemia may cause orthostatic hypotension associated with apathy, fatigue, muscle weakness, anorexia, nausea, and profound thirst. The patient may also develop dizziness, oliguria, sunken eyeballs, poor skin turgor, and dry mucous membranes.

Other causes

Drugs. Certain drugs may cause orthostatic hypotension by reducing circulating blood volume, causing blood vessel dilation, or depressing the sympathetic nervous system. These drugs include antihypertensives (especially guanethidine monosulfate and the initial dosage of prazosin hydrochloride), tricyclic antidepressants, phenothiazines, levodopa, nitrates, monoamine oxidase inhibitors, morphine, bretylium tosylate, and spinal anesthesia. Large doses of diuretics can also cause orthostatic hypotension.

Treatments. Orthostatic hypotension is commonly associated with prolonged bed rest (24 hours or longer). It may also result from sympathectomy, which disrupts normal vasoconstrictive mechanisms.

Nursing considerations

- Monitor intake and output and weigh the patient daily.
- Elevate the head of the bed, and help the patient to a sitting position with feet dangling over the side of the bed; if tolerated, have him sit in a chair for brief periods.
- Evaluate the patient's need for assistive devices, such as a cane or walker.
- Prepare the patient for diagnostic tests, such as hemoglobin level and hematocrit, serum electrolyte and drug levels, urinalysis, 12-lead electrocardiogram, and chest X-ray.

Patient teaching

- Advise the patient to change his position gradually.
- Show the patient how to use the call bell and tell him to call for assistance when getting out of bed or a chair.
- Explain the importance of maintaining an adequate fluid intake.
- Explain prescribed medications and their adverse effects.

Ortolani's sign

Ortolani's sign—a click, clunk, or popping sensation that's felt and commonly heard when a neonate's hip is flexed 90 degrees and abducted—is an indication of developmental dysplasia of the hip (DDH); it results when the femoral head enters or exits the acetabulum. Screening for this sign is an important part of neonatal care because early detection and treatment of DDH improves the neonate's chances of growing with a correctly formed, functional joint.

Ortolani's sign can be elicited only during the first 4 to 6 weeks of life; this is also the optimum time for effective corrective treatment. If treatment is delayed, DDH may cause degenerative hip changes, lordosis, joint malformation, and soft-tissue damage.

Detecting developmental dysplasia of the hip

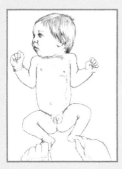

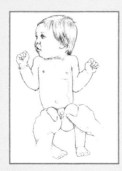

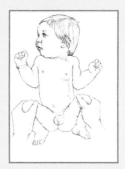

When assessing the neonate, attempt to elicit Ortolani's sign to detect developmental dysplasia of the hip (DDH). Begin by placing the neonate in a supine position with his knees and hips flexed. Observe for symmetry.

Place your hands on the neonate's knees, with your index fingers along his lateral thighs on the greater trochanter. Then raise his knees to a 90-degree angle with his back.

Abduct the neonate's thighs so that the lateral aspect of his knees lies almost flat on the table. If the neonate has a dislocated hip, you'll feel and usually hear a click, clunk, or popping sensation (Ortolani's sign) as the head of the femur moves out of the acetabulum. The neonate may also give a sudden cry of pain. Be sure to distinguish a positive Ortolani's sign from the normal clicks due to rotation of the hip, from signs that don't elicit the sensation of instability, or from simultaneous movement of the knee.

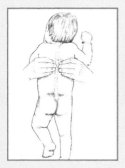

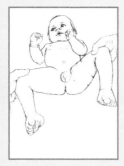

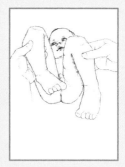

If you elicit Ortolani's sign, look for other signs of DDH.

Flex the neonate's hips to detect limited abduction.

Flex the neonate's knees, and observe for apparent shortening of the femur.

History and physical examination

During assessment for Ortolani's sign, the neonate should be relaxed and lying supine. (See *Detecting developmental dysplasia of the hip*.) After eliciting Ortolani's sign, evaluate the neonate for asymmetrical gluteal folds, limited hip abduction, and unequal leg length.

Medical causes

DDH. With complete dysplasia, the affected leg may appear shorter, or the affected hip may appear more prominent.

Nursing considerations

▪ To maintain a stable joint, abduct the affected hip using a soft splinting device or a plaster hip-spica cast.

Patient teaching

▪ Explain the neonate's condition and its treatments to the parents.
▪ Teach the parents how to keep the affected limb in an abducted position.

Otorrhea

Otorrhea—drainage from the ear—may be bloody (otorrhagia), purulent, clear, or serosanguineous. Its onset, duration, and severity provide clues to the underlying cause. This sign may result from disorders that affect the external ear canal or the middle ear, including allergy, infection, neoplasms, trauma, and collagen diseases. Otorrhea may occur alone or with other symptoms such as ear pain.

History and physical examination

Begin your evaluation by asking the patient when otorrhea began, noting how he recognized it. Did he clean the drainage from deep within the ear canal, or did he wipe it from the auricle? Have him describe the color, consistency, and odor of the drainage. Is it clear, purulent, or bloody? Does it occur in one or both ears? Is it continuous or intermittent? If the patient wears cotton in his ear to absorb the drainage, ask how often he changes it.

Then explore associated otologic symptoms, especially pain. Is there tenderness on movement of the pinna or tragus? Ask about vertigo, which is absent in disorders of the external ear canal. Also ask about tinnitus.

Next, check the patient's medical history for recent upper respiratory infection or head trauma. Also, ask how he cleans his ears and if he's an avid swimmer. Note a history of cancer, dermatitis, or immunosuppressant therapy.

Focus the physical examination on the patient's external ear, middle ear, and tympanic membrane. (If his symptoms are unilateral, examine the uninvolved ear first to avoid cross-contamination.) Inspect the external ear, and apply pressure on the tragus and mastoid area to elicit tenderness. Then insert an otoscope, using the largest speculum that will comfortably fit into the ear canal. If necessary, clean cerumen, pus, or other debris from the canal. Observe for edema, erythema, crusts, or polyps. Inspect the tympanic membrane, which should look like a shiny, pearl-gray cone. Note color changes, perforation, absence of the normal light reflex (a cone of light appearing toward the bottom of the drum), or a bulging membrane.

Next, test hearing acuity. Have the patient occlude one ear while you whisper some common two-syllable words toward the unoccluded ear. Stand behind him so he doesn't read your lips, and ask him to repeat what he heard. Perform the test on the other ear using different words. Then use a tuning fork to perform Weber's and the Rinne tests.

(*See Differentiating conductive from sensorineural hearing loss,* page 304.)

Complete your assessment by palpating the patient's neck and his preauricular, parotid, and postauricular (mastoid) areas for lymphadenopathy. Also, test the function of cranial nerves VII, IX, X, and XI.

Medical causes

Aural polyps. Aural polyps may produce foul, purulent and, perhaps, blood-streaked discharge. If they occlude the external ear canal, the polyps may cause partial hearing loss.

Basilar skull fracture. With a basilar skull fracture, otorrhea may be clear and watery and positive for glucose, representing cerebrospinal fluid (CSF) leakage, or bloody, representing hemorrhage. Occasionally, inspection reveals blood behind the eardrum. Otorrhea may be accompanied by hearing loss, CSF or bloody rhinorrhea, periorbital ecchymosis (raccoon eyes), and mastoid ecchymosis (Battle's sign). Cranial nerve palsies, decreased level of consciousness, and headache are other common findings.

Epidural abscess. With an epidural abscess, profuse, creamy otorrhea is accompanied by steady, throbbing ear pain; fever; and a temporal or temporoparietal headache on the ipsilateral side.

Myringitis (infectious). With acute infectious myringitis, small, reddened, blood-filled blebs erupt in the external ear canal, the tympanic membrane and, occasionally, the middle ear. Spontaneous rupture of these blebs causes serosanguineous otorrhea. Other features include severe ear pain, tenderness over the mastoid process and, rarely, fever and hearing loss.

Chronic infectious myringitis causes purulent otorrhea, pruritus, and gradual hearing loss.

Otitis externa. Acute otitis externa usually causes purulent, yellow, sticky, foul-smelling otorrhea. Inspection may reveal white-green debris in the external ear canal. Associated findings include edema, erythema, pain, and itching of the auricle and external ear canal; severe tenderness with movement of the mastoid, tragus, mouth, or jaw; tenderness and swelling of surrounding nodes; and partial conductive hearing loss. The patient may also develop a low-grade fever and a headache ipsilateral to the affected ear.

Chronic otitis externa usually causes scanty, intermittent otorrhea that may be serous or purulent and possibly foul-smelling. Its primary symptom, however, is itching. Related findings include edema and slight erythema.

Life-threatening malignant otitis externa produces debris in the ear canal, which may build up against the tympanic membrane, causing severe pain that's especially acute during manipulation of the tragus or auricle. Most common in patients with diabetes and immunosuppressed patients, this fulminant bacterial infection may also cause pruritus, tinnitus and, possibly, unilateral hearing loss.

Otitis media. With acute otitis media, rupture of the tympanic membrane produces bloody, purulent otorrhea and relieves continuous or intermittent ear pain. Typically, a conductive hearing loss worsens over several hours.

With acute suppurative otitis media, the patient may also exhibit signs and symptoms of an upper respiratory infection—sore throat, cough, nasal discharge, and headache. Other features include dizziness, fever, nausea, and vomiting.

Chronic otitis media causes intermittent, purulent, foul-smelling otorrhea commonly associated with tympanic membrane perforation. Conductive hearing loss occurs gradually and may be accompanied by pain, nausea, and vertigo.

Trauma. Bloody otorrhea may result from trauma, such as a blow to the external ear, a foreign body in the ear, or barotrauma. Usually, bleeding is minimal or moderate; it may be accompanied by partial hearing loss.

Tumor (malignant). Squamous cell carcinoma of the external ear causes purulent otorrhea with itching; deep, boring ear pain; hearing loss; and, in late stages, facial paralysis.

In squamous cell carcinoma of the middle ear, blood-tinged otorrhea occurs early, typically accompanied by hearing loss on the affected side. Pain and facial paralysis are late features.

Nursing considerations

- Apply warm, moist compresses, heating pads, or hot water bottles to the patient's ears to relieve inflammation and pain.
- Use cotton wicks to gently clean the draining ear or to apply topical drugs.
- Keep eardrops at room temperature because instillation of cold eardrops may cause vertigo.
- If the patient has impaired hearing, ensure that he understands everything that's explained to him, using written messages if necessary.

Patient teaching

- Instruct the patient on safe ways to blow his nose and clean his ears.
- Stress the use of earplugs when swimming.
- Explain signs and symptoms that require medical attention.

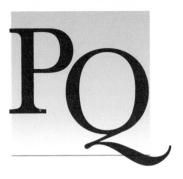

Pallor

Pallor is abnormal paleness or loss of skin color, which may develop suddenly or gradually. Although generalized pallor affects the entire body, it's most apparent on the face, conjunctiva, oral mucosa, and nail beds. Localized pallor commonly affects a single limb.

How easily pallor is detected varies with skin color and the thickness and vascularity of underlying subcutaneous tissue. At times, it's merely a subtle lightening of skin color that may be difficult to detect in dark-skinned persons; sometimes it's evident only on the conjunctiva and oral mucosa.

Pallor may result from decreased peripheral oxyhemoglobin or decreased total oxyhemoglobin. The former reflects diminished peripheral blood flow associated with peripheral vasoconstriction or arterial occlusion or with low cardiac output. (Transient peripheral vasoconstriction may occur with exposure to cold, causing nonpathologic pallor.) The latter usually results from anemia, the chief cause of pallor. (See *How pallor develops.*)

ACTION STAT!

 If generalized pallor suddenly develops, quickly look for signs of shock, such as tachycardia, hypotension, oliguria, and decreased level of consciousness (LOC). Prepare to rapidly infuse fluids or blood. Obtain a blood sample for hemoglobin and serum glucose levels and hematocrit. Keep emergency resuscitation equipment nearby.

History and physical examination

If the patient's condition permits, take a complete history. Does the patient or anyone in his family have a history of anemia or of a chronic disorder that might lead to pallor, such as renal failure, heart failure, or diabetes? Ask about the patient's diet, particularly his intake of red meat and green leafy vegetables.

Then explore the pallor more fully. Find out when the patient first noticed it. Is it constant or intermittent? Does it occur when he's exposed to the cold? Does it occur when he's under emotional stress? Explore associated signs and symptoms, such as dizziness, fainting, orthostasis, weakness and fatigue on exertion, dyspnea, chest pain, palpitations, menstrual irregularities, or loss of libido. If pallor is confined to one or both legs, ask the patient if walking is painful. Do his legs feel cold or numb? If pallor is confined to his fingers, ask about tingling and numbness.

Start the physical examination by taking the patient's vital signs. Be sure to

How pallor develops

Pallor may result from decreased peripheral oxyhemoglobin or decreased total oxyhemoglobin. The chart below illustrates the progression to pallor.

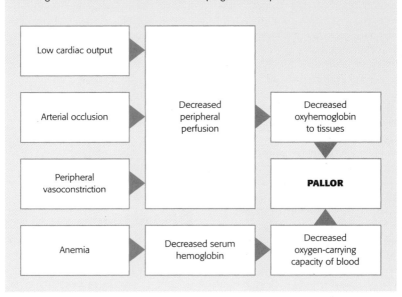

check for orthostatic hypotension. Auscultate the heart for gallops and murmurs and the lungs for crackles. Check the patient's skin temperature—cold extremities commonly occur with vasoconstriction or arterial occlusion. Also, note skin ulceration. Examine the abdomen for splenomegaly. Finally, palpate peripheral pulses. An absent pulse in a pale extremity may indicate arterial occlusion, whereas a weak pulse may indicate low cardiac output.

Medical causes

Anemia. Typically, pallor develops gradually with anemia. The patient's skin may also appear sallow or grayish. Other effects include fatigue, dyspnea, tachycardia, a bounding pulse, an atrial gallop, a systolic bruit over the carotid arteries and, possibly, crackles and bleeding tendencies.

Arterial occlusion (acute). Pallor develops abruptly in the extremity with arterial occlusion, which usually results from an embolus. A line of demarcation develops, separating the cool, pale, cyanotic, and mottled skin below the occlusion from the normal skin above it. Accompanying pallor may be severe pain, intense intermittent claudication, paresthesia, and paresis in the affected extremity. Absent pulses and an increased capillary refill time below the occlusion are also characteristic.

Arterial occlusive disease (chronic). With arterial occlusive disease, pallor is specific to an extremity—usually one leg, but occasionally, both legs or an arm. It develops gradually from obstructive arteriosclerosis or a thrombus and is aggravated by elevating the extremity. Associated findings include intermittent claudication, weakness, cool skin, diminished pulses in the extremity and, possibly, ulceration and gangrene.

Frostbite. Pallor is localized to the frostbitten area, such as the feet, hands, nose, or ears. Typically, the area feels cold, waxy and, perhaps, hard in deep frostbite. The skin doesn't blanch, and sensation may be absent. As the area thaws, the skin turns purplish blue. Blistering and gangrene may then follow if the frostbite is severe.

Orthostatic hypotension. With orthostatic hypotension, pallor occurs abruptly on rising from a recumbent position to a sitting or standing position. A precipitous drop in blood pressure, an increase in heart rate, and dizziness are also characteristic. At times, the patient loses consciousness for several minutes.

Raynaud's disease. Pallor of the fingers upon exposure to cold or stress is a hallmark of Raynaud's disease. Typically, the fingers abruptly turn pale, then cyanotic; with rewarming, they become red and paresthetic. With chronic disease, ulceration may occur.

Shock. Two forms of shock initially cause an acute onset of pallor and cool, clammy skin. With *hypovolemic shock,* other early signs and symptoms include restlessness, thirst, slight tachycardia, and tachypnea. As shock progresses, the skin becomes increasingly clammy, the pulse becomes more rapid and thready, and hypotension develops with narrowing pulse pressure. Other signs and symptoms include oliguria, a subnormal body temperature, and decreased LOC. With *cardiogenic shock,* the signs and symptoms are similar but usually more profound.

Nursing considerations

▪ If the patient has chronic generalized pallor, prepare him for blood studies and, possibly, bone marrow biopsy.

▪ If the patient has localized pallor, he may require arteriography or other diagnostic studies to accurately determine the cause.

▪ When pallor results from low cardiac output, administer blood and fluids as well as a diuretic, a cardiotonic, and an antiarrhythmic as needed.

▪ Monitor the patient's vital signs, intake and output, electrocardiogram results, and hemodynamic status.

Patient teaching

▪ Teach the patient about diagnostic tests and procedures.

▪ Explain the disorder and treatment plan.

Palpitations

Defined as a conscious awareness of one's heartbeat, palpitations are usually felt over the precordium or in the throat or neck. The patient may describe them as pounding, jumping, turning, fluttering, or flopping or as missing or skipping beats. Palpitations may be regular or irregular, fast or slow, paroxysmal or sustained.

Although usually insignificant, palpitations may result from a cardiac or metabolic disorder and from the effects of certain drugs. Nonpathologic palpitations may occur with a newly implanted prosthetic valve because the valve's clicking sound heightens the patient's awareness of his heartbeat. Transient palpitations may accompany emotional stress (such as fright, anger, or anxiety) or physical stress (such as exercise and fever). They can also accompany the use of stimulants, such as tobacco and caffeine.

To help characterize the palpitations, ask the patient to simulate their rhythm by tapping his finger on a hard surface. An irregular "skipped beat" rhythm points to premature ventricular contractions, whereas an episodic racing rhythm that ends abruptly suggests paroxysmal atrial tachycardia.

Action stat!

 If the patient complains of palpitations, ask him about dizziness and shortness of breath. Then inspect for pale, cool, clammy skin. Take the patient's vital signs, noting hypotension and an irregular or abnormal pulse. If these signs are present, suspect cardiac arrhythmia. Place the patient on a cardiac monitor. Insert an I.V. catheter to administer an antiarrhythmic, if needed. Prepare for cardioversion or defibrillation if necessary.

History and physical examination

If the patient isn't in distress, perform a complete cardiac history and physical examination. Ask if he has a cardiovascular or pulmonary disorder, which may produce arrhythmias. Does the patient have a history of hypertension or hypoglycemia? Be sure to obtain a drug history. Has the patient recently started cardiac glycoside therapy? Also, ask about caffeine, tobacco, and alcohol consumption.

Then explore associated symptoms, such as weakness, fatigue, and angina. Finally, auscultate for gallops, murmurs, and abnormal breath sounds.

Medical causes

Anxiety attack (acute). With anxiety, palpitations may be accompanied by diaphoresis, facial flushing, trembling, and an impending sense of doom. Almost invariably, patients hyperventilate, which may lead to dizziness, weakness, and syncope. Other typical findings include tachycardia, precordial pain, shortness of breath, restlessness, and insomnia.

Cardiac arrhythmias. Paroxysmal or sustained palpitations of a cardiac arrhythmias may be accompanied by dizziness, weakness, and fatigue. The patient may also experience an irregular, rapid, or slow pulse rate; decreased blood pressure; confusion; pallor; oliguria; and diaphoresis.

Hypertension. With hypertension, the patient may be asymptomatic or may complain of sustained palpitations alone or with headache, dizziness, tinnitus, "blackouts," and fatigue. His blood pressure typically exceeds 140/90 mm Hg. He may also experience nausea and vomiting, seizures, and decreased level of consciousness.

Hypocalcemia. Typically, hypocalcemia produces palpitations, weakness, and fatigue. It progresses from paresthesia to muscle tension and carpopedal spasms. The patient may also exhibit muscle twitching, hyperactive deep tendon reflexes, chorea, and positive Chvostek's and Trousseau's signs.

Mitral prolapse. Mitral prolapse may cause paroxysmal palpitations accompanied by sharp, stabbing, or aching precordial pain. The hallmark of this disorder, however, is a midsystolic click followed by an apical systolic murmur. Associated signs and symptoms may include dyspnea, dizziness, severe fatigue, a migraine headache, anxiety, paroxysmal tachycardia, crackles, and peripheral edema.

Mitral stenosis. Early features of mitral stenosis typically include sustained palpitations accompanied by exertional dyspnea and fatigue. Auscultation also reveals a loud S_1 or opening snap and a rumbling diastolic murmur at the apex. Patients may also experience related signs and symptoms, such as an atrial gallop and, with advanced mitral stenosis, orthopnea, dyspnea at rest, paroxysmal nocturnal dyspnea, peripheral edema, jugular vein distention, ascites, hepatomegaly, and atrial fibrillation.

Thyrotoxicosis. A characteristic symptom of thyrotoxicosis, sustained palpitations may be accompanied by tachycardia, dyspnea, weight loss despite increased appetite, diarrhea, tremors, nervousness, diaphoresis, heat intolerance and, possibly, exophthalmos and an enlarged thyroid. The patient may also experience an atrial or a ventricular gallop.

Other causes
Drugs. Palpitations may result from drugs that precipitate cardiac arrhythmias or increase cardiac output, such as cardiac glycosides; sympathomimetics, such as cocaine; ganglionic blockers; beta-adrenergic blockers; calcium channel blockers; atropine; thyroid supplements; and minoxidil.

Nursing considerations
- Prepare the patient for diagnostic tests, such as an electrocardiogram and Holter monitoring.
- Maintain a quiet, comfortable environment to minimize anxiety and perhaps decrease palpitations.
- Monitor for signs of reduced cardiac output and cardiac arrhythmias.
- Prepare the patient for cardioversion, if indicated.
- Provide supplemental oxygen.

Patient teaching
- Explain all diagnostic tests and procedures.
- Teach the patient how to reduce anxiety.
- Explain the disorder and treatment plan.

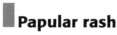

Papular rash

A papular rash consists of small, raised, circumscribed—and perhaps discolored (red to purple)—lesions known as *papules.* It may erupt anywhere on the body in various configurations and may be acute or chronic. Papular rashes characterize many cutaneous disorders; they may also result from allergy and from infectious, neoplastic, and systemic disorders. (To compare papules with other skin lesions, see *Recognizing common skin lesions.*)

History and physical examination
Your first step is to fully evaluate the papular rash: Note its color, configuration, and location on the patient's body. Find out when it erupted. Has the patient noticed changes in the rash since then? Is it itchy or burning, or painful or tender? Has there ever been discharge or drainage from the rash? If so, have the patient describe it. Also, have him describe associated signs and symptoms, such as fevers, headaches, and GI distress.

Next, obtain a medical history, including allergies; previous rashes or skin disorders; infections; childhood diseases; sexual history, including sexually transmitted diseases; and cancers. Has the patient recently been bitten by an insect or rodent or been exposed to anyone with an infectious disease? Finally, obtain a complete drug history.

Medical causes
Acne vulgaris. With acne vulgaris, rupture of enlarged comedones produces inflamed—and perhaps, painful and pruritic—papules, pustules, nodules, or cysts on the face and sometimes the shoulders, chest, and back.

Anthrax (cutaneous). Anthrax begins as a small, painless, or pruritic macular or papular lesion resembling an insect bite. Within 1 or 2 days, it develops into a vesicle and then a painless ulcer with a characteristic black, necrotic cen-

Recognizing common skin lesions

Macule
A small (usually less than 1 cm in diameter), flat blemish or discoloration that can be brown, tan, red, or white and has the same texture as surrounding skin

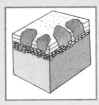

Bulla
A raised, thin-walled blister greater than 0.5 cm in diameter, containing clear or serous fluid

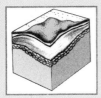

Vesicle
A small (less than 0.5 cm in diameter), thin-walled, raised blister containing clear, serous, purulent, or bloody fluid

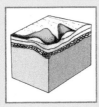

Pustule
A circumscribed, pus- or lymph-filled, elevated lesion that varies in diameter and may be firm or soft and white or yellow

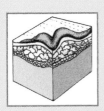

Wheal
A slightly raised, firm lesion of variable size and shape, surrounded by edema; skin may be red or pale

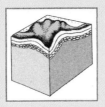

Nodule
A small, firm, circumscribed, elevated lesion 1 or 2 cm in diameter with possible skin discoloration

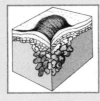

Papule
A small, solid, raised lesion less than 1 cm in diameter, with red to purple skin discoloration

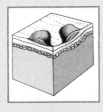

Tumor
A solid, raised mass usually larger than 2 cm in diameter with possible skin discoloration

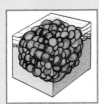

ter. Lymphadenopathy, malaise, headache, or fever may develop.

Dermatomyositis. Gottron's papules—flat, violet-colored lesions on the dorsa of the finger joints and the nape of the neck and shoulders—are pathognomonic of dermatomyositis, as is the dusky lilac discoloration of periorbital tissue and lid margins (heliotrope edema). These signs may be accompanied by a transient, erythematous, macular rash in a malar distribution on the face and sometimes on the scalp, forehead, neck, upper torso, and arms. This rash may be preceded by symmetrical muscle soreness and weakness in the pelvis, upper extremities, shoulders, neck and, possibly, the face (polymyositis).

Follicular mucinosis. With follicular mucinosis, perifollicular papules or plaques are accompanied by prominent alopecia.

Fox-Fordyce disease. Fox-Fordyce disease is marked by pruritic papules on the axillae, pubic area, and areolae associated with apocrine sweat gland inflammation. Sparse hair growth in these areas is also common.

Granuloma annulare. Granuloma annulare produces papules that usually coalesce to form plaques. The papules spread peripherally to form a ring with a normal or slightly depressed center. They usually appear on the feet, legs, hands, or fingers and may be pruritic or asymptomatic.

Human immunodeficiency virus (HIV) infection. Acute infection with the HIV retrovirus typically causes a generalized maculopapular rash. Other signs and symptoms include fever, malaise, sore throat, and headache. Lymphadenopathy and hepatosplenomegaly may also occur.

Kaposi's sarcoma. Kaposi's sarcoma is characterized by purple or blue papules or macules of vascular origin on the skin, mucous membranes, and viscera. These lesions decrease in size with firm pressure and then return to their original size within 10 to 15 seconds. They may become scaly and ulcerate with bleeding.

Lichen planus. Discrete, flat, angular or polygonal, violet papules, commonly marked with white lines or spots, are characteristic of lichen planus. The papules may be linear or coalesce into plaques and usually appear on the lumbar region, genitalia, ankles, anterior tibiae, and wrists. Lesions usually develop first on the buccal mucosa as a lacy network of white or gray threadlike papules

or plaques. Pruritus, distorted fingernails, and atrophic alopecia commonly occur.

Monkeypox. Usually preceded 1 to 3 days by a fever, a papular rash is a characteristic sign of monkeypox. The rash is commonly blisterlike and can follow these stages: vesiculation, postulation, umbilication, and crusting. Typically beginning on the face and spreading to the trunk and extremities, the rash may be either localized or generalized. Other accompanying symptoms in humans include lymphadenopathy, chills, throat pain, and muscle aches.

Mononucleosis (infectious). A maculopapular rash that resembles rubella is an early sign of mononucleosis in 10% of patients. The rash is typically preceded by headache, malaise, and fatigue. It may be accompanied by sore throat, cervical lymphadenopathy, and fluctuating temperature with an evening peak of 101° to 102° F (38.3° to 38.9° C). Splenomegaly and hepatomegaly may also develop.

Necrotizing vasculitis. With necrotizing vasculitis, crops of purpuric, but otherwise asymptomatic, papules are typical. Some patients also develop low-grade fever, headache, myalgia, arthralgia, and abdominal pain.

Pityriasis rosea. Pityriasis rosea begins with an erythematous "herald patch"—a slightly raised, oval lesion about 2 to 6 cm in diameter that may appear anywhere on the body. A few days to weeks later, yellow to tan or erythematous patches with scaly edges appear on the trunk, arms, and legs, commonly erupting along body cleavage lines in a characteristic "pine tree" pattern. These patches may be asymptomatic or slightly pruritic, are 0.5 to 1 cm in diameter, and typically improve with skin exposure.

Polymorphic light eruption. Abnormal reactions to light may produce papular, vesicular, or nodular rashes on sun-exposed areas. Other symptoms include pruritus, headache, and malaise.

Psoriasis. Psoriasis begins with small, erythematous papules on the scalp, chest, elbows, knees, back, buttocks, and genitalia. These papules are sometimes pruritic and painful. Eventually they enlarge and coalesce, forming elevated, red, scaly plaques covered by characteristic silver scales, except in moist areas such as the genitalia. These scales may flake off easily or thicken, covering the plaque. Associated features include pitted fingernails and arthralgia.

Rosacea. Rosacea is characterized by persistent erythema, telangiectasia, and recurrent eruption of papules and pustules on the forehead, malar areas, nose, and chin. Eventually, eruptions occur more frequently and erythema deepens. Rhinophyma may occur in severe cases.

Seborrheic keratosis. With seborrheic keratosis, benign skin tumors begin as small, yellow-brown papules on the chest, back, or abdomen, eventually enlarging and becoming deeply pigmented. However, in blacks, these papules may remain small and affect only the malar part of the face (dermatosis papulosa nigra).

Smallpox (variola major). Initial signs and symptoms of smallpox include a high fever, malaise, prostration, severe headache, a backache, and abdominal pain. A maculopapular rash develops on the mucosa of the mouth, pharynx, face, and forearms and then spreads to the trunk and legs. Within 2 days, the rash becomes vesicular and later pustular. The lesions develop at the same time, appear identical, and are more prominent on the face and extremities. The pustules are round, firm, and deeply embedded in the skin. After 8 or 9 days, the pustules form a crust, and later the scab separates from the skin, leaving a pitted scar. In fatal cases, death results from encephalitis, extensive bleeding, or secondary infection.

Syringoma. With syringoma, adenoma of the sweat glands produces a yellowish or erythematous papular rash on the face (especially the eyelids), neck, and upper chest.

Systemic lupus erythematosus (SLE). SLE is characterized by a "butterfly rash" of erythematous maculopapules or discoid plaques that appears in a malar distribution across the nose and cheeks. Similar rashes may appear elsewhere, especially on exposed body areas. Other cardinal features include photosensitivity and nondeforming arthritis, especially in the hands, feet, and large joints. Common effects are patchy alopecia, mucous membrane ulceration, low-grade or spiking fever, chills, lymphadenopathy, anorexia, weight loss, abdominal pain, diarrhea or constipation, dyspnea, tachycardia, hematuria, headache, and irritability.

Typhus. Initial symptoms of typhus include headache, myalgia, arthralgia, and malaise, followed by an abrupt onset of chills, fever, nausea, and vomiting. A maculopapular rash may be present in some cases.

Other causes

Drugs. Transient maculopapular rashes, usually on the trunk, may accompany reactions to many drugs, including antibiotics, such as tetracycline, ampicillin, cephalosporins, and sulfonamides; benzodiazepines, such as diazepam; lithium; phenylbutazone; gold salts; allopurinol; isoniazid; and salicylates.

Nursing considerations

- Apply cool compresses or an antipruritic lotion.
- Administer an antihistamine for allergic reactions and an antibiotic for infection.

Patient teaching

- Teach the patient appropriate skin care measures.
- Explain ways to reduce itching.
- Discuss signs and symptoms that require medical attention.

Paralysis

Paralysis, the total loss of voluntary motor function, results from severe cortical or pyramidal tract damage. It can occur with a cerebrovascular disorder, degenerative neuromuscular disease, trauma, tumor, or central nervous system infection. Acute paralysis may be an early indicator of a life-threatening disorder such as Guillain-Barré syndrome.

Paralysis can be local or widespread, symmetrical or asymmetrical, transient or permanent, and spastic or flaccid. It's commonly classified according to location and severity as paraplegia (sometimes transient paralysis of the legs), quadriplegia (permanent paralysis of the arms, legs, and body below the level of the spinal lesion), or hemiplegia (unilateral paralysis of varying severity and permanence). Incomplete paralysis with profound weakness (paresis) may precede total paralysis in some patients.

Action stat!

 If paralysis has developed suddenly, suspect trauma or an acute vascular insult. After ensuring that the patient's spine is properly immobilized, quickly determine his level of consciousness (LOC) and take his vital signs. Elevated systolic blood pressure, widening pulse pressure, and bradycardia may signal increasing intracranial pressure (ICP). If possible, elevate the patient's head 30 degrees to decrease ICP, and attempt to keep his head straight and facing forward.

Evaluate the patient's respiratory status, and be prepared to administer oxygen, insert an artificial airway, or provide endotracheal intubation and mechanical ventilation, as needed. To help determine the nature of the patient's injury, ask him for an account of the precipitating events. If he can't respond, try to find an eyewitness.

History and physical examination

If the patient is in no immediate danger, perform a complete neurologic assessment. Start with the history, relying on family members for information if necessary. Ask about the onset, duration, intensity, and progression of paralysis and about the events preceding its development. Focus medical history questions on the incidence of degenerative neurologic or neuromuscular disease, recent infectious illness, sexually transmitted disease, cancer, or recent injury. Explore related signs and symptoms, noting fevers, headaches, vision disturbances, dysphagia, nausea and vomiting, bowel or bladder dysfunction, muscle pain or weakness, and fatigue.

Next, perform a complete neurologic examination, testing cranial nerve (CN), motor, and sensory function and deep tendon reflexes (DTRs). Assess strength in all major muscle groups, and note muscle atrophy. (See *Testing muscle strength,* pages 410 and 411.) Document all findings to serve as a baseline.

Medical causes

Amyotrophic lateral sclerosis (ALS). ALS produces spastic or flaccid paralysis in the body's major muscle groups, eventually progressing to total paralysis. Earlier findings include progressive muscle weakness, fasciculations, and muscle atrophy, usually beginning in the arms and hands. Cramping and hyperreflexia are also common. Involvement of respiratory muscles and the brain stem produces dyspnea and possibly respiratory distress. Progressive cranial nerve paralysis causes dysarthria, dysphagial drooling, choking, and difficulty chewing.

Bell's palsy. Bell's palsy causes transient, unilateral facial muscle paralysis. The affected muscles sag, and eyelid closure is impossible. Other signs include increased tearing, drooling, and a diminished or absent corneal reflex.

Botulism. Botulism can cause rapidly descending muscle weakness that progresses to paralysis within 2 to 4 days after the ingestion of contaminated food. Respiratory muscle paralysis leads to dyspnea and respiratory arrest. Nausea, vomiting, diarrhea, blurred or double vision, bilateral mydriasis, dysarthria, and dysphagia are some early findings.

Brain abscess. Advanced abscess in the frontal or temporal lobe can cause hemiplegia accompanied by other late findings, such as ocular disturbances, unequal pupils, decreased LOC, ataxia, tremors, and signs of infection.

Brain tumor. A tumor affecting the motor cortex of the frontal lobe may cause contralateral hemiparesis that progresses to hemiplegia. The onset is gradual, but paralysis is permanent without treatment. In early stages, a frontal headache and behavioral changes may be the only indicators. Eventually, seizures, aphasia, and signs of increased ICP (decreased LOC and vomiting) develop.

Conversion disorder. Hysterical paralysis, a classic symptom of conversion disorder, is characterized by the loss of voluntary movement with no obvious physical cause. It can affect any muscle group, appears and disappears unpredictably, and may occur with histrionic behavior (manipulative, dramatic, vain, irrational) or a strange indifference.

Encephalitis. Variable paralysis develops in the late stages of encephalitis. Earlier signs and symptoms include rapidly decreasing LOC (possibly coma), fever, headache, photophobia, vomiting, signs of meningeal irritation (nuchal rigidity, positive Kernig's and Brudzinski's signs), aphasia, ataxia, nystagmus, ocular palsies, myoclonus, and seizures.

Guillain-Barré syndrome. Guillain-Barré syndrome is characterized by a rapidly developing, but reversible, ascending paralysis. It commonly begins as leg muscle weakness and progresses symmetrically, sometimes affecting even the cranial nerves, producing dysphagia, nasal speech, and dysarthria. Respiratory muscle paralysis may be life-threatening. Other effects include transient paresthesia, orthostatic hypotension, tachycardia, diaphoresis, and bowel and bladder incontinence.

Head trauma. Cerebral injury can cause paralysis due to cerebral edema and increased ICP. The onset is usually sudden. The location and extent vary, depending on the injury. Associated findings vary, but include decreased LOC; sensory disturbances, such as paresthesia and loss of sensation; headache; blurred or double vision; nausea and vomiting; and focal neurologic disturbances.

Multiple sclerosis (MS). With MS, paralysis commonly waxes and wanes until the later stages, when it may become permanent. Its extent can range from monoplegia to quadriplegia. In most patients, vision and sensory disturbances (paresthesia) are the earliest symptoms. Later findings are widely variable and may include muscle weakness and spasticity, nystagmus, hyperreflexia, an intention tremor, gait ataxia, dysphagia, dysarthria, impotence, and constipation. Urinary frequency, urgency, and incontinence may also occur.

Myasthenia gravis. With myasthenia gravis, profound muscle weakness and abnormal fatigability may produce paralysis of certain muscle groups. Paralysis is usually transient in early stages, but becomes more persistent as the disease progresses. Associated findings depend on the areas of neuromuscular involvement; they include weak eye closure, ptosis, diplopia, lack of facial mobility, dysphagia, nasal speech, and frequent nasal regurgitation of fluids. Neck muscle weakness may cause the patient's jaw to drop and his head to bob. Respiratory muscle involvement can lead to respiratory distress—dyspnea, shallow respirations, and cyanosis.

Parkinson's disease. Tremors, bradykinesia, and lead-pipe or cogwheel rigidity are the classic signs of Parkinson's disease. Extreme rigidity can progress to paralysis, particularly in the extremities. In most cases, paralysis resolves with prompt treatment of the disease.

Peripheral neuropathy. Typically, peripheral neuropathy produces muscle weakness that may lead to flaccid paralysis and atrophy. Related effects include paresthesia, a loss of vibration sensation, hypoactive or absent DTRs, neuralgia, and skin changes such as anhidrosis.

Rabies. Rabies produces progressive flaccid paralysis, vascular collapse, coma, and death within 2 weeks of contact with an infected animal. Prodromal signs and symptoms—fever; headache; hyperesthesia; paresthesia, coldness, and itching at the bite site; photophobia; tachycardia; shallow respirations; and excessive salivation, lacrimation, and perspiration—develop almost immediately. Within 2 to 10 days, a phase of excitement begins, marked by agitation, cranial nerve dysfunction (pupil changes, hoarseness, facial weakness, ocular palsies), tachycardia or bradycardia, cyclic respirations, a high fever, urine retention, drooling, and hydrophobia.

Seizure disorders. Seizures, particularly focal seizures, can cause transient local paralysis (Todd's paralysis). Any part of the body may be affected, although paralysis tends to occur contralateral to the side of the irritable focus.

Spinal cord injury. Complete spinal cord transection results in permanent spastic paralysis below the level of injury. Reflexes may return after spinal shock resolves. Partial transection causes variable paralysis and paresthesia, depending on the location and extent of injury. (See *Understanding spinal cord syndromes.*)

Spinal cord tumors. With a spinal cord tumor, paresis, pain, paresthesia, and variable sensory loss may occur along the nerve distribution pathway served by the affected cord segment. Eventually, these symptoms may progress to spastic paralysis with hyperactive DTRs (unless the tumor is in the cauda equina, which produces hyporeflexia) and, perhaps, bladder and bowel incontinence. Paralysis is permanent without treatment.

Stroke. A stroke involving the motor cortex can produce contralateral paresis or paralysis. The onset may be sudden or gradual, and paralysis may be transient or permanent. Associated signs and symptoms vary widely and may include headache, vomiting, seizures, decreased LOC and mental acuity, dysarthria, dysphagia, ataxia, contralateral paresthesia or sensory loss, apraxia, agnosia, aphasia, vision disturbances, emotional lability, and bowel and bladder dysfunction.

Subarachnoid hemorrhage. Subarachnoid hemorrhage is a potentially life-threatening disorder that can produce sudden paralysis. The condition may be temporary, resolving with de-

Understanding spinal cord syndromes

When a patient's spinal cord is incompletely severed, he experiences partial motor and sensory loss. Most incomplete cord lesions fit into one of the syndromes described below.

Anterior cord syndrome, usually resulting from a flexion injury, causes motor paralysis and loss of pain and temperature sensation below the level of injury. Touch, proprioception, and vibration sensation are usually preserved.

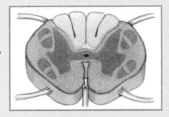

Brown-Séquard syndrome can result from flexion, rotation, or penetration injury. It's characterized by unilateral motor paralysis ipsilateral to the injury and a loss of pain and temperature sensation contralateral to the injury.

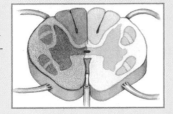

Central cord syndrome is caused by hyperextension or flexion injury. Motor loss is variable and greater in the arms than in the legs; sensory loss is usually slight.

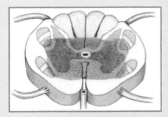

Posterior cord syndrome, produced by a cervical hyperextension injury, causes only a loss of proprioception and light touch sensation. Motor function remains intact.

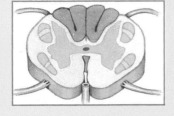

creasing edema, or permanent, if tissue destruction has occurred. Other acute effects are severe headache, mydriasis, photophobia, aphasia, sharply decreased LOC, nuchal rigidity, vomiting, and seizures.

Syringomyelia. Syringomyelia produces segmental paresis, leading to flaccid paralysis of the hands and arms. Reflexes are absent, and loss of pain and temperature sensation is distributed over the neck, shoulders, and arms in a capelike pattern.

Transient ischemic attack (TIA). Episodic TIAs may cause transient unilateral paresis or paralysis accompanied by paresthesia, blurred or double vision, dizziness, aphasia, dysarthria, decreased LOC, and other site-dependent effects.

West Nile encephalitis. Symptoms of West Nile encephalitis include fever, headache, and body aches, which are sometimes accompanied by a skin rash and swollen lymph glands. More severe infections are marked by headache, high fever, neck stiffness, stupor, disorientation, coma, tremors, occasional seizures, paralysis and, rarely, death.

Other causes

Drugs. The therapeutic use of neuromuscular blockers, such as pancuronium or curare, produces paralysis.

Electroconvulsive therapy (ECT). ECT can produce acute, but transient, paralysis.

Nursing considerations

- Provide frequent position changes and meticulous skin care to prevent skin breakdown.
- Administer frequent chest physiotherapy.
- Perform passive range-of-motion exercises to maintain muscle tone.
- Apply splints to prevent contractures and footboards or other devices to prevent footdrop.
- Provide a thickened liquid or soft diet, and keep suction equipment on hand in case aspiration occurs, if the patient has difficulty chewing or swallowing.
- As appropriate, arrange for physical, speech, swallowing, or occupational therapy.

Patient teaching

- Explain all diagnostic tests and procedures.
- Explain the disorder and treatment plan.
- Teach the patient and his family how to prevent complications.

- Provide referrals to social and psychological services.

Paresthesia

Paresthesia is an abnormal sensation or combination of sensations—commonly described as numbness, prickling, or tingling—felt along peripheral nerve pathways; these sensations generally aren't painful. Unpleasant or painful sensations, on the other hand, are termed *dysesthesias*. Paresthesia may develop suddenly or gradually and may be transient or permanent.

A common symptom of many neurologic disorders, paresthesia may also result from a systemic disorder or particular drug. It may reflect damage or irritation of the parietal lobe, thalamus, spinothalamic tract, or spinal or peripheral nerves—the neural circuit that transmits and interprets sensory stimuli.

History and physical examination

First, explore the paresthesia. When did abnormal sensations begin? Have the patient describe their character and distribution. Also, ask about associated signs and symptoms, such as sensory loss and paresis or paralysis. Next, take a medical history, including neurologic, cardiovascular, metabolic, renal, and chronic inflammatory disorders, such as arthritis or lupus. Has the patient recently sustained a traumatic injury or had surgery or an invasive procedure that may have damaged peripheral nerves?

Focus the physical examination on the patient's neurologic status. Assess his level of consciousness (LOC) and cranial nerve function. Test muscle strength and deep tendon reflexes (DTRs) in limbs affected by paresthesia. Systematically evaluate light touch, pain, temperature, vibration, and position sensation. (See

Testing for analgesia, pages 32 and 33.) Also, note skin color and temperature, and palpate pulses.

Medical causes

Arterial occlusion (acute). With acute arterial occlusion, sudden paresthesia and coldness may develop in one or both legs with a saddle embolus. Paresis, intermittent claudication, and aching pain at rest are also characteristic. The extremity becomes mottled with a line of temperature and color demarcation at the level of occlusion. Pulses are absent below the occlusion, and the capillary refill time is increased.

Arteriosclerosis obliterans. Arteriosclerosis obliterans produces paresthesia, intermittent claudication (most common symptom), diminished or absent popliteal and pedal pulses, pallor, paresis, and coldness in the affected leg.

Arthritis. Rheumatoid or osteoarthritic changes in the cervical spine may cause paresthesia in the neck, shoulders, and arms. The lumbar spine occasionally is affected, causing paresthesia in one or both legs and feet.

Brain tumor. Tumors affecting the sensory cortex in the parietal lobe may cause progressive contralateral paresthesia accompanied by agnosia, apraxia, agraphia, homonymous hemianopsia, and a loss of proprioception.

Buerger's disease. With Buerger's disease exposure to cold makes the feet cold, cyanotic, and numb; later, they redden, become hot, and tingle. Intermittent claudication, which is aggravated by exercise and relieved by rest, is also common. Other findings include weak peripheral pulses, migratory superficial thrombophlebitis and, later, ulceration, muscle atrophy, and gangrene.

Diabetes mellitus. Diabetic neuropathy can cause paresthesia with a burning sensation in the hands and feet. Other findings include insidious, permanent anosmia; fatigue; polyuria; polydipsia; weight loss; and polyphagia.

Guillain-Barré syndrome. With Guillain-Barré syndrome, transient paresthesia may precede muscle weakness, which usually begins in the legs and ascends to the arms and facial nerves. Weakness may progress to total paralysis. Other findings include dysarthria, dysphagia, nasal speech, orthostatic hypotension, bladder and bowel incontinence, diaphoresis, tachycardia and, possibly, signs of life-threatening respiratory muscle paralysis.

Head trauma. Unilateral or bilateral paresthesia may occur when head trauma causes a concussion or contusion; however, sensory loss is more common. Other findings include variable paresis or paralysis, decreased LOC, headache, blurred or double vision, nausea and vomiting, dizziness, and seizures.

Herniated disk. Herniation of a lumbar, thoracic, or cervical disk may cause an acute or a gradual onset of paresthesia along the distribution pathways of affected spinal nerves. Other neuromuscular effects include severe pain, muscle spasms, and weakness that may progress to atrophy unless herniation is relieved.

Herpes zoster. An early symptom of herpes zoster, paresthesia occurs in the dermatome supplied by the affected spinal nerve. Within several days, this dermatome is marked by a pruritic, erythematous, vesicular rash associated with sharp, shooting, or burning pain.

Hyperventilation syndrome. Usually triggered by acute anxiety, hyperventilation syndrome may produce transient paresthesia in the hands, feet, and perioral area, accompanied by agitation, vertigo, syncope, pallor, muscle twitching and weakness, carpopedal spasm, and cardiac arrhythmias.

Migraine headache. Paresthesia in the hands, face, and perioral area may herald an impending migraine headache. Other prodromal symptoms include scotomas, hemiparesis, confusion, dizziness, and photophobia. These effects may persist during the characteristic throbbing headache and continue after it subsides.

Multiple sclerosis (MS). With MS, demyelination of the sensory cortex or spinothalamic tract may produce paresthesia—typically one of the earliest symptoms. Like other effects of MS, paresthesia commonly waxes and wanes until the later stages, when it may become permanent. Associated findings include muscle weakness, spasticity, and hyperreflexia.

Peripheral nerve trauma. Injury to a major peripheral nerve can cause paresthesia—commonly dysesthesia—in the area supplied by that nerve. Paresthesia begins shortly after trauma and may be permanent. Other findings are flaccid paralysis or paresis, hyporeflexia, and variable sensory loss.

Peripheral neuropathy. Peripheral neuropathy can cause progressive paresthesia in all extremities. The patient also commonly displays muscle weakness, which may lead to flaccid paralysis and atrophy; a loss of vibration sensation; diminished or absent DTRs; neuralgia; and cutaneous changes, such as glossy, red skin and anhidrosis.

Rabies. Paresthesia, coldness, and itching at the site of an animal bite herald the prodromal stage of rabies. Other prodromal signs and symptoms are fever, headache, photophobia, hyperesthesia, tachycardia, shallow respirations, and excessive salivation, lacrimation, and perspiration.

Raynaud's disease. With Raynaud's disease, exposure to cold or stress makes the fingers turn pale, cold, and cyanotic; with rewarming, they become red and paresthetic. Ulceration may occur in chronic cases.

Seizure disorders. Seizures originating in the parietal lobe usually cause paresthesia of the lips, fingers, and toes. The paresthesia may act as auras that precede tonic-clonic seizures.

Spinal cord injury. Paresthesia may occur in partial spinal cord transection, after spinal shock resolves. It may be unilateral or bilateral, occurring at or below the level of the lesion. Associated sensory and motor loss is variable. (See *Understanding spinal cord syndromes,* page 465.) Spinal cord disorders may be associated with paresthesia on head flexion (Lhermitte's sign).

Spinal cord tumors. Paresthesia, paresis, pain, and sensory loss along nerve pathways served by the affected cord segment result from spinal cord tumors. Eventually, paresis may cause spastic paralysis with hyperactive DTRs (unless the tumor is in the cauda equina, which produces hyporeflexia) and, possibly, bladder and bowel incontinence.

Stroke. Although contralateral paresthesia may occur with stroke, sensory loss is more common. Associated features vary with the artery affected and may include contralateral hemiplegia, decreased LOC, and homonymous hemianopsia.

Systemic lupus erythematosus (SLE). SLE may cause paresthesia, but its primary signs and symptoms include nondeforming arthritis (usually of the hands, feet, and large joints), photosensitivity, and a "butterfly rash" that appears across the nose and cheeks.

Tabes dorsalis. With tabes dorsalis, paresthesia—especially of the legs—is a common, but late, symptom. Other findings include ataxia, loss of proprioception and pain and temperature sensation, absent DTRs, Charcot's joints, Argyll Robertson pupils, incontinence, and impotence.

Transient ischemic attack (TIA).

Paresthesia typically occurs abruptly with a TIA and is limited to one arm or another isolated part of the body. It usually lasts about 10 minutes and is accompanied by paralysis or paresis. Associated findings include decreased LOC, dizziness, unilateral vision loss, nystagmus, aphasia, dysarthria, tinnitus, facial weakness, dysphagia, and an ataxic gait.

Other causes

Drugs. Phenytoin, chemotherapeutic agents (such as vincristine, vinblastine, and procarbazine), D-penicillamine, isoniazid, nitrofurantoin, chloroquine, and parenteral gold therapy may produce transient paresthesia that disappears when the drug is discontinued.

Radiation therapy. Long-term radiation therapy may eventually cause peripheral nerve damage, resulting in paresthesia.

Nursing considerations

- Monitor the patient's neurologic status.
- Help the patient perform activities of daily living, as needed.
- If sensory deficits are present, take measures to protect the patient from injury.

Patient teaching

- Teach the patient safety measures.
- Discuss signs and symptoms that require medical attention.
- Explain the disorder and treatment plan.

Paroxysmal nocturnal dyspnea

Typically dramatic and terrifying to the patient, this sign refers to an attack of dyspnea that abruptly awakens the patient. Common findings include diaphoresis, coughing, wheezing, and chest discomfort. The attack abates after the patient sits up or stands for several minutes, but may recur every 2 or 3 hours.

Paroxysmal nocturnal dyspnea is a sign of left-sided heart failure. It may result from decreased respiratory drive, impaired left ventricular function, enhanced reabsorption of interstitial fluid, or increased thoracic blood volume. All of these pathophysiologic mechanisms cause dyspnea to worsen when the patient lies down.

History and physical examination

Begin by exploring the patient's complaint of dyspnea. Does he have dyspneic attacks only at night or at other times as well, such as after exertion or while sitting down? If so, what type of activity triggers the attack? Does he experience coughing, wheezing, fatigue, or weakness during an attack? Find out if he has a history of lower extremity edema or jugular vein distention. Ask if he sleeps with his head elevated and, if so, on how many pillows or if he sleeps in a reclining chair. Obtain a cardiopulmonary history. Does the patient or a family member have a history of a myocardial infarction, coronary artery disease, or hypertension or of chronic bronchitis, emphysema, or asthma? Has the patient had cardiac surgery?

Next perform a physical examination. Begin by taking the patient's vital signs and forming an overall impression of his appearance. Is he noticeably cyanotic or edematous? Auscultate the lungs for crackles and wheezing and the heart for gallops and arrhythmias.

Medical causes

Left-sided heart failure. Dyspnea—on exertion, during sleep, and eventually even at rest—is an early sign of left-sided heart failure. This sign is characteristically accompanied by Cheyne-Stokes respirations, diaphoresis, weakness, wheezing, and a persistent, nonproductive cough or a cough that produces clear or blood-tinged sputum. As the patient's condition worsens, he develops tachycardia, tachypnea, alternating pulse (commonly initiated by a premature beat), a ventricular gallop, crackles, and peripheral edema.

With advanced left-sided heart failure, the patient may also exhibit severe orthopnea, cyanosis, clubbing, hemoptysis, and cardiac arrhythmias as well as signs and symptoms of shock, such as hypotension, a weak pulse, and cold, clammy skin.

Nursing considerations

- Prepare the patient for diagnostic tests, such as a chest X-ray, echocardiography, exercise electrocardiography, and cardiac blood pool imaging.
- If the hospitalized patient experiences paroxysmal nocturnal dyspnea, assist him to a sitting position or help him walk around the room.
- If necessary, provide supplemental oxygen.
- Keep the patient calm because anxiety can exacerbate dyspnea.

Patient teaching

- Explain signs and symptoms that require immediate medical attention.
- Discuss dietary and fluid restrictions the patient requires.
- Talk about positions that can ease breathing.
- Teach the patient about prescribed medications, their dosage, administration, and adverse effects.

Peau d'orange

Usually a late sign of breast cancer, peau d'orange (orange peel skin) is the edematous thickening and pitting of breast skin. This slowly developing sign can also occur with breast or axillary lymph node infection, erysipelas, or Graves' disease. Its striking orange peel appearance stems from lymphatic edema around deepened hair follicles. (See *Recognizing peau d'orange.*)

History and physical examination

Ask the patient when she first detected peau d'orange. Has she noticed lumps, pain, or other breast changes? Does she have related signs and symptoms, such as fever, malaise, achiness, and weight loss? Is she lactating, or has she recently weaned her infant? Has she noticed any nipple discharge? Has she had previous axillary surgery that might have impaired lymphatic drainage of a breast?

Recognizing peau d'orange

In peau d'orange, the skin appears to be pitted (as shown below). This condition usually indicates late-stage breast cancer.

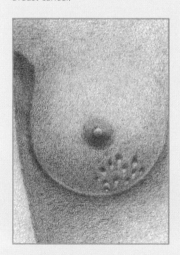

In a well-lit examining room, observe the patient's breasts. Estimate the extent of the peau d'orange and check for erythema. Assess the nipples for discharge, deviation, retraction, dimpling, and cracking. Gently palpate the area of peau d'orange, noting warmth or induration. Then palpate the entire breast, noting fixed or mobile lumps, and the axillary lymph nodes, noting enlargement. Finally, take the patient's temperature.

Medical causes

Breast abscess. Breast abscess causes peau d'orange, malaise, breast tenderness and erythema, and a sudden fever that may be accompanied by shaking chills. A cracked nipple may produce a purulent discharge, and an indurated or palpable soft mass may be present.

Breast cancer. Advanced breast cancer is the most likely cause of peau d'orange, which usually begins in the dependent part of the breast or the areola. Palpation typically reveals a firm, immobile mass that adheres to the skin above the area of peau d'orange. Inspection of the breasts may reveal changes in contour, size, or symmetry. Inspection of the nipples may reveal deviation, erosion, retraction, and a thin and watery, bloody, or purulent discharge. The patient may report a burning and itching sensation in the nipples as well as a sensation of warmth or heat in the breast. Breast pain may occur, but it isn't a reliable indicator of cancer.

Nursing considerations

- Because peau d'orange usually signals advanced breast cancer, provide emotional support for the patient.
- Encourage her to express her fears and concerns.
- Prepare the patient for biopsy, surgery, chemotherapy, or radiation therapy.

Patient teaching

- Explain the underlying cause and treatment plan.
- Explain expected diagnostic tests, such as mammography and breast biopsy.
- Teach the patient how to perform monthly breast self-examinations.
- Discuss signs and symptoms the patient should report.

Pericardial friction rub

Commonly transient, a pericardial friction rub is a scratching, grating, or crunching sound that occurs when two inflamed layers of the pericardium slide over one another. Ranging from faint to loud, this abnormal sound is best heard along the lower left sternal border during deep inspiration. It indicates pericarditis, which can result from an acute infection, a cardiac or renal disorder, postpericardiotomy syndrome, or the use of certain drugs.

Occasionally, a pericardial friction rub can resemble a murmur (See *Pericardial friction rub or murmur?* page 472.) or a pleural friction rub. However, the classic pericardial friction rub has three components. (See *Understanding pericardial friction rubs, page 473.*)

History and physical examination

Obtain a complete medical history, noting especially cardiac dysfunction. Has the patient recently had a myocardial infarction or cardiac surgery? Has he ever had pericarditis or a rheumatic disorder, such as rheumatoid arthritis or systemic lupus erythematosus? Does he have chronic renal failure or an infection? If the patient complains of chest pain, ask him to describe its character and location. What relieves the pain? What worsens it?

Pericardial friction rub or murmur?

Is the sound you hear a pericardial friction rub or a murmur? Here's how to tell. The classic pericardial friction rub has three sound components, which are related to the phases of the cardiac cycle. In some patients, however, the rub's presystolic and early diastolic sounds may be inaudible, causing the rub to resemble the murmur of mitral insufficiency or aortic stenosis and insufficiency.

If you don't detect the classic three-component sound, you can distinguish a pericardial friction rub from a murmur by auscultating again and asking yourself these questions:

How deep is the sound?
A pericardial friction rub usually sounds superficial; a murmur sounds deeper in the chest.

Does the sound radiate?
A pericardial friction rub usually doesn't radiate; a murmur may radiate widely.

Does the sound vary with inspiration or changes in patient position?
A pericardial friction rub is usually loudest during inspiration and is best heard when the patient leans forward. A murmur varies in timing and duration with both factors.

Take the patient's vital signs, noting especially hypotension, tachycardia, an irregular pulse, tachypnea, and fever. Inspect for jugular vein distention, edema, ascites, and hepatomegaly. Auscultate the lungs for crackles. (See *Comparing auscultation findings,* pages 474 and 475.)

Medical causes

Pericarditis. A pericardial friction rub is the hallmark of acute pericarditis. This disorder also causes sharp precordial or retrosternal pain that usually radiates to the left shoulder, neck, and back. The pain worsens when the patient breathes deeply, coughs, or lies flat and, possibly, when he swallows. It abates when he sits up and leans forward. The patient may also develop fever, dyspnea, tachycardia, and arrhythmias.

With chronic constrictive pericarditis, a pericardial friction rub develops gradually and is accompanied by signs of decreased cardiac filling and output, such as peripheral edema, ascites, jugular vein distention on inspiration (Kussmaul's sign), and hepatomegaly. Dyspnea, orthopnea, paradoxical pulse, and chest pain may also occur.

Other causes

Drugs. Procainamide and chemotherapeutic drugs can cause pericarditis.

Nursing considerations
- Monitor the patient's cardiovascular status and cardiac rhythm.
- If the pericardial friction rub disappears, be alert for signs of cardiac tamponade.
- If the patient develops cardiac tamponade, prepare him for pericardiocentesis to prevent cardiovascular collapse.
- Ensure that the patient gets adequate rest.
- Give an anti-inflammatory, antiarrhythmic, diuretic, or antimicrobial to treat the underlying cause.
- If necessary, prepare him for a pericardiectomy to promote adequate cardiac filling and contraction.

Patient teaching

- Teach the patient about the disorder and treatment plan.
- Teach about prescribed medications, including their dosage, administration, and adverse effects.

Peristaltic waves, visible

With intestinal obstruction, peristalsis temporarily increases in strength and frequency as the intestine contracts to force its contents past the obstruction. As a result, visible peristaltic waves may roll across the abdomen. Typically, these waves appear suddenly and vanish quickly because increased peristalsis overcomes the obstruction or the GI tract becomes atonic. Peristaltic waves are best detected by stooping at the patient's side and inspecting his abdominal contour while he's in a supine position.

Visible peristaltic waves may also reflect normal stomach and intestinal contractions in thin patients or in malnourished patients with abdominal muscle atrophy.

History and physical examination

After observing peristaltic waves, collect pertinent history data. Ask about a history of a pyloric ulcer, stomach cancer, or chronic gastritis, which can lead to pyloric obstruction. Also ask about conditions leading to intestinal obstruction, such as intestinal tumors or polyps, gallstones, chronic constipation, and a hernia. Has the patient had recent abdominal surgery? Obtain a complete drug history.

Determine if the patient has related symptoms. Spasmodic abdominal pain, for example, accompanies small-bowel obstruction, whereas colicky pain accompanies pyloric obstruction. Is the

(Text continues on page 476.)

ASSESSMENT TIP

Understanding pericardial friction rubs

The complete, or classic, pericardial friction rub is triphasic. Its three sound components are linked to phases of the cardiac cycle. The *presystolic* component (A) reflects atrial systole and precedes the first heart sound (S_1). The *systolic* component (B) — usually the loudest — reflects ventricular systole and occurs between the S_1 and second heart sound (S_2). The *early diastolic* component (C) reflects ventricular diastole and follows S_2.

Sometimes, the early diastolic component merges with the presystolic component, producing a diphasic to-and-fro sound on auscultation. In other patients, auscultation may detect only one component — a monophasic rub, typically during ventricular systole.

Triphasic rub

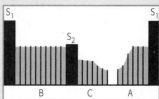

Diphasic rub

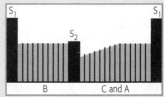

Monophasic rub

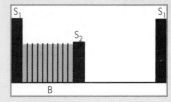

Comparing auscultation findings

During auscultation, you may detect a pleural friction rub, a pericardial friction rub, or crackles — three abnormal sounds that are commonly confused. Use these illustrations to help clarify auscultation findings.

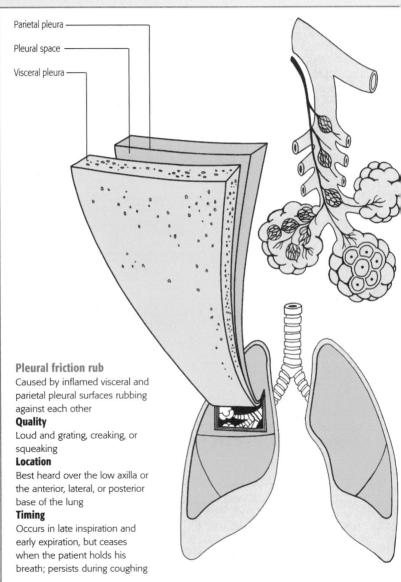

Parietal pleura

Pleural space

Visceral pleura

Pleural friction rub

Caused by inflamed visceral and parietal pleural surfaces rubbing against each other

Quality

Loud and grating, creaking, or squeaking

Location

Best heard over the low axilla or the anterior, lateral, or posterior base of the lung

Timing

Occurs in late inspiration and early expiration, but ceases when the patient holds his breath; persists during coughing

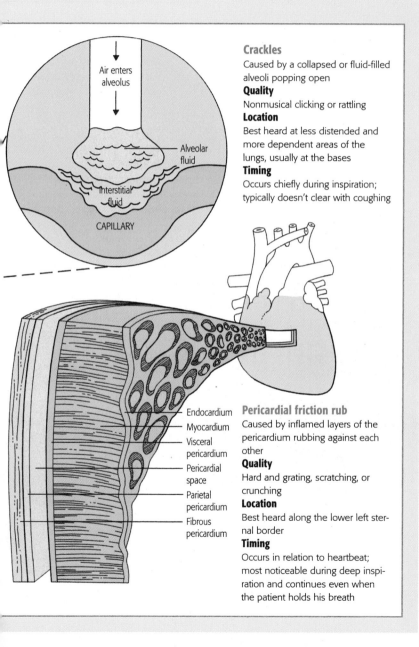

Crackles
Caused by a collapsed or fluid-filled alveoli popping open
Quality
Nonmusical clicking or rattling
Location
Best heard at less distended and more dependent areas of the lungs, usually at the bases
Timing
Occurs chiefly during inspiration; typically doesn't clear with coughing

Pericardial friction rub
Caused by inflamed layers of the pericardium rubbing against each other
Quality
Hard and grating, scratching, or crunching
Location
Best heard along the lower left sternal border
Timing
Occurs in relation to heartbeat; most noticeable during deep inspiration and continues even when the patient holds his breath

patient experiencing nausea and vomiting? If he has vomited, ask about the consistency, amount, and color of the vomitus. Lumpy vomitus may contain undigested food particles; green or brown vomitus may contain bile or fecal matter.

Next, with the patient in a supine position, inspect the abdomen for distention, surgical scars and adhesions, or visible loops of bowel. Auscultate for bowel sounds, noting high-pitched, tinkling sounds. Then jar the patient's bed (or roll the patient from side to side) and auscultate for a succussion splash—a splashing sound in the stomach from retained secretions due to pyloric obstruction. Palpate the abdomen for rigidity and tenderness, and percuss for tympany. Check the skin and mucous membranes for dryness and poor skin turgor, indicating dehydration. Take the patient's vital signs, noting especially tachycardia and hypotension, which indicate hypovolemia.

Medical causes

Large-bowel obstruction. Visible peristaltic waves in the upper abdomen are an early sign of large-bowel obstruction. Obstipation, however, may be the earliest finding. Other characteristic signs and symptoms develop more slowly than in small-bowel obstruction. These include nausea, colicky abdominal pain (milder than in small-bowel obstruction), gradual and eventually marked abdominal distention, and hyperactive bowel sounds.

Pyloric obstruction. With pyloric obstruction, peristaltic waves may be detected in a swollen epigastrium or in the left upper quadrant, usually beginning near the left rib margin and rolling from left to right. Related findings include vague epigastric discomfort or colicky pain after eating, nausea, vomiting,

anorexia, and weight loss. Auscultation reveals a loud succussion splash.

Small-bowel obstruction. Early signs of mechanical obstruction of the small bowel include peristaltic waves rolling across the upper abdomen and intermittent, cramping periumbilical pain. Associated signs and symptoms include nausea, vomiting of bilious or, later, fecal material, and constipation; in partial obstruction, diarrhea may occur. Hyperactive bowel sounds and slight abdominal distention also occur early.

Nursing considerations

- Withhold food and fluids until a definite diagnosis is determined.
- Prepare the patient for abdominal X-rays, computed tomography, and barium studies, which can confirm obstruction.
- If obstruction is confirmed, perform nasogastric suctioning to decompress the stomach and small bowel.
- Provide frequent oral hygiene.
- Frequently monitor the patient's vital signs and intake and output.

Patient teaching

- Teach the patient about any food or fluid restrictions.
- Discuss ways to avoid constipation.
- Explain the disorder and treatment plan.

Photophobia

A common symptom, photophobia is an abnormal sensitivity to light. In many patients, photophobia simply indicates increased eye sensitivity without an underlying disorder. For example, it can stem from wearing contact lenses excessively or using poorly fitted lenses. However, in others, this symptom can result from a systemic disorder, an ocular disorder or trauma, or the use of certain drugs.

History and physical examination

If the patient reports photophobia, find out when it began and how severe it is. Did it follow eye trauma, a chemical splash, or exposure to the rays of a sun lamp? If photophobia results from trauma, avoid manipulating the eyes. Ask the patient about eye pain and have him describe its location, duration, and intensity. Does he have a sensation of a foreign body in his eye? Does he have other signs and symptoms, such as increased tearing and vision changes? Does he have nuchal rigidity and severe headache?

Next, take the patient's vital signs and assess his neurologic status. Assess visual activity, unless the cause is a chemical burn. Follow this with a careful eye examination, inspecting the eyes' external structures for abnormalities. Examine the conjunctiva and sclera, noting their color. Characterize the amount and consistency of any discharge. Then check pupillary reaction to light. Evaluate extraocular muscle function by testing the six cardinal fields of gaze, and test visual acuity in both eyes.

During your assessment, keep in mind that although photophobia can accompany life-threatening meningitis, it isn't a cardinal sign of meningeal irritation.

Medical causes

Burns. With a chemical burn, photophobia and eye pain may be accompanied by erythema and blistering on the face and lids, miosis, diffuse conjunctival injection, and corneal changes. The patient experiences blurred vision and may be unable to keep his eyes open. With an ultraviolet radiation burn, photophobia occurs with moderate to severe eye pain. These symptoms develop about 12 hours after exposure to the rays of a welding arc or sun lamp.

Conjunctivitis. When conjunctivitis affects the cornea, it causes photophobia. Other common findings include conjunctival injection, increased tearing, a foreign-body sensation, a feeling of fullness around the eyes, and eye pain, burning, and itching. Allergic conjunctivitis is distinguished by a stringy eye discharge and milky red injection. Bacterial conjunctivitis tends to cause a copious, mucopurulent, flaky eye discharge that may make the eyelids stick together as well as brilliant red conjunctiva. Fungal conjunctivitis produces a thick, purulent discharge, extreme redness, and crusting, sticky eyelids. Viral conjunctivitis causes copious tearing with little discharge as well as enlargement of the preauricular lymph nodes.

Corneal abrasion. A common finding with corneal abrasion, photophobia is usually accompanied by excessive tearing, conjunctival injection, visible corneal damage, and a foreign-body sensation in the eye. Blurred vision and eye pain may also occur.

Corneal ulcer. A corneal ulcer causes severe photophobia and eye pain aggravated by blinking. Impaired visual acuity may accompany blurring, eye discharge, and sticky eyelids. Conjunctival injection may occur even though the cornea appears white and opaque. A bacterial ulcer may also cause an irregularly shaped corneal ulcer and unilateral pupillary constriction. A fungal ulcer may be surrounded by progressively clearer rings.

Iritis (acute). Severe photophobia may result from acute iritis, along with marked conjunctival injection, moderate to severe eye pain, and blurred vision. The pupil may be constricted and may respond poorly to light.

Keratitis (interstitial). Keratitis is a corneal inflammation that causes photophobia, eye pain, blurred vision, dramatic conjunctival injection, and grayish pink corneas.

Meningitis (acute bacterial). A common symptom of meningitis, photophobia may occur with other signs of meningeal irritation, such as nuchal rigidity, hyperreflexia, and opisthotonos. Brudzinski's and Kernig's signs can be elicited. Fever, an early finding, may be accompanied by chills. Related signs and symptoms may include headache, vomiting, ocular palsies, facial weakness, pupillary abnormalities, and hearing loss. With severe meningitis, seizures may occur along with stupor progressing to coma.

Migraine headache. Photophobia and noise sensitivity are prominent features of a common migraine. Typically severe, this aching or throbbing headache may also cause fatigue, blurred vision, nausea, and vomiting.

Uveitis. Anterior and posterior uveitis can cause photophobia. Typically, anterior uveitis also produces moderate to severe eye pain, severe conjunctival injection, and a small, nonreactive pupil. Posterior uveitis develops slowly, causing visual floaters, eye pain, pupil distortion, conjunctival injection, and blurred vision.

Other causes

Drugs. Mydriatics—such as phenylephrine, atropine, scopolamine, cyclopentolate, and tropicamide—can cause photophobia due to ocular dilation. Amphetamines, cocaine, and ophthalmic antifungals—such as trifluridine, vidarabine, and idoxuridine—can also cause photophobia.

Nursing considerations

- Promote the patient's comfort by darkening the room and telling him to close both eyes. Encourage use of sunglasses.

- Prepare the patient for diagnostic tests, such as corneal scraping and slit-lamp examination.
- Administer eyedrops and ointments, as ordered.

Patient teaching

- Teach the patient how to instill eyedrops or ointments.
- Discuss ways to reduce the discomfort of photophobia.
- Explain the disorder and treatment plan.

Pleural friction rub

Commonly resulting from a pulmonary disorder or trauma, this loud, coarse, grating, creaking, or squeaking sound may be auscultated over one or both lungs during late inspiration or early expiration. It's heard best over the low axilla or the anterior, lateral, or posterior bases of the lung fields with the patient upright. Sometimes intermittent, it may resemble crackles or a pericardial friction rub. (See *Comparing auscultation findings*, pages 474 and 475.)

A pleural friction rub indicates inflammation of the visceral and parietal pleural lining, which causes congestion and edema. The resultant fibrinous exudate covers both pleural surfaces, displacing the fluid that's normally between them and causing the surfaces to rub together.

Action stat!

 When you detect a pleural friction rub, quickly look for signs of respiratory distress: shallow or decreased respirations; crowing, wheezing, or stridor; dyspnea; increased accessory muscle use; intercostal or suprasternal retractions; cyanosis; and nasal flaring. Check for hypotension, tachycardia, and a decreased level of consciousness.

If you detect signs of distress, open and maintain an airway. Endotracheal intubation and supplemental oxygen may be necessary. Insert a large-bore I.V. catheter to deliver drugs and fluids. Elevate the patient's head 30 degrees. Monitor his cardiac status continually, and check his vital signs frequently.

History and physical examination

If the patient isn't in severe distress, explore related symptoms. Find out if he has had chest pain. If so, ask him to describe its location and severity. How long does his chest pain last? Does the pain radiate to his shoulder, neck, or upper abdomen? Does the pain worsen with breathing, movement, coughing, or sneezing? Does the pain abate if he splints his chest, holds his breath, or exerts pressure or lies on the affected side?

Ask the patient about a history of rheumatoid arthritis, a respiratory or cardiovascular disorder, recent trauma, asbestos exposure, or radiation therapy. If he smokes, obtain a history in pack-years.

Characterize the pleural friction rub by auscultating the lungs with the patient sitting upright and breathing deeply and slowly through his mouth. Is the friction rub unilateral or bilateral? Also, listen for absent or diminished breath sounds, noting their location and timing in the respiratory cycle. Do abnormal breath sounds clear with coughing? Observe the patient for clubbing and pedal edema, which may indicate a chronic disorder. Then palpate for decreased chest motion and percuss for flatness or dullness.

Medical causes

Asbestosis. Besides a pleural friction rub, asbestosis may cause exertional dyspnea, cough, chest pain, and crackles. Clubbing is a late sign.

Lung cancer. A pleural friction rub may be heard in the affected area of the lung. Other effects include a cough (with possible hemoptysis), dyspnea, chest pain, weight loss, anorexia, fatigue, clubbing, fever, and wheezing.

Pleurisy. A pleural friction rub occurs early in pleurisy. However, the cardinal symptom is sudden, intense chest pain that's usually unilateral and located in the lower and lateral parts of the chest. Deep breathing, coughing, or thoracic movement aggravates the pain. Decreased breath sounds and inspiratory crackles may be heard over the painful area. Other findings include dyspnea, tachypnea, tachycardia, cyanosis, fever, and fatigue.

Pneumonia (bacterial). A pleural friction rub occurs with bacterial pneumonia, which usually starts with a dry, painful, hacking cough that rapidly becomes productive. Related effects develop suddenly; these include shaking chills, high fever, headache, dyspnea, pleuritic chest pain, tachypnea, tachycardia, grunting respirations, nasal flaring, dullness to percussion, and cyanosis. Auscultation reveals decreased breath sounds and fine crackles.

Pulmonary embolism. A pulmonary embolism can cause a pleural friction rub over the affected area of the lung. Usually, the first symptom is sudden dyspnea, which may be accompanied by angina or unilateral pleuritic chest pain. Other clinical features include a nonproductive cough or a cough that produces blood-tinged sputum, tachycardia, tachypnea, a low-grade fever, restlessness, and diaphoresis. Less common findings include massive hemoptysis, chest splinting, leg edema and, with a large embolus, cyanosis, syncope, and jugular vein distention. Crackles, diffuse wheezing, decreased breath sounds, and signs of circulatory collapse may also occur.

Systemic lupus erythematosus (SLE). With SLE, pulmonary involvement can cause a pleural friction rub, hemoptysis, dyspnea, pleuritic chest pain, and crackles. More characteristic effects of SLE include a butterfly rash, nondeforming joint pain and stiffness, and photosensitivity. Fever, anorexia, weight loss, and lymphadenopathy may also occur.

Tuberculosis (TB)(pulmonary). With pulmonary TB, a pleural friction rub may occur over the affected part of the lung. Early signs and symptoms include weight loss, night sweats, a low-grade fever in the afternoon, malaise, dyspnea, anorexia, and easy fatigability. Progression of the disorder usually produces pleuritic pain, fine crackles over the upper lobes, and a productive cough with blood-streaked sputum. Advanced TB can cause chest retraction, tracheal deviation, and dullness to percussion.

Other causes

Treatments. Thoracic surgery and radiation therapy can cause a pleural friction rub.

Nursing considerations

- Monitor the patient's respiratory status, vital signs, and pulse oximetry.
- If the patient has a persistent dry, hacking cough that tires him, administer an antitussive.
- Administer oxygen and an antibiotic, as ordered.
- Prepare the patient for diagnostic tests, such as chest X-rays, computed tomography, and electrocardiogram.

Patient teaching

- Explain the disorder and treatment plan.
- Discuss pain relief measures, such as splinting the chest.
- Explain signs and symptoms the patient needs to report.
- Review medications the patient will need at home, how to take them correctly, and their possible adverse effects.

Polydipsia

Polydipsia refers to excessive thirst, a common symptom associated with endocrine disorders and certain drugs. It may reflect decreased fluid intake, increased urine output, or excessive loss of water and salt.

History and physical examination

Obtain a medical history. Find out how much fluid the patient drinks each day. How often and how much does he typically urinate? Does the need to urinate awaken him at night? Determine if he or anyone in his family has diabetes or kidney disease. What medications does he use? Has his lifestyle changed recently?

If the patient has polydipsia, take his blood pressure and pulse when he's in supine and standing positions. A decrease of 10 mm Hg in systolic pressure and a pulse rate increase of 10 beats/minute from the supine to the sitting or standing position may indicate hypovolemia. Ask the patient about recent weight loss. Check for signs of dehydration, such as dry mucous membranes and decreased skin turgor.

Medical causes

Diabetes insipidus. Diabetes insipidus characteristically produces polydipsia and may also cause excessive voiding of dilute urine and mild to moderate nocturia. Fatigue and signs of dehydration occur in severe cases.

Diabetes mellitus. Polydipsia is a classic finding with diabetes mellitus—a consequence of the hyperosmolar state. Other characteristic findings include polyuria, polyphagia, nocturia, weakness, fatigue, and weight loss. Signs of dehydration may occur.

Hypercalcemia. As hypercalcemia progresses, the patient develops polydipsia, polyuria, nocturia, constipation, paresthesia and, occasionally, hematuria and pyuria. Severe hypercalcemia can progress quickly to vomiting, decreased level of consciousness, and renal failure. Depression, mental lassitude, and increased sleep requirements are common.

Hypokalemia. Hypokalemia can cause polydipsia, polyuria, and nocturia. Related hypokalemic signs and symptoms include muscle weakness or paralysis, fatigue, decreased bowel sounds, hypoactive deep tendon reflexes, and arrhythmias.

Psychogenic polydipsia. Psychogenic polydipsia causes polydipsia and polyuria. It may occur with any psychiatric disorder, but is more common with schizophrenia. Signs of psychiatric disturbances, such as anxiety or depression, are typical. Other findings include headache, blurred vision, weight gain, edema, elevated blood pressure and, occasionally, stupor and coma. Signs of heart failure may develop with overhydration.

Renal disorders (chronic). Chronic renal disorders, such as glomerulonephritis and pyelonephritis, damage the kidneys, causing polydipsia and polyuria. Associated signs and symptoms include nocturia, weakness, elevated blood pressure, pallor and, in later stages, oliguria.

Sheehan's syndrome. Polydipsia, polyuria, and nocturia occur with Sheehan's syndrome, a disorder of postpartum pituitary necrosis. Other features include fatigue, failure to lactate, amenorrhea, decreased pubic and axillary hair growth, and a reduced libido.

Sickle cell anemia. With sickle cell anemia, as nephropathy develops, polydipsia and polyuria occur. They may be accompanied by abdominal pain and cramps, arthralgia and, occasionally, lower extremity skin ulcers and bone deformities, such as kyphosis and scoliosis.

Other causes

Drugs. Diuretics and demeclocycline may produce polydipsia. Phenothiazines and anticholinergics can cause dry mouth, making the patient so thirsty that he drinks compulsively.

Nursing considerations

- Monitor the patient's intake and output.
- Weigh the patient daily.
- Check the patient's blood pressure and pulse in the supine and standing positions to detect orthostatic hypotension, which may indicate hypovolemia.
- Encourage adequate fluid intake, if appropriate.

Patient teaching

- Explain the underlying disorder and its treatments.
- Teach the patient about diet, exercise, and home blood glucose monitoring, if indicated.

Polyphagia
[Hyperphagia]

Polyphagia refers to voracious or excessive eating. This common symptom can be persistent or intermittent, resulting primarily from endocrine and psychological disorders as well as the use of certain drugs. Depending on the underlying cause, polyphagia may cause weight gain.

History and physical examination

Begin your evaluation by asking the patient about his oral intake within the past 24 hours. (If he easily recalls this information, ask about his intake for the 2 previous days, for a broader view of his dietary habits.) Note the frequency of meals and the amount and types of food eaten. Find out if the patient's eating habits have changed recently. Has he always had a large appetite? Does his overeating alternate with periods of anorexia? Ask about conditions that may trigger overeating, such as stress, depression, or menstruation. Does the patient actually feel hungry, or does he eat simply because food is available? Does he ever vomit or have a headache after overeating?

Explore related signs and symptoms. Has the patient recently gained or lost weight? Does he feel tired, nervous, or excitable? Has he experienced heat intolerance, dizziness, palpitations, diarrhea, or increased thirst or urination? Obtain a complete drug history, including the use of laxatives or enemas.

During the physical examination, weigh the patient. Tell him his current weight, and watch for his reaction. Inspect the skin to detect dryness or poor turgor. Palpate the thyroid for enlargement.

Medical causes

Anxiety. Polyphagia may result from mild to moderate anxiety or emotional stress. Mild anxiety typically produces restlessness, sleeplessness, irritability, repetitive questioning, and constant seeking of attention and reassurance. With moderate anxiety, selective inattention and difficulty concentrating may also occur. Other effects of anxiety may include muscle tension, diaphoresis, GI distress, palpitations, tachycardia, and urinary and sexual dysfunction.

Bulimia. Bulimia causes polyphagia that alternates with self-induced vomiting, fasting, or diarrhea. The patient typically weighs less than normal, but has a morbid fear of obesity. She appears depressed, has low self-esteem, and conceals her overeating.

Diabetes mellitus. With diabetes mellitus, polyphagia occurs with weight loss, polydipsia, and polyuria. It's accompanied by nocturia, weakness, fatigue, and signs of dehydration, such as dry mucous membranes and poor skin turgor.

Premenstrual syndrome (PMS). Appetite changes, typified by food cravings and binges, are common with PMS. Abdominal bloating, the most common associated finding, may occur with behavioral changes, such as depression and insomnia. Headache, paresthesia, and other neurologic symptoms may also occur. Related findings include diarrhea or constipation, edema and temporary weight gain, palpitations, back pain, breast swelling and tenderness, oliguria, and easy bruising.

Other causes

Drugs. Corticosteroids, cyproheptadine, and some hormone supplements may increase appetite, causing weight gain.

Nursing considerations

- Monitor the patient's eating habits and oral intake.
- Monitor the patient's daily weight.
- Provide emotional support.
- Obtain a mental health consult, if indicated.

Patient teaching

- Refer the patient to a registered dietitian or weight loss program for nutritional counseling, if appropriate.
- Explain the underlying disease process and its treatments.

Polyuria

A relatively common sign, polyuria is the daily production and excretion of more than 3 L of urine. It's usually reported by the patient as increased urination, especially when it occurs at night. Polyuria is aggravated by overhydration, consumption of caffeine or alcohol, and excessive ingestion of salt, glucose, or other hyperosmolar substances.

Polyuria usually results from the use of certain drugs, such as a diuretic, or from a psychological, neurologic, or renal disorder. It can reflect central nervous system dysfunction that diminishes or suppresses antidiuretic hormone (ADH) secretion, which regulates fluid balance. Or, when ADH levels are normal, it can reflect renal impairment. In both of these pathophysiologic mechanisms, the renal tubules fail to reabsorb sufficient water, causing polyuria.

History and physical examination

Because the patient with polyuria is at risk for developing hypovolemia, evaluate his fluid status first. Take his vital signs, noting an increased body temperature, tachycardia, and orthostatic hypotension (a 10 mm Hg decrease in systolic blood pressure upon standing and a 10 beats/minute increase in heart rate upon standing). Inspect for dry skin and mucous membranes, decreased skin turgor and elasticity, and reduced perspiration. Is the patient unusually tired or thirsty? Has he recently lost more than 5% of his body weight? If you detect these effects of hypovolemia, you'll need to infuse replacement fluids.

If the patient doesn't display signs of hypovolemia, explore the frequency and pattern of the polyuria. When did it begin? How long has it lasted? Was it precipitated by a certain event? Ask the patient to describe the pattern and amount of his daily fluid intake. Check for a history of visual deficits, headaches, or head trauma, which may precede diabetes insipidus. Also check for a history of urinary tract obstruction, diabetes mellitus, renal disorders, chronic hypokalemia or hypercalcemia, or psychiatric disorders (past and present). Find out the schedule and dosage of any drugs the patient is taking.

Perform a neurologic examination, noting especially any change in the patient's level of consciousness. Then palpate the bladder and inspect the urethral meatus. Obtain a urine specimen and check its specific gravity.

Medical causes

Acute tubular necrosis (ATN). During the diuretic phase of ATN, polyuria of less than 8 L/day gradually subsides after 8 to 10 days. Urine specific gravity (1.010 or less) increases as polyuria subsides. Related findings include weight loss, decreasing edema, and nocturia.

Diabetes insipidus (DI). Polyuria of about 5 L/day with a specific gravity of 1.005 or less is common with DI, although extreme polyuria—up to 30 L/day—occasionally occurs. Polyuria is commonly accompanied by polydipsia, nocturia, fatigue, and signs of dehydration, such as poor skin turgor and dry mucous membranes.

Diabetes mellitus (DM). With DM, polyuria seldom exceeds 5 L/day, and urine specific gravity typically exceeds 1.020. The patient usually reports polydipsia, polyphagia, weight loss, weakness, frequent urinary tract infections and yeast vaginitis, fatigue, and nocturia. The patient may also display signs of dehydration and anorexia.

Glomerulonephritis (chronic). Polyuria gradually progresses to oliguria with chronic glomerulonephritis. Urine output is usually less than 4 L/day; specific gravity is about 1.010. Related GI findings include anorexia, nausea, and vomiting. The patient may experience drowsiness, fatigue, edema, headache, elevated blood pressure, and dyspnea. Nocturia, hematuria, frothy or malodorous urine, and mild to severe proteinuria may occur.

Postobstructive uropathy. After resolution of a urinary tract obstruction, polyuria—usually more than 5 L/day with a specific gravity of less than 1.010—occurs for up to several days before gradually subsiding. Bladder distention and edema may occur with nocturia and weight loss. Occasionally, signs of dehydration appear.

Psychogenic polydipsia. Psychogenic polydipsia usually produces dilute polyuria of 3 to 15 L/day, depending on fluid intake. The patient may appear depressed and have a headache and blurred vision. Weight gain, edema, elevated blood pressure and, occasionally, stupor or coma may develop. With severe overhydration, signs of heart failure may present.

Other causes

Diagnostic tests. Transient polyuria can result from radiographic tests that use contrast media.

Drugs. Diuretics characteristically produce polyuria. Cardiotonics, vitamin D, demeclocycline, phenytoin, lithium, methoxyflurane, and propoxyphene can also produce polyuria.

Nursing considerations

■ Record intake and output, and weigh the patient daily.
■ Monitor the patient's vital signs.
■ Encourage the patient to drink adequate fluids and administer I.V. fluids as necessary.
■ Prepare the patient for serum electrolyte, osmolality, blood urea nitrogen, and creatinine studies to monitor fluid and electrolyte status and for a fluid

deprivation test to determine the cause of polyuria.

Patient teaching

■ Review the underlying disorder and its treatments.
■ Explain the need to replace fluids and monitor weight.
■ Discuss signs and symptoms that require medical attention.

Priapism

A urologic emergency, priapism is a persistent, painful erection that's unrelated to sexual excitation. This relatively rare sign may begin during sleep and appear to be a normal erection, but it may last for several hours or days. It's usually accompanied by a severe, constant, dull aching in the penis. Despite the pain, the patient may be too embarrassed to seek medical help and may try to achieve detumescence through continued sexual activity.

Priapism occurs when the veins of the corpora cavernosa fail to drain correctly, resulting in persistent engorgement of the tissues. Without prompt treatment, penile ischemia and thrombosis occur. In about one-half of all cases, priapism is idiopathic and develops without apparent predisposing factors. Secondary priapism can result from a blood disorder, neoplasm, trauma, or the use of certain drugs.

ACTION STAT!

 If the patient has priapism, apply an ice pack to the penis, administer an analgesic, and insert an indwelling urinary catheter to relieve urine retention. Procedures to remove blood from the corpora cavernosa, such as irrigation and surgery, may be required.

History and physical examination

Ask the patient when the priapism began. Is it continuous or intermittent? Has he had a prolonged erection before? If so, what did he do to relieve it? How long did he remain detumescent? Does he have pain or tenderness when he urinates? Has he noticed changes in sexual function?

Explore the patient's medical history. If he reports sickle cell anemia, find out about factors that could precipitate a crisis, such as dehydration and infection. Ask if he has recently suffered genital trauma, and obtain a thorough drug history. Ask if he has had drugs injected or objects inserted into his penis. Obtain a complete drug history. Note use of medications for erectile dysfunction (ED) (phosphodiesterase inhibitors).

Examine the patient's penis, noting its color and temperature. Check for loss of sensation and signs of infection, such as redness or drainage. Finally, take his vital signs, particularly noting a fever.

Medical causes

Penile cancer. Cancer that exerts pressure on the corpora cavernosa can cause priapism. Usually, the first sign is a painless ulcerative lesion or an enlarging warty growth on the glans or foreskin, which may be accompanied by localized pain, a foul-smelling discharge from the prepuce, a firm lump near the glans, and lymphadenopathy. Later findings include bleeding, dysuria, urine retention, and bladder distention. Phimosis and poor hygiene have been linked to the development of penile cancer.

Sickle cell anemia. With sickle cell anemia, painful priapism can occur without warning, usually on awakening. The patient may have a history of priapism, impaired growth and development, and an increased susceptibility to infection. Related findings include tachycardia, pallor, weakness, hepatomegaly, dyspnea, joint swelling, joint or bone aching, chest pain, fatigue, murmurs, leg ulcers and, possibly, jaundice and gross hematuria.

With sickle cell crisis, signs and symptoms of sickle cell anemia may worsen and others, such as abdominal pain and a low-grade fever, may appear.

Spinal cord injury. With spinal cord injury, the patient may be unaware of the onset of priapism. Related effects depend on the extent and level of injury and may include autonomic signs such as bradycardia.

Stroke. A stroke may cause priapism, but sensory loss and aphasia may prevent the patient from noticing or describing it. Other findings depend on the stroke's location and extent, but may include contralateral hemiplegia, seizures, headache, dysarthria, dysphagia, ataxia, apraxia, and agnosia. Visual deficits include homonymous hemianopsia, blurring, decreased acuity, and diplopia. Urine retention or incontinence, fecal incontinence, constipation, and vomiting may also occur.

Other causes

Drugs. Priapism can result from the use of a phenothiazine, thioridazine, trazodone, an androgenic steroid, an anticoagulant, or an antihypertensive. It may also occur after an intracorporeal injection of papaverine, a common treatment for impotence, or phosphodiesterase inhibitors (used with ED).

Nursing considerations

- Prepare the patient for blood tests to help determine the cause of priapism.
- If he requires surgery, keep his penis flaccid postoperatively by applying a pressure dressing.
- At least once every 30 minutes, inspect the glans for signs of vascular compromise, such as coolness or pallor.

Patient teaching

- Explain the underlying condition and its treatments.
- Tell the patient with sickle cell anemia to report episodes of priapism.

Pruritus

Commonly provoking scratching to gain relief, this unpleasant itching sensation affects the skin, certain mucous membranes, and the eyes. Most severe at night, pruritus may be exacerbated by increased skin temperature, poor skin turgor, local vasodilation, dermatoses, and stress.

The most common symptom of dermatologic disorders, pruritus may also result from a local or systemic disorder or from drug use. Physiologic pruritus, such as pruritic urticarial papules and plaques of pregnancy, may occur in primigravidas late in the third trimester. Pruritus can also stem from emotional upset or contact with skin irritants.

History and physical examination

If the patient reports pruritus, have him describe its onset, frequency, and intensity. If pruritus occurs at night, ask whether it prevents him from falling asleep or awakens him after he falls asleep. (Generally, pruritus related to dermatoses prevents—but doesn't disturb—sleep.) Is the itching localized or generalized? When is it most severe? How long does it last? Is there a relationship to activities (physical exertion, bathing, applying makeup, or the use of perfumes)?

Ask the patient how he cleans his skin and clothes. In particular, look for excessive bathing, harsh soaps, contact allergy, and excessively hot water. Does he have occupational exposure to known skin irritants, such as glass fiber insulation or chemicals? Ask about the patient's general health and the medications he takes (new medications are suspect). Has he recently traveled abroad? Does he have pets? Does anyone else in the house report itching? Does exercise, stress, fear, depression, or illness seem to aggravate the itching? Ask about contact with skin irritants, previous skin disorders, and related symptoms. Obtain a complete drug history. Ask about abdominal pain and the appearance of stools.

Examine the patient for signs of scratching, such as excoriation, purpura, scabs, scars, or lichenification. Look for primary lesions to help confirm dermatoses. Note any jaundice. Check for hepatomegaly or abdominal pain.

Medical causes

Anemia (iron deficiency). Iron deficiency anemia occasionally produces pruritus. Initially producing no symptoms, anemia can later cause exertional dyspnea, fatigue, listlessness, pallor, irritability, headache, tachycardia, poor muscle tone and, possibly, murmurs. Chronic anemia causes spoon-shaped (koilonychia) and brittle nails, cracked mouth corners (cheilosis), a smooth tongue (glossitis), and dysphagia.

Anthrax (cutaneous). Anthrax infection begins as a small, painless or pruritic macular or papular lesion resembling an insect bite. Within 1 or 2 days, it develops into a vesicle and then a painless ulcer with a characteristic black, necrotic center. Lymphadenopathy, malaise, headache, or fever may develop.

Conjunctivitis. All forms of conjunctivitis cause eye itching, burning, and pain along with photophobia, conjunctival injection, a foreign-body sensation, excessive tearing, and a feeling of fullness around the eye. Allergic conjunctivitis may also cause milky redness and a stringy eye discharge. Bacterial conjunctivitis typically causes brilliant redness and a mucopurulent discharge that may make the eyelids stick together. Fungal conjunctivitis produces a thick, purulent discharge and crusting and sticking of the eyelid. Viral conjunctivitis may cause copious tearing—but little discharge—and preauricular lymph node enlargement.

Dermatitis. Several types of dermatitis can cause pruritus accompanied by a skin lesion. Atopic dermatitis begins with intense, severe pruritus and an erythematous rash on dry skin at flexion points (antecubital fossa, popliteal area, and neck). During a flare-up, scratching may produce edema, scaling, and pustules. With chronic atopic dermatitis, lesions may progress to dry, scaly skin with white dermatographia, blanching, and lichenification.

Mild irritants and allergies can cause contact dermatitis, with itchy small vesicles that may ooze and scale and are surrounded by redness. A severe reaction can produce marked localized edema.

Dermatitis herpetiformis, initially causes intense pruritus and stinging. Between 8 and 12 hours later, symmetrically distributed lesions form on the buttocks, shoulders, elbows, and knees. Sometimes, they also form on the neck, face, and scalp. These lesions are erythematous and papular, bullous, or pustular.

Hepatobiliary disease. An important diagnostic clue to liver and gallbladder disease, pruritus is commonly accompanied by jaundice and may be generalized or localized to the palms and soles. Other characteristics include right upper quadrant pain, clay-colored stools, chills and fever, flatus, belching and a bloated feeling, epigastric burning, and bitter fluid regurgitation. Later, liver disease may produce mental changes, ascites, bleeding tendencies, spider angiomas, palmar erythema, dry skin, fetor hepaticus, enlarged superficial abdominal

veins, bilateral gynecomastia, testicular atrophy or menstrual irregularities, and hepatomegaly.

Herpes zoster. With herpes zoster, within 2 to 4 days of a fever and malaise, pruritus, paresthesia or hyperesthesia, and severe, deep pain from cutaneous nerve involvement develop on the trunk or the arms and legs in a dermatome distribution. Up to 2 weeks after initial symptoms, red, nodular skin eruptions appear on the painful areas and become vesicular. About 10 days later, the vesicles rupture and form scabs.

Leukemia (chronic lymphocytic). Pruritus is an uncommon finding in leukemia. More characteristic signs and symptoms include fatigue, malaise, generalized lymphadenopathy, fever, hepatomegaly, splenomegaly, weight loss, pallor, bleeding, and palpitations.

Lichen simplex chronicus. Persistent rubbing and scratching cause localized pruritus and a circumscribed scaling patch with sharp margins. Later, the skin thickens and papules form.

Myringitis (chronic). Myringitis produces pruritus in the affected ear, along with a purulent discharge and gradual hearing loss.

Pediculosis. A prominent symptom of pediculosis, pruritus occurs in the area of infestation. Pediculosis capitis (head lice) may also cause scalp excoriation from scratching, along with matted, foul-smelling, lusterless hair; occipital and cervical lymphadenopathy; and oval, gray-white nits on hair shafts.

Pediculosis corporis (body lice) initially causes small red papules (usually on the shoulders, trunk, or buttocks), which become urticarial from scratching. Later, rashes or wheals may develop. Untreated, pediculosis corporis produces dry, discolored, thickly encrusted, scaly skin with bacterial infection and scarring. In severe cases, it produces headache, fever, and malaise.

With pediculosis pubis (pubic lice), scratching commonly produces skin irritation. Nits or adult lice and erythematous, itching papules may appear in pubic hair or in hair around the anus, abdomen, or thighs.

Pityriasis rosea. Pityriasis rosea occasionally produces mild pruritus that's aggravated by a hot bath or shower. It usually begins with an erythematous herald patch—a slightly raised, oval lesion about 2 to 6 cm in diameter. After a few days or weeks, scaly yellow-tan or erythematous patches erupt on the trunk and extremities and persist for 2 to 6 weeks. Occasionally, these patches are macular, vesicular, or urticarial.

Psoriasis. Pruritus and pain are common in psoriasis. This skin disorder typically begins with small erythematous papules that enlarge or coalesce to form red elevated plaques with silver scales on the scalp, chest, elbows, knees, back, buttocks, and genitals. Nail pitting may occur.

Scabies. Typically, scabies causes localized pruritus that awakens the patient. It may become generalized and persist for up to 2 weeks after treatment. Threadlike lesions several millimeters long appear with a swollen nodule or red papule.

Tinea pedis. Tinea pedis is a fungal infection that causes severe foot pruritus, pain with walking, scales and blisters between the toes, and a dry, scaly squamous inflammation on the entire sole.

Urticaria. With urticaria, extreme pruritus and stinging occur as transient, erythematous or whitish wheals form on the skin or mucous membranes. Prickly sensations typically precede the wheals, which may affect any part of the body and may range from pinpoint to palm-size or larger.

Vaginitis. Vaginitis commonly causes localized pruritus and a foul-smelling vaginal discharge that may be purulent, white or gray, and curdlike. Perineal pain and urinary dysfunction may also occur.

Other causes

Bedbug bites. Typically, bedbug bites produce itching and burning over the ankles and lower legs, along with clusters of purpuric spots.

Drug hypersensitivity. When mild and localized, an allergic reaction to such drugs as penicillin and sulfonamides can cause pruritus, erythema, an urticarial rash, and edema. However, with a severe drug reaction, anaphylaxis may occur.

Nursing considerations

- Administer a topical or oral corticosteroid, an antihistamine, or a tranquilizer, as ordered.
- If the patient doesn't have a localized infection or skin lesions, suspect a systemic disease and prepare him for a complete blood count and differential, erythrocyte sedimentation rate, protein electrophoresis, and radiologic studies.

Patient teaching

- Explain to the patient the cause of pruritus, the treatment plan, and ways to prevent it.
- Teach the patient ways to control pruritus.
- Reinforce the importance of not scratching.

Psoas sign

A positive psoas sign—increased abdominal pain when the patient moves his leg against resistance—indicates direct or reflexive irritation of the psoas muscles. This sign, which can be elicited on the right or left side, usually indi-

Eliciting psoas sign

You can use two techniques to elicit psoas sign in an adult with abdominal pain. With either technique, increased abdominal pain is a positive result, indicating psoas muscle irritation from an inflamed appendix or a localized abscess.

With the patient in a supine position, instruct her to move her flexed left leg against your hand to test for a left psoas sign. Then perform this maneuver on the right leg to test for right psoas sign.

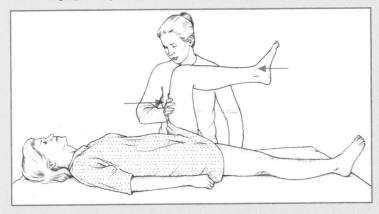

To test for left psoas sign, turn the patient onto her right side. Then instruct her to push her left leg upward from the hip against your hand. Next, turn the patient onto her left side and repeat this maneuver to test for a right psoas sign.

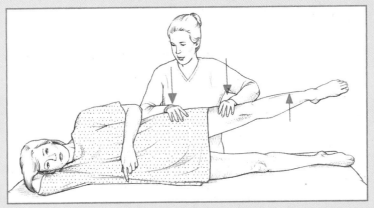

cates appendicitis, but may also occur with localized abscesses. It's elicited in a patient with abdominal or lower back pain *after* completion of an abdominal examination to prevent spurious assessment findings. (See *Eliciting psoas sign*.)

ACTION STAT!

If you elicit a positive psoas sign in a patient with abdominal pain, suspect appendicitis. Quickly check the patient's vital signs, and prepare him for surgery: Explain the procedure, restrict food and fluids, and withhold analgesics, which can mask symptoms. Administer I.V. fluids to prevent dehydration, but don't give a cathartic or an enema, because it can cause the appendix to rupture, leading to peritonitis.

Check for Rovsing sign by deeply palpating the patient's left lower quadrant. If he reports pain in the right lower quadrant, the sign is positive, indicating peritoneal irritation.

Medical causes

Appendicitis. An inflamed retrocecal appendix can cause a positive right psoas sign. Early epigastric and periumbilical pain disappears, only to worsen and localize in the right lower quadrant. This pain also worsens with walking or coughing. Related findings include nausea and vomiting, abdominal rigidity and rebound tenderness, and constipation or diarrhea. Fever, tachycardia, retractive respirations, anorexia, and malaise may also occur. If the appendix ruptures, additional findings may include sudden, severe pain, followed by signs of peritonitis, such as hypoactive or absent bowel sounds, a high fever, and boardlike abdominal rigidity. A positive obturator sign may also be evident.

Retroperitoneal abscess. After a lower retroperitoneal infection, an iliac or lumbar abscess can produce a positive right or left psoas sign and fever. An iliac abscess causes iliac or inguinal pain that may radiate to the hip, thigh, flank, or knee; a tender mass in the lower abdomen or groin may be palpable. A lumbar abscess usually produces back tenderness and spasms on the affected side with a palpable lumbar mass; a tender abdominal mass without back pain may occur instead.

Nursing considerations

- Monitor the patient's vital signs to detect complications, such as pain extension along fascial planes in the abdomen, thigh, hip, subphrenic spaces, mediastinum, and pleural cavities, and peritonitis.
- Promote patient comfort by helping with position changes.
- Prepare the patient for diagnostic tests, such as electrolyte studies, complete blood count, abdominal X-rays, and computed tomography scans.

Patient teaching

- Teach the patient about his underlying condition and its treatments.
- Discuss signs and symptoms that require immediate medical attention.

Psychotic behavior

Psychotic behavior reflects an inability or unwillingness to recognize and acknowledge reality and to relate with others. It may begin suddenly or insidiously, progressing from vague complaints of fatigue, insomnia, or headaches to withdrawal, social isolation, and preoccupation with certain issues, resulting in gross impairment in functioning.

Various behaviors together or separately can constitute psychotic behavior. These include delusions, illusions, hallucinations, bizarre language, and perseveration. Delusions are persistent beliefs that have no basis in reality or in the patient's knowledge or experience such as delusions of grandeur. Illusions are misinterpretations of external sensory stimuli such as a mirage in the desert. In contrast, hallucinations are sensory perceptions that don't result from external stimuli. Bizarre language reflects a communication disruption. It can range from echolalia (purposeless repetition of a word or phrase) and clang association (repetition of words or phrases that sound similar) to neologisms (creation and use of words whose meaning only the patient knows). Perseveration, a persistent verbal or motor response, may indicate organic brain disease. Motor changes include inactivity, excessive activity, and repetitive movements.

History and physical examination

Because the patient's behavior can make it difficult—or potentially dangerous—to obtain pertinent information, conduct the interview in a calm, safe, and well-lit room. Provide enough personal space to avoid threatening or agitating the patient. Ask him to describe his problem and circumstances that may have precipitated it. Obtain a drug history, noting especially the use of an antipsychotic, and explore his use of alcohol and other drugs, such as cocaine, indicating duration of use and amount and when it was last taken. Ask about recent illnesses or accidents.

As the patient talks, watch for cognitive, linguistic, or perceptual abnormalities such as delusions. Do thoughts and actions seem to match? Look for unusual gestures, posture, gait, tone of voice, and mannerisms. Does the patient appear to be responding to stimuli? For example, is he looking around the room?

Interview the patient's family. Which family members does he seem closest to? How does the family describe the patient's relationships, communication patterns, and role? Has a family member ever been hospitalized for psychiatric or emotional illness? Ask about the patient's compliance with his drug regimen.

Finally, evaluate the patient's environment, educational and employment history, and socioeconomic status. Are community services available? How does the patient spend his leisure time? Does he have friends? Has he ever had a close emotional relationship?

Medical causes

Organic disorders. Various organic disorders, such as alcohol withdrawal syndrome, cocaine or amphetamine intoxication, cerebral hypoxia, and nutritional disorders, can produce psychotic behavior. Endocrine disorders, such as adrenal dysfunction, and severe infections, such as encephalitis, can also cause psychotic behavior. Neurologic causes include Alzheimer's disease and other dementias.

Psychiatric disorders. Psychotic behavior usually occurs with bipolar disorder, personality disorder, schizophrenia, and some pervasive developmental disorders.

Other causes

Drugs. Certain drugs can cause psychotic behavior. (See *Psychotic behavior: An adverse drug effect,* pages 492 and 493.) However, almost any drug can provoke psychotic behavior as a rare, severe adverse or idiosyncratic reaction.

Surgery. Postoperative delirium and depression may produce psychotic behavior.

Nursing considerations

- Frequently evaluate the patient's orientation to reality.
- Help him develop a conception of reality by calling him by his preferred name, telling him your name, describing where he is, and using clocks and calendars. (See *Controlling psychotic behavior,* page 493.)
- Encourage the patient to become involved in structured activities; however, if he's nonverbal or incoherent, be sure to spend time with him.

Psychotic behavior: An adverse drug effect

Certain drugs can cause psychotic behavior and other psychiatric signs and symptoms, ranging from depression to violent behavior. Usually, these effects occur during therapy and resolve when the drug is discontinued. If the patient is receiving one of these common drugs and exhibits the behavior described, the dosage may have to be changed or another drug may have to be substituted.

Drug	Psychiatric signs and symptoms
albuterol	Hallucinations, paranoia
alprazolam	Anger, hostility
amantadine	Visual hallucinations, nightmares
asparaginase	Confusion, depression, paranoia
atropine and anticholinergics	Auditory, visual, and tactile hallucinations; memory loss; delirium; fear; paranoia
bromocriptine	Mania, delusions, sudden relapse of schizophrenia, paranoia, aggressive behavior
cardiac glycosides	Paranoia, euphoria, amnesia, visual hallucinations
cimetidine	Hallucinations, paranoia, confusion, depression, delirium
clonidine	Delirium, hallucinations, depression
corticosteroids (prednisone, corticotropin, cortisone)	Mania, catatonia, depression, confusion, paranoia, hallucinations
cycloserine	Anxiety, depression, confusion, paranoia, hallucinations
dapsone	Insomnia, agitation, hallucinations
diazepam	Suicidal thoughts, rage, hallucinations, depression
disopyramide	Agitation, paranoia, auditory and visual hallucinations, panic
disulfiram	Delirium, auditory hallucinations, paranoia, depression
indomethacin	Hostility, depression, paranoia, hallucinations
lidocaine	Disorientation, hallucinations, paranoia
methyldopa	Severe depression, amnesia, paranoia, hallucinations
propranolol	Severe depression, hallucinations, paranoia, confusion

Psychotic behavior: An adverse drug effect *(continued)*

Drug	Psychiatric signs and symptoms
thyroid hormones	Mania, hallucinations, paranoia
vincristine	Hallucinations

DO'S & DON'TS

Controlling psychotic behavior

A patient who displays psychotic behavior may be terrified and unable to differentiate between himself and his environment. To control his behavior and to prevent injury to the patient, staff, and others, follow these guidelines.

Do's

■ Remove potentially dangerous objects, such as belts or metal utensils, from the patient's environment.
■ Help the patient discern what's real and unreal in an honest and genuine way.
■ Be straightforward, concise, and non-threatening when speaking to the patient. Discuss simple, concrete subjects.
■ Positively reinforce the patient's perceptions of reality, and correct his misperceptions in a matter-of-fact way.
■ Move the patient to a safer, less-stimulating environment.
■ Provide one-on-one care if the patient's behavior is extremely bizarre, disturbing to other patients, or dangerous to himself.
■ Medicate the patient appropriately.

Don'ts

■ *Never* argue with the patient, but also don't support his misperceptions.
■ Don't leave the patient if he's frightened; stay with him.
■ Don't touch the patient to provide reassurance *unless* you've done this before and know that it's safe.
■ Don't discuss theories or philosophical issues with the patient.

■ Refer the patient for psychiatric evaluation.
■ Administer an antipsychotic or other drugs, as needed, and prepare him for transfer to a mental health center, if necessary.
■ Monitor the patient's eating and elimination habits.

■ Ensure patient and health care worker safety.

Patient teaching
■ Explain the importance of structured activities.
■ Discuss the patient's medications and how to take them correctly.

Ptosis

Ptosis is the excessive drooping of one or both upper eyelids. This sign can be constant, progressive, or intermittent and unilateral or bilateral. When it's unilateral, it's easy to detect by comparing the eyelids' relative positions. When it's bilateral or mild, it's difficult to detect—the eyelids may be abnormally low, covering the upper part of the iris or even part of the pupil instead of overlapping the iris slightly. Other clues include a furrowed forehead or a tipped-back head—both of these help the patient see under his drooping lids. With severe ptosis, the patient may not be able to raise his eyelids voluntarily. Because ptosis can resemble enophthalmos, exophthalmometry may be required.

Ptosis can be classified as congenital or acquired. Classification is important for proper treatment. Congenital ptosis results from levator muscle underdevelopment or disorders of the third cranial (oculomotor) nerve. Acquired ptosis may result from trauma to or inflammation of these muscles and nerves or from certain drugs, a systemic disease, an intracranial lesion, or a life-threatening aneurysm. However, the most common cause is advanced age, which reduces muscle elasticity and produces senile ptosis.

History and physical examination

Ask the patient when he first noticed his drooping eyelid. Also, ask him if it has worsened or improved since he first noticed it. Find out if he has recently suffered a traumatic eye injury. (If he has, avoid manipulating the eye to prevent further damage.) Ask about eye pain or headaches, and determine its location and severity. Has the patient experienced vision changes? If so, have him describe them. Obtain a drug history, noting especially the use of a chemotherapeutic drug.

Assess the degree of ptosis, and check for eyelid edema, exophthalmos, deviation, and conjunctival injection. Evaluate extraocular muscle function by testing the six cardinal fields of gaze. Carefully examine the pupils' size, color, shape, and reaction to light, and test visual acuity.

Keep in mind that ptosis occasionally indicates a life-threatening condition. For example, sudden unilateral ptosis can herald a cerebral aneurysm.

Medical causes

Botulism. Acute cranial nerve dysfunction as a result of botulism infection causes hallmark signs of ptosis, dysarthria, dysphagia, and diplopia. Other findings include a dry mouth, a sore throat, weakness, vomiting, diarrhea, hyporeflexia, and dyspnea.

Cerebral aneurysm. An aneurysm that compresses the oculomotor nerve can cause sudden ptosis, along with diplopia, a dilated pupil, and an inability to rotate the eye. These may be the first signs of this life-threatening disorder. A ruptured aneurysm typically produces a sudden severe headache, nausea, vomiting, and decreased level of consciousness (LOC). Other findings include nuchal rigidity, back and leg pain, fever, restlessness, irritability, occasional seizures, blurred vision, hemiparesis, sensory deficits, dysphagia, and visual defects.

Lacrimal gland tumor. A lacrimal gland tumor commonly produces mild to severe ptosis, depending on the tumor's size and location. It may also cause brow elevation, exophthalmos, eye deviation and, possibly, eye pain.

Myasthenia gravis. Commonly the first sign of myasthenia gravis, gradual bilateral ptosis may be mild to severe and is accompanied by weak eye closure and diplopia. Other characteristics include muscle weakness and fatigue, which eventually may lead to paralysis. Depending on the muscles affected, other findings may include masklike facies, difficulty chewing or swallowing, dyspnea, and cyanosis.

Ocular muscle dystrophy. With ocular muscle dystrophy, bilateral ptosis progresses slowly to complete eyelid closure. Related signs and symptoms include progressive external ophthalmoplegia and muscle weakness and atrophy of the upper face, neck, trunk, and limbs.

Ocular trauma. Trauma to the nerve or muscles that control the eyelids can cause mild to severe ptosis. Depending on the damage, eye pain, lid swelling, ecchymosis, and decreased visual acuity may also occur.

Parry-Romberg syndrome. Unilateral ptosis and facial hemiatrophy occur with Parry-Romberg syndrome. Other signs include miosis, sluggish pupil reaction to light, enophthalmos, different-colored irises, ocular muscle paralysis, nystagmus, and neck, shoulder, trunk, and extremity atrophy.

Other causes

Drugs. Vinca alkaloids can produce ptosis.

Lead poisoning. With lead poisoning, ptosis usually develops over 3 to 6 months. Other findings include anorexia, nausea, vomiting, diarrhea, colicky abdominal pain, a lead line in the gums, decreased LOC, tachycardia, hypotension and, possibly, irritability and peripheral nerve weakness.

Nursing considerations

- If the patient has decreased visual acuity, orient him to his surroundings.
- Provide special spectacle frames that suspend the eyelid by traction with a wire crutch.

- Prepare the patient for diagnostic studies, such as the Tensilon test and slit-lamp examination.

Patient teaching

- Prepare the patient for surgery, if needed.
- Discuss the underlying disorder and its treatments.

Pulse, absent or weak

An absent or a weak pulse may be generalized or affect only one extremity. When generalized, this sign is an important indicator of such life-threatening conditions as shock and arrhythmia. Localized loss or weakness of a pulse that's normally present and strong may indicate acute arterial occlusion, which could require emergency surgery. However, the pressure of palpation may temporarily diminish or obliterate superficial pulses, such as the posterior tibial or the dorsal pedal. Thus, bilateral weakness or absence of these pulses doesn't necessarily indicate an underlying disorder. (See *Evaluating peripheral pulses,* page 496.)

History and physical examination

If you detect an absent or a weak pulse, quickly palpate the remaining arterial pulses to distinguish between localized or generalized loss or weakness. If localized, ask whether the patient has experienced or is presently experiencing pain in that area. Assess the limb for color and temperature. Then quickly check the patient's other vital signs, evaluate his cardiopulmonary status, and obtain a brief history. Based on your findings, proceed with emergency interventions. (See *Managing an absent or a weak pulse,* pages 498 and 499.)

Evaluating peripheral pulses

The rate, amplitude, and symmetry of peripheral pulses provide important clues to cardiac function and the quality of peripheral perfusion. To gather these clues, palpate peripheral pulses lightly with the pads of your index, middle, and ring fingers, as space permits.

Rate
Count all pulses for at least 30 seconds (60 seconds when recording vital signs). The normal rate is between 60 and 100 beats/minute.

Amplitude
Palpate the blood vessel during ventricular systole. Describe pulse amplitude by using a scale such as the one below:
  4+ = bounding
  3+ = increased
  2+ = normal
  1+ = weak, thready
  0 = absent.
Use a stick figure to easily document the location and amplitude of all pulses.

Symmetry
Simultaneously palpate pulses (except for the carotid pulse) on both sides of the patient's body, and note inequality. Always assess peripheral pulses methodically, moving from the arms to the legs.

Medical causes
Aortic aneurysm (dissecting). When a dissecting aneurysm affects circulation to the innominate, left common carotid, subclavian, or femoral artery, it causes weak or absent arterial pulses distal to the affected area. Absent or diminished pulses occur in 50% of patients with proximal dissection and usually involve the brachiocephalic vessels. Pulse deficits are much less common in patients with distal dissection and tend to involve the left subclavian and femoral arteries. Tearing pain usually develops suddenly in the chest and neck and may radiate to the upper and lower back and abdomen. Other findings include syncope, loss of consciousness, weakness or transient paralysis of the legs or arms, the diastolic murmur of aortic insufficiency, systemic hypotension, and mottled skin below the waist.

Aortic arch syndrome (Takayasu's arteritis). Aortic arch syndrome produces weak or abruptly absent carotid pulses and unequal or absent radial pulses. These signs are usually preceded by malaise, night sweats, pallor, nausea, anorexia, weight loss, arthralgia, and Raynaud's phenomenon. Other findings include neck, shoulder, and chest pain; paresthesia; intermittent claudication; bruits; vision disturbances; dizziness; and syncope. If the carotid artery is involved, diplopia and transient blindness may occur.

Aortic bifurcation occlusion (acute). Aortic bifurcation occlusion produces abrupt absence of all leg pulses. The patient reports moderate to severe pain in the legs and, less commonly, in the abdomen, lumbosacral area, or perineum. Also, his legs are cold, pale, numb, and flaccid.

Aortic stenosis. With aortic stenosis, the carotid pulse is sustained but weak. Dyspnea (especially on exertion or paroxysmal nocturnal), chest pain, and syncope dominate the clinical picture. The patient commonly has an atrial gallop. Other findings include a harsh systolic ejection murmur, crackles, palpitations, fatigue, and narrowed pulse pressure.

Arrhythmias. Cardiac arrhythmias may produce generalized weak pulses accompanied by cool, clammy skin.

Other findings reflect the arrhythmia's severity and may include hypotension, chest pain, dyspnea, dizziness, and decreased level of consciousness (LOC).

Arterial occlusion. With acute occlusion, arterial pulses distal to the obstruction are unilaterally weak and then absent. The affected limb is cool, pale, and cyanotic, with an increased capillary refill time, and the patient complains of moderate to severe pain and paresthesia. A line of color and temperature demarcation develops at the level of obstruction. Varying degrees of limb paralysis may also occur, along with intense intermittent claudication. With chronic occlusion, occurring with disorders such as arteriosclerosis and Buerger's disease, pulses in the affected limb weaken gradually.

Cardiac tamponade. Life-threatening cardiac tamponade causes a weak, rapid pulse accompanied by these classic findings: paradoxical pulse, jugular vein distention, hypotension, and muffled heart sounds. Narrowed pulse pressure, pericardial friction rub, and hepatomegaly may also occur. The patient may appear anxious, restless, and cyanotic and may have chest pain, clammy skin, dyspnea, and tachypnea.

Coarctation of the aorta. Findings of coarctation of the aorta include bounding pulses in the arms and neck, with decreased pulsations and systolic pulse pressure in the lower extremities.

Peripheral vascular disease. Peripheral vascular disease causes a weakening and loss of peripheral pulses. The patient complains of aching pain distal to the occlusion that worsens with exercise and abates with rest. The skin feels cool and shows decreased hair growth. Impotence may occur in male patients with occlusion in the descending aorta or femoral areas.

Pulmonary embolism. Pulmonary embolism causes a generalized weak, rapid pulse. It may also cause an abrupt onset of chest pain, tachycardia, dyspnea, apprehension, syncope, diaphoresis, and cyanosis. Acute respiratory findings include tachypnea, dyspnea, decreased breath sounds, crackles, a pleural friction rub, and a cough—possibly with blood-tinged sputum.

Shock. With *anaphylactic shock,* pulses become rapid and weak and then uniformly absent within seconds or minutes after exposure to an allergen. This is preceded by hypotension, anxiety, restlessness, feelings of doom, intense itching, a pounding headache and, possibly, urticaria.

With *cardiogenic shock,* peripheral pulses are absent and central pulses are weak, depending on the degree of vascular collapse. Pulse pressure is narrow. A drop in systolic blood pressure to 30 mm Hg below baseline, or a sustained reading below 80 mm Hg, produces poor tissue perfusion. Resulting signs include cold, pale, clammy skin; tachycardia; rapid, shallow respirations; oliguria; restlessness; confusion; and obtundation.

With *hypovolemic shock,* all pulses in the extremities become weak and then uniformly absent, depending on the severity of hypovolemia. As shock progresses, remaining pulses become thready and more rapid. Early signs of hypovolemic shock include restlessness, thirst, tachypnea, and cool, pale skin. Late signs include hypotension with narrowing pulse pressure, clammy skin, a drop in urine output to less than 25 ml/hour, confusion, decreased LOC and, possibly, hypothermia.

With *septic shock,* all pulses in the extremities first become weak. Depending on the degree of vascular collapse, pulses may then become uniformly absent. Shock is heralded by chills, a sudden

(Text continues on page 500.)

Managing an absent or a weak pulse

An absent or a weak pulse can result from any one of several life-threatening disorders. Your evaluation and interventions will vary, depending on whether the weak or absent pulse is generalized or localized to one extremity. They'll also depend on associated signs and symptoms. Use the flowchart below to help you establish priorities for successfully managing this emergency.

Weak or absent pulse ▶ Localized to one extremity

Generalized

Patient is confused and restless; has hypotension and cool, pale, clammy skin.

Patient has a history of trauma, possibly with external bleeding, and reports thirst.	Patient has a history of myocardial infarction (MI) or heart failure.	Patient has a history of recent cardiac surgery or catheterization, chest trauma, pericardial effusion, or anticoagulant therapy.	Patient has a history of MI or chronic heart or lung disease.
Check for flat jugular veins, low urine output, and narrowed pulse pressure.	Check for distended jugular veins, ventricular gallop (S_3), crackles, and narrowed pulse pressure.	Check for distended jugular veins, pulsus paradoxus, and muffled heart sounds.	Check for irregular heart rate, severe tachycardia, and bradycardia.
If your examination reveals these findings, suspect *hypovolemic shock.*	If your examination reveals these findings, suspect *cardiogenic shock.*	If your examination reveals these findings, suspect *cardiac tamponade.*	If your examination reveals these findings, suspect *arrhythmia.*

Administer oxygen by nasal cannula, and insert an I.V. catheter for fluid infusion. Begin cardiac monitoring, and check the patient's vital signs every 5 to 15 minutes. A central venous pressure (CVP) line, an arterial line, or a pulmonary artery catheter (PAC) may have to be inserted. Be prepared for emergency resuscitation, if necessary.

Anticipate colloid or crystalloid replacement, as well as the need for transfusion.	Anticipate administering nitroprusside, dopamine, and dobutamine.	Anticipate pericardiocentesis.	Anticipate administering antiarrhythmics or delivering cardioversion therapy, or both.

Examine affected extremity for cool, mottled skin and pain.

If your examination reveals these findings suspect *arterial occlusive disease.*

Prepare the patient for diagnostic tests to confirm or rule out arterial occlusion, such as arteriography, aortography, or Doppler ultrasonography. Don't elevate the affected extremity. Insert an I.V. catheter in an unaffected arm or leg, and administer heparin or a thrombotic, as required. Anticipate preparing the patient for emergency embolectomy or peripheral angioplasty.

Patient has a history of trauma, congenital heart disease, or hypertension and reports severe, tearing chest pain.

Check for pulse quality and blood pressure variation between extremities.

If your examination reveals these findings, suspect *dissecting aortic aneurysm* or *aortic coarctation.*

Patient has a history of severe infection — frequent gram-negative, urinary, or respiratory infection.

Check for fever, chills, and widened pulse pressure.

If your examination reveals these findings, suspect *septic shock.*

Patient has a history of an insect sting, drug ingestion, or exposure to another possible allergen.

Check for urticaria, wheezing or stridor, and dyspnea.

If your examination reveals these findings, suspect *anaphylactic shock.*

Patient has history of venous stasis or deep vein thrombosis and reports sharp, substernal chest pain.

Check for dyspnea, crackles, pleural friction rub, and hemoptysis.

If your examination reveals these findings, suspect *pulmonary embolism.*

Administer oxygen by nasal cannula, and insert an I.V. catheter for fluid infusion. Begin cardiac monitoring, and check the patient's vital signs every 5 to 15 minutes. A CVP line, an arterial line, or a PAC may have to be inserted. Be prepared for emergency resuscitation, if necessary.

Anticipate preparing the patient for surgery and administering an antihypertensive or nitroprusside.

Anticipate administering antibiotics and vasopressors.

Anticipate emergency endotracheal (ET) intubation or cricothyrotomy and administration of epinephrine.

Anticipate possible ET intubation and anticoagulant or thrombolytic therapy.

fever and, possibly, nausea, vomiting, and diarrhea. Typically, the patient experiences tachycardia, tachypnea, and flushed, warm, and dry skin. As shock progresses, he develops thirst, hypotension, anxiety, restlessness, and confusion. Then pulse pressure narrows and the skin becomes cold, clammy, and cyanotic. The patient experiences severe hypotension, oliguria or anuria, respiratory failure, and coma.

Thoracic outlet syndrome. A patient with thoracic outlet syndrome may develop gradual or abrupt weakness or loss of the pulses in the arms, depending on how quickly vessels in the neck compress. These pulse changes commonly occur after the patient works with his hands above his shoulders, lifts a weight, or abducts his arm. Paresthesia and pain occur along the ulnar distribution of the arm and disappear as soon as the patient returns his arm to a neutral position. The patient may also have asymmetrical blood pressure and cool, pale skin.

Other causes
Treatments. Localized absent pulse may occur distal to arteriovenous shunts for dialysis or following orthopedic injury or repair.

Nursing considerations
- Monitor the patient's vital signs to detect untoward changes in his condition.
- Monitor weight, intake and output, and central venous pressure.
- Monitor pulses and limb appearances.

Patient teaching
- Explain the signs and symptoms that require medical attention.
- Discuss activities to avoid that reduce circulation.
- Explain the underlying disorder and treatment plan.

Pulse, bounding

Produced by large waves of pressure as blood ejects from the left ventricle with each contraction, a bounding pulse is strong and easily palpable and may be visible over superficial peripheral arteries. It's characterized by regular, recurrent expansion and contraction of the arterial walls and isn't obliterated by the pressure of palpation. A healthy person develops a bounding pulse during exercise, pregnancy, and periods of anxiety. However, this sign also results from fever and certain endocrine, hematologic, and cardiovascular disorders that increase the basal metabolic rate.

History and physical examination
After you detect a bounding pulse, check the patient's vital signs and temperature, and then auscultate the heart and lungs for abnormal sounds, rates, or rhythms. Ask the patient if he has noticed weakness, fatigue, shortness of breath, or other health changes. Review his medical history for hyperthyroidism, anemia, or a cardiovascular disorder, and ask about his use of alcohol.

Medical causes
Alcoholism (acute). Vasodilation produces a rapid, bounding pulse and flushed face. An odor of alcohol on the breath and an ataxic gait are common. Other findings include hypothermia, bradypnea, labored and loud respirations, nausea, vomiting, diuresis, a decreased level of consciousness, and seizures.

Aortic insufficiency. Sometimes called a *water-hammer pulse,* the bounding pulse associated with aortic insufficiency is characterized by rapid, forceful expansion of the arterial pulse followed by rapid contraction. Widened pulse pressure also occurs. This disorder may produce findings associated with left-sided heart failure and cardiovascular collapse, such as weakness, severe dyspnea, hypotension, an S_3, and tachycardia. Additional findings include pallor, chest pain, palpitations, or strong, abrupt carotid pulsations. The patient may also experience pulsus bisferiens, an early systolic murmur, a murmur heard over the femoral artery during systole and diastole, and a high-pitched diastolic murmur that starts with the second heart sound. An apical diastolic rumble (Austin Flint murmur) may also occur, especially with heart failure. Most patients with chronic aortic insufficiency remain asymptomatic until their 40s or 50s, when exertional dyspnea, increased fatigue, orthopnea and, eventually, paroxysmal nocturnal dyspnea, angina, and syncope may develop.

Febrile disorder. Fever can cause a bounding pulse and tachycardia. Accompanying findings reflect the specific disorder causing the fever.

Thyrotoxicosis. Thyrotoxicosis produces a rapid, full, bounding pulse. Associated findings include tachycardia, palpitations, an S_3 or S_4 gallop, weight loss despite increased appetite, and heat intolerance. The patient may also develop diarrhea, an enlarged thyroid, dyspnea, tremors, nervousness, chest pain, exophthalmos, and signs of cardiovascular collapse. His skin will be warm, moist, and diaphoretic, and he may be hypersensitive to heat.

Nursing considerations

- Prepare the patient for diagnostic laboratory and radiographic studies.
- If a bounding pulse is accompanied by a rapid or irregular heartbeat, you may need to place the patient on a cardiac monitor for further evaluation.
- Provide for rest periods.
- Administer iron supplements, if indicated.

Patient teaching

- Explain signs and symptoms that require medical attention.
- Explain the underlying disorder and treatment plan.

Pulse pressure, narrowed

Pulse pressure, the difference between systolic and diastolic blood pressures, is measured by sphygmomanometry or intra-arterial monitoring. Normally, systolic pressure exceeds diastolic by about 40 mm Hg. Narrowed pressure—a difference of less than 30 mm Hg—occurs when peripheral vascular resistance increases, cardiac output declines, or intravascular volume markedly decreases.

With conditions that cause mechanical obstruction, such as aortic stenosis, pulse pressure is directly related to the severity of the underlying condition. Usually a late sign, narrowed pulse pressure alone doesn't signal an emergency, even though it commonly occurs with shock and other life-threatening disorders.

History and physical examination

After you detect a narrowed pulse pressure, check for other signs of heart failure, such as hypotension, tachycardia, dyspnea, jugular vein distention, pulmonary crackles, and decreased urine output. Also check for changes in skin temperature or color, the strength of peripheral pulses, and the patient's level of consciousness (LOC). Auscultate the heart for murmurs. Ask about a history of chest pain, dizziness, or syncope. Obtain a complete drug history.

Medical causes

Cardiac tamponade. In cardiac tamponade, a life-threatening disorder, pulse pressure narrows by 10 to 20 mm Hg.

Paradoxical pulse, jugular vein distention, hypotension, and muffled heart sounds are classic. The patient may be anxious, restless, and cyanotic, with clammy skin and chest pain. He may exhibit dyspnea, tachypnea, decreased LOC, and a weak, rapid pulse. A pericardial friction rub and hepatomegaly may also occur.

Heart failure. Narrowed pulse pressure occurs relatively late with heart failure and may accompany tachypnea, palpitations, dependent edema, steady weight gain despite nausea and anorexia, chest tightness, slowed mental response, hypotension, diaphoresis, pallor, and oliguria. Assessment reveals a ventricular gallop, inspiratory crackles and, possibly, a tender, palpable liver. Later, dullness develops over the lung bases, and hemoptysis, cyanosis, marked hepatomegaly, and marked pitting edema may occur.

Shock. With *anaphylactic shock,* narrowed pulse pressure occurs late, preceded by a rapid, weak pulse that soon becomes uniformly absent. Within seconds or minutes after exposure to an allergen, the patient experiences hypotension, anxiety, restlessness, and feelings of doom, along with intense itching, a pounding headache and, possibly, urticaria. Other findings include dyspnea, stridor, and hoarseness; chest or throat tightness; skin flushing; nausea, abdominal cramps, and urinary incontinence; and seizures.

With *cardiogenic shock,* narrowed pulse pressure occurs relatively late. Typically, peripheral pulses are absent and central pulses are weak. A drop in systolic pressure to 30 mm Hg below baseline, or a sustained reading below 80 mm Hg not attributable to medication, produces poor tissue perfusion. Poor perfusion produces tachycardia; tachypnea; cold, pale, clammy skin;

cyanosis; oliguria; restlessness; confusion; and obtundation.

With *hypovolemic shock,* narrowed pulse pressure occurs as a late sign. All peripheral pulses become first weak and then uniformly absent. Deepening shock leads to hypotension, urine output of less than 25 ml/hour, confusion, decreased LOC and, possibly, hypothermia.

With *septic shock,* narrowed pulse pressure is a relatively late sign. All peripheral pulses become first weak and then uniformly absent. As shock progresses, the patient exhibits oliguria, thirst, anxiety, restlessness, confusion, and hypotension. Extremities become cool and cyanotic; the skin becomes cold and clammy. In time, he develops severe hypotension, persistent oliguria or anuria, respiratory failure, and coma.

Nursing considerations

- Monitor the patient closely for changes in the pulse rate or quality and for hypotension or diminished LOC.
- Prepare the patient for diagnostic studies, such as echocardiography, to detect valvular heart disease or cardiac tamponade secondary to a pericardial effusion.

Patient teaching

- Explain the underlying disorder and its treatments.
- Discuss any food and fluid restrictions.
- Stress the importance of rest periods to reduce fatigue.

Pulse pressure, widened

Pulse pressure is the difference between systolic and diastolic blood pressures. Normally, systolic pressure is about 40 mm Hg higher than diastolic pressure. Widened pulse pressure—a difference of more than 50 mm Hg—commonly occurs as a physiologic response to a fever, hot weather, exercise, anxiety, anemia, or pregnancy. However, it can also result from certain neurologic disorders—especially life-threatening increased intracranial pressure (ICP)—or from cardiovascular disorders that cause blood backflow into the heart with each contraction such as aortic insufficiency. Widened pulse pressure can easily be identified by monitoring arterial blood pressure and is commonly detected during routine sphygmomanometric recordings.

Action stat!

If the patient's level of consciousness (LOC) is decreased, and you suspect that his widened pulse pressure results from increased ICP, check his vital signs. Maintain a patent airway, and prepare to hyperventilate the patient with a handheld resuscitation bag to help reduce partial pressure of carbon dioxide levels and, thus, ICP. Perform a thorough neurologic examination to serve as a baseline for assessing subsequent changes. Use the Glasgow Coma Scale to evaluate the patient's LOC. (See *Glasgow Coma Scale*, page 363.) Also, check cranial nerve function—especially in cranial nerves III, IV, and VI—and assess pupillary reactions, reflexes, and muscle tone. Insertion of an ICP monitor may be necessary. If you don't suspect increased ICP, ask about associated symptoms, such as chest pain, shortness of breath, weakness, fatigue, or syncope. Check for edema, and auscultate for murmurs.

Medical causes

Aortic insufficiency. With acute aortic insufficiency, pulse pressure widens progressively as the valve deteriorates, and a bounding pulse and an atrial or a ventricular gallop develop. These signs may be accompanied by chest pain; palpitations; pallor; strong, abrupt carotid pulsations; pulsus bisferiens; and signs of heart failure, such as crackles, dyspnea, and jugular vein distention. Auscultation may reveal several murmurs, such as an early diastolic murmur (common) and an apical diastolic rumble (Austin Flint murmur).

Arteriosclerosis. With arteriosclerosis, reduced arterial compliance causes progressive widening of pulse pressure, which becomes permanent without treatment of the underlying disorder. This sign is preceded by moderate hypertension and accompanied by signs of vascular insufficiency, such as claudication and angina.

Febrile disorder. Fever can cause widened pulse pressure. Accompanying symptoms vary depending on the specific disorder causing the fever.

Increased ICP. Widening pulse pressure is an intermediate to late sign of increased ICP. Although decreased LOC is the earliest and most sensitive indicator of this life-threatening condition, the onset and progression of widening pulse pressure also parallel rising ICP. (A gap of 50 mm Hg can signal a rapid deterioration in the patient's condition.) Assessment reveals Cushing's triad: bradycardia, hypertension, and respiratory pattern changes. Other findings include headache, vomiting, and impaired or unequal motor movement. The patient may also exhibit vision disturbances, such as blurring or photophobia, and pupillary changes.

Nursing considerations
- If the patient displays increased ICP, continually evaluate his neurologic status.
- Be alert for restlessness, confusion, unresponsiveness, or decreased LOC.
- Watch for subtle changes in the patient's condition.

Patient teaching

- Explain diagnostic tests, such as blood studies, computed tomography scan, and magnetic resonance imaging.
- Explain the underlying disorder and treatment plan.

Pulse rhythm abnormality

An abnormal pulse rhythm is an irregular expansion and contraction of the peripheral arterial walls. It may be persistent or sporadic and rhythmic or arrhythmic. Detected by palpating the radial or carotid pulse, an abnormal rhythm is typically reported first by the patient, who complains of palpitations. This important finding reflects an underlying cardiac arrhythmia, which may range from benign to life-threatening. Arrhythmias are commonly associated with cardiovascular, renal, respiratory, metabolic, and neurologic disorders as well as the effects of drugs, diagnostic tests, and treatments. (See *Abnormal pulse rhythm: A clue to cardiac arrhythmias*, pages 506 to 509.)

ACTION STAT!

 If you detect an abnormal pulse rhythm, quickly look for signs of reduced cardiac output, such as decreased level of consciousness (LOC), hypotension, or dizziness. Promptly obtain an electrocardiogram (ECG) and possibly a chest X-ray, and begin cardiac monitoring. Insert an I.V. catheter for administration of emergency cardiac drugs and fluids, and give oxygen by nasal cannula or mask. Closely monitor the patient's vital signs, pulse quality, and cardiac rhythm because accompanying bradycardia or tachycardia may result in deterioration of cardiac output. Keep emergency intubation, cardioversion, defibrillation, and suction equipment handy.

History and physical examination

If the patient's condition permits, ask if he's experiencing pain. If so, find out about its onset and location. Does the pain radiate? Ask about a history of heart disease and treatment for arrhythmias. Obtain a drug history and check the patient's compliance. Also, ask about caffeine or alcohol intake. Digoxin toxicity, cessation of an antiarrhythmic, and the use of quinidine, a sympathomimetic (such as epinephrine), caffeine, or alcohol may cause arrhythmias.

Next, check the patient's apical and peripheral arterial pulses. An apical rate exceeding a peripheral arterial rate indicates a pulse deficit, which may also cause associated signs and symptoms of low cardiac output. Evaluate heart sounds: A long pause between S_1 (*lub*) and S_2 (*dub*) may indicate a conduction defect. A faint or absent S_1 and an easily audible S_2 may indicate atrial fibrillation or flutter. You may hear the two heart sounds close together on certain beats—possibly indicating premature atrial contractions—or other variations in heart rate or rhythm. Take the patient's apical and radial pulses while you listen for heart sounds. With some arrhythmias, such as premature ventricular contractions, you may hear the beat with your stethoscope but not feel it over the radial artery. This indicates an ineffective contraction that failed to produce a peripheral pulse. Next, count the apical pulse for 60 seconds, noting the frequency of skipped peripheral beats. Place the patient on a cardiac monitor and obtain an ECG to evaluate the cardiac rhythm. Report your findings to the practitioner.

Medical causes

Arrhythmias. An abnormal pulse rhythm may be the only sign of a cardiac arrhythmia. The patient may complain of palpitations, a fluttering heartbeat, or weak and skipped beats. Pulses may be weak and rapid or slow. Depending on the specific arrhythmia, dull chest pain or discomfort and hypotension may occur. Associated findings, if any, reflect decreased cardiac output. Neurologic findings, for example, include confusion, dizziness, light-headedness, decreased LOC and, sometimes, seizures. Other findings include decreased urine output, dyspnea, tachypnea, pallor, and diaphoresis.

Nursing considerations

- Monitor cardiac rhythm and obtain a 12-lead ECG.
- Prepare the patient for cardioversion, if indicated .
- Check vital signs frequently to detect hypertension or hypotension, tachypnea, and dyspnea. Also, monitor intake, output, daily weight, and pulse oximetry.
- Collect blood samples for serum electrolyte, cardiac markers, complete blood count, and drug level studies. Prepare the patient for a chest X-ray.
- Obtain a previous ECG with which to compare current findings.

Patient teaching

- Explain the importance of keeping a diary of activities and any symptoms that develop to correlate with the incidence of arrhythmias.
- Instruct the patient to avoid tobacco and caffeine.
- Teach the patient how to take his pulse.
- Reinforce signs and symptoms that require prompt medical attention.
- Explain the underlying disorder and treatment plan.

- Teach the patient about prescribed medications, including dosage, administration, and possible adverse effects.

Pulsus alternans

A sign of severe left-sided heart failure, pulsus alternans (alternating pulse) is a beat-to-beat change in the size and intensity of a peripheral pulse. Although pulse rhythm remains regular, strong and weak contractions alternate. (See *Comparing arterial pressure waves,* page 510.) An alteration in the intensity of heart sounds and of existing heart murmurs may accompany this sign.

Pulsus alternans is thought to result from the change in stroke volume that occurs with beat-to-beat alteration in the left ventricle's contractility. Recumbency or exercise increases venous return and reduces the abnormal pulse, which typically disappears with treatment for heart failure. Rarely, a patient with normal left ventricular function has pulsus alternans, but the abnormal pulse seldom persists for more than 10 to 12 beats.

Although most easily detected by sphygmomanometry, pulsus alternans can be detected by palpating the brachial, radial, or femoral artery when systolic pressure varies from beat to beat by more than 20 mm Hg. Because the small changes in arterial pressure that occur during normal respirations may obscure this abnormal pulse, you'll need to have the patient hold his breath during palpation. Apply *light* pressure to avoid obliterating the weaker pulse.

When using a sphygmomanometer to detect pulsus alternans, inflate the cuff 10 to 20 mm Hg above the systolic pressure as determined by palpation, and then slowly deflate it. At first, you'll hear only the strong beats. With further deflation, all beats will become audible

(Text continues on page 511.)

Abnormal pulse rhythm: A clue to cardiac arrhythmias

An abnormal pulse rhythm may be your only clue that the patient has a cardiac arrhythmia, but this sign doesn't help you pinpoint the specific type of arrhythmia. For that, you need a cardiac monitor or an electrocardiogram (ECG) machine. These devices record the electrical current generated by the heart's conduction system and display this information on an oscilloscope screen or a strip-chart recorder. Besides rhythm disturbances, they can identify conduction defects and electrolyte imbalances.

The ECG strips below show some common cardiac arrhythmias that can cause abnormal pulse rhythms.

Arrhythmia

Sinus arrhythmia

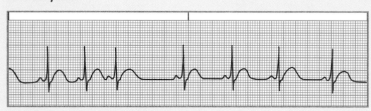

Premature atrial contractions (PACs)

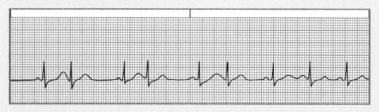

Paroxysmal atrial tachycardia

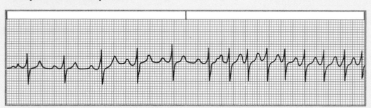

Pulse rhythm and rate	Clinical implications
Irregular rhythm; fast, slow, or normal rate	■ Reflex vagal tone inhibition (heart rate increases with inspiration and decreases with expiration) related to normal respiratory cycle ■ May result from drugs, as in digoxin toxicity ■ Occurs most commonly in children and young adults
Irregular rhythm during PACs; fast, slow, or normal rate	■ Occasional PAC may be normal ■ Isolated PACs indicate atrial irritation — for example, from anxiety or excessive caffeine intake. Increasing PACs may herald other atrial arrhythmias. ■ May result from heart failure, chronic obstructive pulmonary disease (COPD), or use of a cardiac glycoside, aminophylline, or medications that prolong the absolute refractory period of the sinoatrial node
Regular rhythm with abrupt onset and termination of arrhythmia; heart rate exceeding 160 beats/minute	■ May occur in otherwise healthy persons who are suffering from physical or psychological stress, hypoxia, or digoxin toxicity; who use marijuana; or who consume excessive amounts of caffeine or other stimulants ■ May precipitate angina or heart failure

(continued)

Abnormal pulse rhythm: A clue to cardiac arrhythmias *(continued)*

Atrial fibrillation

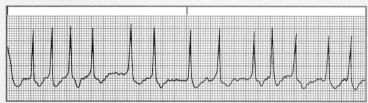

Premature junctional contractions (PJCs)

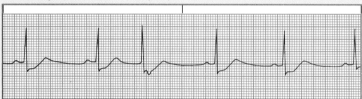

Second-degree atrioventricular (AV) heart block, Mobitz Type I (Wenckebach)

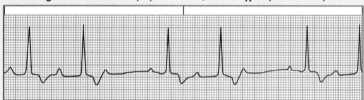

Second-degree AV heart block, Mobitz Type II

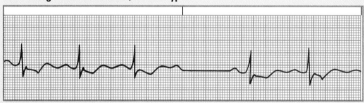

Premature ventricular contractions (multifocal)

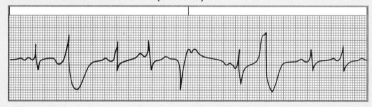

Pulse rhythm and rate	Clinical implications
Irregular rhythm; atrial rate may exceed 400 beats/minute; ventricular rate varies	■ May result from heart failure, COPD, hypertension, sepsis, pulmonary embolus, mitral valve disease, digoxin toxicity (rarely), atrial irritation, postcoronary bypass, or valve replacement surgery ■ Because atria don't contract, preload isn't consistent, so cardiac output changes with each beat. Emboli may also result.
Irregular rhythm during PJCs; fast, slow, or normal rate	■ May result from myocardial infarction (MI) or ischemia, excessive caffeine intake, and most commonly digoxin toxicity (from enhanced automaticity)
Irregular ventricular rhythm; fast, slow, or normal rate	■ Usually transient; may progress to complete heart block ■ May result from inferior wall MI, digoxin or quinidine toxicity, vagal stimulation, electrolyte imbalance, or arteriosclerotic heart disease
Irregular ventricular rhythm; slow or normal rate	■ May progress to complete heart block ■ May result from degenerative disease of conduction system, ischemia of AV node in an anterior MI, anteroseptal infarction, electrolyte imbalance, or digoxin or quinidine toxicity
Usually irregular rhythm with a long pause after the premature beat; fast, slow, or normal rate	■ Arise from different ventricular sites or from the same site with changing patterns of conduction ■ May result from caffeine or stress, alcohol ingestion, myocardial ischemia or infarction, myocardial irritation by pacemaker electrodes, hypocalcemia, hypercalcemia, digoxin toxicity, or exercise

Comparing arterial pressure waves

The waveforms shown here help differentiate a normal arterial pulse from pulsus alternans and pulsus paradoxus.

Normal arterial pulse

The percussion wave in a *normal arterial pulse* reflects ejection of blood into the aorta (early systole). The tidal wave is the peak of the pulse wave (later systole), and the dicrotic notch marks the beginning of diastole.

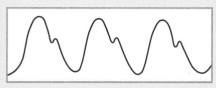

Pulsus alternans

Pulsus alternans is a beat-to-beat alteration in pulse size and intensity. Although the rhythm of pulsus alternans is regular, the volume varies. If you take the blood pressure of a patient with this abnormality, you'll first hear a loud Korotkoff sound and then a soft sound, continually alternating. Pulsus alternans commonly accompanies states of poor contractility that occur with left-sided heart failure.

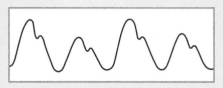

Pulsus bisferiens

Pulsus bisferiens is a double-beating pulse with two systolic peaks. The first beat reflects pulse pressure and the second reverberation from the periphery. Pulsus bisferiens commonly occurs with aortic insufficiency (aortic stenosis, aortic regurgitation), hypertrophic cardiomyopathy, or high cardiac output states.

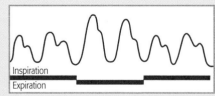

Pulsus paradoxus

Pulsus paradoxus is an exaggerated decline in blood pressure during inspiration, resulting from an increase in negative intrathoracic pressure. Pulsus paradoxus that exceeds 10 mm Hg is considered abnormal and may result from cardiac tamponade, constrictive pericarditis, or severe lung disease.

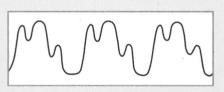

Inspiration
Expiration

and palpable, and then equally intense. (The difference between this point and the peak systolic level is commonly used to determine the degree of pulsus alternans.) When the cuff is removed, pulsus alternans returns.

Occasionally, the weak beat is so small that no palpable pulse is detected at the periphery. This produces total pulsus alternans, an apparent halving of the pulse rate.

ACTION STAT!

 Pulsus alternans indicates a critical change in the patient's status. When you detect it, be sure to quickly check his other vital signs. Closely evaluate the patient's heart rate, respiratory pattern, and blood pressure. Also, auscultate for a ventricular gallop and increased crackles.

Medical causes

Left-sided heart failure. With left-sided heart failure, pulsus alternans is commonly initiated by a premature beat and is almost always associated with a ventricular gallop. Other findings include hypotension and cyanosis. Possible respiratory findings include exertional and paroxysmal nocturnal dyspnea, orthopnea, tachypnea, Cheyne-Stokes respirations, hemoptysis, and crackles. Fatigue and weakness are common.

Nursing considerations

■ If left-sided heart failure develops suddenly, prepare the patient for pulmonary artery catheter insertion and transfer to an intensive or cardiac care unit.
■ Elevate the head of his bed to promote respiratory excursion and increase oxygenation.
■ Administer oxygen and diuretics, as ordered.

Patient teaching

■ Explain the underlying disorder and its treatments.
■ Discuss lifestyle changes that the patient needs to adopt.
■ Teach about prescribed medications, including dosage, administration, and possible adverse effects.

Pulsus bisferiens

A biferious pulse is a hyperdynamic, double-beating pulse characterized by two systolic peaks separated by a midsystolic dip. Both peaks may be equal or either may be larger; usually, however, the first peak is taller or more forceful than the second. The first peak (percussion wave) is believed to be the pulse pressure; the second (tidal wave), reverberation from the periphery. Pulsus bisferiens occurs in conditions in which a large blood volume is rapidly ejected from the left ventricle, as in aortic insufficiency. The pulse can be palpated in peripheral arteries or observed on an arterial pressure wave recording.

To detect pulsus bisferiens, *lightly* palpate the carotid, brachial, radial, or femoral artery. (The pulse is easiest to palpate in the carotid artery.) At the same time, listen to the patient's heart sounds to determine if the two palpable peaks occur during systole. If they do, you'll feel the double pulse between S_1 and S_2. (See *Comparing arterial pressure waves,* page 510.)

History and physical examination

After you detect a biferious pulse, review the patient's history for cardiac disorders. Next, find out what medication he's taking, if any, and ask if he has other illnesses. Also, ask about the development of associated signs and symptoms, such as dyspnea, chest pain, or fatigue. Find out how long he has had these

Managing the patient with hypertrophic cardiomyopathy

A primary disease of the cardiac muscle, hypertrophic cardiomyopathy is characterized by disproportionate, asymmetric thickening of the interventricular septum in relation to the free wall of the ventricle. With hypertrophic cardiomyopathy, cardiac output may be low, normal, or high, depending on whether stenosis is obstructive or nonobstructive.

The natural history of hypertrophic cardiomyopathy varies. Some patients may remain asymptomatic for years. The dyspnea that results is primarily due to markedly impaired diastolic compliance rather than systolic dysfunction. Sudden death, especially during exercise, may be the initial event, as has occurred with certain athletes.

Do's

■ Administer anticoagulants to the patient with atrial fibrillation and prepare him for cardioversion, as appropriate.
■ Administer medications, such as beta-adrenergic blockers, as ordered.
■ Prepare the patient for surgery, such as ventricular myotomy, valve replacement, or heart transplant, if medications fail to control symptoms.
■ Prepare the patient for a permanent pacemaker or implantable defibrillator, if indicated.
■ Space activities and provide for rest periods.
■ Teach the patient about the need for prophylactic antibiotics before dental work.

Don'ts

■ Don't administer angiotensin-converting enzyme inhibitors, nitroglycerin, digoxin, and diuretics because they can worsen the obstruction.
■ Caution the patient to avoid strenuous physical activity.
■ Caution the patient to avoid Valsalva's maneuver or sudden position changes.

symptoms and if they change with activity or rest. Then take his vital signs and auscultate for abnormal heart or breath sounds.

Medical causes

Aortic insufficiency. Aortic insufficiency may cause exertional dyspnea, worsening fatigue, orthopnea and, eventually, andparoxysmal nocturnal dyspnea.

Acute aortic insufficiency may produce signs and symptoms of left-sided heart failure and cardiovascular collapse, such as weakness, severe dyspnea, hypotension, a ventricular gallop, and tachycardia. Additional findings include chest pain, palpitations, pallor, and strong, abrupt carotid pulsations. The patient may also exhibit widened pulse pressure and one or more murmurs, especially an apical diastolic rumble (Austin Flint murmur).

High cardiac output states. Pulsus bisferiens commonly occurs with high output states, such as anemia, thyrotoxicosis, fever, and exercise. Associated findings vary with the underlying cause and may include moderate tachycardia, a cervical venous hum, and widened pulse pressure.

Hypertrophic obstructive cardiomyopathy. About 40% of patients with hypertrophic obstructive cardiomyopathy have pulsus bisferiens because of a pressure gradient in the left ventricular outflow tract. Recorded more often than it's palpated, the pulse rises rapidly, and the first wave is the more forceful one. Associated findings include a systolic murmur, dyspnea, angina, fatigue, and syncope.

Nursing considerations

- Prepare the patient for diagnostic tests, such as an electrocardiogram, chest X-ray, cardiac catheterization, or angiography. (See *Managing the patient with hypertrophic cardiomyopathy.*)
- Schedule regular rest periods.
- Monitor intake and output and daily weight.

Patient teaching

- Explain the underlying disorder and its treatments.
- Discuss signs and symptoms that require prompt medical attention.

Pulsus paradoxus

Pulsus paradoxus, or paradoxical pulse, is an exaggerated decline in blood pressure during inspiration. Normally, systolic pressure falls less than 10 mm Hg during inspiration. In pulsus paradoxus, it falls more than 10 mm Hg. (See *Comparing arterial pressure waves,* page 510.) When systolic pressure falls more than 20 mm Hg, the peripheral pulses may be barely palpable or may disappear during inspiration.

Pulsus paradoxus is thought to result from an exaggerated inspirational increase in negative intrathoracic pressure. Normally, systolic pressure drops during inspiration because of blood pooling in the pulmonary system. This, in turn, reduces left ventricular filling and stroke volume and transmits negative intrathoracic pressure to the aorta. Conditions associated with large intrapleural pressure swings, such as asthma, or those that reduce left-sided heart filling, such as pericardial tamponade, produce pulsus paradoxus.

To accurately detect and measure pulsus paradoxus, use a sphygmomanometer or an intra-arterial monitoring device. Inflate the blood pressure cuff 10 to 20 mm Hg beyond the peak systolic pressure. Then deflate the cuff at a rate of 2 mm Hg/second until you hear the first Korotkoff sound during expiration. Note the systolic pressure. As you continue to slowly deflate the cuff, observe the patient's respiratory pattern. If pulsus paradoxus is present, the Korotkoff sounds will disappear with inspiration and return with expiration. Continue to deflate the cuff until you hear Korotkoff sounds during inspiration and expiration and, again, note the systolic pressure. Subtract this reading from the first one to determine the degree of pulsus paradoxus. A difference of more than 10 mm Hg is abnormal.

You can also detect pulsus paradoxus by palpating the radial pulse over several cycles of slow inspiration and expiration. Marked pulse diminution during inspiration indicates pulsus paradoxus. When you check for pulsus paradoxus, remember that irregular heart rhythms and tachycardia cause variations in pulse amplitude and must be ruled out before true pulsus paradoxus can be identified.

ACTION STAT!

 Pulsus paradoxus may signal cardiac tamponade—a life-threatening complication of pericardial effusion that occurs when sufficient blood or fluid accumulates to compress the heart. When you detect pulsus paradoxus, quickly take the patient's vital signs. Check for additional signs and symptoms of cardiac tamponade, such as dyspnea, tachypnea, diaphoresis, jugular vein distention, tachycardia, narrowed pulse pressure, and hypotension. Emergency pericardiocentesis to aspirate blood or fluid from the pericardial sac may be necessary. Evaluate the effectiveness of pericardiocentesis by measuring the degree of pulsus paradoxus; it should decrease after aspiration.

History and physical examination

If the patient doesn't have signs of cardiac tamponade, find out if he has a history of chronic cardiac or pulmonary disease. Ask about the development of associated signs and symptoms, such as a cough or chest pain. Then auscultate for abnormal breath sounds.

Medical causes

Cardiac tamponade. Pulsus paradoxus commonly occurs with cardiac tamponade, but it may be difficult to detect if intrapericardial pressure rises abruptly and profound hypotension occurs. With severe tamponade, assessment also reveals these classic findings: hypotension, diminished or muffled heart sounds, and jugular vein distention. Related findings include chest pain, a pericardial friction rub, narrowed pulse pressure, anxiety, restlessness, clammy skin, and hepatomegaly. Characteristic respiratory signs and symptoms include dyspnea, tachypnea, and cyanosis; the patient typically sits up and leans forward to facilitate breathing.

If cardiac tamponade develops gradually, pulsus paradoxus may be accompanied by weakness, anorexia, and weight loss. The patient may also report chest pain, but he won't have muffled heart sounds or severe hypotension.

Chronic obstructive pulmonary disease (COPD). The wide fluctuations in intrathoracic pressure that characterize COPD produce pulsus paradoxus and possibly tachycardia. Other findings vary, but may include dyspnea, tachypnea, wheezing, a productive or nonproductive cough, accessory muscle use, barrel chest, and clubbing. The patient may show labored, pursed-lip breathing after exertion or even at rest. He typically sits up and leans forward to facilitate breathing. Auscultation reveals decreased breath sounds, rhonchi, and crackles. Weight loss, cyanosis, and edema may occur.

Pericarditis (chronic constrictive). Pulsus paradoxus can occur in up to 50% of patients with pericarditis. Other findings include a pericardial friction rub, chest pain, exertional dyspnea, orthopnea, hepatomegaly, and ascites. Patients also exhibit peripheral edema and Kussmaul's sign—jugular vein distention that becomes more prominent on inspiration.

Pulmonary embolism (massive). Decreased left ventricular filling and stroke volume with massive pulmonary embolism produce pulsus paradoxus as well as syncope and severe apprehension, dyspnea, tachypnea, and pleuritic chest pain. The patient appears cyanotic, with jugular vein distention. He may succumb to circulatory collapse, with hypotension and a weak, rapid pulse. Pulmonary infarction may produce hemoptysis along with decreased breath sounds and a pleural friction rub over the affected area.

Nursing considerations
- Prepare the patient for an echocardiogram to visualize cardiac motion and to help determine the causative disorder.
- Monitor vital signs and frequently check the degree of paradox because an increase in the degree of paradox may

indicate recurring or worsening cardiac tamponade or impending respiratory arrest in severe COPD.
- Provide respiratory treatments, such as chest physiotherapy, to avert the need for endotracheal intubation.

Patient teaching
- Teach the patient about the underlying disorder and its treatments.
- Explain self-care techniques to the patient with COPD, such as pursed-lip, diaphragmatic breathing; coughing and deep-breathing exercises; and proper use of home oxygen equipment.

Pupils, nonreactive

Nonreactive (fixed) pupils fail to constrict in response to light or to dilate when the light is removed. The development of a unilateral or bilateral nonreactive response indicates an important change in the patient's condition and may signal a life-threatening emergency and possibly brain death. It also occurs with the use of certain optic drugs.

To evaluate pupillary reaction to light, first test the patient's direct light reflex. Darken the room, and cover one of the patient's eyes while you hold open the opposite eyelid. Using a bright penlight, bring the light toward the patient from the side and shine it directly into his opened eye. If normal, the pupil will promptly constrict. Next, test the consensual light reflex. Hold the patient's eyelids open and shine the light into one eye while watching the pupil of the opposite eye. If normal, both pupils will promptly constrict. Repeat both procedures in the opposite eye. A unilateral or bilateral nonreactive response indicates dysfunction of cranial nerves (CNs) II and III, which mediate the pupillary light reflex. (See *Innervation of direct and consensual light reflexes*, page 516.)

ACTION STAT!

If the patient is unconscious and develops unilateral or bilateral nonreactive pupils, quickly take his vital signs. Be alert for decerebrate or decorticate posture, bradycardia, elevated systolic blood pressure, widened pulse pressure, and the development of other changes in the patient's condition. A unilateral dilated, nonreactive pupil may be an early sign of uncal brain herniation. Emergency surgery to decrease intracranial pressure (ICP) may be necessary. If the patient isn't already being treated for increased ICP, insert an I.V. catheter to administer a diuretic, an osmotic, or a corticosteroid. You may also need to start the patient on controlled hyperventilation.

History and physical examination

If the patient is conscious, obtain a brief history. Ask him what type of eyedrops he's using, if any, and when they were last instilled. Also ask if he's experiencing pain and, if so, try to determine its location, intensity, and duration. Check the patient's visual acuity in both eyes. Then test the pupillary reaction to accommodation: Normally, both pupils constrict equally as the patient shifts his glance from a distant to a near object.

Next, hold a penlight at the side of each eye and examine the cornea and iris for abnormalities. Measure intraocular pressure (IOP) with a tonometer, or estimate IOP by placing your second and third fingers over the patient's closed eyelid. If the eyeball feels rock-hard, suspect elevated IOP. Ophthalmoscopic and slit-lamp examinations of the eye will need to be performed. If the patient has experienced ocular trauma, don't manipulate the affected eye. After the examination, be sure to cover the af-

Innervation of direct and consensual light reflexes

Two reactions—direct and consensual—constitute the pupillary light reflex. Normally, when a light is shined directly onto the retina of one eye, the parasympathetic nerves are stimulated to cause brisk constriction of that pupil—the *direct light reflex.* The pupil of the opposite eye also constricts—the *consensual light reflex.*

The optic nerve (cranial nerve [CN] II) mediates the afferent arc of this reflex from each eye, whereas the oculomotor nerve (CN III) mediates the efferent arc to both eyes. A nonreactive or sluggish response in one or both pupils indicates dysfunction of these cranial nerves, usually due to degenerative disease of the central nervous system.

The illustration shows the nerves involved in testing direct light and consensual light reflexes.

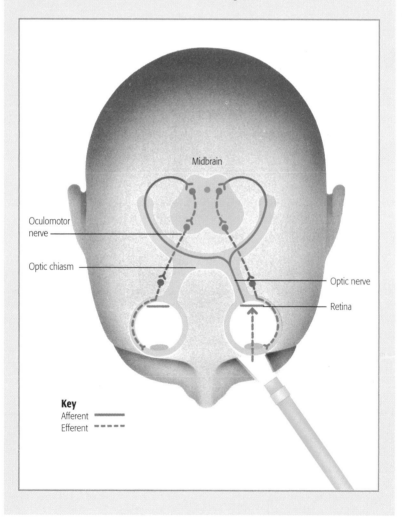

fected eye with a protective metal shield, but don't let the shield rest on the globe.

Medical causes

Botulism. Bilateral mydriasis and nonreactive pupils usually appear 12 to 36 hours after eating tainted food. Other early findings include blurred vision, diplopia, ptosis, strabismus, and extraocular muscle palsies, along with anorexia, nausea, vomiting, diarrhea, and dry mouth. Vertigo, deafness, hoarseness, a nasal voice, dysarthria, and dysphagia follow. Progressive muscle weakness and absent deep tendon reflexes usually evolve over 2 to 4 days, resulting in severe constipation and paralysis of respiratory muscles with respiratory distress.

Encephalitis. As encephalitis progresses, initially sluggish pupils become dilated and nonreactive. Decreased accommodation and other symptoms of cranial nerve palsies, such as dysphagia, develop. Within 48 hours after onset, encephalitis causes decreased level of consciousness, high fever, headache, vomiting, and nuchal rigidity. Aphasia, ataxia, nystagmus, hemiparesis, and photophobia may occur with seizures.

Glaucoma (acute angle-closure). With acute angle-closure glaucoma, an ophthalmic emergency, examination reveals a moderately dilated, nonreactive pupil in the affected eye. Conjunctival injection, corneal clouding, and decreased visual acuity also occur. The patient experiences a sudden onset of blurred vision, followed by excruciating pain in and around the affected eye. He commonly reports seeing halos around white lights at night. Severely elevated IOP commonly induces nausea and vomiting.

Oculomotor nerve palsy. Commonly, the first signs of oculomotor nerve palsy are a dilated, nonreactive pupil and loss of the accommodation reaction.

These findings may occur in one or both eyes, depending on whether the palsy is unilateral or bilateral. Among the causes of total CN III palsy is life-threatening brain herniation. Central herniation causes bilateral midposition nonreactive pupils, whereas uncal herniation initially causes a unilateral dilated, nonreactive pupil. Other common findings include diplopia, ptosis, outward deviation of the eye, and an inability to elevate or adduct the eye. Additional findings depend on the underlying cause of the palsy.

Uveitis. A small, nonreactive pupil that appears suddenly with severe eye pain, conjunctival injection, and photophobia typifies anterior uveitis. With posterior uveitis, similar features develop insidiously, along with blurred vision and a distorted pupil shape.

Other causes

Drugs. Instillation of a topical mydriatic and a cycloplegic may induce a temporarily nonreactive pupil in the affected eye. Opiates, such as heroin and morphine, cause pinpoint pupils with a minimal light response that can be seen only with a magnifying glass. Atropine poisoning produces widely dilated, nonreactive pupils.

Nursing considerations
- If the patient is conscious, monitor his pupillary light reflex to detect changes.
- If he's unconscious, close his eyes to prevent corneal exposure using tape to secure the eyelids, if needed.
- Monitor neurologic status.

Patient teaching
- Explain the underlying disorder and treatment plan.
- Teach proper methods for instilling eye drops.
- Explain methods of reducing photophobia.

■ Stress the importance of follow-up care to check IOP.

Pupils, sluggish

A sluggish pupillary reaction is an abnormally slow pupillary response to light. It can occur in one pupil or both, unlike the normal reaction, which is always bilateral. A sluggish reaction accompanies degenerative disease of the central nervous system and diabetic neuropathy. It can occur normally in elderly people, whose pupils become smaller and less responsive with age.

To assess pupillary reaction to light, first test the patient's direct light reflex. Darken the room, and cover one of the patient's eyes while you hold open the opposite eyelid. Using a bright penlight, bring the light toward the patient from the side and shine it directly into his opened eye. If normal, the pupil will promptly constrict. Next, test the consensual light reflex. Hold both of the patient's eyelids open, and shine the light into one eye while watching the pupil of the opposite eye. If normal, both pupils will promptly constrict. Repeat both procedures to test light reflexes in the opposite eye. A sluggish reaction in one or both pupils indicates dysfunction of cranial nerves II and III, which mediate the pupillary light reflex. (See *Innervation of direct and consensual light reflexes,* page 516.)

History and physical examination

If the patient is conscious, obtain a brief history. Ask about eyedrops or vision disturbances. Find out if the patient has had fever or complaints of headache or neck pain. Next, determine the patient's visual function. Start by testing visual acuity in both eyes. Then test the pupillary reaction to accommodation; the pupils should constrict equally as the patient shifts his glance from a distant to a near object.

Next, hold a penlight at the side of each eye and examine the cornea and iris for irregularities, scars, and foreign bodies. Measure intraocular pressure (IOP) with a tonometer, or estimate IOP by placing your fingers over the patient's closed eyelid. If the eyeball feels rockhard, suspect elevated IOP. Also, ophthalmoscopic and slit-lamp examinations of the eye will need to be performed. Check the patient's neurologic status. Note decreased LOC, headache, or nuchal rigidity.

Medical causes

Adie's syndrome. Adie's syndrome produces an abrupt onset of unilateral mydriasis and a sluggish pupillary response that may progress to a nonreactive response. The patient may complain of blurred vision and cramplike eye pain. Eventually, both eyes may be affected. Musculoskeletal assessment also reveals hypoactive or absent deep tendon reflexes in the arms and legs.

Encephalitis. Encephalitis initially produces a bilateral sluggish pupillary response. Later, pupils become dilated and nonreactive, and decreased accommodation may occur, along with other cranial nerve palsies, such as dysphagia and facial weakness. Within 24 to 48 hours after onset, encephalitis causes a decreased level of consciousness, headache, a high fever, vomiting, and nuchal rigidity. Also, aphasia, ataxia, nystagmus, hemiparesis, and photophobia may occur. The patient may exhibit seizure activity and myoclonic jerks.

Herpes zoster. Herpes zoster affecting the nasociliary nerve causes a sluggish pupillary response. Examination of the conjunctiva reveals follicles. Additional ocular findings include a serous discharge, absence of tears, ptosis, and extraocular muscle palsy.

Iritis (acute). With iritis, the affected eye exhibits a sluggish pupillary response and conjunctival injection. The pupil may remain constricted; if posterior synechiae have formed, the pupil will also be irregularly shaped. The patient reports a sudden onset of eye pain and photophobia and may also have blurred vision.

Myotonic dystrophy. With myotonic dystrophy, sluggish pupillary reaction may be accompanied by lid lag, ptosis, miosis and, possibly, diplopia. The patient may develop decreased visual acuity from cataract formation. Muscular weakness and atrophy and testicular atrophy may occur.

Tertiary syphilis. A sluggish pupillary reaction (especially in Argyll Robertson pupils) occurs in the late stage of neurosyphilis, along with marked weakness of the extraocular muscles, visual field defects and, possibly, cataractous changes in the lens. The patient may complain of orbital rim pain, which worsens at night. He may also exhibit lid edema, decreased visual acuity, and exophthalmos. Tertiary lesions appear on the skin and mucous membranes. Liver, respiratory, cardiovascular, and additional neurologic dysfunction may also occur.

Wernicke's disease. Initially, Wernicke's disease produces an intention tremor accompanied by a sluggish pupillary reaction. Later, pupils may become nonreactive. Additional ocular findings include diplopia, gaze paralysis, nystagmus, ptosis, decreased visual acuity, and conjunctival injection. The patient may also exhibit orthostatic hypotension, tachycardia, ataxia, apathy, and confusion.

Nursing considerations

- Perform interventions to treat the underlying disorder.
- If vision is affected, provide for the patient's safety.
- Monitor for eye pain and changes in vision.
- Monitor neurologic status, if indicated.

Patient teaching

- Explain the underlying disorder and treatment plan.
- Stress the importance of regular ophthalmologic examinations.
- Discuss methods to reduce photophobia.
- Teach self-care for diabetes, if needed.

Purpura

Purpura is the extravasation of red blood cells from the blood vessels into the skin, subcutaneous tissue, or mucous membranes. It's characterized by discoloration that's easily visible through the epidermis, usually purplish or brownish red. Purpuric lesions include petechiae, ecchymoses, and hematomas. (See *Identifying purpuric lesions*, page 520.) Purpura differs from erythema in that it doesn't blanch with pressure because it involves blood in the tissues, not just dilated vessels.

Purpura results from damage to the endothelium of small blood vessels, a coagulation defect, ineffective perivascular support, capillary fragility and permeability, or a combination of these factors. These faulty hemostatic factors, in turn, can result from thrombocytopenia or another hematologic disorder, an invasive procedure or, of course, the use of an anticoagulant.

Additional causes are nonpathologic. Purpura can be a consequence of aging, when loss of collagen decreases connective tissue support of upper skin blood vessels. In an elderly or cachectic person, skin atrophy and inelasticity and loss of subcutaneous fat increase susceptibility to minor trauma, causing purpu-

Identifying purpuric lesions

Purpuric lesions fall into three categories: petechiae, ecchymoses, and hematomas.

Petechiae
Petechiae are painless, round, pinpoint lesions, 1 to 3 mm in diameter. Caused by extravasation of red blood cells into cutaneous tissue, these red or purple lesions usually arise on dependent portions of the body. They appear and fade in crops and can group to form ecchymoses.

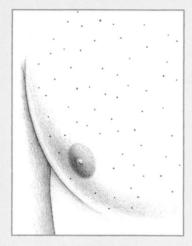

Ecchymoses
Ecchymoses, another form of blood extravasation, are larger than petechiae. These purple, blue, or yellow-green bruises vary in size and shape and can arise anywhere on the body as a result of trauma. Ecchymoses usually appear on the arms and legs of patients with bleeding disorders.

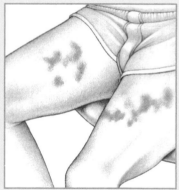

Hematomas
Hematomas are palpable ecchymoses that are painful and swollen. Usually the result of trauma, superficial hematomas are red, whereas deep hematomas are blue. Hematomas commonly exceed 1 cm in diameter, but their size varies widely.

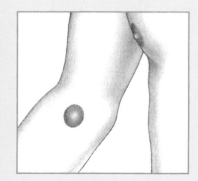

ra to appear along the veins of the forearms, hands, legs, and feet. Prolonged coughing or vomiting can produce crops of petechiae in loose face and neck tissue. Violent muscle contraction, as occurs in seizures or weight lifting, sometimes results in localized ecchymoses from increased intraluminal pressure and rupture. A high fever, which increases capillary fragility, can also produce purpura.

History and physical examination

Ask the patient when he first noticed the lesion and whether he has noticed other lesions on his body. Does he or his family have a history of bleeding disorders or easy bruising? Find out what medications he's taking, if any, and ask him to describe his diet. Ask about recent trauma or transfusions and the development of associated signs, such as epistaxis, bleeding gums, hematuria, and hematochezia. Also ask about systemic complaints that may suggest infection, such as a fever. If the patient is female, ask about heavy menstrual flow.

Inspect the patient's entire skin surface to determine the type, size, location, distribution, and severity of purpuric lesions. Also inspect the mucous membranes. Remember that the same mechanisms that cause purpura can also cause internal hemorrhage, although purpura isn't a cardinal indicator of this condition.

Medical causes

Autoerythrocyte sensitivity. With autoerythrocyte sensitivity, painful ecchymoses appear either singly or in groups, usually preceded by local itching, burning, or pain. Common associated findings include epistaxis, hematuria, hematemesis, and menometrorrhagia. Abdominal pain, diarrhea, nausea,

vomiting, syncope, headache, and chest pain are also common.

Disseminated intravascular coagulation (DIC). DIC can cause varying degrees of purpura, depending on its severity and underlying cause. Rarely, the patient develops life-threatening purpura fulminans, with symmetrical cutaneous and subcutaneous lesions on the arms and legs. Or, he may have cutaneous oozing, hematemesis, or bleeding from incision or needle insertion sites. Other findings include acrocyanosis; nausea; dyspnea; seizures; severe muscle, back, and abdominal pain; and signs of acute tubular necrosis such as oliguria.

Dysproteinemias. With multiple myeloma, petechiae and ecchymoses accompany other bleeding tendencies: hematemesis, epistaxis, gum bleeding, and excessive bleeding after surgery. Similar findings occur with cryoglobulinemia, which may also produce malignant maculopapular purpura. Hyperglobulinemia typically begins insidiously with occasional outbreaks of purpura over the lower legs and feet. These outbreaks eventually become more frequent and extensive, involving the entire lower leg and possibly the trunk. The purpura usually occurs after prolonged standing or exercise and may be heralded by skin burning or stinging. Leg edema, knee or ankle pain, and a low-grade fever may precede or accompany the purpura, which gradually fades over 1 or 2 weeks. Persistent pigmentation develops after repeated outbreaks.

Ehlers-Danlos syndrome (EDS). Besides petechiae, EDS is marked by easy bruising, epistaxis, gum bleeding, hematuria, melena, menorrhagia, and excessive bleeding after surgery. EDS characteristically produces soft, velvety, hyperelastic skin; hyperextensible joints; increased skin and blood vessel fragility;

and repeated dislocations of the temporomandibular joint.

Idiopathic thrombocytopenic purpura (ITP). Chronic ITP typically begins insidiously, with scattered petechiae that are usually found on the distal arms and legs. Deep-lying ecchymoses may also occur. Other findings include epistaxis, easy bruising, hematuria, hematemesis, and menorrhagia.

Leukemia. Leukemia produces widespread petechiae on the skin, mucous membranes, retina, and serosal surfaces that persist throughout the course of the disease. Confluent ecchymoses are uncommon. The patient may also exhibit swollen and bleeding gums, epistaxis, and other bleeding tendencies. Lymphadenopathy and splenomegaly are common.

Acute leukemias also produce severe prostration and a high fever and may cause dyspnea, tachycardia, palpitations, and abdominal or bone pain. Confusion, headache, seizures, vomiting, papilledema, and nuchal rigidity may occur late in the disease. Chronic leukemias begin insidiously with minor bleeding tendencies, malaise, fatigue, pallor, a low-grade fever, anorexia, and weight loss.

Myeloproliferative disorders. Myeloproliferative disorders, which include polycythemia vera, paradoxically can cause hemorrhage accompanied by ecchymoses and ruddy cyanosis. The oral mucosa takes on a deep purplish red hue, and slight trauma causes swollen gums to bleed. Other findings include pruritus, urticaria, and such nonspecific signs and symptoms as lethargy, weakness, fatigue, and weight loss. The patient typically complains of a headache, a sensation of fullness in the head, and rushing in the ears; dizziness and vertigo; dyspnea; paresthesia of the fingers; double or blurred vision and scotoma; and epigastric distress. He may also experience intermittent claudication, hypertension, hepatosplenomegaly, and impaired mentation.

Systemic lupus erythematosus (SLE). SLE may produce purpura accompanied by other cutaneous findings, such as scaly patches on the scalp, face, neck, and arms; diffuse alopecia; telangiectasia; urticaria; and ulceration. The characteristic butterfly rash appears in the disorder's acute phase. Common associated signs and symptoms include nondeforming joint pain and stiffness, Raynaud's phenomenon, seizures, psychotic behavior, photosensitivity, fever, anorexia, weight loss, and lymphadenopathy.

Thrombotic thrombocytopenic purpura. Generalized purpura, hematuria, vaginal bleeding, jaundice, and pallor are among the usual presenting signs and symptoms in thrombotic thrombocytopenic purpura. Most patients have fever, and some also experience fatigue, weakness, headache, nausea, abdominal pain, arthralgia, and hepatosplenomegaly. Possible neurologic effects include seizures, paresthesia, cranial nerve palsies, vertigo, and an altered level of consciousness. Renal failure may also occur.

Trauma. Traumatic injury can cause local or widespread purpura.

Other causes

Diagnostic tests. Invasive procedures, such as venipuncture and arterial catheterization, may produce local ecchymoses and hematomas due to extravasated blood.

Drugs. The anticoagulants heparin and warfarin can produce purpura.

Surgery and other procedures. Any procedure that disrupts circulation, coagulation, or platelet activity or production can cause purpura. These include pulmonary and cardiac surgery, radiation therapy, chemotherapy, hemodialysis, multiple blood transfusions with platelet-poor blood, and the use of plasma expanders such as dextran.

Nursing considerations

■ Prepare the patient for diagnostic tests, including a peripheral blood smear, bone marrow examination, and blood tests to determine platelet count, bleeding and coagulation times, capillary fragility, clot retraction, prothrombin time, partial thromboplastin time, and fibrinogen levels.

■ If the patient has a hematoma, apply pressure and cold compresses initially to help reduce bleeding and swelling. After the first 24 hours, apply hot compresses to help speed blood absorption.

Patient teaching

■ Explain the underlying cause and treatment plan.

■ Reassure the patient that purpuric lesions aren't permanent and will fade if the underlying cause can be successfully treated.

■ Warn the patient not to use cosmetic fade creams or other products in an attempt to reduce pigmentation.

▌Pustular rash

A pustular rash is made up of crops of pustules—a visible collection of pus within or beneath the epidermis, commonly in a hair follicle or sweat pore. These lesions vary greatly in size and shape and can be generalized or localized to the hair follicles or sweat glands. (See *Recognizing common skin lesions,* page 459.) Pustules can result from a skin or systemic disorder, the use of certain drugs, or exposure to a skin irritant. For example, people who have been swimming in salt water commonly develop a papulopustular rash under the bathing suit or elsewhere on the body from irritation by sea organisms. Al-

though many pustular lesions are sterile, a pustular rash usually indicates an infection. A vesicular eruption, or even acute contact dermatitis, can become pustular if secondary infection occurs.

History and physical examination

Have the patient describe the appearance, location, and onset of the first pustular lesion. Did another type of skin lesion precede the pustule? Find out how the lesions spread. Ask what medications the patient takes and if he has applied topical medication to his rash. If so, what type and when did he last apply it? Find out if he has a family history of a skin disorder.

Examine the entire skin surface, noting if it's dry, oily, moist, or greasy. Record the exact location and distribution of the skin lesions and their color, shape, and size.

Medical causes

Acne vulgaris. Pustules typify inflammatory lesions of acne vulgaris, which is accompanied by papules, nodules, cysts, open comedones (blackheads), and closed comedones (whiteheads). Lesions commonly appear on the face, shoulders, back, and chest. Other findings include pain on pressure, pruritus, and burning. Chronic recurrent lesions produce scars.

Blastomycosis. Blastomycosis is a fungal infection that produces small, painless, nonpruritic macules or papules that can enlarge to well-circumscribed, verrucous, crusted, or ulcerated lesions edged by pustules. Localized infection may cause only one lesion; systemic infection may cause many lesions on the hands, feet, face, and wrists. Blastomycosis also produces signs of pulmonary infection, such as pleuritic chest pain and a dry, hacking or productive cough with occasional hemoptysis.

Folliculitis. Folliculitis is a bacterial infection of hair follicles that produces individual pustules, each pierced by a hair and possibly accompanied by pruritus. "Hot tub" folliculitis produces pustules on areas covered by a bathing suit.

Furunculosis. A furuncle is an acute, deep-seated, red, hot, tender abscess that evolves from a staphylococcal folliculitis. Furuncles usually begin as small, tender red pustules at the base of hair follicles. They're likely to occur on the face, neck, forearm, groin, axillae, buttocks, and legs or areas that are prone to repeated friction. The pustules usually remain tense for 2 to 4 days and then become fluctuant. Rupture discharges pus and necrotic material. Then pain subsides, but erythema and edema may persist.

Impetigo contagiosa. Impetigo contagiosa, a vesiculopustular eruptive disorder that occurs in nonbullous and bullous forms, is usually caused by streptococci or staphylococci. Vesicles form and break, and a crust forms from the exudate: a thick, yellow crust in streptococcal impetigo and a thin, clear crust in staphylococcal impetigo. Both forms usually produce painless itching.

Pustular miliaria. Pustular miliaria causes pustular lesions that begin as tiny erythematous papulovesicles located at sweat pores. Diffuse erythema may radiate from the lesion. The rash and associated burning and pruritus worsen with sweating.

Pustular psoriasis. Small vesicles form and eventually become pustules with pustular psoriasis. The patient may report pruritus, burning, and pain. Localized pustular psoriasis usually affects the hands and feet. Generalized pustular psoriasis may erupt suddenly in a patient with psoriasis, psoriatic arthritis, or exfoliative psoriasis; although rare, this form of psoriasis can occasionally be fatal.

Rosacea. Rosacea commonly produces telangiectasia with acute episodes of pustules, papules, and edema. Characterized by persistent erythema, rosacea may begin as a flush covering the forehead, malar region, nose, and chin. Intermittent episodes gradually become more persistent, and the skin—instead of returning to its normal color—develops varying degrees of erythema.

Scabies. Threadlike channels or burrows under the skin characterize scabies, which can also produce pustules, vesicles, and excoriations. The lesions are a few millimeters long, with a swollen nodule or red papule that contains the itch mite.

Smallpox (variola major). Initial signs and symptoms of smallpox include high fever, malaise, prostration, severe headache, backache, and abdominal pain. A maculopapular rash develops on the mucosa of the mouth, pharynx, face, and forearms and then spreads to the trunk and legs. Within 2 days, the rash becomes vesicular and later pustular. The lesions develop at the same time, appear identical, and are more prominent on the face and extremities. The pustules are round, firm, and deeply embedded in the skin. After 8 or 9 days, the pustules form a crust and, later, the scab separates from the skin, leaving a pitted scar. In fatal cases, death results from encephalitis, extensive bleeding, or secondary infection.

Varicella zoster. When immunity to varicella declines, the virus reactivates along a dermatome, producing extremely painful and pruritic vesicles and pustules (herpes zoster, or shingles). Even with resolution of the rash, patients may experience chronic pain (postherpetic neuralgia) that may persist for months.

Other causes

Drugs. Bromides and iodides commonly cause a pustular rash. Other drug causes include corticotropin, corticosteroids, dactinomycin, trimethadione, lithium, phenytoin, phenobarbital, isoniazid, hormonal contraceptives, androgens, and anabolic steroids.

Nursing considerations
- Observe wound and skin isolation procedures until infection is ruled out by a Gram stain or culture and sensitivity test of the pustule's contents.
- If the organism is infectious, don't allow drainage to touch unaffected skin.
- Give medications to relieve pain and itching, and encourage the patient to express his feelings.

Patient teaching
- Explain the underlying disorder and treatment plan.
- Explain methods to prevent the spread of infection.
- Discuss ways to relieve pain and itching.

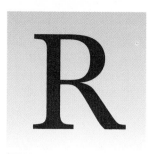

Raccoon eyes

Raccoon eyes are bilateral periorbital ecchymoses that don't result from facial soft-tissue trauma. Usually an indicator of basilar skull fracture, this sign develops when damage at the time of a fracture tears the meninges and causes the venous sinuses to bleed into the arachnoid villi and the cranial sinuses. Raccoon eyes may be the only indicator of a basilar skull fracture, which isn't always visible on skull X-rays. Their appearance signals the need for careful assessment to detect underlying trauma because a basilar skull fracture can injure cranial nerves, blood vessels, and the brain stem. Raccoon eyes can also occur after a craniotomy if the surgery causes a meningeal tear.

History and physical examination

After raccoon eyes are detected, check the patient's vital signs and try to find out when the head injury occurred and the nature of the head injury. (See *Recognizing raccoon eyes.*) Then evaluate the extent of underlying trauma.

Start by evaluating the patient's level of consciousness (LOC) using the Glasgow Coma Scale. Next, evaluate cranial

Recognizing raccoon eyes

It's usually easy to differentiate raccoon eyes from the "black eye" associated with facial trauma. Raccoon eyes (shown below) are always bilateral. They develop 2 to 3 days after a closed-head injury that results in a basilar skull fracture. In contrast, the periorbital ecchymosis that occurs with facial trauma can affect one eye or both. It usually develops within hours of injury.

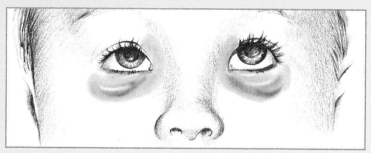

nerve (CN) function, especially CN I (olfactory), III (oculomotor), IV (trochlear), VI (abducens), and VII (facial). If the patient's condition permits, also test his visual acuity and gross hearing. Note irregularities in the facial or skull bones as well as swelling, localized pain, Battle's sign, or face or scalp lacerations. Check for ecchymoses over the mastoid bone. Inspect for hemorrhage or cerebrospinal fluid (CSF) leakage from the nose or ears.

Also, test drainage with a sterile 4″ × 4″ gauze pad, and note whether you find a halo sign—a circle of clear fluid that surrounds the drainage, indicating CSF. Also, use a glucose reagent stick to test clear drainage for glucose. An abnormal test result indicates CSF because mucus doesn't contain glucose.

Medical causes

Basilar skull fracture. A basilar skull fracture produces raccoon eyes after head trauma that doesn't involve the orbital area. Associated signs and symptoms vary with the fracture site and may include pharyngeal hemorrhage, epistaxis, rhinorrhea, otorrhea, and a bulging tympanic membrane from blood or CSF. The patient may experience difficulty hearing, headache, nausea, vomiting, cranial nerve palsies, and altered LOC. He may also exhibit a positive Battle's sign.

Other causes

Surgery. Raccoon eyes occurring after a craniotomy may indicate a meningeal tear and bleeding into the sinuses.

Nursing considerations

- Keep the patient on complete bed rest.
- Perform frequent neurologic evaluations to reevaluate the patient's LOC.
- Check the patient's vital signs frequently; be alert for such changes as bradypnea, bradycardia, hypertension, and fever.

- To avoid worsening a dural tear, instruct the patient not to blow his nose, cough vigorously, or strain.
- If otorrhea or rhinorrhea is present, don't attempt to stop the flow; instead, place a sterile, loose gauze pad under the nose or ear to absorb drainage.
- Monitor the amount of drainage and test it with a glucose reagent strip to confirm or rule out CSF leakage.
- To prevent further tearing of the mucous membranes and infection, never suction or pass a nasogastric tube through the patient's nose.
- Observe the patient for signs and symptoms of meningitis, such as fever, photophobia, and nuchal rigidity, and expect to administer a prophylactic antibiotic.
- Prepare the patient for diagnostic tests, such as skull X-ray and a computed tomography scan.
- If the dural tear doesn't heal spontaneously, prepare the patient for contrast cisternography to locate the tear, possibly followed by corrective surgery, as ordered.

Patient teaching

- Explain the disorder and treatment plan.
- Explain the signs and symptoms of neurologic deterioration that require immediate medical attention.
- Explain activity limitations.

Rebound tenderness
[Blumberg's sign]

A reliable indicator of peritonitis, rebound tenderness is intense, elicited abdominal pain caused by the rebound of palpated tissue. The tenderness may be localized, as in an abscess, or generalized, as in perforation of an intra-abdominal organ. Rebound tenderness usually occurs with abdominal pain, tenderness, and rigidity. When a patient

Eliciting rebound tenderness

To elicit rebound tenderness, help the patient into a supine position, and push your fingers deeply and steadily into his abdomen (as shown). Then quickly release the pressure. Pain that results from the rebound of palpated tissue—rebound tenderness—indicates peritoneal inflammation or peritonitis.

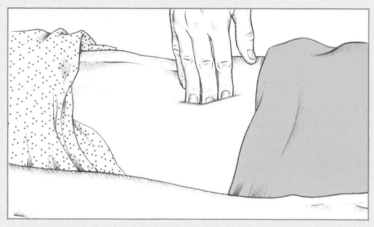

You can also elicit this symptom on a miniature scale by percussing the patient's abdomen lightly and indirectly (as shown). Better still, simply ask the patient to cough. This allows you to elicit rebound tenderness without having to touch the patient's abdomen and may also increase his cooperation because he won't associate exacerbation of his pain with your actions.

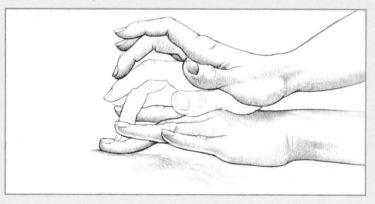

has sudden, severe abdominal pain, this symptom is usually elicited to detect peritoneal inflammation.

A C T I O N   S T A T !

 If you elicit rebound tenderness in a patient who's experiencing constant, severe abdominal pain, quickly take his vital signs. Insert a large-bore I.V. catheter, and begin administering I.V. fluids. Also insert an indwelling urinary catheter, and monitor intake and output. Give supplemental oxygen as needed, and continue to monitor the patient for signs of shock, such as hypotension and tachycardia.

History and physical examination

If the patient's condition permits, ask him to describe the events that led up to the tenderness. Does movement, exertion, or another activity relieve or aggravate the tenderness? Also, ask about other signs and symptoms, such as nausea and vomiting, fever, or abdominal bloating or distention. Inspect the abdomen for distention, visible peristaltic waves, and scars. Then auscultate for bowel sounds and characterize their motility. Palpate for associated rigidity or guarding, and percuss the abdomen, noting tympany. (See *Eliciting rebound tenderness.*)

Medical causes

Peritonitis. With peritonitis, a life-threatening disorder, rebound tenderness is accompanied by sudden and severe abdominal pain, which may be either diffuse or localized. Because movement worsens the patient's pain, he usually lies still on his back with his knees flexed or in a fetal position. Typically, he displays weakness, pallor, excessive sweating, and cold skin. He may also display hypoactive or absent bowel sounds; tachypnea; nausea and vomiting; abdominal distention, rigidity, and guarding; positive psoas and obturator signs; and a fever of 103° F (39.4° C) or higher. Inflammation of the diaphragmatic peritoneum may cause shoulder pain and hiccups.

Nursing considerations

- Promote comfort by having the patient flex his knees or assume semi-Fowler's position.
- Administer an analgesic, antiemetic, and an antipyretic, as ordered.
- Because of decreased intestinal motility and the probability that the patient will have surgery, don't give oral drugs or fluids.
- Obtain blood samples and urine and feces specimens for laboratory testing, and prepare the patient for chest and abdominal X-rays, sonograms, and computed tomography scans.
- Administer an antibiotic I.V., as ordered.
- Insert a nasogastric tube, if indicated.

Patient teaching

- Explain the disorder and treatment plan.
- Explain signs and symptoms that should be reported immediately.
- Instruct the patient in postoperative care.

▌Rectal pain

A common symptom of anorectal disorders, rectal pain is discomfort that arises in the anorectal area. Although the anal canal is separated from the rest of the rectum by the internal sphincter, the patient may refer to all local pain as rectal pain.

Because the mucocutaneous border of the anal canal and the perianal skin contains somatic nerve fibers, lesions in this area are especially painful. This pain may result from or be aggravated by diarrhea, constipation, or passage of hardened stools. It may also be aggravated by intense pruritus and continued scratching associated with drainage of mucus, blood, or fecal matter that irritates the skin and nerve endings.

History and physical examination

Begin by taking the patient's history. Ask him to describe the pain. Is it sharp or dull, burning or knifelike? How often does it occur? Ask if the pain is worse during or immediately after defecation. Does the patient avoid having bowel movements because of anticipated pain? Find out what alleviates the pain.

Be sure to ask appropriate questions about the development of associated signs and symptoms. For example, does the patient experience bleeding along with rectal pain? If so, find out how frequently this occurs and whether the blood appears on the toilet tissue, on the surface of the stools, or in the toilet bowl. Is the blood bright or dark red? Also, ask whether the patient has noticed other drainage, such as mucus or pus, and whether he's experiencing constipation or diarrhea. Ask when he last had a bowel movement. Obtain a dietary and drug history.

Then inspect the rectal area for bleeding; abnormal drainage, such as pus; or protrusions, such as skin tags or thrombosed hemorrhoids. Also, check for inflammation and other lesions. A rectal examination may be necessary.

Medical causes

Abscess (perirectal). A perirectal abscess can occur in various locations in the rectum and anus, causing pain in the perianal area. Typically, a superficial abscess produces constant, throbbing local pain that's exacerbated by sitting or walking. The local pain associated with a deeper abscess may begin insidiously, commonly high in the rectum or even in the lower abdomen, and is accompanied by an indurated anal mass. The patient may also develop associated signs and symptoms, such as fever, malaise, anal swelling and inflammation, purulent drainage, and local tenderness.

Anal fissure. An anal fissure causes sharp rectal pain on defecation. The patient typically experiences a burning sensation and gnawing pain that can continue up to 4 hours after defecation. Fear of provoking this pain may lead to acute constipation. The patient may also develop anal pruritus and extreme tenderness and may report finding spots of blood on the toilet tissue after defecation.

Anorectal fistula. Anorectal fistula causes rectal pain to develop when a tract formed between the anal canal and skin temporarily seals. It persists until drainage resumes. Other chief complaints include pruritus and drainage of pus, blood, mucus and, occasionally, stools.

Hemorrhoids. Thrombosed or prolapsed hemorrhoids cause rectal pain that may worsen during defecation and abate after it. The patient's fear of provoking the pain may lead to constipation. Usually, rectal pain is accompanied by severe itching. Internal hemorrhoids may also produce mild, intermittent bleeding that characteristically occurs as spotting on the toilet tissue or on the stool surface. External hemorrhoids are visible outside the anal sphincter.

Nursing considerations

- Apply analgesic ointment or suppositories.
- Administer a stool softener if needed.
- If the rectal pain results from prolapsed hemorrhoids, apply cold compresses to help shrink protruding hemorrhoids, prevent thrombosis, and reduce pain.
- If the patient's condition permits, place him in Trendelenburg's position with his buttocks elevated to further relieve pain.
- Prepare the patient for an anoscopic examination and proctosigmoidoscopy to determine the cause of the rectal pain, if indicated.

■ Because the patient may feel embarrassed, provide emotional support and as much privacy as possible.

Patient teaching
■ Explain the disorder and treatment plan.
■ Instruct the patient on measures to ease discomfort.
■ Discuss proper diet and fluid intake.
■ Explain the use of stool softeners.

Respirations, grunting

Characterized by a deep, low-pitched grunting sound at the end of each breath, grunting respirations are a chief sign of respiratory distress in infants and children. They may be soft and heard only on auscultation, or loud and clearly audible without a stethoscope. Typically, the intensity of grunting respirations reflects the severity of respiratory distress. The grunting sound coincides with closure of the glottis, an effort to increase end-expiratory pressure in the lungs and prolong alveolar gas exchange, thereby enhancing ventilation and perfusion.

Grunting respirations indicate intrathoracic disease with lower respiratory involvement. Though most common in children, they sometimes occur in adults who are in severe respiratory distress. Whether they occur in children or adults, grunting respirations demand immediate medical attention.

Action stat!

 If the patient exhibits grunting respirations, quickly place him in a comfortable position and check for signs of respiratory distress: wheezing; tachypnea (a minimum respiratory rate of 60 breaths/minute in infants, 40 breaths/minute in children ages 1 to 5, 30 breaths/minute in children older than age 5, or 20 breaths/minute in adults); accessory muscle use; substernal, subcostal, or intercostal retractions; nasal flaring; tachycardia (a minimum of 160 beats/minute in infants, 120 to 140 beats/minute in children ages 1 to 5, 120 beats/minute in children older than age 5, or 100 beats/minute in adults); cyanotic lips or nail beds; hypotension (less than 80/40 mm Hg in infants, less than 80/50 mm Hg in children ages 1 to 5, less than 90/55 mm Hg in children older than age 5, or less than 90/60 mm Hg in adults); and decreased level of consciousness.

If you detect any of these signs, monitor oxygen saturation, and administer oxygen and prescribed medications such as a bronchodilator. Have emergency equipment available and prepare to intubate the patient if necessary. Obtain arterial blood gas analysis to determine oxygenation status.

History and physical examination
After addressing the child's respiratory status, ask his parents when the grunting respirations began. If the patient is a premature infant, find out his gestational age. Ask the parents if anyone in the home has recently had an upper respiratory tract infection. Has the child had signs and symptoms of such an infection, such as a runny nose, cough, low-grade fever, or anorexia? Does he have a history of frequent colds or upper respiratory tract infections? Does he have a history of respiratory syncytial virus? Ask the parents to describe changes in the child's activity level or feeding pattern to determine if the child is lethargic or less alert than usual.

Begin the physical examination by auscultating the lungs, especially the lower lobes. Note diminished or abnormal sounds, such as crackles or sibilant rhonchi, which may indicate mucus or fluid buildup. Characterize the color, amount, and consistency of any discharge or sputum. Note the characteristics of the cough, if any. Note the respiratory rate. Assess accessory muscle use for breathing and cyanosis.

Medical causes

Asthma. Grunting respirations may be apparent during a severe asthma attack, usually triggered by an upper respiratory tract infection or an allergic response. As the attack progresses, dyspnea, audible wheezing, chest tightness, and coughing occur. Patients may have a silent chest if air movement is poor. Immediate bronchodilator therapy is needed.

Heart failure. A late sign of left-sided heart failure, grunting respirations accompany increasing pulmonary edema. Associated features include a productive cough, crackles, jugular vein distention, and chest wall retractions. Cyanosis may also be evident, depending on the underlying congenital cardiac defect.

Pneumonia. Life-threatening bacterial pneumonia causes grunting respirations accompanied by high fever, tachypnea, a productive cough, anorexia, and lethargy. Auscultation reveals diminished breath sounds, scattered crackles, and sibilant rhonchi over the affected lung. As the disorder progresses, the patient may also develop severe dyspnea, substernal and subcostal retractions, nasal flaring, cyanosis, and increasing lethargy. Some infants display GI signs, such as vomiting, diarrhea, and abdominal distention.

Respiratory distress syndrome. The result of lung immaturity in a premature infant (less than 37 weeks' gestation) usually of low birth weight, this syndrome initially causes audible expiratory grunting along with intercostal, subcostal, or substernal retractions; tachycardia; and tachypnea. Later, as respiratory distress tires the infant, apnea or irregular respirations replace the grunting. Severe respiratory distress is characterized by cyanosis, frothy sputum, dramatic nasal flaring, lethargy, bradycardia, and hypotension. Eventually, the infant becomes unresponsive. Auscultation reveals harsh, diminished breath sounds and crackles over the base of the lungs on deep inspiration. Oliguria and peripheral edema may also occur.

Nursing considerations

- Closely monitor the patient's respiratory status.
- Keep emergency equipment nearby in case respiratory distress worsens.
- Administer oxygen.
- Continually monitor arterial blood gas levels and deliver the minimum amount of oxygen possible to avoid causing retinopathy of prematurity from excessively high oxygen levels.
- Begin inhalation therapy with a bronchodilator.
- Administer an I.V. antimicrobial if the patient has pneumonia.
- Perform chest physical therapy as necessary.
- Prepare the patient for chest X-rays or computed tomography scan.

Patient teaching

- Explain the disorder and treatment plan.
- Explain all procedures to the patient or his parents and provide emotional support.
- Teach techniques for home respiratory care and therapy.
- Give instructions on the proper use of prescribed drugs.
- Explain the signs and symptoms to report.

Respirations, shallow

Respirations are shallow when a diminished volume of air enters the lungs during inspiration. In an effort to obtain enough air, the patient with shallow respirations usually breathes at an accelerated rate. However, as he tires or as his muscles weaken, this compensatory increase in respirations diminishes, leading to inadequate gas exchange and such signs as dyspnea, cyanosis, confusion, agitation, loss of consciousness, and tachycardia.

Shallow respirations may develop suddenly or gradually and may last briefly or become chronic. They're a key sign of respiratory distress and neurologic deterioration. Causes include inadequate central respiratory control over breathing, neuromuscular disorders, increased resistance to airflow into the lungs, respiratory muscle fatigue or weakness, voluntary alterations in breathing, decreased activity from prolonged bed rest, and pain.

A<small>CTION</small> S<small>TAT</small>!

If you observe shallow respirations, be alert for impending respiratory failure or arrest. Is the patient severely dyspneic? Agitated or frightened? Look for signs of airway obstruction. If the patient is choking, perform four back blows and then four abdominal thrusts to try to expel the foreign object. Use suction if secretions occlude the patient's airway. If the patient is also wheezing, check for stridor, nasal flaring, and accessory muscle use. Administer oxygen with a face mask or handheld resuscitation bag. Attempt to calm the patient. Administer I.V. epinephrine.

If the patient loses consciousness, insert an artificial airway and prepare for endotracheal intubation and ventilatory support. Measure his tidal volume and minute volume to determine the need for mechanical ventilation. (See *Measuring lung volumes,* page 534.) Check arterial blood gas (ABG) levels, heart rate, blood pressure, and oxygen saturation. Tachycardia, increased or decreased blood pressure, poor minute volume, and deteriorating ABG levels or oxygen saturation signal the need for intubation and mechanical ventilation.

History and physical examination

If the patient isn't in severe respiratory distress, begin with the history. Ask about chronic illness and surgery or trauma. Has he had a tetanus booster in the past 10 years? Does he have asthma, allergies, or a history of heart failure or vascular disease? Does he have a chronic respiratory disorder or respiratory tract infection, tuberculosis, or a neurologic or neuromuscular disease? Does he smoke? Obtain a drug history as well, and explore the possibility of drug abuse.

Ask about the patient's shallow respirations: When did they begin? How long do they last? What makes them subside? What aggravates them? Ask about changes in appetite, weight, activity level, and behavior.

Perform the physical examination by first assessing the patient's level of consciousness (LOC) and his orientation to time, place, and person. Observe spontaneous movements, and test muscle strength and deep tendon reflexes. Next, inspect the chest for deformities or abnormal movements such as intercostal retractions. Inspect the extremities for cyanosis and digital clubbing.

Now, palpate for expansion and diaphragmatic tactile fremitus, and percuss for hyperresonance or dullness. Auscultate for diminished, absent, or adventitious breath sounds and for ab-

Measuring lung volumes

Use a Wright respirometer to measure tidal volume (the amount of air inspired with each breath) and minute volume (the volume of air inspired in a minute—or tidal volume multiplied by respiratory rate). You can connect the respirometer to an intubated patient's airway via an endotracheal tube (shown here) or a tracheostomy tube. If the patient isn't intubated, connect the respirometer to a face mask, making sure the seal over the patient's mouth and nose is airtight.

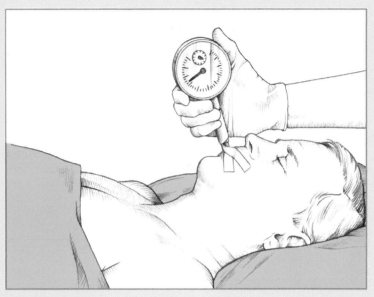

normal or distant heart sounds. Do you note peripheral edema? Finally, examine the abdomen for distention, tenderness, or masses.

Medical causes

Acute respiratory distress syndrome (ARDS). Initially, ARDS produces rapid, shallow respirations and dyspnea. Hypoxemia leads to intercostal and suprasternal retractions, diaphoresis, and fluid accumulation, causing rhonchi and crackles. As hypoxemia worsens, the patient exhibits more difficulty breathing, restlessness, apprehension, decreased LOC, cyanosis and, possibly, tachycardia.

Amyotrophic lateral sclerosis (ALS). Respiratory muscle weakness in ALS causes progressive shallow respirations. Exertion may result in increased weakness and respiratory distress. ALS initially produces upper extremity muscle weakness and wasting, which in several years affect the trunk, neck, tongue, and muscles of the larynx, pharynx, and lower extremities. Associated signs and symptoms include muscle cramps and atrophy, hyperreflexia, slight spasticity of the legs, coarse fasciculations of the affected muscle, impaired speech, and difficulty chewing and swallowing.

Asthma. With asthma, bronchospasm and hyperinflation of the lungs cause rapid, shallow respirations. In adults, mild persistent signs and symptoms may worsen during severe attacks. Related respiratory effects include wheezing, rhonchi, a dry cough, dyspnea, prolonged expirations, intercostal and supraclavicular retractions on inspiration, nasal flaring, and accessory muscle use. Chest tightness, tachycardia, diaphoresis, and flushing or cyanosis may occur.

Atelectasis. With atelectasis, decreased lung expansion or pleuritic pain causes a sudden onset of rapid, shallow respirations. Other signs and symptoms include a dry cough, dyspnea, tachycardia, anxiety, cyanosis, and diaphoresis. Examination reveals dullness to percussion, decreased breath sounds and vocal fremitus, inspiratory lag, and substernal or intercostal retractions.

Bronchiectasis. Bronchiectasis causes increased secretions that obstruct airflow in the lungs, leading to shallow respirations and a productive cough with copious, foul-smelling, mucopurulent sputum (a classic finding). Other findings include hemoptysis, wheezing, rhonchi, coarse crackles during inspiration, and late-stage clubbing. The patient may complain of weight loss, fatigue, exertional weakness and dyspnea on exertion, fever, malaise, and halitosis.

Coma. In a coma, rapid, shallow respirations result from neurologic dysfunction or restricted chest movement.

Emphysema. With emphysema, increased breathing effort causes muscle fatigue, leading to chronic shallow respirations. The patient may also display dyspnea, anorexia, malaise, tachypnea, diminished breath sounds, cyanosis, pursed-lip breathing, accessory muscle use, barrel chest, a chronic productive cough, and clubbing (a late sign).

Flail chest. With flail chest, decreased air movement results in rapid, shallow respirations, paradoxical chest wall motion from rib instability, tachy-

cardia, hypotension, ecchymoses, cyanosis, and pain over the affected area.

Guillain-Barré syndrome. With Guillain-Barré syndrome, progressive ascending paralysis causes a rapid or progressive onset of shallow respirations in this syndrome. Muscle weakness begins in the lower limbs and extends finally to the face. Associated findings include paresthesia, dysarthria, a diminished or an absent corneal reflex, nasal speech, dysphagia, ipsilateral loss of facial muscle control, and flaccid paralysis.

Multiple sclerosis (MS). With MS, muscle weakness causes progressive shallow respirations. Early features include diplopia, blurred vision, and paresthesia. Other possible findings are nystagmus, constipation, paralysis, spasticity, hyperreflexia, intention tremor, an ataxic gait, dysphagia, dysarthria, urinary dysfunction, impotence, and emotional lability.

Myasthenia gravis. Progression of myasthenia gravis causes respiratory muscle weakness marked by shallow respirations, dyspnea, and cyanosis. Other effects include fatigue, weak eye closure, ptosis, diplopia, and difficulty chewing and swallowing.

Pleural effusion. With pleural effusion, restricted lung expansion causes shallow respirations, beginning suddenly or gradually. Other findings include a nonproductive cough, weight loss, dyspnea, and pleuritic chest pain. Examination reveals a pleural friction rub, tachycardia, tachypnea, decreased chest motion, flatness to percussion, egophony, decreased or absent breath sounds, and decreased tactile fremitus.

Pneumothorax. Pneumothorax causes a sudden onset of shallow respirations and dyspnea. Related effects include tachycardia; tachypnea; sudden sharp, severe chest pain (commonly unilateral) that worsens with movement; a nonproductive cough; cyanosis; accessory muscle use; asymmetrical chest expansion; anxiety; restlessness; hyperresonance or tympany on the affected side; subcutaneous crepitation; decreased vocal fremitus; and diminished or absent breath sounds on the affected side.

Pulmonary edema. Pulmonary vascular congestion causes rapid, shallow respirations. Early signs and symptoms include exertional dyspnea, paroxysmal nocturnal dyspnea, a nonproductive cough, tachycardia, tachypnea, dependent crackles, and a ventricular gallop. Severe pulmonary edema produces more rapid, labored respirations; widespread crackles; a productive cough with frothy, bloody sputum; worsening tachycardia; arrhythmias; cold, clammy skin; cyanosis; hypotension; and a thready pulse.

Pulmonary embolism. Pulmonary embolism causes sudden, rapid, shallow respirations and severe dyspnea with angina or pleuritic chest pain. Other clinical features include tachycardia, tachypnea, a nonproductive cough or a productive cough with blood-tinged sputum, a low-grade fever, restlessness, diaphoresis, a pleural friction rub, crackles, diffuse wheezing, dullness to percussion, decreased breath sounds, and signs of circulatory collapse. Less-common findings are massive hemoptysis, chest splinting, leg edema, and (with a large embolism) cyanosis, syncope, and jugular vein distention.

Other causes

Drugs. Opioids, sedatives and hypnotics, tranquilizers, neuromuscular blockers, magnesium sulfate, and anesthetics can produce slow, shallow respirations.

Surgery. After abdominal or thoracic surgery, pain associated with chest splinting and decreased chest wall motion may cause shallow respirations.

Nursing considerations

- Prepare the patient for diagnostic tests, such as ABG analysis, drug levels, pulmonary function tests, chest X-rays, bronchoscopy, and computed tomography scan.
- Position the patient as upright as possible to ease his breathing.
- If he's taking a drug that depresses respirations, follow all precautions, and monitor him closely.
- Ensure adequate hydration, and use humidification as needed to thin secretions and to relieve inflamed, dry, or irritated airway mucosa.
- Administer humidified oxygen, a bronchodilator, a mucolytic, an expectorant, or an antibiotic, as ordered.
- Perform tracheal suctioning, as needed, to clear secretions.
- Turn the patient frequently.
- Administer chest physiotherapy, incentive spirometry, or intermittent positive-pressure breathing, as ordered.
- Monitor for increasing lethargy, which may indicate rising carbon dioxide levels.
- Have emergency equipment at the patient's bedside.

Patient teaching

- Explain the disorder and treatment plan.
- Explain the importance of coughing and deep breathing.
- Teach the postoperative patient to splint his incision while coughing.
- Explain all procedures to the patient.

Respirations, stertorous

Characterized by a harsh, rattling, or snoring sound, stertorous respirations usually result from the vibration of relaxed oropharyngeal structures during sleep or coma, causing partial airway obstruction. Less commonly, these respirations result from retained mucus in the upper airway.

This common sign occurs in about 10% of healthy individuals; however, it's especially prevalent in middle-aged men who are obese. It may be aggravated by the use of alcohol or a sedative before bed, which increases oropharyngeal flaccidity, and by sleeping in the supine position, which allows the relaxed tongue to slip back into the airway. The major pathologic causes of stertorous respirations are obstructive sleep apnea and life-threatening upper airway obstruction associated with an oropharyngeal tumor or with uvular or palatal edema. This obstruction may also occur during the postictal phase of a generalized seizure when mucus secretions or a relaxed tongue blocks the airway.

Occasionally, stertorous respirations are mistaken for stridor, which is another sign of upper airway obstruction. However, stridor indicates laryngeal or tracheal obstruction, whereas stertorous respirations signal higher airway obstruction.

ACTION STAT!

 If you detect stertorous respirations, check the patient's mouth and throat for edema, redness, masses, or foreign objects. If edema is marked, quickly take the patient's vital signs, including oxygen saturation. Observe him for signs and symptoms of respiratory distress, such as dyspnea, tachypnea, accessory muscle use, intercostal muscle retractions, and cyanosis. Elevate the head of the bed 30 degrees to help ease breathing and reduce edema. Then administer supplemental oxygen by nasal cannula or face mask, and prepare to intubate the patient, perform a tracheostomy, and provide mechanical

ventilation. Insert an I.V. catheter for fluid and drug administration, if prescribed, and begin cardiac monitoring.

History and physical examination

If you detect stertorous respirations while the patient is sleeping, observe his breathing pattern for 3 to 4 minutes. Do noisy respirations cease when he turns on his side and recur when he assumes a supine position? Watch carefully for periods of apnea and note their length.

If the patient isn't in severe respiratory distress, begin with the history. Question the patient about his snoring habits. Is his partner frequently awakened by his snoring? Does the snoring improve if the patient sleeps with the window open? Does he talk in his sleep or sleepwalk? Ask about signs of sleep deprivation, such as personality changes, headaches, daytime somnolence, or decreased mental acuity.

Perform the physical examination by first assessing the patient's level of consciousness and his orientation to time, place, and person. Observe spontaneous movements, and test muscle strength and deep tendon reflexes. Next, inspect the chest for deformities or abnormal movements such as intercostal retractions. Inspect the extremities for cyanosis and digital clubbing.

Now, palpate for expansion and diaphragmatic tactile fremitus, and percuss for hyperresonance or dullness. Auscultate for diminished, absent, or adventitious breath sounds and for abnormal or distant heart sounds. Do you note peripheral edema? Finally, examine the abdomen for distention, tenderness, or masses.

Medical causes
Airway obstruction. Regardless of its cause, partial airway obstruction may

lead to stertorous respirations accompanied by wheezing, dyspnea, tachypnea and, later, intercostal retractions and nasal flaring. If the obstruction becomes complete, the patient abruptly loses his ability to talk and displays diaphoresis, tachycardia, and inspiratory chest movement but absent breath sounds. Severe hypoxemia rapidly ensues, resulting in cyanosis, loss of consciousness, and cardiopulmonary collapse.

Obstructive sleep apnea. Loud and disruptive snoring is a major characteristic of obstructive sleep apnea, which commonly affects people who are obese. Typically, the snoring alternates with periods of sleep apnea, which usually end with loud gasping sounds. Alternating tachycardia and bradycardia may occur.

Episodes of snoring and apnea recur in a cyclic pattern throughout the night. Sleep disturbances, such as somnambulism and talking during sleep, may also occur. Some patients display hypertension and ankle edema. Most awaken in the morning with a generalized headache, feeling tired and unrefreshed. The most common complaint is excessive daytime sleepiness. Lack of sleep may cause depression, hostility, and decreased mental acuity.

Other causes

Endotracheal (ET) intubation, suction, or surgery. ET intubation, suction, or surgery may cause significant palatal or uvular edema, resulting in stertorous respirations.

Nursing considerations

■ Monitor the patient's respiratory status carefully.
■ Administer a corticosteroid or an antibiotic, as ordered.
■ Administer cool, humidified oxygen to reduce palatal and uvular inflammation and edema.

■ Prepare the patient for laryngoscopy and bronchoscopy (to rule out airway obstruction) or formal sleep studies, as necessary.

Patient teaching

■ Explain the disorder and treatment plan.
■ Discuss with the patient the importance of weight loss and smoking cessation.
■ Demonstrate the use of a positive airway pressure device, if indicated.
■ Teach the patient how to elevate his head while sleeping.

Retractions, costal and sternal

A cardinal sign of respiratory distress in infants and children, retractions are visible indentations of the soft tissue covering the chest wall. They may be suprasternal (directly above the sternum and clavicles), intercostal (between the ribs), subcostal (below the lower costal margin of the rib cage), or substernal (just below the xiphoid process). Retractions may be mild or severe, producing barely visible to deep indentations.

Normally, infants and young children use abdominal muscles for breathing, unlike older children and adults, who use the diaphragm. When breathing requires extra effort, accessory muscles assist respiration, especially inspiration. Retractions typically accompany accessory muscle use.

ACTION STAT!

 If you detect retractions in a child, check quickly for other signs of respiratory distress, such as cyanosis, tachypnea, tachycardia, and decreased oxygen saturation. Also, prepare the child for suctioning, artificial airway insertion, and oxygen administration.

History and physical examination

If the child's condition permits, ask his parents about his medical history. Was he born prematurely? Was he born with a low birth weight? Was the delivery complicated? Ask about recent signs of an upper respiratory tract infection, such as runny nose, cough, and low-grade fever. How often has the child had respiratory problems during the past year? Does he participate in a day care program or have school-aged siblings? Has he been in contact with anyone who has had a cold, the flu, or other respiratory ailments? Did he ever have respiratory syncytial virus? Did he aspirate food, liquid, or a foreign body? Inquire about a personal or family history of allergies or asthma.

Observe the depth and location of the retractions. Also, note the rate, depth, and quality of respirations. Look for accessory muscle use, nasal flaring during inspiration, or grunting during expiration. If the child has a cough, record its characteristics as well as the color, consistency, amount, and odor of any sputum. Note whether the child appears restless or lethargic. Finally, auscultate the child's lungs to detect abnormal breath sounds. (See *Observing retractions,* page 540.)

Medical causes

Asthma. Intercostal and suprasternal retractions may accompany an asthma attack. They're preceded by dyspnea, wheezing, a hacking cough, and pallor. Related features include cyanosis or flushing, crackles, rhonchi, diaphoresis, tachycardia, tachypnea, a frightened, anxious expression and, in patients with severe distress, nasal flaring.

Epiglottiditis. Epiglottiditis is a life-threatening bacterial infection that may precipitate severe respiratory distress with suprasternal, substernal, and intercostal retractions; stridor; nasal flaring; cyanosis; and tachycardia. Early features include a sudden onset of a barking cough and high fever, a sore throat, hoarseness, dysphagia, drooling, dyspnea, and restlessness. The child becomes panicky as edema makes breathing difficult. Total airway occlusion may occur in 2 to 5 hours.

Heart failure. Usually linked to a congenital heart defect in children, heart failure may cause intercostal and substernal retractions along with nasal flaring, progressive tachypnea, and—in severe respiratory distress—grunting respirations, edema, and cyanosis. Other findings include a productive cough, crackles, jugular vein distention, tachycardia, right upper quadrant pain, anorexia, and fatigue.

Laryngotracheobronchitis (acute). With laryngotracheobronchitis, substernal and intercostal retractions typically follow a low to moderate fever, runny nose, poor appetite, a barking cough, hoarseness, and inspiratory stridor. Associated signs and symptoms include tachycardia; shallow, rapid respirations; restlessness; irritability; and pale, cyanotic skin.

Pneumonia (bacterial). Pneumonia begins with signs and symptoms of acute infection, such as a high fever and lethargy, which are followed by subcostal and intercostal retractions, nasal flaring, dyspnea, tachypnea, grunting respirations, cyanosis, and a productive cough. Auscultation may reveal diminished breath sounds, scattered crackles, and sibilant rhonchi over the affected lung. GI effects may include vomiting, diarrhea, and abdominal distention.

Respiratory distress syndrome. Substernal and subcostal retractions are an

Observing retractions

When you observe retractions in infants and children, be sure to note their exact location—an important clue to the cause and severity of respiratory distress. For example, subcostal and substernal retractions usually result from lower respiratory tract disorders; suprasternal retractions, from upper respiratory tract disorders.

Mild intercostal retractions alone may be normal. However, intercostal retractions accompanied by subcostal and substernal retractions may indicate moderate respiratory distress. Deep suprasternal retractions typically indicate severe distress.

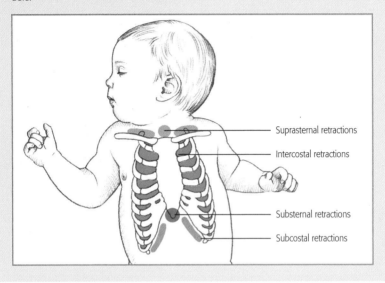

Suprasternal retractions

Intercostal retractions

Substernal retractions

Subcostal retractions

early sign of respiratory distress syndrome, a life-threatening syndrome, which affects premature neonates shortly after birth. Associated early signs include tachypnea, tachycardia, and expiratory grunting. As respiratory distress worsens, intercostal and suprasternal retractions typically occur, and apnea or irregular respirations replace grunting. Other effects include nasal flaring, cyanosis, lethargy, and eventual unresponsiveness as well as bradycardia and hypotension. Auscultation may detect crackles over the lung bases on deep inspiration and harsh, diminished breath sounds. Oliguria and peripheral edema may occur.

Nursing considerations
■ Monitor vital signs frequently.
■ Keep suction equipment and emergency equipment at the bedside.
■ If the infant weighs less than 15 lb (6.8 kg), place him in an oxygen hood; if he weighs more, place him in a cool mist tent instead.
■ Perform chest physical therapy with postural drainage to help mobilize and drain excess lung secretions.
■ Administer a bronchodilator or steroid, as ordered.

■ Prepare the child for chest X-rays, cultures, pulmonary function tests, and arterial blood gas analysis.

Patient teaching

■ Explain the procedures to the child's parents, and have them calm and comfort him.
■ Explain the disorder and treatment plan.
■ Teach the patient and his family about medications.
■ Tell them how to provide a humidified environment.
■ Stress the importance of ensuring adequate hydration.

Rhinorrhea

Common and rarely serious, rhinorrhea is the free discharge of thin nasal mucus. It can be self-limiting or chronic, resulting from a nasal, sinus, or systemic disorder or from a basilar skull fracture. Rhinorrhea can also result from sinus or cranial surgery, excessive use of vasoconstricting nose drops or sprays, or inhalation of an irritant, such as tobacco smoke, dust, and fumes. Depending on the cause, the discharge may be clear, purulent, bloody, or serosanguineous.

History and physical examination

Begin the history by asking the patient if the discharge runs from both nostrils. Is the discharge intermittent or persistent? Did it begin suddenly or gradually? Does the position of his head affect the discharge? Does anything make it better? Does anything make it worse?

Next, ask the patient to characterize the discharge. Is it watery, bloody, purulent, or foul smelling? Is it copious or scanty? Does the discharge worsen or improve with the time of day? Also, find out if the patient is using medications, especially nose drops or nasal sprays.

Has he been exposed to nasal irritants at home or at work? Does he experience seasonal allergies? Did he recently experience a head injury?

Examine the patient's nose, checking airflow from each nostril. Evaluate the size, color, and condition of the turbinate mucosa (normally pale pink). Note if the mucosa is red, unusually pale, blue, or gray. Then examine the area beneath each turbinate. (See *Using a nasal speculum,* page 542.) Be sure to palpate over the frontal, ethmoid, and maxillary sinuses for tenderness.

To differentiate nasal mucus from cerebrospinal fluid (CSF), collect a small amount of drainage on a glucose test strip. If CSF (which contains glucose) is present, the test result will be abnormal. Finally, using a nonirritating substance, be sure to test for anosmia.

Medical causes

Basilar skull fracture. With a basilar skull fracture, a tear in the dura can lead to cerebrospinal rhinorrhea, which increases when the patient lowers his head. Other findings include epistaxis, otorrhea, and a bulging tympanum from blood or fluid. A basilar fracture may also cause headache, facial paralysis, nausea and vomiting, impaired eye movement, ocular deviation, vision and hearing loss, depressed level of consciousness, Battle's sign, and raccoon eyes.

Nasal or sinus tumors. Nasal tumors can produce an intermittent, unilateral bloody or serosanguineous discharge that may be purulent and foul smelling. Nasal congestion, postnasal drip, and headache may also occur. In advanced stages, paranasal sinus tumors may cause a cheek mass or eye displacement, facial paresthesia or pain, and nasal obstruction.

Rhinitis. *Allergic rhinitis* produces an episodic, profuse watery discharge. (A

Using a nasal speculum

To visualize the interior of the nares, use a nasal speculum and a good light source such as a penlight. Hold the speculum in the palm of one hand and the penlight in the other hand. Have the patient tilt her head back slightly and rest it against a wall or other firm support, if possible. Insert the speculum blades about ½" (1.3 cm) into the nasal vestibule, as shown.

Place your index finger on the tip of the patient's nose for stability. Carefully open the speculum blades. Shine the light source in the direction of the nares. Now, inspect the nares. The mucosa should be pink to light red. Note any discharge, masses, lesions, or mucosal swellings. Check the nasal septum for perforation, bleeding, or crusting. Bluish turbinates suggest allergy. A rounded, elongated projection suggests a polyp.

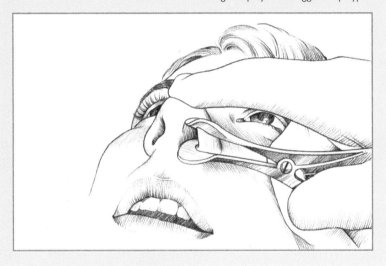

mucopurulent discharge indicates infection.) Typical associated signs and symptoms include increased lacrimation; nasal congestion; itchy eyes, nose, and throat; postnasal drip; recurrent sneezing; mouth breathing; an impaired sense of smell; and a frontal or temporal headache. Also, the turbinates are pale and engorged; the mucosa, pale and boggy.

With *atrophic rhinitis,* the nasal discharge is scanty, purulent, and foul smelling. Nasal obstruction is common, and the crusts may bleed on removal. The mucosa is pale pink and shiny.

With *vasomotor rhinitis,* a profuse and watery nasal discharge accompanies chronic nasal obstruction, sneezing, recurrent postnasal drip, and pale, swollen turbinates. The nasal septum is pink; the mucosa, blue.

Sinusitis. With *acute sinusitis,* a thick and purulent nasal discharge leads to a purulent postnasal drip that results in throat pain and halitosis. The patient may also experience nasal congestion, severe pain and tenderness over the involved sinuses, fever, headache, and malaise.

With *chronic sinusitis,* the nasal discharge is usually scanty, thick, and intermittently purulent. Nasal congestion and low-grade discomfort or pressure over the involved sinuses can be persistent or recurrent. The patient may also be suffering from a chronic sore throat and nasal polyps.

With *chronic fungal sinusitis,* the clinical picture resembles that of chronic bacterial sinusitis. However, some cases—especially in patients who are immunocompromised—may progress rapidly to exophthalmos, blindness, intracranial extension and, eventually, death.

Upper respiratory infection. With the common cold, an initially watery nasal discharge may become thicker and mucopurulent. Related findings include sneezing, nasal congestion, a dry and hacking cough, a sore throat, mouth breathing, and a transient loss of smell and taste. The patient may also experience malaise, fatigue, myalgia, arthralgia, a slight headache, dry lips, and a red upper lip and nose.

Other causes

Drugs. Nasal sprays or nose drops containing vasoconstrictors may cause rebound rhinorrhea (rhinitis medicamentosa) if used longer than 5 days.

Surgery. Cerebrospinal rhinorrhea may occur after sinus or cranial surgery.

Nursing considerations

■ Prepare the patient for X-rays of the sinuses or skull (if you suspect a skull fracture) or a computed tomography scan.

■ Administer an antihistamine, a decongestant, an analgesic, or an antipyretic, as ordered.

Patient teaching

■ Explain the disorder and treatment plan.

■ Advise the patient to drink plenty of fluids to thin secretions.

■ Explain the proper use of over-the-counter sprays.

 # Rhonchi

Rhonchi are continuous adventitious breath sounds detected by auscultation. They're usually louder and lower pitched than crackles—more like a hoarse moan or a deep snore—though they may be described as rattling, sonorous, bubbling, rumbling, or musical. However, sibilant rhonchi, or wheezes, are high-pitched.

Rhonchi are heard over large airways such as the trachea. They can occur in a patient with a pulmonary disorder when air flows through passages that have been narrowed by secretions, a tumor or foreign body, bronchospasm, or mucosal thickening. The resulting vibration of airway walls produces the rhonchi.

History and physical examination

If you auscultate rhonchi, take the patient's vital signs, including oxygen saturation, and be alert for signs of respiratory distress. Characterize the patient's respirations as rapid or slow, shallow or deep, and regular or irregular. Inspect the chest, noting accessory muscle use. Is the patient audibly wheezing or gurgling? Auscultate for other abnormal breath sounds, such as crackles and a pleural friction rub. If you detect these sounds, note their location. Are breath sounds diminished or absent? Next, percuss the chest. If the patient has a cough, note its frequency and characterize its sound. If it's productive, examine the sputum for color, odor, consistency, amount, and blood.

Ask related questions: Does the patient smoke? If so, obtain a history in pack-years. Has he recently lost weight or felt tired or weak? Does he have asthma or another pulmonary disorder? Is he taking any prescribed or over-the-counter medication?

During the examination, keep in mind that thick or excessive secretions, bronchospasm, or inflammation of mucous membranes may lead to airway obstruction. If necessary, suction the patient and keep equipment available for inserting an artificial airway. Keep a bronchodilator available to treat bronchospasm.

Medical causes

Asthma. An asthma attack can cause rhonchi, crackles and, commonly, wheezing. Other features include apprehension, a dry cough that later becomes productive, prolonged expirations, and intercostal and supraclavicular retractions on inspiration. The patient may also exhibit increased accessory muscle use, nasal flaring, tachypnea, tachycardia, diaphoresis, and flushing or cyanosis.

Bronchiectasis. Bronchiectasis causes lower-lobe rhonchi and crackles, which coughing may help relieve. Its classic sign is a cough that produces mucopurulent, foul-smelling and, possibly, bloody sputum. Other findings include fever, weight loss, exertional dyspnea, fatigue, malaise, halitosis, weakness, and late-stage clubbing.

Bronchitis. *Acute tracheobronchitis* produces sonorous rhonchi and wheezing due to bronchospasm or increased mucus in the airways. Related findings include chills, a sore throat, a low-grade fever (rising up to 102° F [38.9° C] in those with severe illness), muscle and back pain, and substernal tightness. A cough becomes productive as secretions increase.

With *chronic bronchitis,* auscultation may reveal scattered rhonchi, coarse crackles, wheezing, high-pitched piping sounds, and prolonged expirations. An early hacking cough later becomes productive. The patient also displays exertional dyspnea, increased accessory muscle use, barrel chest, cyanosis, tachypnea, and clubbing (a late sign).

Pneumonia. Bacterial pneumonia can cause rhonchi and a dry cough that later becomes productive. Related signs and symptoms—shaking chills, high fever, myalgia, headache, pleuritic chest pain, tachypnea, tachycardia, dyspnea, cyanosis, diaphoresis, decreased breath sounds, and fine crackles—develop suddenly.

Pulmonary coccidioidomycosis. Pulmonary coccidioidomycosis causes rhonchi and wheezing. Other features include cough with fever, occasional chills, pleuritic chest pain, a sore throat, headache, a backache, malaise, marked weakness, anorexia, hemoptysis, and an itchy macular rash.

Other causes

Diagnostic tests. Pulmonary function tests or bronchoscopy can loosen secretions and mucus, causing rhonchi.

Respiratory therapy. Respiratory therapy may produce rhonchi from loosened secretions and mucus.

Nursing considerations

- To ease the patient's breathing, place him in semi-Fowler's position.
- Administer an antibiotic, a bronchodilator, and an expectorant, as ordered.
- Provide humidification to thin secretions, relieve inflammation, and prevent drying.
- Perform pulmonary physiotherapy with postural drainage and percussion to loosen secretions.
- Use tracheal suctioning, if necessary, to help the patient clear secretions and to promote oxygenation and comfort.
- Promote coughing, deep breathing, and incentive spirometry.

- Prepare the patient for diagnostic tests, such as arterial blood gas analysis, pulmonary function studies, sputum analysis, and chest X-rays.

Patient teaching
- Explain the disorder and treatment plan.
- Demonstrate deep-breathing and coughing techniques.
- Explain to the patient the need for increased fluid intake.

S

Scotoma

A scotoma is an area of partial or complete blindness within an otherwise normal or slightly impaired visual field. Usually located within the central 30-degree area, the defect ranges from absolute blindness to a barely detectable loss of visual acuity. Typically, the patient can pinpoint the scotoma's location in the visual field. (See *Locating scotomas.*)

A scotoma can result from a retinal, choroid, or optic nerve disorder. It can be classified as absolute, relative, or scintillating. An absolute scotoma refers to the total inability to see all sizes of test objects used in mapping the visual field. A relative scotoma, in contrast, refers to the ability to see only large test objects. A scintillating scotoma refers to the flashes or bursts of light commonly seen during a migraine headache.

History and physical examination

Explore the patient's medical history, noting especially eye disorders, vision problems, or chronic systemic disorders. Find out if he takes medications or uses eyedrops.

Identify and characterize the scotoma, using such visual field tests as the tangent screen examination, the Goldmann perimeter test, and the automated perimetry test. Two other visual field tests—confrontation testing and the Amsler grid—may also help in identifying a scotoma.

Next, test the patient's visual acuity and inspect his pupils for size, equality, and reaction to light. An ophthalmoscopic examination and measurement of intraocular pressure are necessary.

Medical causes

Chorioretinitis. Inflammation of the choroid and retina produces a paracentral scotoma. Ophthalmoscopic examination reveals clouding and cells in the vitreous, subretinal hemorrhage, and neovascularization. The patient may have photophobia along with blurred vision.

Macular degeneration. Any degenerative process or disorder affecting the fovea centralis results in a central scotoma. Ophthalmoscopic examination reveals changes in the macular area. The patient may notice subtle changes in visual acuity, in color perception, and in the size and shape of objects.

Optic neuritis. Inflammation, degeneration, or demyelination of the optic nerve produces a central, circular, or centrocecal scotoma. The scotoma may be unilateral with involvement of one nerve, or bilateral with involvement of both nerves. It can vary in size, density, and symmetry. The patient may report

Locating scotomas

Scotomas, or "blind spots," are classified according to the affected area of the visual field. The normal scotoma—shown in the temporal region of the right eye—appears in black in all the illustrations.

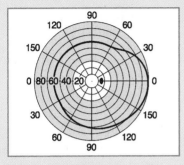

The *normally present scotoma* represents the position of the optic nerve head in the visual field. It appears between 10 and 20 degrees on this chart of the normal visual field.

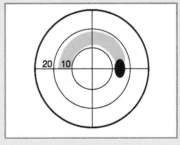

A *paracentral scotoma* affects an area of the visual field that's nasal or temporal to the point of central fixation.

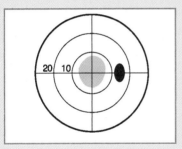

A *central scotoma* involves the point of central fixation. It's always associated with decreased visual acuity.

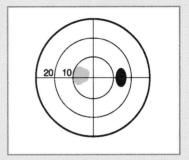

An *arcuate scotoma* arches around the fixation point, usually ending on the nasal side of the visual field.

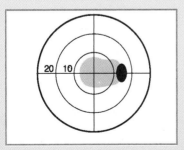

A *centrocecal scotoma* involves the point of central fixation and the area between the blind spot and the fixation point.

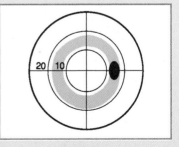

An *annular scotoma* forms a circular defect around the fixation point. It's common with retinal pigmentary degeneration.

severe vision loss or blurring, lasting up to 3 weeks, and pain—especially with eye movement. Common ophthalmoscopic findings include hyperemia of the optic disk, retinal vein distention, blurred disk margins, and filling of the physiologic cup.

Retinal pigmentary degeneration. Retinal pigmentary degeneration causes premature retinal cell changes leading to cell death. One disorder, retinitis pigmentosa, initially involves loss of peripheral rods; the resulting annular scotoma progresses concentrically until only a central field of vision (tunnel vision) remains. The earliest symptom—impaired night vision—appears during adolescence. Associated signs include narrowing of the retinal blood vessels and pallor of the optic disk. Eventually, with invasion of the macula, blindness may occur.

Nursing considerations

- Take measures to provide for the patient's safety.
- Administer the prescribed drugs.

Patient teaching

- Teach the patient with a disorder involving the fovea centralis (or the area surrounding it) to periodically use the Amsler grid to detect progression of macular degeneration.
- Emphasize the importance of compliance with drug therapy.
- Explain the underlying disorder and its treatments.
- Discuss assistive devices available to help the patient.
- Teach signs and symptoms that require immediate medical attention.

▎Scrotal swelling

Scrotal swelling occurs when a condition affecting the testicles, epididymis, or scrotal skin produces edema or a mass; the penis may be involved. Scrotal swelling can affect males of any age. It can be unilateral or bilateral and painful or painless.

The sudden onset of painful scrotal swelling suggests torsion of a testicle or testicular appendages, especially in a prepubescent male. This emergency requires immediate surgery to untwist and stabilize the spermatic cord or to remove the appendage.

ACTION STAT!

 If severe pain accompanies scrotal swelling, ask the patient when the swelling began. Using a Doppler stethoscope, evaluate blood flow to the testicle. If it's decreased or absent, suspect testicular torsion and prepare the patient for surgery. Withhold food and fluids, insert an I.V. catheter, and apply an ice pack to the scrotum to reduce pain and swelling. An attempt may be made to untwist the cord manually, but even if this is successful, the patient may still require surgery for stabilization.

History and physical examination

If the patient isn't in distress, proceed with the history. Ask about injury to the scrotum, urethral discharge, cloudy urine, increased urinary frequency, and dysuria. Is the patient sexually active? When was his last sexual contact? Does he have a history of sexually transmitted disease? Find out about recent illnesses, particularly mumps. Does he have a history of prostate surgery or prolonged catheterization? Does changing his body position or level of activity affect the swelling?

Take the patient's vital signs, especially noting fever, and palpate his abdomen for tenderness. Then examine the entire genital area. Assess the scrotum with the patient in a supine position and standing. Note its size and color. Is the swelling unilateral or bilateral? Do you see signs of trauma or bruising? Are there rashes or lesions present? Gently palpate the scrotum for a cyst or lump. Note especially tenderness or increased firmness. Check the testicles' position in the scrotum. Finally, transilluminate the scrotum to distinguish a fluid-filled cyst from a solid mass. (A solid mass can't be transilluminated.)

Medical causes

Epididymal cysts. Located in the head of the epididymis, epididymal cysts produce painless scrotal swelling.

Epididymitis. Key features of epididymitis are pain, extreme tenderness, and swelling in the groin and scrotum. The patient waddles to avoid pressure on the groin and scrotum during walking. He may have a high fever, malaise, a urethral discharge and cloudy urine, and lower abdominal pain on the affected side. His scrotal skin may be hot, red, dry, flaky, and thin.

Hydrocele. With a hydrocele, fluid accumulation produces gradual scrotal swelling that's usually painless. The scrotum may be soft and cystic or firm and tense. Palpation reveals a round, nontender scrotal mass.

Idiopathic scrotal edema. Swelling occurs quickly with idiopathic scrotal edema and usually disappears within 24 hours. The affected testicle is pink.

Orchitis (acute). Mumps, syphilis, or tuberculosis may precipitate orchitis, which causes sudden painful swelling of one or, at times, both testicles. Related findings include a hot, reddened scrotum; a fever of up to 104° F (40° C); chills; lower abdominal pain; nausea; vomiting; and extreme weakness. Urinary signs are usually absent.

Scrotal trauma. Blunt trauma causes scrotal swelling with bruising and severe pain. The scrotum may appear dark or bluish.

Spermatocele. Spermatocele is a usually painless cystic mass that lies above and behind the testicle and contains opaque fluid and sperm. Its onset may be acute or gradual. Less than 1 cm in diameter, it's movable and may be transilluminated.

Testicular torsion. Most common before puberty, testicular torsion is a urologic emergency that causes scrotal swelling; sudden, severe pain; and, possibly, elevation of the affected testicle within the scrotum. It may also cause nausea and vomiting.

Testicular tumor. Typically painless, smooth, and firm, a testicular tumor produces swelling and a sensation of excessive weight in the scrotum.

Torsion of a hydatid of Morgagni. Torsion of this small, pea-size cyst severs its blood supply, causing a hard, painful swelling on the testicle's upper pole.

Other causes

Surgery. An effusion of blood from surgery can produce a hematocele, leading to scrotal swelling.

Nursing considerations
- Place the patient on bed rest.
- Administer an antibiotic, if ordered.
- Provide adequate fluids, fiber, and stool softeners.
- Place a rolled towel between the patient's legs and under the scrotum for elevation to help reduce severe swelling.
- Apply ice packs to the scrotum.
- Administer an analgesic to relieve pain.
- Prepare the patient for needle aspiration of fluid-filled cysts and other diagnostic tests, such as lung tomography and a computed tomography scan of the abdomen, to rule out malignant tumors.

Patient teaching

■ Explain the disorder and treatment plan.

■ For mild or moderate swelling, advise the patient to wear a loose-fitting athletic supporter lined with a soft cotton dressing.

■ Tell the patient to use a sitz bath and apply heat or ice packs to decrease inflammation.

Seizures, absence

Absence seizures are benign, generalized seizures thought to originate subcortically. These brief episodes of unconsciousness usually last 3 to 20 seconds and can occur 100 or more times per day, causing periods of inattention. Absence seizures usually begin between ages 4 and 12. Their first sign may be deteriorating schoolwork and behavior. The cause of these seizures is unknown.

Absence seizures occur without warning. The patient suddenly stops all purposeful activity and stares blankly ahead, as if he were daydreaming. Absence seizures may produce automatisms, such as repetitive lip smacking, or mild clonic or myoclonic movements, including mild jerking of the eyelids. The patient may drop an object that he's holding, and muscle relaxation may cause him to drop his head or arms or to slump. After the attack, the patient resumes activity, typically unaware of the episode.

Absence status, a rare form of absence seizure, occurs as a prolonged absence seizure or as repeated episodes of these seizures. Usually not life-threatening, it occurs most commonly in patients who have previously experienced absence seizures.

History and physical examination

If you suspect a patient is having an absence seizure, evaluate its occurrence and duration by reciting a series of numbers and then asking him to repeat them after the attack ends. If the patient has had an absence seizure, he can't do this. Alternatively, if the seizures are occurring within minutes of each other, ask the patient to count for about 5 minutes. He'll stop counting during a seizure and resume when it's over. Look for accompanying automatisms. Find out if the family has noticed a change in behavior or deteriorating schoolwork.

Next, perform a complete neurologic examination.

Medical causes

Idiopathic epilepsy. Some forms of absence seizure are accompanied by learning disabilities.

Other causes

Drugs. Drugs that lower the threshold for seizures, such as alcohol, cocaine, penicillin in high doses, isoniazid, and phenothiazines may trigger seizures in patients with preexisting epilepsy.

Nursing considerations

■ Administer an anticonvulsant, as ordered.

■ Assess neurologic status, noting episodes of possible absence seizures.

Patient teaching

■ Teach the patient and family about the condition and its treatments.

■ Explain signs and symptoms that require immediate attention.

■ Emphasize the importance of follow-up medical care.

■ Discuss the need to wear medical identification.

Seizures, complex partial

A complex partial seizure occurs when a focal seizure begins in the temporal lobe and causes a partial alteration of consciousness—usually confusion. Psychomotor seizures can occur at any age, but their incidence usually increases during adolescence and adulthood. Two-thirds of patients also have generalized seizures.

An aura—usually a complex hallucination, illusion, or sensation—typically precedes a psychomotor seizure. The hallucination may be audiovisual (images with sounds), auditory (abnormal or normal sounds or voices from the patient's past), or olfactory (unpleasant smells, such as rotten eggs or burning materials). Other types of auras include sensations of déjà vu, unfamiliarity with surroundings, or depersonalization. The patient may become fearful or anxious, experience lip smacking, or have an unpleasant feeling in the epigastric region that rises toward the chest and throat. The patient usually recognizes the aura and lies down before losing consciousness.

A period of unresponsiveness follows the aura. The patient may experience automatisms, appear dazed and wander aimlessly, perform inappropriate acts (such as undressing in public), be unresponsive, utter incoherent phrases, or (rarely) go into a rage or tantrum. After the seizure, the patient is confused, drowsy, and doesn't remember the seizure. Behavioral automatisms rarely last longer than 5 minutes, but postseizure confusion, agitation, and amnesia may persist.

Between attacks, the patient may exhibit slow and rigid thinking, outbursts of anger and aggressiveness, tedious conversation, a preoccupation with naive philosophical ideas, a diminished libido, mood swings, and paranoid tendencies.

History and physical examination

If you witness a complex partial seizure, never attempt to restrain the patient. Instead, lead him gently to a safe area. (*Exception:* Don't approach him if he's angry or violent.) Calmly encourage him to sit down, and remain with him until he's fully alert. After the seizure, ask him if he experienced an aura. Record all observations and findings. Obtain a history. Has the patient experienced a seizure in the past? Has he had a recent head injury? Has he experienced any fever, headaches, or periods of confusion? Obtain a complete drug history. Take his vital signs and perform a complete neurologic examination.

Medical causes

Brain abscess. If the brain abscess is in the temporal lobe, complex partial seizures commonly occur after the abscess disappears. Related problems may include headache, nausea, vomiting, generalized seizures, and decreased level of consciousness (LOC). The patient may also develop central facial weakness, auditory receptive aphasia, hemiparesis, and ocular disturbances.

Head trauma. Severe trauma to the temporal lobe (especially from a penetrating injury) can produce complex partial seizures months or years later. The seizures may decrease in frequency and eventually stop. Head trauma also causes generalized seizures and behavior and personality changes.

Herpes simplex encephalitis. Herpes simplex virus commonly attacks the temporal lobe, resulting in complex partial seizures. Other features include fever, headache, coma, and generalized seizures.

Temporal lobe tumor. Complex partial seizures may be the first sign of a temporal lobe tumor. Other signs and symptoms include headache, pupillary changes, and mental dullness. Increased intracranial pressure may cause decreased LOC, vomiting and, possibly, papilledema.

Nursing considerations

- After the seizure, remain with the patient to reorient him to his surroundings and to protect him from injury.
- Keep the patient in bed until he's fully alert, and remove harmful objects from the area.
- Prepare the patient for diagnostic tests, such as EEG, computed tomography scan, or magnetic resonance imaging.

Patient teaching

- Explain the disorder and its treatment.
- Offer emotional support to the patient and his family, and teach them how to cope with seizures.
- Discuss with the patient and his family safety measures to take during a seizure.
- Emphasize compliance with drug therapy.
- Stress the importance of carrying medical identification.

Seizures, generalized tonic-clonic

Like other types of seizures, generalized tonic-clonic seizures are caused by the paroxysmal, uncontrolled discharge of central nervous system neurons, leading to neurologic dysfunction. Unlike most other types of seizures, however, this cerebral hyperactivity isn't confined to the original focus or to a localized area but extends to the entire brain.

A generalized tonic-clonic seizure may begin with or without an aura. As seizure activity spreads to the subcortical structures, the patient loses consciousness, falls, and may utter a loud cry that's precipitated by air rushing from the lungs through the vocal cords. His body stiffens (tonic phase), and then undergoes rapid, synchronous muscle jerking and hyperventilation (clonic phase). Tongue biting, incontinence, diaphoresis, profuse salivation, and signs of respiratory distress may also occur. The seizure usually stops after 2 to 5 minutes. The patient then regains consciousness but displays confusion. He may complain of headache, fatigue, muscle soreness, and arm and leg weakness.

Generalized tonic-clonic seizures usually occur singly. The patient may be asleep or awake and active. (See *What happens during a generalized tonic-clonic seizure.*) Possible complications include respiratory arrest due to airway obstruction from secretions, status epilepticus (occurring in 5% to 8% of patients), head or spinal injuries and bruises, Todd's paralysis and, rarely, cardiac arrest. Life-threatening status epilepticus is marked by prolonged seizure activity or by rapidly recurring seizures with no intervening periods of recovery. It's most commonly triggered by the abrupt discontinuation of anticonvulsant therapy.

Generalized seizures may be caused by a brain tumor, vascular disorder, head trauma, infection, metabolic defect, drug or alcohol withdrawal syndrome, exposure to toxins, or a genetic defect. Generalized seizures may also result from a focal seizure. With recurring seizures, or epilepsy, the cause may be unknown.

ACTION STAT!

 If you witness the beginning of the patient's seizure, first check his airway, breathing, and circulation, and ensure that the cause isn't asystole or an obstructed airway. Stay with the patient and ensure a patent air-

What happens during a generalized tonic-clonic seizure

Before the seizure

Prodromal signs and symptoms, such as myoclonic jerks, a throbbing headache, and mood changes, may occur over several hours or days. The patient may have premonitions of the seizure. For example, he may report an *aura*, such as seeing a flashing light or smelling a characteristic odor.

During the seizure

If a generalized seizure begins with an aura, this indicates that irritability in a specific area of the brain quickly became widespread. Common auras include palpitations, epigastric distress rapidly rising to the throat, head or eye turning, and sensory hallucinations.

Next, *loss of consciousness* occurs as a sudden discharge of intense electrical activity overwhelms the brain's subcortical center. The patient falls and experiences brief, bilateral myoclonic contractures. Air forced through spasmodic vocal cords may produce a birdlike, piercing cry.

During the *tonic phase,* skeletal muscles contract for 10 to 20 seconds. The patient's eyelids are drawn up, his arms are flexed, and his legs are extended. His mouth opens wide, then snaps shut; he may bite his tongue. His respirations cease because of respiratory muscle spasm, and initial pallor of the skin and mucous membranes (the result of impaired venous return) changes to cyanosis secondary to apnea. The patient arches his back and slowly lowers his arms (as shown below). Other effects include dilated, nonreactive pupils; greatly increased heart rate and blood pressure; increased salivation and tracheobronchial secretions; and profuse diaphoresis.

During the *clonic phase,* lasting about 60 seconds, mild trembling progresses to violent contractures or jerks. Other motor activity includes facial grimaces (with possible tongue biting) and violent expiration of bloody, foamy saliva from clonic contractures of thoracic cage muscles. Clonic jerks slowly decrease in intensity and frequency. The patient is still apneic.

After the seizure

The patient's movements gradually cease, and he becomes unresponsive to external stimuli. Other post-seizure features include stertorous respirations from increased tracheobronchial secretions, equal or unequal pupils (but becoming reactive), and urinary incontinence due to brief muscle relaxation. After about 5 minutes, the patient's level of consciousness increases, and he appears confused and disoriented. His muscle tone, heart rate, and blood pressure return to normal.

After several hours' sleep, the patient awakens exhausted and may have a headache, sore muscles, and amnesia about the seizure.

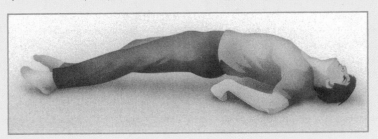

way. Focus your care on observing the seizure and protecting the patient. Place a towel under his head to prevent injury, loosen his clothing, and move any sharp or hard objects out of his way. Never try to restrain the patient or force a hard object into his mouth; you might chip his teeth or fracture his jaw. Only at the start of the ictal phase can you safely insert a soft object into his mouth.

If possible, turn the patient to one side *during* the seizure to allow secretions to drain and to prevent aspiration. Otherwise, do this at the end of the clonic phase when respirations return. (If they fail to return, check for airway obstruction and suction the patient if necessary. Cardiopulmonary resuscitation, endotracheal intubation, and mechanical ventilation may be needed.)

Protect the patient after the seizure by providing a safe area in which he can rest. As he awakens, reassure and reorient him. Check his vital signs and neurologic status. Be sure to carefully record these data and your observations during the seizure.

If the seizure lasts longer than 4 minutes or if a second seizure occurs before full recovery from the first, suspect status epilepticus. Establish an airway, insert an I.V. catheter, give supplemental oxygen, and begin cardiac monitoring. Draw blood for appropriate studies. Turn the patient on his side, with his head in a semi-dependent position, to drain secretions and prevent aspiration. Periodically turn him to the opposite side, check his arterial blood gas levels for hypoxemia, and administer oxygen by mask, increasing the flow rate if necessary. Administer diazepam or lorazepam by slow I.V. push, repeated two or three times at 10- to 20-minute intervals, to stop the seizures. If the patient isn't known to have epilepsy, an I.V. bolus of dextrose 50% (50 ml) with thiamine (100 mg) may be ordered. Dextrose may stop the seizures if the patient has hypoglycemia.

History and physical examination

If you didn't witness the patient's seizure, obtain a description from his companion. Ask when the seizure started and how long it lasted. Did the patient report unusual sensations before the seizure began? Did the seizure start in one area of the body and spread, or did it affect the entire body right away? Did the patient fall on a hard surface? Did his eyes or head turn? Did he turn blue? Did he lose bladder control? Did he have other seizures before recovering?

If the patient may have sustained a head injury, observe him closely for loss of consciousness, unequal or nonreactive pupils, and focal neurologic signs. Does he complain of headache and muscle soreness? Is he increasingly difficult to arouse when you check on him at 20-minute intervals? Examine his arms, legs, and face (including tongue) for injury, residual paralysis, or limb weakness.

Next, obtain a history. Has the patient ever had generalized or focal seizures before? If so, do they occur frequently? Do other family members also have them? Is the patient receiving drug therapy? Is he compliant? Also, ask about sleep deprivation and emotional or physical stress at the time the seizure occurred.

Next, assess the patient's level of consciousness (LOC) and proceed with a complete neurologic examination.

Medical causes

Brain abscess. Generalized seizures may occur in the acute stage of a brain abscess formation or after the abscess disappears. Depending on the size and location of the abscess, a decreased LOC varies from drowsiness to deep stupor. Early signs and symptoms reflect increased intracranial pressure (ICP) and include a constant headache, nausea, vomiting, and focal seizures. Typical later features include ocular disturbances, such as nystagmus, impaired vision, and unequal pupils. Other findings vary with the abscess site but may include aphasia, hemiparesis, abnormal behavior, and personality changes.

Brain tumor. Generalized seizures may occur with a brain tumor, depending on it's location and type. Other findings include a slowly decreasing LOC, a morning headache, dizziness, confusion, focal seizures, vision loss, motor and sensory disturbances, aphasia, and ataxia. Later findings include papilledema, vomiting, increased systolic blood pressure, widening pulse pressure and, eventually, a decorticate posture.

Chronic renal failure. End-stage renal failure produces the rapid onset of twitching, trembling, myoclonic jerks, and generalized seizures. Related signs and symptoms include anuria or oliguria, fatigue, malaise, irritability, decreased mental acuity, muscle cramps, peripheral neuropathies, anorexia, and constipation or diarrhea. Integumentary effects include skin color changes (yellow, brown, or bronze), pruritus, and uremic frost. Other effects include an ammonia breath odor, nausea and vomiting, ecchymoses, petechiae, GI bleeding, mouth and gum ulcers, hypertension, and Kussmaul's respirations.

Eclampsia. Generalized seizures are a hallmark of eclampsia. Related findings include a severe frontal headache, nausea and vomiting, vision disturbances, increased blood pressure, a fever of up to 104° F (40° C), peripheral edema, and sudden weight gain. The patient may also exhibit oliguria, irritability, hyperactive deep tendon reflexes (DTRs), and decreased LOC.

Encephalitis. Seizures are an early sign of encephalitis, indicating a poor prognosis; they may also occur after recovery as a result of residual damage. Other findings include fever, headache, photophobia, nuchal rigidity, neck pain, vomiting, aphasia, ataxia, hemiparesis, nystagmus, irritability, cranial nerve palsies (causing facial weakness, ptosis, and dysphagia), and myoclonic jerks.

Epilepsy (idiopathic). In most cases, the cause of recurrent seizures is unknown.

Head trauma. With severe head trauma, generalized seizures may occur at the time of injury. (Months later, focal seizures may occur.) Severe head trauma may also cause decreased LOC, leading to coma; soft-tissue injury of the face, head, or neck; clear or bloody drainage from the mouth, nose, or ears; facial edema; bony deformity of the face, head, or neck; Battle's sign; and a lack of response to oculocephalic and oculovestibular stimulation. Motor and sensory deficits may occur along with altered respirations. Examination may reveal signs of increasing ICP, such as a decreased response to painful stimuli, nonreactive pupils, bradycardia, increased systolic pressure, and widening pulse pressure. If the patient is conscious, he may exhibit visual deficits, behavioral changes, and headache.

Hepatic encephalopathy. Generalized seizures may occur late in hepatic encephalopathy. Associated late-stage findings in the comatose patient include fetor hepaticus, asterixis, hyperactive DTRs, and a positive Babinski's sign.

Hypoglycemia. Generalized seizures usually occur with severe hypoglycemia, accompanied by blurred or double vision, motor weakness, hemiplegia, trembling, excessive diaphoresis, tachycardia, myoclonic twitching, and decreased LOC.

Hyponatremia. Seizures may develop when the serum sodium level falls below 125 mEq/L, especially if the sodium loss is rapid. Hyponatremia also causes orthostatic hypotension, headache, muscle twitching and weakness, fatigue, oliguria or anuria, cold and clammy skin, decreased skin turgor, irritability, lethargy, confusion, and stupor or coma. Excessive thirst, tachycardia, nausea, vomiting, and abdominal cramps may also occur. Severe hyponatremia may cause cyanosis and vasomotor collapse, with a thready pulse.

Hypoparathyroidism. Chronic hypoparathyroidism produces neuromuscular irritability and hyperactive DTRs. Worsening tetany causes generalized seizures.

Hypoxic encephalopathy. Besides generalized seizures, hypoxic encephalopathy may produce myoclonic jerks and coma. Later, if the patient has recovered, dementia, visual agnosia, choreoathetosis, and ataxia may occur.

Neurofibromatosis. Multiple brain lesions from neurofibromatosis cause focal and generalized seizures. Inspection reveals café-au-lait spots, multiple skin tumors, scoliosis, and kyphoscoliosis. Related findings include dizziness, ataxia, monocular blindness, and nystagmus.

Stroke. Seizures (focal more commonly than generalized) may occur within 6 months of an ischemic stroke. Associated signs and symptoms vary with the location and extent of brain damage. They include decreased LOC, contralateral hemiplegia, dysarthria, dysphagia, ataxia, unilateral sensory loss, apraxia, agnosia, and aphasia. The patient may also develop visual deficits, memory loss, poor judgment, personality changes, emotional lability, urine retention or urinary incontinence, constipation, headache, and vomiting.

Other causes

Arsenic poisoning. Besides generalized seizures, arsenic poisoning may cause a garlicky breath odor, increased salivation, and generalized pruritus. GI effects include diarrhea, nausea, vomiting, and severe abdominal pain. Related effects include diffuse hyperpigmentation; sharply defined edema of the eyelids, face, and ankles; paresthesia of the extremities; alopecia; irritated mucous membranes; weakness; muscle aches; and peripheral neuropathy.

Barbiturate withdrawal. In chronically intoxicated patients, barbiturate withdrawal may produce generalized seizures 2 to 4 days after the last dose. Status epilepticus is possible.

Diagnostic tests. Contrast agents used in radiologic tests may cause generalized seizures.

Drugs. Toxic blood levels of some drugs, such as theophylline, lidocaine, meperidine, penicillins, and cimetidine, may cause generalized seizures. Phenothiazines, tricyclic antidepressants, amphetamines, isoniazid, and vincristine may cause seizures in patients with preexisting epilepsy.

Nursing considerations

- Institute seizure precautions.
- Closely monitor the patient after the seizure for recurring seizure activity.
- Prepare him for a computed tomography scan or magnetic resonance imaging and EEG.
- Administer anticonvulsants, as ordered, and monitor drug levels.

Patient teaching

- Explain the disorder and treatment plan.
- Teach the family how to observe and record seizure activity.

- Emphasize the importance of compliance with drug therapy and follow-up appointments.
- Tell the patient to carry medical identification.

Seizures, simple partial

Resulting from an irritable focus in the cerebral cortex, simple partial seizures typically last about 30 seconds and don't alter the patient's level of consciousness (LOC). The type and pattern reflect the location of the irritable focus. Simple partial seizures may be classified as motor (including jacksonian seizures and epilepsia partialis continua) or somatosensory (including visual, olfactory, and auditory seizures).

A *focal motor seizure* is a series of unilateral clonic (muscle jerking) and tonic (muscle stiffening) movements of one part of the body. The patient's head and eyes characteristically turn away from the hemispheric focus—usually the frontal lobe near the motor strip. A tonic-clonic contraction of the trunk or extremities may follow.

A *jacksonian motor seizure* typically begins with a tonic contraction of a finger, the corner of the mouth, or one foot. Clonic movements follow, spreading to other muscles on the same side of the body, moving up the arm or leg, and eventually involving the whole side. Alternatively, clonic movements may spread to the opposite side, becoming generalized and leading to loss of consciousness. In the postictal phase, the patient may experience paralysis (Todd's paralysis) in the affected limbs, usually resolving within 24 hours.

Epilepsia partialis continua causes clonic twitching of one muscle group, usually in the face, arm, or leg. Twitching occurs every few seconds and persists for hours, days, or months without spreading. Spasms usually affect the distal arm and leg muscles more than the proximal ones; in the face, they affect the corner of the mouth, one or both eyelids and, occasionally, the neck or trunk muscles unilaterally.

A *focal somatosensory seizure* affects a localized body area on one side. Usually, this type of seizure initially causes numbness, tingling, or crawling or "electric" sensations; occasionally, it causes pain or burning sensations in the lips, fingers, or toes. A visual seizure involves sensations of darkness or of stationary or moving lights or spots, usually red at first, then blue, green, and yellow. It can affect both visual fields or the visual field on the side opposite the lesion. The irritable focus is in the occipital lobe. In contrast, the irritable focus in an auditory or olfactory seizure is in the temporal lobe. (See *Body functions affected by focal seizures,* page 558.)

History and physical examination

Be sure to record the patient's seizure activity in detail; your data may be critical in locating the lesion in the brain. Does the patient turn his head and eyes? If so, to what side? Where does movement first start? Does it spread? Because a partial seizure may become generalized, you'll need to watch closely for loss of consciousness, bilateral tonicity and clonicity, cyanosis, tongue biting, and urinary incontinence. (See "Seizures, generalized tonic-clonic," page 552.)

After the seizure, ask the patient to describe exactly what he remembers, if anything, about the seizure. Check the patient's LOC, and test for residual deficits (such as weakness in the involved extremity) and sensory disturbances.

Then obtain a history. Ask the patient what happened before the seizure. Can he describe an aura or did he recog-

Body functions affected by focal seizures

The site of the irritable focus determines which body functions are affected by a focal seizure, as shown in this illustration.

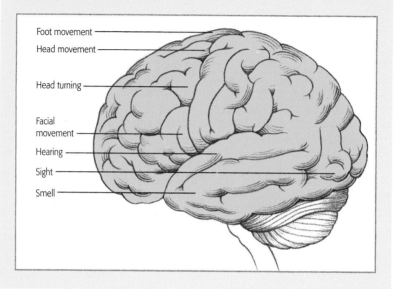

nize its onset? If so, how—by a smell, a vision disturbance, or a sound or visceral phenomenon such as an unusual sensation in his stomach? How does this seizure compare with others he has had?

Also, explore fully any history—recent or remote—of head trauma. Check for a history of stroke or recent infection, especially with fever, headache, or stiff neck.

Perform a complete neurologic examination.

Medical causes

Brain abscess. Seizures can occur in the acute stage of a brain abscess formation or after resolution of the abscess. A decreased LOC varies from drowsiness to deep stupor. Early signs and symptoms reflect increased intracranial pressure and include a constant, intractable headache; nausea; and vomiting. Later signs and symptoms include ocular disturbances, such as nystagmus, decreased visual acuity, and unequal pupils. Other findings vary according to the abscess site and may include aphasia, hemiparesis, and personality changes.

Brain tumor. Focal seizures are commonly the earliest indicators of a brain tumor. The patient may report a morning headache, dizziness, confusion, vision loss, and motor and sensory disturbances. He may also develop aphasia, generalized seizures, ataxia, decreased LOC, papilledema, vomiting, increased systolic blood pressure, and widening pulse pressure. Eventually, he may assume a decorticate posture.

Head trauma. Any head injury can cause seizures, but penetrating wounds are characteristically associated with focal seizures. The seizures usually begin 3 to 15 months after injury, decrease in frequency after several years, and eventually stop. The patient may develop generalized seizures and decreased LOC that may progress to coma.

Stroke. A major cause of seizures, a stroke may induce focal seizures up to 6 months after its onset. Related effects depend on the type and extent of the stroke, but may include decreased LOC, contralateral hemiplegia, dysarthria, dysphagia, ataxia, unilateral sensory loss, apraxia, agnosia, and aphasia. A stroke may also cause visual deficits, memory loss, poor judgment, personality changes, emotional lability, headache, urinary incontinence or urine retention, and vomiting. It may result in generalized seizures.

Nursing considerations

- Institute seizure precautions.
- Stay with the patient during seizure activity and reassure him.
- Monitor neurologic status.
- Prepare the patient for such diagnostic tests as a computed tomography scan and EEG.

Patient teaching

- Explain the disorder and treatment plan.
- Explain that no emergency care is necessary during a focal seizure, unless it progresses to a generalized seizure. (See "Seizures, generalized tonic-clonic," page 552.)
- Teach the family how to record seizures.
- Tell the patient to carry medical identification.

▌Setting-sun sign
[Sunset eyes]

Setting-sun sign refers to the downward deviation of an infant's or a young child's eyes as a result of pressure on cranial nerves III, IV, and VI. With this late and

ominous sign of increased intracranial pressure (ICP), both eyes are rotated downward, typically revealing an area of sclera above the irises; occasionally, the irises appear to be forced outward. Pupils are sluggish, responding to light unequally. (See *Identifying setting-sun sign*.)

The infant with increased ICP is typically irritable and lethargic and feeds poorly. Changes in the level of consciousness (LOC), lower-extremity spasticity, and opisthotonos may also be obvious. Increased ICP typically results from space-occupying lesions—such as tumors—or from an accumulation of fluid in the brain's ventricular system, as occurs with hydrocephalus. It also results from intracranial bleeding or cere-

---

 ASSESSMENT TIP

Identifying setting-sun sign

With this late sign of increased intracranial pressure in an infant or a young child, pressure on cranial nerves III, IV, and VI forces the eyes downward, revealing a rim of sclera above the irises.

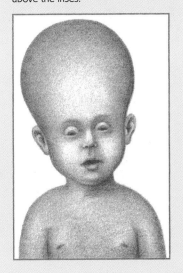

bral edema. Other signs include a globular appearance of the head, a loss of upgaze, and distended scalp veins.

Setting-sun sign may be intermittent—for example, it may disappear when the infant is upright because this position slightly reduces ICP. The sign may be elicited in a healthy infant younger than age 4 weeks by suddenly changing his head position, and in a healthy infant up to age 9 months by shining a bright light into his eyes and removing it quickly.

History and physical examination

If you observe setting-sun sign in an infant, evaluate his neurologic status; then obtain a brief history from his parents. Has the infant experienced a fall or even a minor trauma? When did this sign appear? Ask about early nonspecific signs of increasing ICP: Has the infant's sucking reflex diminished? Is he irritable, restless, or unusually tired? Does he cry when moved? Is his cry high-pitched? Has he vomited recently?

Next, perform a physical examination, keeping in mind that neurologic responses are primarily reflexive during early infancy. Assess the infant's LOC. Is he awake, irritable, or lethargic? Keeping in mind his age and level of development, try to determine his ability to reach for a bright object or turn toward the sound of a music box. Observe his posture for normal flexion and extension or opisthotonos. Examine muscle tone, and observe for seizure automatisms.

Examine the infant's anterior fontanel for bulging, measure his head circumference and compare it with previous results, and observe his breathing pattern. (Cheyne-Stokes respirations may accompany increased ICP.) Also, check his pupillary response to light: Unilateral or bilateral dilation occurs as ICP rises. Finally, elicit reflexes that are diminished in increased ICP, especially Moro reflex. Keep endotracheal (ET) intubation equipment available.

Medical causes

Increased ICP. Transient or intermittent setting-sun sign usually occurs late in the infant with increased ICP. He may have bulging, widened fontanels, an increased head circumference, and widened sutures. He may also exhibit decreased LOC, behavioral changes, a high-pitched cry, pupillary abnormalities, and impaired motor movement as ICP increases. Other findings include increased systolic pressure, widened pulse pressure, bradycardia, changes in breathing pattern, vomiting, and seizures as ICP increases.

Nursing considerations

- Monitor the patient's vital signs and neurologic status.
- Elevate the head of the crib to at least 30 degrees, and monitor intake and output.
- Monitor ICP, restrict fluids, and insert an I.V. catheter to administer a diuretic.
- For severely increased ICP, prepare for ET intubation and mechanical hyperventilation to reduce serum carbon dioxide levels and constrict cerebral vessels.
- Anticipate therapy to induce a barbiturate coma or hypothermia therapy to lower the metabolic rate.
- Maintain a calm environment.
- Perform nursing duties judiciously because procedures may further increase ICP.
- Encourage the parents' help in calming the infant, and offer them emotional support.

Patient teaching

- Explain the underlying condition and its treatment to the patient's parents.

- Prepare the child and his family for surgical management of increased ICP and hydrocephalus, as appropriate.

Skin, clammy

Clammy skin—moist, cool, and usually pale—is a sympathetic response to stress, which triggers release of the hormones epinephrine and norepinephrine. These hormones cause cutaneous vasoconstriction and secretion of cold sweat from eccrine glands, particularly on the palms, forehead, and soles.

Clammy skin typically accompanies shock, acute hypoglycemia, anxiety reactions, arrhythmias, and heat exhaustion. It also occurs as a vasovagal reaction to severe pain associated with nausea, anorexia, epigastric distress, hyperpnea, tachypnea, weakness, confusion, tachycardia, and pupillary dilation or a combination of these findings. Marked bradycardia and syncope may follow.

History and physical examination

If you detect clammy skin, remember that rapid evaluation and intervention are paramount. (See *Clammy skin: A key finding,* page 562.) Ask the patient if he has a history of type 1 diabetes mellitus or a cardiac disorder. Is he taking medications, especially an antiarrhythmic? Is he experiencing pain, chest pressure, nausea, or epigastric distress? Does he feel weak? Does he have a dry mouth? Does he have diarrhea or increased urination?

Next, take the patient's vital signs and pulse oximetry. Examine the pupils for dilation and check his level of consciousness. Note respiratory rate. Assess for respiratory distress. Auscultate the heart and lungs. Place the patient on a cardiac monitor and assess heart

rhythm. Also, check for abdominal distention and increased muscle tension.

Medical causes

Anxiety. An acute anxiety attack commonly produces cold, clammy skin on the forehead, palms, and soles. Other features include pallor, a dry mouth, tachycardia or bradycardia, palpitations, and hypertension or hypotension. The patient may also develop tremors, breathlessness, headache, muscle tension, nausea, vomiting, abdominal distention, diarrhea, increased urination, and sharp chest pain.

Arrhythmias. Cardiac arrhythmias may produce generalized cool, clammy skin along with mental status changes, dizziness, and hypotension.

Cardiogenic shock. Generalized cool, moist, pale skin accompanies confusion, restlessness, hypotension, tachycardia, tachypnea, narrowing pulse pressure, cyanosis, and oliguria.

Heat exhaustion. In the acute stage of heat exhaustion, generalized cold, clammy skin accompanies an ashen appearance, headache, confusion, syncope, giddiness and, possibly, a subnormal temperature, with mild heat exhaustion. The patient may exhibit a rapid and thready pulse, nausea, vomiting, tachypnea, oliguria, thirst, muscle cramps, and hypotension.

Hypoglycemia (acute). Generalized cool, clammy skin or diaphoresis may accompany irritability, tremors, palpitations, hunger, headache, tachycardia, and anxiety. Central nervous system disturbances include blurred vision, diplopia, confusion, motor weakness, hemiplegia, and coma. These signs and symptoms typically resolve after the patient is given glucose.

Hypovolemic shock. With hypovolemic shock, generalized pale, cold, clammy skin accompanies a subnormal

▬▬ Action stat!

 Clammy skin: A key finding

Be alert for clammy skin because it commonly accompanies emergency conditions, such as shock, acute hypoglycemia, and arrhythmias. To know what to do, review these typical clinical situations.

You detect clammy skin in a patient who appears anxious and restless.

▼

Quickly take his vital signs, noting tachypnea, hypotension, and a weak, irregular pulse. If present:

▼

Suspect shock.

▼

Place the patient in a supine position in bed. Elevate his legs 20 to 30 degrees to promote perfusion to vital organs.

▼

Insert an I.V. catheter for administration of drugs, fluids, or blood. Also, give supplemental oxygen and begin cardiac monitoring.

You detect clammy skin and possible tremors in a patient who appears irritable, anxious, and confused. He may also be difficult to arouse and report persistent hunger.

▼

Quickly take his vital signs, which will typically be normal. A vagal reaction to the stress of hypoglycemia may cause hypotension and tachycardia. If present:

▼

Suspect acute hypoglycemia.

▼

Immediately draw blood for glucose studies, and test a drop with a glucose reagent strip. Insert an I.V. catheter, and give a 50-ml bolus of dextrose 50%. Also, begin cardiac monitoring.

You detect clammy skin in a patient with changes in mental status such as confusion.

▼

Quickly take his vital signs, noting hypotension and changes in pulse rate and rhythm. If present:

▼

Suspect an arrhythmia.

▼

Insert an I.V. catheter and administer an antiarrhythmic. Also, give supplemental oxygen and begin cardiac monitoring.

---

body temperature, hypotension with narrowing pulse pressure, tachycardia, tachypnea, and a rapid, thready pulse. Other findings are flat neck veins, an increased capillary refill time, decreased urine output, confusion, and decreased level of consciousness.

Septic shock. The cold shock stage causes generalized cold, clammy skin. Associated findings include a rapid and thready pulse, severe hypotension, persistent oliguria or anuria, and respiratory failure.

Nursing considerations
- Take the patient's vital signs frequently.
- Monitor the patient's intake and output.
- Provide measures to correct the underlying condition. For example, if clammy skin occurs with an anxiety reaction or

pain, offer the patient emotional support, administer pain medication, and provide a quiet environment.

Patient teaching
- Explain the underlying disorder and its treatment.
- Orient the patient to the intensive care unit.
- Explain any diagnostic tests or procedures.

Skin, mottled

Mottled skin is patchy discoloration indicating primary or secondary changes of the deep, middle, or superficial dermal blood vessels. It can result from a hematologic, immune, or connective tissue disorder; chronic occlusive arterial disease; dysproteinemia; immobility; exposure to heat or cold; or shock. Mottled skin can be a normal reaction such as the diffuse mottling that occurs when exposure to cold causes venous stasis in cutaneous blood vessels (cutis marmorata).

Mottling that occurs with other signs and symptoms usually affects the extremities, typically indicating restricted blood flow. For example, livedo reticularis, a characteristic network pattern of reddish blue discoloration, occurs when vasospasm of the mid-dermal blood vessels slows local blood flow in dilated superficial capillaries and small veins. Shock causes mottling from systemic vasoconstriction.

History and physical examination
Mottled skin may indicate an emergency condition requiring rapid evaluation and intervention. (See *Mottled skin: Knowing what to do*.) However, if the patient isn't in distress, obtain a history. Ask if the mottling began suddenly or gradually. What precipitated it? How long has he had it? Does anything make it better? Does anything make it worse? Does the patient have other symptoms, such as pain, numbness, or tingling in an extremity? If so, do they disappear with temperature changes?

Take the patient's vital signs. Observe the patient's skin color, and palpate his arms and legs for skin texture, swelling, and temperature differences between ex-

---

ACTION STAT!

 ## Mottled skin: Knowing what to do

If the patient's skin is pale, cool, clammy, and mottled at the elbows and knees or all over, he may be developing *hypovolemic* shock. Quickly take his vital signs, and be sure to note tachycardia or a weak, thready pulse. Observe the neck for flattened veins. Does the patient appear anxious?

If you detect these signs and symptoms, place the patient in a supine position in bed with his legs elevated 20 to 30 degrees. Administer oxygen by nasal cannula or face mask, and begin cardiac monitoring. Insert a large-bore I.V. catheter for rapid fluid or blood product administration, and prepare to insert a central catheter or a pulmonary artery catheter. Also prepare to insert an indwelling urinary catheter to monitor urine output.

Localized mottling in a pale, cool extremity that the patient says feels painful, numb, and tingling may signal acute arterial occlusion. Immediately check the patient's distal pulses: If they're absent or diminished, you'll need to insert an I.V. catheter in an unaffected extremity, and prepare the patient for arteriography or immediate surgery.

tremities. Check the capillary refill time. Also, palpate for the presence (or absence) of pulses and for their quality. Note breaks in the skin, muscle appearance, and hair distribution. Also, assess motor and sensory function.

Medical causes

Acrocyanosis. With acrocyanosis, anxiety or exposure to cold can cause vasospasm in small cutaneous arterioles. This results in persistent symmetrical blue and red mottling of the affected hands, feet, and nose.

Arterial occlusion (acute). Initial signs of acute arterial occlusion include skin temperature and color changes. Pallor may change to blotchy cyanosis and livedo reticularis. Color and temperature demarcation develop at the level of obstruction. Other effects include sudden onset of pain in the extremity and, possibly, paresthesia, paresis, and a sensation of cold in the affected area. Examination reveals diminished or absent pulses, cool extremities, an increased capillary refill time, pallor, and diminished reflexes.

Arteriosclerosis obliterans. Atherosclerotic buildup narrows intra-arterial lumina, resulting in reduced blood flow through the affected artery. Obstructed blood flow to the extremities (most commonly the legs) produces such peripheral signs and symptoms as leg pallor, cyanosis, blotchy erythema, and livedo reticularis. Related findings include intermittent claudication (most common symptom), diminished or absent pedal pulses, and leg coolness. Other symptoms include coldness and paresthesia.

Buerger's disease. Buerger's disease produces unilateral or asymmetrical color changes and mottling, particularly livedo networking in the lower extremities. It also typically causes intermittent claudication and erythema along ex-

tremity blood vessels. During exposure to cold, the feet are cold, cyanotic, and numb; later they're hot, red, and tingling. Other findings include impaired peripheral pulses and peripheral neuropathy. Buerger's disease is typically exacerbated by smoking.

Cryoglobulinemia. Cryoglobulinemia causes patchy livedo reticularis, petechiae, and ecchymoses. Other findings include fever, chills, urticaria, melena, skin ulcers, epistaxis, Raynaud's phenomenon, eye hemorrhages, hematuria, and gangrene.

Hypovolemic shock. Vasoconstriction from hypovolemic shock commonly produces skin mottling, initially in the knees and elbows. As shock worsens, mottling becomes generalized. Early signs include a sudden onset of pallor, cool skin, restlessness, thirst, tachypnea, and slight tachycardia. As shock progresses, associated findings include cool, clammy skin; a rapid, thready pulse; hypotension; narrowed pulse pressure; decreased urine output; subnormal temperature; confusion; and decreased level of consciousness.

Livedo reticularis (idiopathic or primary). With livedo reticularis, symmetrical, diffuse mottling can involve the hands, feet, arms, legs, buttocks, and trunk. Initially, networking is intermittent and most pronounced on exposure to cold or stress; eventually, mottling persists even with warming.

Periarteritis nodosa. Skin findings in periarteritis nodosa include asymmetrical, patchy livedo reticularis, palpable nodules along the path of medium-sized arteries, erythema, purpura, muscle wasting, ulcers, gangrene, peripheral neuropathy, fever, weight loss, and malaise.

Polycythemia vera. Polycythemia vera produces livedo reticularis, hemangiomas, purpura, rubor, ulcerative nodules, and scleroderma-like lesions. Other symptoms include headache, a vague feeling of fullness in the head, dizziness, vertigo, vision disturbances, dyspnea, and aquagenic pruritus.

Systemic lupus erythematosus (SLE). SLE can cause livedo reticularis, most commonly on the outer arms. Other signs and symptoms include a butterfly rash, nondeforming joint pain and stiffness, photosensitivity, Raynaud's phenomenon, patchy alopecia, seizures, fever, anorexia, weight loss, lymphadenopathy, and emotional lability.

Other causes

Drugs. Vasoconstrictors administered at a high dose can cause mottling of the extremities.

Immobility. Prolonged immobility may cause bluish mottling, most noticeably in dependent extremities.

Thermal exposure. Prolonged thermal exposure, as from a heating pad or hot water bottle, may cause erythema ab igne—a localized, reticulated, brown-to-red mottling.

Nursing considerations

- Provide care to treat the patient's underlying condition.
- Monitor vital signs, especially noting blood pressure.
- Monitor the patient's skin for changes in the mottled appearance.
- Monitor pulses, noting the strength of impulse.

Patient teaching

- Teach the patient to avoid tight clothing and overexposure to cold or to heating devices, such as hot water bottles and heating pads.
- Discuss treatment of the underlying condition.

Skin, scaly

Scaly skin results when cells of the uppermost skin layer (stratum corneum) desiccate and shed, causing excessive accumulation of loosely adherent flakes of normal or abnormal keratin. Normally, skin cell loss is imperceptible; the appearance of scale indicates increased cell proliferation secondary to altered keratinization.

Scaly skin varies in texture from fine and delicate to branlike, coarse, or stratified. Scales are typically dry, brittle, and shiny, but they can be greasy and dull. Their color ranges from whitish gray, yellow, or brown to a silvery sheen.

Usually benign, scaly skin occurs with fungal, bacterial, and viral infections (cutaneous or systemic), lymphomas, and lupus erythematosus; it's also common in those with inflammatory skin disease. A form of scaly skin—generalized fine desquamation—commonly follows prolonged febrile illness, sunburn, and thermal burns. Red patches of scaly skin that appear or worsen in winter may result from dry skin (or from actinic keratosis, common in elderly patients). Certain drugs also cause scaly skin. Aggravating factors include cold, heat, immobility, and frequent bathing.

History and physical examination

Begin the history by asking how long the patient has had scaly skin and whether he has had it before. Where did it first appear? Did a lesion or skin eruption, such as erythema, precede it? Has the patient used a new or different topical skin product recently? How often does he bathe? Has he had recent joint pain, illness, or malaise? Ask the patient about work exposure to chemicals, use of prescribed drugs, and a family history of skin disorders. Find out what kinds of soap, detergents, dryer sheets, cosmetics, skin lotion, and hair preparations he uses.

Next, examine the entire skin surface. Is it dry, oily, moist, or greasy? Observe the general pattern of skin lesions, and record their location. Note their color, shape, and size. Are they thick or fine? Do they itch? Does the patient have other lesions besides scaly skin? Examine the mucous membranes of his mouth, lips, and nose, and inspect his ears, hair, and nails. Then assess the skin over the remaining areas of the body.

Medical causes

Bowen's disease. Bowen's disease causes painless, erythematous plaques that are raised and indurated with a thick, hyperkeratotic scale and, possibly, ulcerated centers.

Dermatitis. Exfoliative dermatitis begins with rapidly developing generalized erythema. Desquamation with fine scales or thick sheets of all or most of the skin surface may cause life-threatening hypothermia. Other possible complications include cardiac output failure and septicemia. Systemic signs and symptoms include a low-grade fever, chills, malaise, lymphadenopathy, and gynecomastia.

With *nummular dermatitis,* round, pustular lesions commonly ooze purulent exudate, itch severely, and rapidly become encrusted and scaly. Lesions appear on the extensor surfaces of the limbs, posterior trunk, and buttocks.

Seborrheic dermatitis begins with erythematous, scaly papules that progress to larger, dry or moist, greasy scales with yellowish crusts. This disorder primarily involves the center of the face, the chest and scalp and, possibly, the genitalia, axillae, and perianal regions. Pruritus occurs with scaling.

Dermatophytosis. Tinea capitis produces lesions with reddened, slightly elevated borders and a central area of dense scaling; these lesions may become inflamed and pus-filled (kerions). Patchy alopecia and itching may also occur. *Tinea pedis* causes scaling and blisters between the toes. The squamous type produces diffuse, fine, branlike scales. Adherent and silvery white, they're most prominent in skin creases and may affect the entire dorsum of the foot. *Tinea corporis* produces crusty lesions. As they enlarge, their centers heal, causing the classic ringworm shape.

Lymphoma. Hodgkin's disease and non-Hodgkin's lymphoma commonly cause scaly rashes. *Hodgkin's disease* may cause pruritic scaling dermatitis that begins in the legs and spreads to the entire body. Remissions and recurrences are common. Small nodules and diffuse pigmentation are related signs. This disease typically produces painless enlargement of the peripheral lymph nodes. Other signs and symptoms include fever, fatigue, weight loss, malaise, and hepatosplenomegaly.

Non-Hodgkin's lymphoma initially produces erythematous patches with some scaling that later become interspersed with nodules. Pruritus and discomfort are common; later, tumors and ulcers form. Progression produces nontender lymphadenopathy.

Parapsoriasis (chronic). Parapsoriasis produces small or moderate-sized maculopapular, erythematous eruptions, with a thin, adherent scale on the trunk, hands, and feet. Removal of the scale reveals a shiny brown surface.

Pityriasis. Pityriasis rosea, an acute, benign, and self-limiting disorder, produces widespread scales. It begins with an erythematous, raised, oval herald patch anywhere on the body. A few days or weeks later, yellow-tan or erythematous patches with scaly edges erupt on the trunk and limbs and sometimes on the face, hands, and feet. Pruritus also occurs.

Pityriasis rubra pilaris, an uncommon disorder, initially produces seborrheic scaling on the scalp, progressing to the face and ears. Later, scaly red patches develop on the palms and soles, becoming diffuse, thick, fissured, hyperkeratotic, and painful. Lesions also appear on the hands, fingers, wrists, and forearms and then on wide areas of the trunk, neck, and limbs.

Psoriasis. Silvery white, micaceous scales cover erythematous plaques that have sharply defined borders. Psoriasis usually appears on the scalp, chest, elbows, knees, back, buttocks, and genitalia. Associated signs and symptoms include nail pitting, pruritus, arthritis, and sometimes pain from dry, cracked, encrusted lesions.

Systemic lupus erythematosus (SLE). SLE produces a bright-red maculopapular eruption, sometimes with scaling. Patches are sharply defined and involve the nose and malar regions of the face in a butterfly pattern—a primary sign. Similar characteristic rashes appear on other body surfaces; scaling occurs along the lower lip or anterior hair line. Other primary signs and symptoms include photosensitivity and joint pain and stiffness. Vasculitis (leading to infarctive lesions, necrotic leg ulcers, or digital gangrene), Raynaud's phenomenon, patchy alopecia, and mucous membrane ulcers can also occur.

 ## Managing the patient with psoriasis

Psoriasis is a chronic, recurrent disease, marked by epidermal proliferation. Its lesions, which appear as erythematous papules and plaques covered with silver scales, vary widely in severity and distribution. Although this disorder commonly affects young adults, it may strike at any age, including during infancy. Psoriasis is characterized by recurring partial remissions and exacerbations. Flare-ups are commonly related to specific systemic and environmental factors but may be unpredictable; they can usually be controlled with therapy.

Do's

■ Administer creams, ointments, methotrexate, ultraviolet light, oatmeal baths, and other treatments, as ordered.
■ If a medication has been applied to scales to soften them, use a soft brush to remove them.
■ Watch for adverse reactions to treatments, especially allergic reactions to anthralin, atrophy and acne from steroids, and burning, itching, nausea, and squamous cell epitheliomas.
■ Initially evaluate the patient on methotrexate weekly, then monthly for red blood cell, white blood cell, and platelet counts because cytotoxins may cause hepatic or bone marrow toxicity.

Don'ts

■ If the patient is receiving anthralin, never put an occlusive dressing over this medication.
■ Tell the patient not to scrub the skin vigorously, to prevent Köbner's phenomenon (the development of lesions at the site of injury).
■ Caution the patient receiving therapy to stay out of the sun on the day of treatment, and to protect his eyes with sunglasses that screen UVA for 24 hours after treatment.
■ Because stressful situations can exacerbate psoriasis, help the patient learn positive coping techniques.

Tinea versicolor. Tinea versicolor typically produces macular hypopigmented, fawn-colored, or brown patches of varying sizes and shapes. All are slightly scaly. Lesions commonly affect the upper trunk, arms, and lower abdomen; sometimes the neck; and, rarely, the face.

Other causes

Drugs. Many drugs—including penicillins, sulfonamides, barbiturates, quinidine, diazepam, phenytoin, and isoniazid—can produce scaling patches.

Nursing considerations

- If scaling results from corticosteroid therapy, wean the patient off the drug. (See *Managing the patient with psoriasis*, page 567.)
- Prepare the patient for such diagnostic tests as a Wood's light examination, skin scraping, and skin biopsy.
- Administer lotions and creams, as prescribed.

Patient teaching

- Instruct the patient in proper skin care.
- Explain the underlying disorder and its treatment.

Skin turgor, decreased

Skin turgor—the skin's elasticity—is determined by observing the time required for the skin to return to its normal position after being stretched or pinched. With decreased turgor, pinched skin "holds" for up to 30 seconds, and then slowly returns to its normal contour. Skin turgor is commonly assessed over the hand, arm, or sternum—areas normally free from wrinkles and with wide variations in tissue thickness. (See *Evaluating skin turgor*.)

Decreased skin turgor results from dehydration, or volume depletion, which moves interstitial fluid into the vascular bed to maintain circulating blood volume, leading to slackness in the skin's dermal layer. It's a normal finding in elderly patients and in people who have lost weight rapidly; it also occurs with disorders affecting the GI, renal, endocrine, and other systems.

History and physical examination

If your examination reveals decreased skin turgor, ask the patient about food and fluid intake and fluid loss. Has he recently experienced prolonged fluid loss from vomiting, diarrhea, draining wounds, or increased urination? Has he recently had a fever with sweating? Is the patient taking a diuretic? If so, how often? Does he frequently use alcohol? How much fluid, especially water, does he ingest daily?

Next, take the patient's vital signs. Note if his systolic blood pressure is abnormally low (90 mm Hg or less) when he's in a supine position, if it drops 15 to 20 mm Hg or more when he stands, or if his pulse increases by 10 beats/ minute when he sits or stands. If you detect these signs of orthostatic hypotension or resting tachycardia, insert an I.V. catheter for fluid administration.

Evaluate the patient's level of consciousness for confusion, disorientation, and signs of profound dehydration. Inspect his oral mucosa, the furrows of his tongue (especially under the tongue), and his axillae for dryness. Also, check his jugular veins for flatness, and monitor his urine output.

Medical causes

Cholera. Cholera is characterized by abrupt watery diarrhea and vomiting, which leads to severe water and electrolyte loss. These imbalances cause the

Evaluating skin turgor

To evaluate skin turgor in an adult, pick up a fold of skin over the sternum or the arm, as shown below left. (In an infant, roll a fold of loosely adherent skin on the abdomen between your thumb and forefinger.) Then release it. Normal skin will immediately return to its previous contour. In decreased skin turgor, the skin fold will "hold," or "tent," as shown below right, for up to 30 seconds.

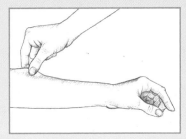 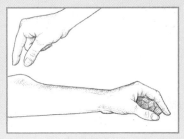

following symptoms: decreased skin turgor, thirst, weakness, muscle cramps, oliguria, tachycardia, and hypotension. Without treatment, death can occur within hours.

Dehydration. Decreased skin turgor commonly occurs with moderate to severe dehydration. Associated findings include dry oral mucosa, decreased perspiration, resting tachycardia, orthostatic hypotension, a dry and furrowed tongue, increased thirst, weight loss, oliguria, fever, and fatigue. As dehydration worsens, other findings include enophthalmos, lethargy, weakness, confusion, delirium or obtundation, anuria, and shock. Hypotension persists even when the patient lies down.

Nursing considerations

■ Turn the patient every 2 hours to prevent skin breakdown.
■ Monitor the patient's intake and output, administer I.V. fluids, and frequently offer oral fluids.
■ Weigh the patient daily.

■ Monitor the patient for signs of electrolyte imbalance; monitor laboratory values.

Patient teaching

■ Explain the disorder and treatment.
■ Explain to the patient the importance of fluid replacement.
■ Explain signs and symptoms the patient needs to report.

Splenomegaly

Because it occurs with various disorders and in up to 5% of normal adults, splenomegaly—an enlarged spleen— isn't a diagnostic sign by itself. Usually, however, it points to infection, trauma, or a hepatic, autoimmune, neoplastic, or hematologic disorder.

Because the spleen functions as the body's largest lymph node, splenomegaly can result from any process that triggers lymphadenopathy. For example, it may reflect reactive hyperplasia (a response to infection or inflammation), proliferation or infiltration of neoplastic cells, extramedullary hemopoiesis, phagocytic cell proliferation, increased blood cell destruction, or vascular congestion associated with portal hypertension.

Splenomegaly may be detected by light palpation under the left costal margin. (See *Palpating for splenomegaly*.) However, because this technique isn't always advisable or effective, splenomegaly may need to be confirmed by a computed tomography or radionuclide scan.

 If the patient has a history of abdominal or thoracic trauma, don't palpate the abdomen because this may aggravate internal bleeding. Instead, examine him for left upper quadrant pain and signs of shock, such as tachycardia and tachypnea. If you detect these signs, suspect splenic rupture. Insert an I.V. catheter for emergency fluid and blood replacement, and administer oxygen. Also, catheterize the patient to evaluate urine output, and begin cardiac monitoring. Prepare the patient for possible surgery.

History and physical examination

If you detect splenomegaly during a routine physical examination, begin by exploring associated signs and symptoms. Ask the patient if he has been unusually tired lately. Does he frequently have colds, sore throats, or other infections? Does he bruise easily? Ask about left upper quadrant pain, abdominal fullness, and early satiety. Finally, examine the patient's skin for pallor and ecchymoses, and palpate his axillae, groin, and neck for lymphadenopathy.

Medical causes

Brucellosis. With severe cases of brucellosis, splenomegaly is a major sign.

Typically, brucellosis begins insidiously with fatigue, headache, backache, anorexia, arthralgia, fever, chills, sweating, and malaise. Later, it may cause hepatomegaly, lymphadenopathy, weight loss, and vertebral or peripheral nerve pain on pressure.

Cirrhosis. About one-third of patients with advanced cirrhosis develop moderate to marked splenomegaly. Among other late findings are jaundice, hepatomegaly, leg edema, hematemesis, and ascites. Signs of hepatic encephalopathy—such as asterixis, fetor hepaticus, slurred speech, and decreased level of consciousness that may progress to coma—are also common. Besides jaundice, skin effects may include severe pruritus, poor tissue turgor, spider angiomas, palmar erythema, pallor, and signs of bleeding tendencies. Endocrine effects may include menstrual irregularities or testicular atrophy, gynecomastia, and a loss of chest and axillary hair. The patient may also develop a fever and right upper abdominal pain that's aggravated by sitting up or leaning forward.

Felty's syndrome. Splenomegaly is characteristic in Felty's syndrome. Associated findings are joint pain and deformity, sensory or motor loss, rheumatoid nodules, palmar erythema, lymphadenopathy, and leg ulcers.

Histoplasmosis. Acute disseminated histoplasmosis commonly produces splenomegaly and hepatomegaly. It may also cause lymphadenopathy, jaundice, fever, anorexia, emaciation, and signs and symptoms of anemia, such as weakness, fatigue, pallor, and malaise. Occasionally, the patient's tongue, palate, epiglottis, and larynx become ulcerated, resulting in pain, hoarseness, and dysphagia.

Leukemia. Moderate to severe splenomegaly is an early sign of acute and chronic leukemia. With chronic granulocytic leukemia, splenomegaly is

Palpating for splenomegaly

Detecting splenomegaly requires skillful and gentle palpation to avoid rupturing the enlarged spleen. Follow these steps carefully:

■ Place the patient in the supine position, and stand at her right side. Place your left hand under the left costovertebral angle, and push lightly to move the spleen forward. Then press your right hand gently under the left front costal margin.

■ Have the patient take a deep breath and then exhale. As she exhales, move your right hand along the tissue contours under the border of the ribs, feeling for the spleen's edge. The enlarged spleen should feel like a firm mass that bumps against your fingers. Remember to begin palpation low enough in the abdomen to catch the edge of a massive spleen.

■ Grade the splenomegaly as slight (½" to 1½" [1 to 4 cm] below the costal margin), moderate (1½" to 3" [4 to 8 cm] below the costal margin), or great (greater than or equal to 3" [8 cm] below the costal margin).

■ Reposition the patient on her right side with her hips and knees flexed slightly to move the spleen forward. Then repeat the palpation procedure.

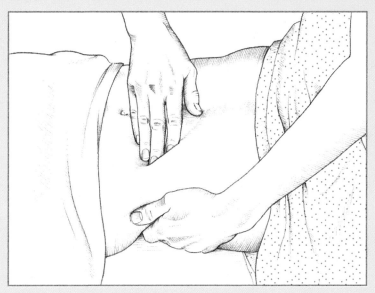

sometimes painful. Accompanying it may be hepatomegaly, lymphadenopathy, fatigue, malaise, pallor, fever, gum swelling, bleeding tendencies, weight loss, anorexia, and abdominal, bone, and joint pain. At times, acute leukemia also causes dyspnea, tachycardia, and palpitations. With advanced disease, the patient may display confusion, headache, vomiting, seizures, papilledema, and nuchal rigidity.

Mononucleosis (infectious). A common sign of mononucleosis, splenomegaly is most pronounced during the second and third weeks of the illness. Typically, it's accompanied by a triad of signs and symptoms: a sore throat, cervical lymphadenopathy, and fluctuating temperature with an evening peak of 101° to 102° F (38.3° to 38.9° C). Occasionally, hepatomegaly, jaundice, and a maculopapular rash may also occur.

Pancreatic cancer. Pancreatic cancer may cause moderate to severe splenomegaly if tumor growth compresses the splenic vein. Other characteristic findings include abdominal or back pain, anorexia, nausea and vomiting, weight loss, GI bleeding, jaundice, pruritus, skin lesions, emotional lability, weakness, and fatigue. Palpation may reveal a tender abdominal mass and hepatomegaly; auscultation reveals a bruit in the periumbilical area and left upper quadrant.

Polycythemia vera. Late in polycythemia vera, the spleen may become markedly enlarged, resulting in easy satiety, abdominal fullness, and left upper quadrant or pleuritic chest pain. Signs and symptoms accompanying splenomegaly are widespread and numerous. The patient may exhibit deep, purplish red oral mucous membranes, headache, dyspnea, dizziness, vertigo, weakness, and fatigue. He may also develop finger and toe paresthesia, impaired mentation, tinnitus, blurred or double vision, scotoma, increased blood pressure, and intermittent claudication. Other signs and symptoms include pruritus, urticaria, ruddy cyanosis, epigastric distress, weight loss, hepatomegaly, and bleeding tendencies.

Sarcoidosis. Sarcoidosis may produce splenomegaly and hepatomegaly, possibly accompanied by vague abdominal discomfort. Its other signs and symptoms vary with the affected body system, but may include a nonproductive cough, dyspnea, malaise, fatigue, arthralgia, myalgia, weight loss, lymphadenopathy, skin lesions, an irregular

pulse, impaired vision, dysphagia, and seizures.

Splenic rupture. Splenomegaly may result from massive hemorrhage with splenic rupture. The patient may also experience left upper quadrant pain, abdominal rigidity, and Kehr's sign.

Thrombotic thrombocytopenic purpura. Thrombotic thrombocytopenic purpura may produce splenomegaly and hepatomegaly accompanied by fever, generalized purpura, jaundice, pallor, vaginal bleeding, and hematuria. Other effects include fatigue, weakness, headache, pallor, abdominal pain, and arthralgia. Eventually, the patient develops signs of neurologic deterioration and renal failure.

Nursing considerations

- Prepare the patient for diagnostic studies, such as a complete blood count, blood cultures, and radionuclide and computed tomography scans of the spleen.
- Monitor vital signs.
- Provide measures to treat the underlying disorder.
- Take measures to avoid infection.

Patient teaching

- Explain the underlying disorder and treatment plan.
- Discuss with the patient ways to avoid infection.
- Emphasize the importance of complying with drug therapy.

Stools, clay-colored

Pale, putty-colored stools usually result from hepatic, gallbladder, or pancreatic disorders. Normally, bile pigments give stools their characteristic brown color. However, hepatocellular degeneration or biliary obstruction may interfere with the formation or release of these pigments into the intestine, resulting in clay-colored stools. These stools are commonly associated with jaundice and dark "cola-colored" urine.

History and physical examination

After documenting when the patient first noticed clay-colored stools, explore associated signs and symptoms, such as abdominal pain, nausea and vomiting, fatigue, anorexia, weight loss, and dark urine. Does the patient have trouble digesting fatty foods or heavy meals? Does he bruise easily?

Next, review the patient's medical history for gallbladder, hepatic, or pancreatic disorders. Has he ever had biliary surgery? Has he recently undergone barium studies? (Barium lightens stool color for several days.) Also, ask about antacid use because large amounts may lighten stool color. Ask about recent appetite and any weight loss. Note a history of alcoholism or exposure to other hepatotoxic substances.

After assessing the patient's general appearance, take his vital signs and check his skin and eyes for jaundice. Then examine the abdomen: inspect for distention and ascites, and auscultate for hypoactive bowel sounds. Percuss and palpate for masses and rebound tenderness. Finally, obtain urine and stool specimens for laboratory analysis.

Medical causes

Bile duct cancer. Commonly a presenting sign of bile duct cancer, clay-colored stools may be accompanied by jaundice, pruritus, anorexia and weight loss, upper abdominal pain, bleeding tendencies, and a palpable mass.

Biliary cirrhosis. Clay-colored stools typically follow unexplained pruritus that worsens at bedtime, weakness, fatigue, weight loss, and vague abdominal pain; these features may be present for

years. Associated findings include jaundice, hyperpigmentation, and signs of malabsorption, such as nocturnal diarrhea, steatorrhea, purpura, and bone and back pain due to osteomalacia. The patient may also develop firm, nontender hepatomegaly; hematemesis; ascites; edema; and xanthomas on his palms, soles, and elbows.

Cholangitis (sclerosing). Characterized by fibrosis of the bile ducts, cholangitis, a chronic inflammatory disorder, may cause clay-colored stools, chronic or intermittent jaundice, pruritus, right upper quadrant pain, chills, and fever.

Cholelithiasis. Calculi in the biliary tract may cause clay-colored stools when they obstruct the common bile duct (choledocholithiasis). However, if the obstruction is intermittent, the stools may alternate between normal and clay colored. Associated symptoms include dyspepsia and—in sudden, severe obstruction—characteristic biliary colic. This right upper quadrant pain intensifies over several hours, may radiate to the epigastrium or shoulder blades, and is unrelieved by antacids. The pain is accompanied by tachycardia, restlessness, nausea, intolerance to certain foods, vomiting, upper abdominal tenderness, fever, chills, and jaundice.

Hepatic cancer. Before clay-colored stools develop with hepatic cancer, the patient usually experiences weight loss, weakness, and anorexia. Later, he may develop nodular, firm hepatomegaly, jaundice, right upper quadrant pain, ascites, dependent edema, and fever. A bruit, hum, or rubbing sound may be heard on auscultation if the cancer involves a large part of the liver.

Hepatitis. With *viral hepatitis,* clay-colored stools signal the start of the icteric phase and are typically followed by jaundice within 1 to 5 days. Associated signs include mild weight loss and dark urine as well as continuation of some preicteric findings, such as anorexia and tender hepatomegaly. During the icteric phase, the patient may become irritable and develop right upper quadrant pain, splenomegaly, enlarged cervical lymph nodes, and severe pruritus. After jaundice disappears, the patient continues to experience fatigue, flatulence, abdominal pain or tenderness, and dyspepsia, although his appetite usually returns and hepatomegaly subsides. The posticteric phase generally lasts from 2 to 6 weeks, with full recovery in 6 months.

With *cholestatic nonviral hepatitis,* clay-colored stools occur with other signs of viral hepatitis.

Pancreatic cancer. Common bile duct obstruction associated with pancreatic cancer may cause clay-colored stools. Classic associated features include abdominal or back pain, jaundice, pruritus, nausea and vomiting, anorexia, weight loss, fatigue, weakness, and fever. Other possible effects include diarrhea, skin lesions (especially on the legs), emotional lability, splenomegaly, and signs of GI bleeding. Auscultation may reveal a bruit in the periumbilical area and left upper quadrant.

Pancreatitis (acute). Pancreatitis may cause clay-colored stools, dark urine, and jaundice. Typically, it also causes severe epigastric pain that radiates to the back and is aggravated by lying down. Associated findings include nausea and vomiting, fever, abdominal rigidity and tenderness, hypoactive bowel sounds, and crackles at the lung bases. With severe pancreatitis, findings include marked restlessness, tachycardia, mottled skin, and cold, sweaty extremities.

Other causes

Biliary surgery. Biliary surgery may cause bile duct stricture, resulting in clay-colored stools.

Nursing considerations

- Prepare the patient for diagnostic tests, such as liver enzyme and serum bilirubin levels, hepatitis panels, sonograms, a computed tomography scan, endoscopy, retrograde cholangiopancreatography, and stool analysis.
- Provide for rest periods.
- Administer vaccines for hepatitis A and B.

Patient teaching

- Explain the disorder and treatment plan.
- Discuss with the patient ways to reduce abdominal pain.
- Explain any dietary modifications.
- Emphasize the importance of rest.
- Stress the importance of avoiding alcohol.

▐ Stridor

A loud, harsh, musical respiratory sound, stridor results from a partial to near complete obstruction of the trachea or larynx. Usually heard during inspiration, this sign may also occur during expiration in severe upper airway obstruction. It may begin as low-pitched "croaking" and progress to high-pitched "crowing" as respirations become more vigorous.

Life-threatening upper airway obstruction can stem from foreign-body aspiration, increased secretions, an intraluminal tumor, localized edema or muscle spasms, and external compression by a tumor or aneurysm.

ACTION STAT!

 If you detect stridor, quickly check the patient's vital signs, including oxygen saturation, and examine him for other signs of partial airway obstruction—choking or gagging, tachypnea, dyspnea, shallow respirations, intercostal retractions, nasal flaring, tachycardia, cyanosis, and diaphoresis. (Be aware that abrupt cessation of stridor signals complete obstruction in which the patient has inspiratory chest movement but absent breath sounds. Unable to talk, he quickly becomes lethargic and loses consciousness.)

If you detect signs of airway obstruction, try to clear the airway with back blows or abdominal thrusts. Next, administer oxygen by nasal cannula or face mask, or prepare the patient for emergency endotracheal (ET) intubation or tracheostomy and mechanical ventilation. (See *Emergency endotracheal intubation,* page 576.) Have equipment ready to suction aspirated vomitus or blood through the ET or tracheostomy tube. Connect the patient to a cardiac monitor, and position him in Fowler's position to ease his breathing.

History and physical examination

When the patient's condition permits, obtain a patient history from him or a family member. First, find out when the stridor began. Has he had it before? Does he have an upper respiratory tract infection? If so, how long has he had it?

Ask about a history of allergies, tumors, and respiratory and vascular disorders. Note recent exposure to smoke or noxious fumes or gases. Next, explore associated signs and symptoms. Does stridor occur with pain or cough?

Then examine the patient's mouth for excessive secretions, foreign matter, inflammation, and swelling. Assess his neck for swelling, masses, subcutaneous crepitation, and scars. Observe the patient's chest for delayed, decreased, or asymmetrical chest expansion. Auscultate for wheezes, rhonchi, crackles, rubs, and other abnormal breath sounds. Percuss for dullness, tympany, or flatness.

Finally, note burns or signs of trauma, such as ecchymoses and lacerations.

Medical causes

Airway trauma. Local trauma to the upper airway commonly causes acute obstruction, resulting in the sudden onset of stridor. Accompanying this sign are dysphonia, dysphagia, hemoptysis, cyanosis, accessory muscle use, intercostal retractions, nasal flaring, tachypnea, progressive dyspnea, and shallow respirations. Palpation may reveal subcutaneous crepitation in the neck or upper chest.

Anaphylaxis. With a severe allergic reaction, upper airway edema and laryngospasm cause stridor and other signs and symptoms of respiratory distress: nasal flaring, wheezing, accessory muscle use, intercostal retractions, and dyspnea. The patient may also develop nasal congestion and profuse, watery rhinorrhea. Typically, these respiratory effects are preceded by a feeling of impending doom or fear, weakness, diaphoresis, sneezing, nasal pruritus, urticaria, erythema, and angioedema. Common associated findings include chest or throat tightness, dysphagia and, possibly, signs of shock, such as hypotension, tachycardia, and cool, clammy skin.

Anthrax (inhalation). Initial signs and symptoms of anthrax are flulike and include fever, chills, weakness, cough, and chest pain. The disease generally occurs in two stages with a period of recovery after the initial symptoms. The second stage develops abruptly with rapid deterioration marked by stridor, fever, dyspnea, and hypotension generally leading to death within 24 hours. Radiologic findings include mediastinitis and symmetric mediastinal widening.

Hypocalcemia. With hypocalcemia, laryngospasm can cause stridor. Other findings include paresthesia, carpopedal

Emergency endotracheal intubation

For a patient with stridor, you may have to assist with emergency endotracheal (ET) intubation to establish a patent airway and administer mechanical ventilation. Just follow these essential steps:
■ Gather the necessary equipment.
■ Explain the procedure to the patient.
■ Place the patient flat on his back with a small blanket or pillow under his head. This position aligns the axis of the oropharynx, posterior pharynx, and trachea.
■ Check the cuff on the ET tube for leaks.
■ After intubation, inflate the cuff, using the minimal leak technique.
■ Check tube placement by auscultating for bilateral breath sounds and using a capnometer; observe the patient for chest expansion and feel for warm exhalations at the ET tube's opening.
■ Insert an oral airway or bite block.
■ Secure the tube and airway with an ET tube holder or tape.
■ Suction secretions from the patient's mouth and the ET tube as needed.
■ Administer oxygen or initiate mechanical ventilation (or both).

After the patient has been intubated, suction secretions as needed and check cuff pressure once every shift (correcting any air leaks with the minimal leak technique). Provide mouth care every 2 to 3 hours and as needed. Prepare the patient for a chest X-ray to confirm tube placement.

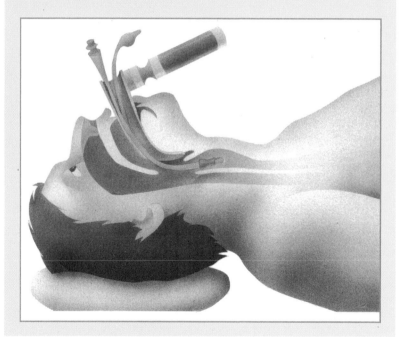

spasm, and positive Chvostek's and Trousseau's signs.

Inhalation injury. Within 48 hours after inhalation of smoke or noxious fumes, the patient may develop laryngeal edema and bronchospasms, resulting in stridor. Associated signs and symptoms include singed nasal hairs, orofacial burns, coughing, hoarseness, sooty sputum, crackles, rhonchi, wheezes, and other signs and symptoms of respiratory distress, such as dyspnea, accessory muscle use, intercostal retractions, and nasal flaring.

Mediastinal tumor. Commonly producing no symptoms at first, a mediastinal tumor may eventually compress the trachea and bronchi, resulting in stridor. Its other effects include hoarseness, a brassy cough, a tracheal shift or tug, dilated neck veins, swelling of the face and neck, stertorous respirations, and suprasternal retractions on inspiration. The patient may also report dyspnea, dysphagia, and pain in the chest, shoulder, or arm.

Retrosternal thyroid. Retrosternal thyroid causes stridor, dysphagia, cough, hoarseness, and tracheal deviation. It can also cause signs of thyrotoxicosis.

Other causes

Diagnostic tests. Bronchoscopy or laryngoscopy may precipitate laryngospasm and stridor.

Foreign body aspiration. Sudden stridor is characteristic in foreign body aspiration, a life-threatening situation. Related findings include an abrupt onset of dry, paroxysmal coughing; gagging or choking; hoarseness; tachycardia; wheezing; dyspnea; tachypnea; intercostal muscle retractions; diminished breath sounds; cyanosis; and shallow respirations. The patient typically appears anxious and distressed.

Treatments. After prolonged intubation, the patient may exhibit laryngeal edema and stridor when the tube is removed. Aerosol therapy with epinephrine may reduce stridor. Reintubation may be necessary in some cases. Neck surgery, such as thyroidectomy, may cause laryngeal paralysis and stridor.

Nursing considerations
- Monitor the patient's vital signs closely.
- Prepare him for diagnostic tests, such as arterial blood gas analysis and chest X-rays.
- Administer oxygen and monitor airway and ventilation.
- Provide emotional support.

Patient teaching
- Explain the underlying disorder and treatment.
- Explain to the patient all procedures and treatments.
- Stay with the patient and talk to him in a calm voice to reduce anxiety.

Syncope

A common neurologic sign, syncope (or *fainting*) refers to a transient loss of consciousness associated with impaired cerebral blood supply or cerebral hypoxia. It usually occurs abruptly and lasts for seconds to minutes. An episode of syncope usually starts as a feeling of light-headedness. A patient can usually prevent an episode of syncope by lying down or sitting with his head between his knees. Typically, the patient lies motionless with his skeletal muscles relaxed but sphincter muscles controlled. However, the depth of unconsciousness varies—some patients can hear voices or see blurred outlines; others are unaware of their surroundings.

In many ways, syncope simulates death: The patient is strikingly pale with a slow, weak pulse, hypotension, and almost imperceptible breathing. If severe hypotension lasts for 20 seconds or longer, the patient may also develop convulsive, tonic-clonic movements.

Syncope may result from cardiac and cerebrovascular disorders, hypoxemia, and postural changes in the presence of autonomic dysfunction. It may also follow vigorous coughing (tussive syncope) and emotional stress, injury, shock, or pain (vasovagal syncope, or common fainting). Hysterical syncope may also follow emotional stress but isn't accompanied by other vasodepressor effects.

 If you see a patient faint, ensure the ABCs—a patent airway, breathing, and circulation—and take his vital signs. Then place the patient in a supine position, elevate his legs, and loosen tight clothing. Be alert for tachycardia, bradycardia, or an irregular pulse. Place him on a cardiac monitor to detect arrhythmias. If an arrhythmia appears, give oxygen and insert an I.V. catheter for medication or fluid administration. Be ready to begin cardiopulmonary resuscitation, if indicated. Cardioversion, defibrillation, or insertion of a temporary pacemaker may be required.

History and physical examination

If the patient reports a fainting episode, gather information about the episode from him and his family. Did he feel weak, light-headed, nauseous, or sweaty just before he fainted? Did he get up quickly from a chair or from lying down? During the fainting episode, did he have muscle spasms or incontinence? How long was he unconscious? When he regained consciousness, was he alert or confused? Did he have a headache? Has he fainted before? If so, how often does it occur? Obtain a complete drug history.

Next, take the patient's vital signs and examine him for any injuries that may have occurred during his fall. Place him on a cardiac monitor and assess his heart rhythm for abnormalities. Assess cardiac and respiratory status. Monitor pulse oximetry. Perform a neurologic examination.

Medical causes

Aortic arch syndrome. With aortic arch syndrome, syncope, weak or abruptly absent carotid pulses, and unequal or absent radial pulses may occur. Early signs and symptoms include night sweats, pallor, nausea, anorexia, weight loss, arthralgia, and Raynaud's phenomenon. He may also develop hypotension in the arms; neck, shoulder, and chest pain; paresthesia; intermittent claudication; bruits; vision disturbances; and dizziness.

Aortic stenosis. A cardinal late sign of aortic stenosis, syncope is accompanied by exertional dyspnea and angina. Related findings include marked fatigue, orthopnea, paroxysmal nocturnal dyspnea, palpitations, and diminished carotid pulses. Typically, auscultation reveals atrial and ventricular gallops as well as a harsh, crescendo-decrescendo systolic ejection murmur that's loudest at the right sternal border of the second intercostal space.

Cardiac arrhythmias. Any arrhythmia that decreases cardiac output and impairs cerebral circulation may cause syncope. Other effects—such as palpitations, pallor, confusion, diaphoresis, dyspnea, and hypotension—usually develop first. However, with Adams-Stokes syndrome, syncope may occur without warning. During syncope, the patient develops asystole, which may precipitate spasm and myoclonic jerks if prolonged. He also displays an ashen pallor that progresses to cyanosis, incontinence, a bilateral Babinski's reflex, and fixed pupils.

Hypoxemia. Regardless of its cause, severe hypoxemia may produce syncope. Common related effects include confusion, tachycardia, restlessness, and incoordination.

Orthostatic hypotension. Syncope occurs when the patient rises quickly from a recumbent position. Look for a drop of 10 to 20 mm Hg or more in systolic or diastolic blood pressure as well as tachycardia, pallor, dizziness, blurred vision, nausea, and diaphoresis.

Transient ischemic attack (TIA). Marked by transient neurologic deficits, TIAs may produce syncope and decreased level of consciousness. Other findings vary with the affected artery, but may include vision loss, nystagmus, aphasia, dysarthria, unilateral numbness, hemiparesis or hemiplegia, tinnitus, facial weakness, dysphagia, and a staggering or an uncoordinated gait.

Other causes

Drugs. Quinidine may cause syncope—and possibly sudden death—associated with ventricular fibrillation. Prazosin may cause severe orthostatic hypotension and syncope, usually after the first dose. Occasionally, griseofulvin, levodopa, and indomethacin can produce syncope.

Nursing considerations

- Monitor the patient's vital signs closely.
- Prepare him for an electrocardiogram and Holter monitor, carotid duplex, carotid Doppler, and electrophysiology studies.
- Take measures to provide for patient safety.

Patient teaching

- Explain the underlying disorder and treatment plan.
- Encourage the patient to pace his activities.
- Teach the patient measures to take if he feels faint.
- Tell the patient to rise slowly from a lying or sitting to a standing position.

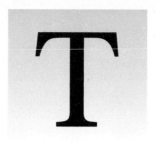

Tachycardia

Easily detected by counting the apical, carotid, or radial pulse, tachycardia is a heart rate greater than 100 beats/ minute. The patient with tachycardia usually complains of palpitations or of a "racing" heart. This common sign normally occurs in response to emotional or physical stress, such as excitement, exercise, pain, anxiety, and fever. It may also result from the use of stimulants, such as caffeine and tobacco. However, tachycardia may be an early sign of a life-threatening disorder, such as cardiogenic, hypovolemic, or septic shock. It may also result from a cardiovascular, respiratory, or metabolic disorder or from the effects of certain drugs, tests, or treatments. (See *What happens in tachycardia.*)

ACTION STAT!

After detecting tachycardia, take the patient's other vital signs and determine his level of consciousness (LOC). If the patient has increased or decreased blood pressure and is drowsy or confused, administer oxygen and begin cardiac monitoring. Perform electrocardiography (ECG) to assess cardiac rhythm. Insert an I.V. catheter for fluid, blood product, and drug administration, and gather emergency resuscitation equipment.

History and physical examination

If the patient's condition permits, take a focused history. Find out if he has had palpitations in the past. If so, how were they treated? Explore associated symptoms. Is the patient dizzy or short of breath? Is he weak or fatigued? Is he experiencing episodes of syncope or chest pain? Next, ask about a history of trauma, diabetes, or cardiac, pulmonary, or thyroid disorders. Also, obtain an alcohol and drug history, including prescription, over-the-counter, and illicit drugs.

Inspect the patient's skin for pallor or cyanosis. Assess pulses, noting peripheral edema. Finally, auscultate the heart and lungs for abnormal sounds or rhythms.

Medical causes

Acute respiratory distress syndrome (ARDS). Besides tachycardia, ARDS causes crackles, rhonchi, dyspnea, tachypnea, nasal flaring, and grunting respirations. Other findings include cyanosis, anxiety, decreased LOC, and abnormal chest X-ray findings.

Adrenocortical insufficiency. With adrenocortical insufficiency, tachycardia commonly occurs with a weak pulse as well as progressive weakness and fatigue, which may become so severe that the patient requires bed rest. Other signs and symptoms include abdominal pain, nausea and vomiting, altered bowel habits, weight loss, orthostatic hypotension, irritability, bronze skin, decreased libido, and syncope. Some patients report an enhanced sense of taste, smell, and hearing.

Anaphylactic shock. With life-threatening anaphylactic shock, tachycardia and hypotension develop within minutes after exposure to an allergen, such as penicillin or an insect sting. Typically, the patient is visibly anxious and has severe pruritus, perhaps with urticaria and a pounding headache. Other findings may include flushed and clammy skin, cough, dyspnea, nausea, abdominal cramps, seizures, stridor, change or loss of voice associated with laryngeal edema, and urinary urgency and incontinence.

Anemia. Tachycardia and bounding pulse are characteristics of anemia. Associated signs and symptoms include fatigue, pallor, dyspnea and, possibly, bleeding tendencies. Auscultation may reveal an atrial gallop, a systolic bruit over the carotid arteries, and crackles.

Aortic insufficiency. Accompanying tachycardia with aortic insufficiency are a "water-hammer" bounding pulse and a large, diffuse apical heave. With severe insufficiency, widened pulse pressure occurs. Auscultation reveals a hallmark diastolic murmur that starts with the second heart sound; is decrescendo, high-pitched, and blowing; and is heard best at the left sternal border of the second and third intercostal spaces. An atrial or ventricular gallop, an early systolic murmur, an Austin Flint murmur (apical diastolic rumble), or Duroziez's sign (a murmur over the femoral artery during systole and diastole) may also be heard. Other findings include angina, dyspnea, palpitations, strong and abrupt carotid pulsations, pallor, and signs of heart failure, such as crackles and jugular vein distention.

What happens in tachycardia

Tachycardia represents the heart's effort to deliver more oxygen to body tissues by increasing the rate at which blood passes through the vessels. This sign can reflect overstimulation within the sinoatrial node, the atrium, the atrioventricular node, or the ventricles.

Because heart rate affects cardiac output (cardiac output = heart rate × stroke volume), tachycardia can lower cardiac output by reducing ventricular filling time and stroke volume (the output of each ventricle at every contraction). As cardiac output plummets, arterial pressure and peripheral perfusion decrease. Tachycardia further aggravates myocardial ischemia by increasing the heart's demand for oxygen while reducing the duration of diastole—the period of greatest coronary flow.

Aortic stenosis. Typically, aortic stenosis causes tachycardia, a weak, thready pulse, and an atrial gallop. Its chief features are exertional dyspnea, angina, dizziness, and syncope. Aortic stenosis also causes a harsh, crescendo-decrescendo systolic ejection murmur that's loudest at the right sternal border of the second intercostal space. Other findings include palpitations, crackles, and fatigue.

Cardiac arrhythmias. Tachycardia may occur with an irregular heart rhythm. The patient may be hypotensive and report dizziness, palpitations, weakness, and fatigue. Depending on his heart rate, he may also exhibit tachypnea, decreased LOC, and pale, cool, clammy skin.

Cardiac contusion. Cardiac contusion may cause tachycardia, substernal pain, dyspnea, and palpitations. Assessment may detect sternal ecchymoses and a pericardial friction rub.

Cardiac tamponade. With life-threatening cardiac tamponade, tachycardia is commonly accompanied by paradoxical pulse, dyspnea, and tachypnea. The patient is visibly anxious and restless and has cyanotic, clammy skin and distended jugular veins. He may develop muffled heart sounds, pericardial friction rub, chest pain, hypotension, narrowed pulse pressure, and hepatomegaly.

Cardiogenic shock. With cardiogenic shock, tachycardia is accompanied by a weak, thready pulse; narrowing pulse pressure; hypotension; tachypnea; cold, pale, clammy, and cyanotic skin; oliguria; restlessness; and altered LOC.

Cholera. Cholera causes abrupt watery diarrhea and vomiting, which leads to severe fluid and electrolyte loss, causing tachycardia, thirst, weakness, muscle cramps, decreased skin turgor, oliguria, and hypotension. Without treatment, death can occur within hours.

Chronic obstructive pulmonary disease (COPD). Although the clinical picture varies widely with COPD, tachycardia is a common sign. Other characteristic findings include cough, tachypnea, dyspnea, pursed-lip breathing, accessory muscle use, cyanosis, diminished breath sounds, rhonchi, crackles, and wheezing. Clubbing and barrel chest are usually late findings.

Diabetic ketoacidosis. Life-threatening diabetic ketoacidosis commonly produces tachycardia and a thready pulse. Its cardinal sign, however, is Kussmaul's respirations—abnormally rapid, deep breathing. Other signs and symptoms of acidosis include fruity breath odor, orthostatic hypotension, generalized weakness, anorexia, nausea, vomiting, and abdominal pain. The patient's LOC may vary from lethargy to coma.

Heart failure. Especially common with left-sided heart failure, tachycardia may be accompanied by a ventricular gallop, fatigue, dyspnea (exertional and paroxysmal nocturnal), orthopnea, and leg edema. Eventually, the patient develops widespread signs and symptoms, such as palpitations, narrowed pulse pressure, hypotension, tachypnea, crackles, dependent edema, weight gain, slowed mental response, diaphoresis, pallor and, possibly, oliguria. Late signs include hemoptysis, cyanosis, and marked hepatomegaly and pitting edema.

Hyperosmolar hyperglycemic non-ketotic syndrome (HHNS). With HHNS, a rapidly deteriorating LOC is commonly accompanied by tachycardia, hypotension, tachypnea, seizures, oliguria, and severe dehydration with poor skin turgor and dry mucous membranes.

Hypertensive crisis. Life-threatening hypertensive crisis is characterized by tachycardia, tachypnea, diastolic blood pressure that exceeds 120 mm Hg, and systolic blood pressure that may exceed 200 mm Hg. Typically, the patient develops pulmonary edema with jugular vein distention, dyspnea, and pink, frothy sputum. Related findings include chest pain, severe headache, drowsiness, confusion, anxiety, tinnitus, epistaxis, muscle twitching, seizures, nausea, and vomiting. Focal neurologic signs, such as paresthesia, may also occur.

Hypoglycemia. A common sign of hypoglycemia, tachycardia accompanies hypothermia, nervousness, trembling, fatigue, malaise, weakness, headache, hunger, nausea, diaphoresis, and moist, clammy skin. Central nervous system effects include blurred or double vision, motor weakness, hemiplegia, seizures, and decreased LOC.

Hypovolemia. Tachycardia occurs with hypovolemia. Associated findings include hypotension, decreased skin turgor, sunken eyeballs, thirst, syncope, and dry skin and tongue.

Hypovolemic shock. Mild tachycardia, an early sign of life-threatening hypovolemic shock, may be accompanied by tachypnea, restlessness, thirst, and pale, cool skin. As shock progresses, the patient's skin becomes clammy and his pulse becomes increasingly rapid and thready. He may also develop hypotension, narrowed pulse pressure, oliguria, subnormal body temperature, and decreased LOC.

Neurogenic shock. Tachycardia or bradycardia may accompany tachypnea, apprehension, oliguria, variable body temperature, decreased LOC, and warm, dry skin.

Orthostatic hypotension. Tachycardia accompanies the characteristic signs and symptoms of orthostatic hypotension, which include dizziness, syncope, pallor, blurred vision, diaphoresis, and nausea.

Pneumothorax. Life-threatening pneumothorax causes tachycardia and other signs and symptoms of distress, such as severe dyspnea and chest pain, tachypnea, and cyanosis. Related findings include dry cough, subcutaneous crepitation, absent or decreased breath sounds, cessation of normal chest movement on the affected side, and decreased vocal fremitus.

Pulmonary embolism. With pulmonary embolism, tachycardia is usually preceded by sudden dyspnea, angina, or pleuritic chest pain. Common associated signs and symptoms include weak peripheral pulses, cyanosis, tachypnea, low-grade fever, restlessness, diaphoresis, and a dry cough or a cough with blood-tinged sputum.

Thyrotoxicosis. Tachycardia is a classic feature of thyrotoxicosis—a thyroid disorder. Others include an enlarged thyroid, nervousness, heat intolerance, weight loss despite increased appetite, diaphoresis, diarrhea, tremors, and palpitations. Although also considered characteristic, exophthalmos is sometimes absent.

Because thyrotoxicosis affects virtually every body system, its associated features are diverse and numerous. Some examples include full and bounding pulse, widened pulse pressure, dyspnea, anorexia, nausea, vomiting, altered bowel habits, hepatomegaly, and muscle weakness, fatigue, and atrophy. The patient's skin is smooth, warm, and flushed; his hair is fine and soft and may gray prematurely or fall out. The female patient may have a reduced libido and oligomenorrhea or amenorrhea; the male patient may exhibit a reduced libido and gynecomastia.

Other causes

Diagnostic tests. Cardiac catheterization and electrophysiologic studies may induce transient tachycardia.

Drugs and alcohol. Various drugs affect the nervous system, circulatory system, or heart muscle, resulting in tachycardia. Examples of these include sympathomimetics; phenothiazines; anticholinergics, such as atropine; thyroid drugs; vasodilators, such as hydralazine; acetylcholinesterase inhibitors, such as captopril; nitrates, such as nitroglycerin; alpha-adrenergic blockers, such as phentolamine; and beta-adrenergic bronchodilators, such as albuterol. Excessive caffeine intake and alcohol intoxication may also cause tachycardia.

Surgery and pacemakers. Cardiac surgery and pacemaker malfunction or wire irritation may cause tachycardia.

Nursing considerations

- Monitor the patient's cardiovascular status and vital signs closely.
- Administer medications or fluids to control heart rate.

■ Prepare the patient for diagnostic tests, such as a thyroid panel, electrolyte and hemoglobin levels, hematocrit, pulmonary function studies, 12-lead ECG, if appropriate, an ambulatory ECG.

Patient teaching

■ Educate the patient about the possibility of the tachyarrhythmia recurring.
■ Explain that an antiarrhythmic and an internal defibrillator or ablation therapy may be indicated for symptomatic tachycardia.
■ Discuss the underlying cause of the tachycardia and its treatments.
■ Explain medications, their proper dosage and administration, and possible adverse effects.

Tachypnea

A common sign of cardiopulmonary disorders, tachypnea is an abnormally fast respiratory rate—greater than 20 breaths/minute. Tachypnea may reflect the need to increase minute volume—the amount of air breathed each minute. Under these circumstances, it may be accompanied by an increase in tidal volume—the volume of air inhaled or exhaled per breath—resulting in hyperventilation. Tachypnea, however, may also reflect stiff lungs or overloaded ventilatory muscles, in which case tidal volume may actually be reduced.

Tachypnea may result from reduced arterial oxygen tension or arterial oxygen content, decreased perfusion, or increased oxygen demand. Heightened oxygen demand, for example, may result from fever, exertion, anxiety, and pain. It may also occur as a compensatory response to metabolic acidosis or may result from pulmonary irritation, stretch receptor stimulation, or a neurologic disorder that upsets medullary respiratory control.

ACTION STAT!

 After detecting tachypnea, quickly evaluate cardiopulmonary status; obtain a set of vital signs with oxygen saturation; and check for cyanosis, chest pain, dyspnea, tachycardia, and hypotension. If the patient has paradoxical chest movement, suspect flail chest and immediately splint his chest with your hands or with sandbags. Administer supplemental oxygen by nasal cannula or face mask and, if possible, place the patient in semi-Fowler's position to help ease his breathing. Endotracheal intubation and mechanical ventilation may be necessary if respiratory failure occurs. Insert an I.V. catheter for fluid and drug administration and begin cardiac monitoring.

History and physical examination

If the patient's condition permits, obtain a medical history. Find out when the tachypnea began. Did it follow activity? Has he had it before? Does the patient have a history of asthma, chronic obstructive pulmonary disease (COPD), or any other pulmonary or cardiac conditions? Then have him describe associated signs and symptoms, such as diaphoresis, chest pain, and recent weight loss. Is he anxious about anything, or does he have a history of anxiety attacks? Obtain a complete drug and alcohol history.

Begin the physical examination by taking the patient's vital signs, including oxygen saturation and observing his overall behavior. Does he seem restless, confused, or fatigued? Then auscultate the chest for abnormal heart and breath sounds. If the patient has a productive cough, record the color, amount, and consistency of sputum. Finally, check for jugular vein distention, and examine the skin for pallor, cyanosis, edema, and warmth or coolness.

Medical causes

Acute respiratory distress syndrome (ARDS). With life-threatening ARDS, tachypnea and apprehension may be the earliest features. Tachypnea gradually worsens as fluid accumulates in the patient's lungs, causing them to stiffen. It's accompanied by accessory muscle use, grunting expirations, suprasternal and intercostal retractions, crackles, and rhonchi. Eventually, ARDS produces hypoxemia, resulting in tachycardia, dyspnea, cyanosis, respiratory failure, and shock.

Anaphylactic shock. With anaphylactic shock, tachypnea develops within minutes after exposure to an allergen, such as penicillin or insect venom. Accompanying signs and symptoms include anxiety, a pounding headache, skin flushing, intense pruritus and, possibly, diffuse urticaria. The patient may exhibit widespread edema, affecting the eyelids, lips, tongue, hands, feet, and genitalia. Other findings include cool, clammy skin; a rapid, thready pulse; cough; dyspnea; stridor; and a change or loss of voice associated with laryngeal edema.

Asthma. Tachypnea is common with life-threatening asthma attacks, which commonly occur at night. These attacks usually begin with mild wheezing and a dry cough that progresses to mucus expectoration. Eventually, the patient becomes apprehensive and develops prolonged expirations, intercostal and supraclavicular retractions on inspiration, accessory muscle use, severe audible wheezing, rhonchi, flaring nostrils, tachycardia, diaphoresis, and flushing or cyanosis.

Bronchitis (chronic). Mild tachypnea may occur in chronic bronchitis but it isn't typically a predominant sign. Usually, chronic bronchitis begins with a dry, hacking cough, which later produces copious amounts of sputum. Other characteristics include dyspnea, prolonged expirations, wheezing, scattered rhonchi, accessory muscle use, and cyanosis. Clubbing and barrel chest are late signs.

Cardiac arrhythmias. Depending on the patient's heart rate and type of arrhythmia, tachypnea may occur along with hypotension, dizziness, palpitations, weakness, and fatigue. The patient's level of consciousness (LOC) may be decreased.

Cardiac tamponade. With life-threatening cardiac tamponade, tachypnea may accompany tachycardia, dyspnea, and paradoxical pulse. Related findings include muffled heart sounds, pericardial friction rub, chest pain, hypotension, narrowed pulse pressure, and hepatomegaly. The patient is noticeably anxious and restless. His skin is clammy and cyanotic, and his jugular veins are distended.

Cardiogenic shock. Tachypnea occurs with cardiogenic shock along with cold, pale, clammy, cyanotic skin; hypotension; tachycardia; narrowed pulse pressure; a ventricular gallop; oliguria; decreased LOC; and jugular vein distention.

Emphysema. Emphysema commonly produces tachypnea accompanied by exertional dyspnea. It may also cause anorexia, malaise, peripheral cyanosis, pursed-lip breathing, accessory muscle use, and chronic productive cough. Percussion yields a hyperresonant tone; auscultation reveals wheezing, crackles, and diminished breath sounds. Clubbing and barrel chest are late signs.

Flail chest. Tachypnea usually appears early with life-threatening flail chest. Other findings include paradoxical chest wall movement, rib bruises and palpable fractures, localized chest pain, hypotension, and diminished breath sounds. The patient may also develop signs of respiratory distress, such as dyspnea and accessory muscle use.

Hyperosmolar hyperglycemic nonketotic syndrome (HHNS). With HHNS, rapidly deteriorating LOC occurs with tachypnea, tachycardia, hypotension, seizures, oliguria, and signs of dehydration.

Hypovolemic shock. An early sign of life-threatening hypovolemic shock, tachypnea is accompanied by cool, pale skin; restlessness; thirst; and mild tachycardia. As shock progresses, the patient's skin becomes clammy; his pulse is increasingly rapid and thready. Other findings include hypotension, narrowed pulse pressure, oliguria, subnormal body temperature, and decreased LOC.

Hypoxia. Lack of oxygen from any cause increases the rate (and commonly the depth) of breathing. Associated symptoms are related to the cause of the hypoxia.

Interstitial fibrosis. With interstitial fibrosis, tachypnea develops gradually and may become severe. Associated features include exertional dyspnea, pleuritic chest pain, a paroxysmal dry cough, crackles, late inspiratory wheezing, cyanosis, fatigue, and weight loss. Clubbing is a late sign.

Lung abscess. With lung abscess, tachypnea is usually paired with dyspnea and accentuated by fever. However, the chief sign is a productive cough with copious amounts of purulent, foul-smelling, usually bloody sputum. Other findings include chest pain, halitosis, diaphoresis, chills, fatigue, weakness, anorexia, weight loss, and clubbing.

Mesothelioma (malignant). Commonly related to asbestos exposure, this pleural mass initially produces tachypnea and dyspnea on mild exertion. Other classic symptoms are persistent, dull chest pain and aching shoulder pain that progresses to arm weakness and paresthesia. Later signs and symptoms include cough, insomnia associated with pain, clubbing, and dullness over the malignant mesothelioma.

Neurogenic shock. Tachypnea is characteristic in neurogenic shock. It's commonly accompanied by apprehension, bradycardia or tachycardia, oliguria, fluctuating body temperature, and decreased LOC that may progress to coma. The patient's skin is warm, dry, and perhaps flushed. He may experience nausea and vomiting.

Plague (Yersinia pestis). The onset of the pneumonic form of plague is usually sudden with chills, fever, headache, and myalgia. Pulmonary signs and symptoms include tachypnea, productive cough, chest pain, dyspnea, hemoptysis, and increasing respiratory distress and cardiopulmonary insufficiency. The pneumonic form may be contracted from person-to-person direct contact via the respiratory system. This would also be the form contracted in biological warfare from aerosolization and inhalation of the organism.

Pneumonia (bacterial). A common sign of pneumonia, tachypnea is usually preceded by a painful, hacking, dry cough that rapidly becomes productive. Other signs and symptoms quickly follow, including high fever, shaking chills, headache, dyspnea, pleuritic chest pain, tachycardia, grunting respirations, nasal flaring, and cyanosis. Auscultation reveals diminished breath sounds and fine crackles; percussion yields a dull tone.

Pneumothorax. Tachypnea, a common sign of life-threatening pneumothorax, is typically accompanied by severe, sharp, and commonly unilateral chest pain that's aggravated by chest movement. Associated signs and symptoms include dyspnea, tachycardia, accessory muscle use, asymmetrical chest expansion, dry cough, cyanosis, anxiety, and restlessness. Examination of the affected lung reveals hyperresonance or tympany, subcutaneous crepitation, decreased vocal fremitus, and diminished or absent breath sounds on the affected side. The patient with tension pneumothorax also develops a deviated trachea.

Pulmonary edema. An early sign of life-threatening pulmonary edema, tachypnea is accompanied by exertional dyspnea, paroxysmal nocturnal dyspnea and, later, orthopnea. Other features include a dry cough, crackles, tachycardia, and a ventricular gallop. With severe pulmonary edema, respirations become increasingly rapid and labored, tachycardia worsens, and crackles become more diffuse. The patient's cough also produces frothy, bloody sputum. Signs of shock—such as hypotension, thready pulse, and cold, clammy skin—may also occur.

Pulmonary embolism (acute). Tachypnea occurs suddenly with pulmonary embolism and is usually accompanied by dyspnea. Other signs include angina or pleuritic chest pain, tachycardia, a dry or productive cough with blood-tinged sputum, low-grade fever, restlessness, and diaphoresis. Less-common signs include massive hemoptysis, chest splinting, leg edema, and—with a large embolus—jugular vein distention and syncope. Other findings include pleural friction rub, crackles, diffuse wheezing, dullness on percussion, diminished breath sounds, and signs of shock, such as hypotension and a weak, rapid pulse.

Septic shock. With septic shock, tachypnea; sudden fever; chills; flushed, warm, yet dry skin; and possibly nausea, vomiting, and diarrhea occur. Tachycardia and normal or slightly decreased blood pressure may also develop. As this life-threatening type of shock progresses, the patient may display anxiety; restlessness; decreased LOC; hypotension; cool, clammy, and cyanotic skin; rapid,

thready pulse; thirst; and oliguria that may progress to anuria.

Other causes

Drugs. Tachypnea may result from an overdose of salicylates.

Foreign body aspiration. A dry, paroxysmal cough with rapid, shallow respirations is characteristic of life-threatening partial upper airway obstruction caused by foreign body aspiration. Other signs and symptoms include dyspnea, gagging or choking, intercostal retractions, nasal flaring, cyanosis, decreased or absent breath sounds, hoarseness, and stridor or coarse wheezing. Typically, the patient appears frightened and distressed. A complete obstruction may rapidly cause asphyxia and death.

Nursing considerations

- Monitor the patient's vital signs and LOC closely.
- Keep suction and emergency equipment nearby.
- Prepare to intubate the patient and to provide mechanical ventilation if necessary.
- Prepare the patient for diagnostic studies, such as arterial blood gas analysis, blood cultures, chest X-rays, computed tomography scan, pulmonary function tests, and an electrocardiogram.

Patient teaching

- Explain the underlying disorder and treatment plan.
- Teach the patient about stress reduction techniques.
- Demonstrate breathing techniques, such as deep-breathing or pursed-lip breathing, as appropriate.
- Explain home respiratory care.

▌Throat pain

Throat pain—commonly known as a *sore throat*—refers to discomfort in any part of the pharynx: the nasopharynx, the oropharynx, or the hypopharynx. This common symptom ranges from a sensation of scratchiness to severe pain. It's commonly accompanied by ear pain because cranial nerves IX and X innervate the pharynx as well as the middle and external ear. (See *Anatomy of the throat.*)

Throat pain may result from infection, trauma, allergy, cancer, or a systemic disorder. It may also follow surgery and endotracheal intubation. Nonpathologic causes include dry mucous membranes associated with mouth breathing and laryngeal irritation associated with alcohol consumption, inhaling smoke or chemicals such as ammonia, and vocal strain.

History and physical examination

Ask the patient when he first noticed the pain, and have him describe it. Has he had throat pain before? How was it treated? Is it accompanied by fever, ear pain, or dysphagia? Review the patient's medical history for throat problems, allergies, and systemic disorders.

Next, carefully examine the pharynx, noting redness, exudate, or swelling. Examine the oropharynx and the nasopharynx. Laryngoscopic examination of the hypopharynx may be required. (If necessary, spray the soft palate and pharyngeal wall with a local anesthetic to prevent gagging.) Observe the tonsils for redness, swelling, or exudate. Obtain an exudate specimen for culture. Then examine the nose. Also, check the patient's ears, especially if he reports ear pain. Finally, palpate the neck and oropharynx for nodules or lymph node enlargement.

Medical causes

Agranulocytosis. With agranulocytosis, throat pain may accompany other signs and symptoms of infection, such as fever, chills, and headache. Typically, it follows progressive fatigue and weakness. Other findings include nausea and vomiting, anorexia, and bleeding tendencies. Rough-edged ulcers with gray or black membranes may appear on the gums, palate, or perianal area.

Avian influenza. Throat pain, muscle aches, cough, and fever are common early symptoms of avian influenza. The most virulent of these viruses, avian influenza A (H5N1), may also cause pneumonia, acute respiratory distress, and other life-threatening complications.

Bronchitis (acute). Acute bronchitis may produce lower throat pain associated with fever, chills, cough, and muscle and back pain. Auscultation reveals rhonchi, wheezing and, at times, crackles.

Chronic fatigue syndrome. Chronic fatigue syndrome is characterized by incapacitating fatigue. Associated findings include throat pain, myalgia, and cognitive dysfunction.

Contact ulcers. Common in men with stressful jobs, contact ulcers appear symmetrically on the posterior vocal cords, resulting in sore throat. The pain is aggravated by talking and may be accompanied by referred ear pain and, occasionally, hemoptysis. Typically, the patient also has a history of chronic throat clearing or acid reflux.

Gastroesophageal reflux disease (GERD). With GERD, an incompetent gastroesophageal sphincter allows gastric juices to enter the hypopharynx and irritate the larynx, causing chronic throat pain and hoarseness. The arytenoids may also appear red and swollen, resulting in a sensation of a lump in the throat.

Influenza. Patients with the flu commonly complain of throat pain, fever with chills, headache, weakness, malaise, muscle aches, cough and, occasionally, hoarseness and rhinorrhea.

Anatomy of the throat

The throat, or pharynx, is divided into three areas: the nasopharynx (the soft palate and the posterior nasal cavity), the oropharynx (the area between the soft palate and the upper edge of the epiglottis), and the hypopharynx (the area between the epiglottis and the level of the cricoid cartilage). A disorder affecting any of these areas may cause throat pain. Pinpointing the causative disorder begins with accurate assessment of the throat structures illustrated here.

Frontal view

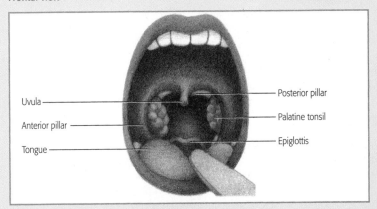

Cross-sectional view

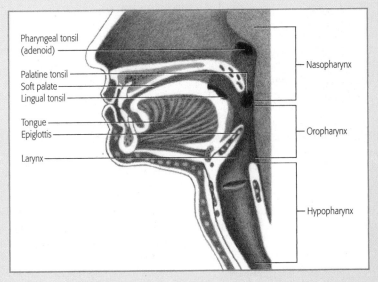

Laryngeal cancer. With extrinsic laryngeal cancer, the chief symptom is pain or burning in the throat when drinking citrus juice or hot liquids or a lump in the throat; with intrinsic laryngeal cancer, the chief symptom is hoarseness that persists for longer than 3 weeks. Later signs and symptoms of metastasis include dysphagia, dyspnea, cough, enlarged cervical lymph nodes, and pain that radiates to the ear.

Monkeypox. Early symptoms of this rare viral disease include throat pain, fever, lymphadenopathy, chills, myalgia, and rash. The virus exhibits some similarities to smallpox, but its symptoms tend to be milder.

Mononucleosis (infectious). Throat pain is one of the three classic findings in this infection. The other two classic signs are cervical lymphadenopathy and fluctuating temperature with an evening peak of 101° to 102° F (38.3° to 38.9° C). Splenomegaly and hepatomegaly may also develop.

Necrotizing ulcerative gingivitis (acute). Also known as *trench mouth,* necrotizing ulcerative gingivitis usually begins abruptly with throat pain and tender gums that ulcerate and bleed. A gray exudate may cover the gums and pharyngeal tonsils. Related signs and symptoms include a foul taste in the mouth, halitosis, cervical lymphadenopathy, headache, malaise, and fever.

Peritonsillar abscess. A complication of bacterial tonsillitis, this abscess typically causes severe throat pain that radiates to the ear. Accompanying the pain may be dysphagia, drooling, dysarthria, halitosis, fever with chills, malaise, and nausea. The patient usually tilts his head toward the side of the abscess. Examination may also reveal a deviated uvula, trismus, and tender cervical lymphadenopathy.

Pharyngitis. Whether bacterial, fungal, or viral, pharyngitis may cause throat pain and localized erythema and edema. *Bacterial pharyngitis* begins abruptly with a unilateral throat pain. Associated signs and symptoms include

dysphagia, fever, malaise, headache, abdominal pain, myalgia, and arthralgia. Inspection reveals an exudate on the tonsil or tonsillar fossae, uvular edema, soft palate erythema, and tender cervical lymph nodes.

Also known as *thrush, fungal pharyngitis* causes diffuse throat pain—commonly described as a burning sensation—accompanied by pharyngeal erythema and edema. White plaques mark the pharynx, tonsil, tonsillar pillars, base of the tongue, and oral mucosa; scraping these plaques uncovers a hemorrhagic base.

With *viral pharyngitis,* findings include diffuse throat pain, malaise, fever, and mild erythema and edema of the posterior oropharyngeal wall. Tonsillary enlargement may be present along with anterior cervical lymphadenopathy.

Sinusitis (acute). Sinusitis may cause throat pain with purulent nasal discharge and postnasal drip, resulting in halitosis. Other effects include headache, malaise, cough, fever, and facial pain and swelling associated with nasal congestion.

Tongue cancer. With tongue cancer, the patient experiences localized throat pain that may occur around a raised white lesion or ulcer. The pain may radiate to the ear and be accompanied by dysphagia.

Tonsillar cancer. Throat pain is the presenting symptom in tonsillar cancer. Unfortunately, the cancer is usually quite advanced before the appearance of this symptom. The pain may radiate to the ear and is accompanied by a superficial ulcer on the tonsil or one that extends to the base of the tongue.

Tonsillitis. With *acute tonsillitis,* mild to severe throat pain is usually the first symptom. The pain may radiate to the ears and be accompanied by dysphagia and headache. Related findings include malaise, fever with chills, halitosis, myalgia, arthralgia, and tender cervical lymphadenopathy. Examination reveals edematous, reddened tonsils with a purulent exudate.

Chronic tonsillitis causes mild throat pain, malaise, and tender cervical lymph nodes. The tonsils appear smooth, pink and, possibly, enlarged, with purulent debris in the crypts. Halitosis and a foul taste in the mouth are other common findings.

Unilateral or bilateral throat pain just above the hyoid bone occurs with *lingual tonsillitis*. The lingual tonsils appear red and swollen and are covered with exudate. Other findings include a muffled voice, dysphagia, and tender cervical lymphadenopathy on the affected side.

Upper respiratory infection (URI). With a URI, throat pain may accompany coughing, sneezing, nasal congestion, rhinorrhea, fatigue, headache, myalgia, and arthralgia.

Uvulitis. Uvulitis may cause throat pain or a sensation of something in the throat. The uvula is usually swollen and red but, in *allergic uvulitis,* it's pale.

Other causes
Foreign body aspiration. A foreign body lodged in the palatine or lingual tonsil and pyriform sinus may produce localized throat pain. The pain may persist after the foreign body is dislodged until mucosal irritation resolves.

Treatments. Endotracheal intubation and local surgery, such as tonsillectomy and adenoidectomy, commonly cause throat pain.

Nursing considerations
- Provide analgesic sprays or lozenges to relieve throat pain.
- Prepare the patient for throat culture, complete blood count, and a Monospot test.

Patient teaching
- Explain the underlying disorder and treatment plan.
- Explain the importance of taking the full course of antibiotics, as ordered.
- Discuss ways to soothe the throat.

Thyroid enlargement

An enlarged thyroid can result from inflammation, physiologic changes, iodine deficiency, thyroid tumors, and drugs. Depending on the medical cause, hyperfunction or hypofunction may occur with resulting excess or deficiency, respectively, of the hormone thyroxine. If no infection is present, enlargement is usually slow and progressive. An enlarged thyroid that causes visible swelling in the front of the neck is called a *goiter.*

History and physical examination
The patient's history commonly reveals the cause of thyroid enlargement. Important data includes a family history of thyroid disease, onset of thyroid enlargement, any previous irradiation of the thyroid or the neck, recent infections, and the use of thyroid replacement drugs.

Begin the physical examination by inspecting the patient's trachea for midline deviation. Although you can usually see the enlarged gland, you should always palpate it. To palpate the thyroid gland, you'll need to stand behind the patient. Give the patient a cup of water, and have him extend his neck slightly. Place the fingers of both hands on the patient's neck, just below the cricoid cartilage and just lateral to the trachea. Tell the patient to take a sip of water and swallow. The thyroid gland should rise as he swallows. Use your fingers to palpate laterally and downward to feel the whole thyroid gland. Palpate over the midline to feel the isthmus of the thyroid.

During palpation, be sure to note the size, shape, and consistency of the gland, and the presence or absence of nodules. Using the bell of a stethoscope, listen over the lateral lobes for a bruit. The bruit is often continuous.

Medical causes

Hypothyroidism. Hypothyroidism causes an enlarged thyroid. Additional signs and symptoms include weight gain despite anorexia; fatigue; cold intolerance; constipation; menorrhagia; slowed intellectual and motor activity; dry, pale, cool skin; dry, sparse hair; and thick, brittle nails. Eventually, the face assumes a dull expression with periorbital edema.

Iodine deficiency. A deficiency of iodine in the food or water of a particular area may cause an *endemic goiter.* Associated signs and symptoms of an endemic goiter include dysphagia, dyspnea, and tracheal deviation. This condition is uncommon in developed countries with iodized salt.

Thyroiditis. Autoimmune thyroiditis usually produces no symptoms other than thyroid enlargement.

Thyrotoxicosis. Signs and symptoms of thyrotoxicosis include an enlarged thyroid, nervousness; heat intolerance; fatigue; weight loss despite increased appetite; diarrhea; sweating; palpitations; tremors; smooth, warm, flushed skin; fine, soft hair; exophthalmos; nausea and vomiting due to increased GI motility and peristalsis; and, in females, oligomenorrhea or amenorrhea.

Tumors. An enlarged thyroid may result from a malignant tumor or a nonmalignant tumor (such as an adenoma). Associated signs and symptoms include hoarseness, loss of voice, and dysphagia.

Thyroid tissue contained in ovarian dermoid tumors can function autonomously or in combination with thyrotoxicosis. Pituitary tumors that secrete thyroid-stimulating hormone (TSH), a rare type, are the only cause of normal or high TSH levels in association with thyrotoxicosis. Finally, high levels of human chorionic gonadotropin, as seen in trophoblastic tumors and pregnant women, can cause thyrotoxicosis.

Other causes

Goitrogens. Goitrogens are drugs—such as lithium, sulfonamides, phenylbutazone, and para-aminosalicylic acid—and substances in foods that decrease thyroxine production. Foods containing goitrogens include peanuts, cabbage, soybeans, strawberries, spinach, rutabagas, and radishes.

Nursing considerations

- Prepare the patient for diagnostic tests, which may include needle aspiration, ultrasound, and radioactive thyroid scanning.
- Prepare the patient for surgery or radiation therapy, if necessary.
- Provide specific interventions, depending on whether the patient is hypothyroid or has thyroiditis.
- Provide postoperative care for the patient who has undergone thyroidectomy.

Patient teaching

- Explain the underlying disorder and treatment plan.
- Explain the signs and symptoms of hypothyroidism to report.
- Explain posttreatment precautions to the patient undergoing radioactive iodine therapy.
- Teach thyroid hormone replacement therapy and signs of thyroid hormone overdose to report.

Tics

A tic is an involuntary, repetitive movement of a specific group of muscles—usually those of the face, neck, shoulders, trunk, and hands. This sign typically occurs suddenly and intermittently. It may involve a single isolated movement, such as lip smacking, grimacing, blinking, sniffing, tongue thrusting, throat clearing, hitching up one shoulder, or protruding the chin. Or, it may involve a complex set of movements. Mild tics, such as twitching of an eyelid, are especially common. Tics differ from minor seizures in that tics aren't associated with transient loss of consciousness or amnesia.

Tics are usually psychogenic and may be aggravated by stress or anxiety. Psychogenic tics commonly begin between ages 5 and 10 as voluntary, coordinated, and purposeful actions that the child feels compelled to perform to decrease anxiety. Unless the tics are severe, the child may be unaware of them. The tics may subside as the child matures, or they may persist into adulthood. However, tics are also associated with one rare affliction—Tourette's syndrome, which typically begins during childhood.

History and physical examination

Begin by asking the parents how long the child has had the tic. How often does it occur? Can they identify any precipitating or exacerbating factors? Can the patient control the tics with conscious effort? Ask about stress in the child's life such as difficult schoolwork. Next, carefully observe the tic. Is it a purposeful or involuntary movement? Note whether it's localized or generalized, and describe it in detail.

Medical causes

Tourette's syndrome. Tourette's syndrome typically begins with a tic that involves the face or neck. Indications include both motor and vocal tics that may involve the muscles of the shoulders, arms, trunk, and legs. The tics may be associated with violent movements and outbursts of obscenities (coprolalia). The patient snorts, barks, and grunts and may emit explosive sounds, such as hissing, when he speaks. He may involuntarily repeat another person's words (echolalia) or movements (echopraxia). At times, this syndrome subsides spontaneously or undergoes a prolonged remission, but it may persist throughout life.

Nursing considerations

■ Administer drugs, as indicated, to control tics.
■ Provide referrals for psychotherapy, as indicated.

Patient teaching

■ Explain the disorder and treatment plan.
■ Help the patient identify and eliminate any avoidable stress.
■ Discuss with the patient positive ways to deal with his anxiety.
■ Offer emotional support to the patient and family.

Tinnitus

Tinnitus literally means ringing in the ears, although many other abnormal sounds fall under this term. For example, tinnitus may be described as the sound of escaping air, running water, the inside of a seashell, or as a sizzling, buzzing, or humming noise. Occasionally, it's described as a roaring or musical sound. This common symptom may be unilateral or bilateral and constant or intermittent. Although the brain may adjust to or suppress constant tinnitus, tinnitus may be so disturbing that some patients contemplate suicide as their only source of relief.

Tinnitus can be classified in several ways. Subjective tinnitus is heard only by the patient; objective tinnitus is also heard by the observer who places a stethoscope near the patient's affected ear. Tinnitus aurium refers to noise that the patient hears in his ears; tinnitus cerebri, to noise that he hears in his head.

Tinnitus is usually associated with neural injury within the auditory pathway, resulting in altered, spontaneous firing of sensory auditory neurons. Commonly resulting from an ear disorder, tinnitus may also stem from a cardiovascular or systemic disorder or from the effects of drugs. Nonpathologic causes of tinnitus include acute anxiety and presbycusis.

History and physical examination

Ask the patient to describe the sound he hears, including its onset, pattern, pitch, location, and intensity. Ask whether it's accompanied by other symptoms, such as vertigo, headache, or hearing loss. Next, take a health history, including a complete drug history.

Inspect the patient's ears and examine the tympanic membrane. To check for hearing loss, perform the Weber and Rinne tuning fork tests.

Also, auscultate for bruits in the neck. Then compress the jugular or carotid artery to see if this affects the tinnitus. Finally, examine the nasopharynx for masses that might cause eustachian tube dysfunction and tinnitus.

Medical causes

Acoustic neuroma. An early symptom of acoustic neuroma, unilateral tinnitus precedes unilateral sensorineural hearing loss and vertigo. Facial paralysis, headache, nausea, vomiting, and papilledema may also occur.

Atherosclerosis of the carotid artery. With atherosclerosis of the carotid artery, the patient has constant tinnitus that can be stopped by applying pressure over the carotid artery. Auscultation over the upper part of the neck, on the auricle, or near the ear on the affected side may detect a bruit. Palpation may reveal a weak carotid pulse.

Cervical spondylosis. With degenerative cervical spondylosis, osteophytic growths may compress the vertebral arteries, resulting in tinnitus. Typically, a stiff neck and pain aggravated by activity accompany tinnitus. Other features include brief vertigo, nystagmus, hearing loss, paresthesia, weakness, and pain that radiates down the arms.

Eustachian tube patency. Normally, the eustachian tube remains closed, except during swallowing. However, persistent patency of this tube can cause tinnitus, audible breath sounds, loud and distorted voice sounds, and a sense of fullness in the ear. Examination with a pneumatic otoscope reveals movement of the tympanic membrane with respirations. At times, breath sounds can be heard with a stethoscope placed over the auricle.

Glomus jugulare (tympanicum tumor). A pulsating sound is usually the first symptom of this tumor. Other early features include a reddish blue mass behind the tympanic membrane and progressive conductive hearing loss. Later, total unilateral deafness is accompanied by ear pain and dizziness. Otorrhagia may also occur if the tumor breaks through the tympanic membrane.

Hypertension. Bilateral, high-pitched tinnitus may occur with severe hypertension. Diastolic blood pressure exceeding 120 mm Hg may also cause a severe, throbbing headache, restlessness, nausea, vomiting, blurred vision, seizures, and decreased level of consciousness.

Labyrinthitis (suppurative). With labyrinthitis, tinnitus may accompany sudden, severe attacks of vertigo, unilateral or bilateral sensorineural hearing loss, nystagmus, dizziness, nausea, and vomiting.

Ménière's disease. Ménière's disease is characterized by attacks of tinnitus, vertigo, a feeling of fullness or blockage in the ear, and fluctuating sensorineural hearing loss. These attacks last from 10 minutes to several hours; they occur over a few days or weeks and are followed by a remission. Severe nausea, vomiting, diaphoresis, and nystagmus may also occur during attacks.

Ossicle dislocation. Acoustic trauma, such as a slap on the ear, may dislocate the ossicle, resulting in tinnitus and sensorineural hearing loss. Bleeding from the middle ear may also occur.

Otitis externa (acute). Although not a major complaint with otitis externa, tinnitus may result if debris in the external ear canal impinges on the tympanic membrane. More typical findings include pruritus, foul-smelling purulent discharge, and severe ear pain that's aggravated by manipulation of the tragus or auricle, teeth clenching, mouth opening, and chewing. The external ear canal typically appears red and edematous and may be occluded by debris, causing partial hearing loss.

Otitis media. Otitis media may cause tinnitus and conductive hearing loss. However, its more typical features include ear pain, a red and bulging tympanic membrane, high fever, chills, and dizziness.

Otosclerosis. With otosclerosis, the patient may describe ringing, roaring, or whistling tinnitus or a combination of these sounds. He may also report progressive hearing loss, which may lead to bilateral deafness, and vertigo.

Presbycusis. Presbycusis produces tinnitus and a progressive, symmetrical, bilateral sensorineural hearing loss, usually of high-frequency tones.

Tympanic membrane perforation. With tympanic membrane perforation, tinnitus and hearing loss go hand-in-hand. Tinnitus is usually the chief complaint in a small perforation; hearing loss is usually the chief complaint in a larger perforation. These symptoms typically develop suddenly and may be accompanied by pain, vertigo, and a feeling of fullness in the ear. If the patient has had otitis media, the perforation will cause drainage and relief of pain.

Other causes

Drugs and alcohol. An overdose of salicylates commonly causes reversible tinnitus. Quinine, alcohol, and indomethacin may also cause reversible tinnitus. Common drugs that may cause irreversible tinnitus include the aminoglycoside antibiotics (especially kanamycin, streptomycin, and gentamicin) and vancomycin.

Noise. Chronic exposure to noise, especially high-pitched sounds, can damage the ear's hair cells, causing tinnitus and a bilateral hearing loss. These symptoms may be temporary or permanent.

Nursing considerations

- Treat the underlying disorder.
- Have the patient use a hearing aid, as prescribed, to amplify environmental sounds, thereby obscuring tinnitus.

Patient teaching

- Explain the underlying disorder and treatment plan.
- Educate the patient about strategies for adapting to the tinnitus, including biofeedback and masking devices.

■ Provide information about avoiding excessive noise, ototoxic agents, and other factors that may cause cochlear damage.

 Tracheal deviation

Normally, the trachea is located at the midline of the neck—except at the bifurcation, where it shifts slightly toward the right. Visible deviation from its normal position signals an underlying condition that can compromise pulmonary function and possibly cause respiratory distress. A hallmark of life-threatening tension pneumothorax, tracheal deviation occurs with disorders that produce mediastinal shift due to asymmetrical thoracic volume or pressure. A nonlesion pneumothorax can produce tracheal deviation to the ipsilateral side. (See *Detecting slight tracheal deviation*.)

A C T I O N   S T A T !

 If you detect tracheal deviation, be alert for signs and symptoms of respiratory distress (tachypnea, dyspnea, decreased or absent breath sounds, stridor, nasal flaring, accessory muscle use, asymmetrical chest expansion, restlessness, and anxiety). If possible, place the patient in semi-Fowler's position to aid respiratory excursion and improve oxygenation. Give supplemental oxygen, and intubate the patient if necessary. Insert an I.V. catheter for fluid and drug administration. Palpate for subcutaneous crepitation in the neck and chest, a sign of tension pneumothorax. Obtain a chest X-ray. Chest tube insertion may be necessary to release trapped air or fluid and to restore normal intrapleural and intrathoracic pressure gradients.

History and physical examination

If the patient doesn't display signs of distress, ask about a history of pulmonary or cardiac disorders, surgery, trauma, or infection. If he smokes, determine how much. Ask about associated signs and symptoms, especially breathing difficulty, pain, and cough.

Then perform a physical examination. Inspect the chest wall for symmetry during ventilation. Check pulse oximetry and vital signs. Auscultate the lungs for breath sounds. Note signs of respiratory distress. Place the patient on a cardiac monitor and assess heart sounds. Palpate the chest and abdomen for abnormalities.

Medical causes

Atelectasis. Extensive lung collapse can produce tracheal deviation toward the affected side. Respiratory findings include dyspnea, tachypnea, pleuritic chest pain, dry cough, dullness on percussion, decreased vocal fremitus and breath sounds, inspiratory lag, and substernal or intercostal retraction.

Hiatal hernia. Intrusion of abdominal viscera into the pleural space causes tracheal deviation toward the unaffected side. The degree of attendant respiratory distress depends on the extent of herniation. Other effects include pyrosis, regurgitation or vomiting, and chest or abdominal pain.

Kyphoscoliosis. Kyphoscoliosis can cause rib cage distortion and mediastinal shift, producing tracheal deviation toward the compressed lung. Respiratory effects include dry coughing, dyspnea, asymmetrical chest expansion and, possibly, asymmetrical breath sounds. Backache and fatigue are also common.

Mediastinal tumor. Typically producing no symptoms in its early stages, a mediastinal tumor, when large, can

Detecting slight tracheal deviation

Although gross tracheal deviation is visible, detection of slight deviation requires palpation and perhaps even an X-ray. Try palpation first.

With the tip of your index finger, locate the patient's trachea by palpating between the sternocleidomastoid muscles. Then compare the trachea's position to an imaginary line drawn vertically through the suprasternal notch. Any deviation from midline is usually considered abnormal.

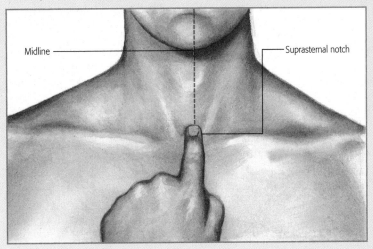

Midline ———

——— Suprasternal notch

press against the trachea and nearby structures, causing tracheal deviation and dysphagia. Other late findings include stridor, dyspnea, brassy cough, hoarseness, and stertorous respirations with suprasternal retraction. The patient may experience shoulder, arm, or chest pain as well as edema of the neck, face, or arm. His neck and chest wall veins may be dilated.

Pulmonary tuberculosis (TB). With a large cavitation resulting from TB, tracheal deviation toward the affected side accompanies asymmetrical chest excursion, dullness on percussion, increased tactile fremitus, amphoric breath sounds, and inspiratory crackles. Insidious early effects include fatigue, anorexia, weight loss, fever, chills, and night sweats. Productive cough, hemoptysis,

pleuritic chest pain, and dyspnea develop as the disease progresses.

Retrosternal thyroid. Retrosternal thyroid can displace the trachea. The gland is felt as a movable neck mass above the suprasternal notch. Dysphagia, cough, hoarseness, and stridor are common. Signs of thyrotoxicosis may be present.

Tension pneumothorax. Tension pneumothorax is an acute, life-threatening condition that produces tracheal deviation toward the unaffected side. It's marked by a sudden onset of respiratory distress with sharp chest pain, dry cough, severe dyspnea, tachycardia, wheezing, cyanosis, accessory muscle use, nasal flaring, air hunger, and asymmetrical chest movement. Restless and anxious, the patient may also develop subcutaneous crepitation in the neck and upper chest, decreased vocal fremitus, decreased or absent breath sounds on the affected side, jugular vein distention, and hypotension.

Thoracic aortic aneurysm. Thoracic aortic aneurysm usually causes the trachea to deviate to the right. Highly variable associated findings may include stridor, dyspnea, wheezing, brassy cough, hoarseness, and dysphagia. Edema of the face, neck, or arm may occur with distended chest wall and jugular veins. The patient may also experience substernal, neck, shoulder, or lower back pain, possibly with paresthesia or neuralgia.

Nursing considerations

- Monitor the patient's respiratory and cardiac status.
- Administer oxygen if needed.
- Make sure that emergency equipment is readily available.
- Give analgesics for comfort, if needed.
- Prepare the patient for diagnostic tests, such as chest X-rays, bronchoscopy, an electrocardiogram, and arterial blood gas analysis.
- Assist with insertion of a large bore needle into the pleural space or a thoracostomy tube for tension pneumothorax.

Patient teaching

- Explain the underlying disorder and treatment plan.
- Teach the patient how to perform coughing and deep-breathing exercises.
- Explain signs and symptoms of respiratory difficulty to report immediately.

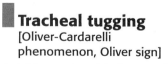

Tracheal tugging
[Oliver-Cardarelli phenomenon, Oliver sign]

A visible recession of the larynx and trachea that occurs in synchrony with car-

diac systole, tracheal tugging commonly results from an aneurysm or a tumor near the aortic arch and may signal dangerous compression or obstruction of major airways. The tugging movement, best observed with the patient's neck hyperextended, reflects abnormal transmission of aortic pulsations because of compression and distortion of the heart, esophagus, great vessels, airways, and nerves.

ACTION STAT!

If you observe tracheal tugging, examine the patient for signs of respiratory distress, such as tachypnea, stridor, accessory muscle use, cyanosis, and agitation. If the patient is in distress, check airway patency. Administer oxygen, and prepare to intubate the patient if necessary. Insert an I.V. catheter for fluid and drug access, and begin cardiac monitoring.

History and physical examination

If the patient isn't in distress, obtain a pertinent history. Ask about associated symptoms, especially pain, and about history of cardiovascular disease, cancer, chest surgery, or trauma.

Then examine the patient's neck and chest for abnormalities. Palpate the neck for masses, enlarged lymph nodes, abnormal arterial pulsations, and tracheal deviation. Percuss and auscultate the lung fields for abnormal sounds, auscultate the heart for murmurs, and auscultate the neck and chest for bruits. Palpate the chest for a thrill.

Medical causes

Aortic arch aneurysm. A large aneurysm can distort and compress surrounding tissues and structures, producing tracheal tugging. The cardinal sign of this aneurysm is severe pain in the substernal area, sometimes radiating to the back or side of the chest. A sudden increase in pain may herald impending rupture—a medical emergency. Depending on the aneurysm's site and size, associated findings may include a visible pulsatile mass in the first or second intercostal space or suprasternal notch, a diastolic murmur of aortic insufficiency, and an aortic systolic murmur and thrill in the absence of any peripheral signs of aortic stenosis. Dyspnea and stridor may occur with hoarseness, dysphagia, brassy cough, and hemoptysis. Jugular vein distention may also develop along with edema of the face, neck, or arm. Compression of the left main bronchus can cause atelectasis of the left lung.

Hodgkin's disease. A tumor that develops adjacent to the aortic arch can cause tracheal tugging. Initial signs and symptoms include usually painless cervical lymphadenopathy, sustained or remittent fever, fatigue, malaise, pruritus, night sweats, and weight loss. Swollen lymph nodes may become tender and painful. Later findings include dyspnea and stridor; dry cough; dysphagia; jugular vein distention; edema of the face, neck, or arm; hepatosplenomegaly; hyperpigmentation, jaundice, or pallor; and neuralgia.

Thymoma. Thymoma is a rare tumor that can cause tracheal tugging if it develops in the anterior mediastinum. Cough, chest pain, dysphagia, dyspnea, hoarseness, a palpable neck mass, jugular vein distention, and edema of the face, neck, or upper arm are common findings.

Nursing considerations

- Place the patient in semi-Fowler's position to ease respiration and administer oxygen if needed.
- Administer a cough suppressant and prescribed pain medications.

- Be alert for signs of respiratory depression.
- Prepare the patient for diagnostic procedures, which may include chest X-rays, computed tomography scan, lymphangiography, aortography, bone marrow biopsy, liver biopsy, echocardiography, and a complete blood count.

Patient teaching

- Explain to the patient the underlying condition and its treatments.
- Discuss positions that will ease his breathing.

Tremors

The most common type of involuntary muscle movement, tremors are regular rhythmic oscillations that result from alternating contraction of opposing muscle groups. They're typical signs of extrapyramidal or cerebellar disorders and can also result from certain drugs.

Tremors can be characterized by their location, amplitude, and frequency. They're classified as resting, intention, or postural. Resting tremors occur when an extremity is at rest and subside with movement. They include the classic pill-rolling tremor of Parkinson's disease. Conversely, intention tremors occur only with movement and subside with rest. Postural (or action) tremors appear when an extremity or the trunk is actively held in a particular posture or position. A common type of postural tremor is called an *essential tremor.*

Tremorlike movements may also be elicited, such as asterixis—the characteristic flapping tremor seen in hepatic failure. (See "Asterixis," page 54.)

Stress or emotional upset tends to aggravate a tremor. Alcohol commonly diminishes postural tremors.

History and physical examination

Begin the patient history by asking the patient about the tremor's onset (sudden or gradual) and about its duration, progression, and any aggravating or alleviating factors. Does the tremor interfere with the patient's normal activities? Does he have other symptoms? Ask the patient and his family and friends about behavioral changes or memory loss.

Explore the patient's personal and family medical history for a neurologic (especially seizures), endocrine, or metabolic disorder. Obtain a complete drug history, noting especially the use of phenothiazines. Also, ask about alcohol use.

Assess the patient's overall appearance and demeanor, noting mental status. Test range of motion and strength in all major muscle groups while observing for chorea, athetosis, dystonia, and other involuntary movements. Check deep tendon reflexes and, if possible, observe the patient's gait.

Medical causes

Alcohol withdrawal syndrome.
Acute alcohol withdrawal after long-term dependence may first be manifested by resting and intention tremors that appear as soon as 7 hours after the last drink and progressively worsen. Other early signs and symptoms include diaphoresis, tachycardia, elevated blood pressure, anxiety, restlessness, irritability, insomnia, headache, nausea, and vomiting. Severe withdrawal may produce profound tremors, agitation, confusion, hallucinations and, possibly, seizures.

Alkalosis. Severe alkalosis may produce a severe intention tremor along with twitching, carpopedal spasms, agitation, diaphoresis, and hyperventilation. The patient may complain of dizziness, tinnitus, palpitations, and peripheral and circumoral paresthesia.

Benign familial essential tremor.
Benign familial essential tremor produces a bilateral essential tremor that typically begins in the fingers and hands and may spread to the head, jaw, lips, and tongue. Laryngeal involvement may result in a quavering voice.

Cerebellar tumor. An intention tremor is a cardinal sign of cerebellar tumor; related findings may include ataxia, nystagmus, incoordination, muscle weakness and atrophy, and hypoactive or absent deep tendon reflexes.

Graves' disease. Fine tremors of the hand, nervousness, weight loss, fatigue, palpitations, dyspnea, and increased heat intolerance are some of the typical signs of Graves' disease. It's also characterized by an enlarged thyroid (goiter) and exophthalmos.

Hypercapnia. Elevated partial pressure of carbon dioxide may result in a rapid, fine intention tremor. Other common findings include headache, fatigue, blurred vision, weakness, lethargy, and decreasing level of consciousness (LOC).

Hypoglycemia. Acute hypoglycemia may produce a rapid, fine intention tremor accompanied by confusion, weakness, tachycardia, diaphoresis, and cold, clammy skin. Early patient complaints typically include a mild generalized headache, profound hunger, nervousness, and blurred or double vision. The tremor may disappear as hypoglycemia worsens and hypotonia and decreased LOC become evident.

Multiple sclerosis (MS). An intention tremor that waxes and wanes may be an early sign of MS. Commonly, vision and sensory impairments are the earliest findings. Associated effects vary greatly and may include nystagmus, muscle weakness, paralysis, spasticity, hyperreflexia, ataxic gait, dysphagia, and dysarthria. Constipation, urinary frequency and urgency, incontinence, impotence, and emotional lability may also occur.

Parkinson's disease. Tremors, a classic early sign of Parkinson's disease, usually begin in the fingers and may eventually affect the foot, eyelids, jaw, lips, and tongue. The slow, regular, rhythmic resting tremor takes the form of flexion-extension or abduction-adduction of the fingers or hand, or pronation-supination of the hand. Flexion-extension of the fingers combined with abduction-adduction of the thumb yields the characteristic pill-rolling tremor.

Leg involvement produces flexion-extension foot movement. Lightly closing the eyelids causes them to flutter. The jaw may move up and down, and the lips may purse. The tongue, when protruded, may move in and out of the mouth in tempo with tremors elsewhere in the body. The rate of the tremor holds constant over time, but its amplitude varies.

Other characteristic findings include cogwheel or lead-pipe rigidity, bradykinesia, propulsive gait with forward-leaning posture, monotone voice, masklike facies, drooling, dysphagia, dysarthria, and occasionally oculogyric crisis (eyes fix upward, with involuntary tonic movements) or blepharospasm (eyelids close completely).

Thalamic syndrome. *Central midbrain syndromes* are heralded by contralateral ataxic tremors and other abnormal movements, along with Weber's syndrome (oculomotor palsy with contralateral hemiplegia), paralysis of vertical gaze, and stupor or coma.

Anteromedial-inferior thalamic syndrome produces varying combinations of tremor, deep sensory loss, and hemiataxia. However, the main effect of this syndrome may be an extrapyramidal dysfunction, such as hemiballismus or hemichoreoathetosis.

Thyrotoxicosis. Neuromuscular effects of thyrotoxicosis include a rapid, fine intention tremor of the hands and tongue, along with clonus, hyperreflexia, and Babinski's reflex. Other common signs and symptoms include tachycardia, cardiac arrhythmias, palpitations, anxiety, dyspnea, diaphoresis, heat intolerance, weight loss despite increased appetite, diarrhea, an enlarged thyroid and, possibly, exophthalmos.

Wernicke's disease. An intention tremor is an early sign of Wernicke's disease. Other features include ocular abnormalities (such as gaze paralysis and nystagmus), ataxia, apathy, and confusion. Orthostatic hypotension and tachycardia may also develop.

West Nile encephalitis. This brain infection causes fever, headache, and body aches, commonly accompanied by a rash and swollen lymph glands. More severe infections are marked by headache, high fever, neck stiffness, stupor, disorientation, coma, tremors, occasional seizures, paralysis and, rarely, death.

Other causes

Drugs. Phenothiazines (particularly piperazine derivatives such as fluphenazine) and other antipsychotics may cause resting and pill-rolling tremors. Less commonly, metoclopramide and metyrosine also cause these tremors. Lithium toxicity, sympathomimetics (such as terbutaline and pseudoephedrine), amphetamines, and phenytoin can all cause tremors that disappear with dose reduction.

Nursing considerations

■ Assist the patient with activities of daily living, as necessary.
■ Provide the patient with a safe environment.

Patient teaching

- Explain the underlying disorder and treatment plan.
- Discuss ways for the patient to be as independent as possible.
- Instruct the patient on the use of assistive devices.

▌Tunnel vision
[Gun barrel vision, tubular vision]

Resulting from severe constriction of the visual field that leaves only a small central area of sight, tunnel vision is typically described as the sensation of looking through a tunnel or gun barrel. It may be unilateral or bilateral and usually de-

Comparing tunnel vision with normal vision

The patient with tunnel vision experiences drastic constriction of his peripheral visual field. The illustrations here convey the extent of this constriction, comparing test findings for normal and tunnel vision.

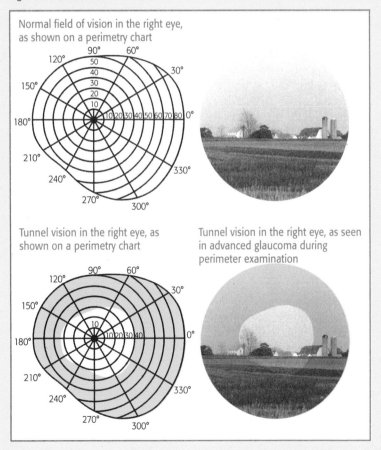

Normal field of vision in the right eye, as shown on a perimetry chart

Tunnel vision in the right eye, as shown on a perimetry chart

Tunnel vision in the right eye, as seen in advanced glaucoma during perimeter examination

velops gradually. (See *Comparing tunnel vision with normal vision.*) This abnormality results from chronic open-angle glaucoma and advanced retinal degeneration. Tunnel vision may also result from laser photocoagulation therapy, which aims to correct retinal detachment. Also a common complaint of malingerers, tunnel vision can be verified or discounted by visual field examination performed by an ophthalmologist.

History and physical examination

Ask the patient when he first noticed a loss of peripheral vision, and have him describe the progression of vision loss. Ask him to describe in detail exactly what and how far he can see peripherally. Explore the patient's personal and family history for ocular problems, especially progressive blindness that began at an early age.

To rule out malingering, observe the patient as he walks. A patient with severely limited peripheral vision typically bumps into objects (and may even have bruises), whereas the malingerer manages to avoid them.

If your examination findings suggest tunnel vision, refer the patient to an ophthalmologist for further evaluation.

Medical causes

Chronic open-angle glaucoma. With chronic open-angle glaucoma, bilateral tunnel vision occurs late and slowly progresses to complete blindness. Other late findings include mild eye pain, halo vision, and reduced visual acuity (especially at night) that isn't correctable with glasses.

Retinal pigmentary degeneration. Retinal pigmentary degeneration disorders, a group of hereditary disorders such as retinitis pigmentosa, produces an annular scotoma that progresses concentrically, causing tunnel vision and

eventually resulting in complete blindness, usually by age 50. Impaired night vision, the earliest symptom, typically appears during the first or second decade of life. An ophthalmoscopic examination may reveal narrowed retinal blood vessels and a pale optic disk.

Nursing considerations
■ To protect the patient from injury, remove all potentially dangerous objects and orient him to his surroundings.
■ Prepare the patient for diagnostic procedures, such as tonometry, perimeter examination, and visual field testing.

Patient teaching
■ Explain the underlying disorder and treatment plan.
■ Because vision impairment is frightening, reassure the patient, and clearly explain diagnostic procedures.
■ Teach the patient how to compensate for tunnel vision to avoid bumping into objects.

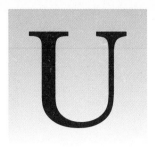

Urethral discharge

Urethral discharge is an excretion from the urinary meatus that may be purulent, mucoid, or thin; sanguineous or clear; and scant or profuse. It usually develops suddenly, most commonly in men with a prostate infection.

History and physical examination

Ask the patient when he first noticed the discharge, and have him describe its color, consistency, and quantity. Does he experience pain or burning on urination? Does he have difficulty initiating a urine stream? Does he experience urinary frequency? Ask the patient about other associated signs and symptoms, such as fever, chills, and perineal fullness. Explore his history for prostate problems, sexually transmitted disease, or urinary tract infection. Ask the patient if he has had recent sexual contacts or a new sexual partner. Obtain a complete drug history.

Inspect the patient's urethral meatus for inflammation and swelling. Using proper technique, obtain a culture specimen. (See *Collecting a urethral discharge specimen.*) Then obtain a urine specimen for urinalysis, culture, and possibly a three-glass urine specimen. (See *Performing the three-glass urine test,* page 613.) In the male patient, the prostate gland may have to be palpated.

Medical causes

Prostatitis. *Acute prostatitis* is characterized by purulent urethral discharge. Initial signs and symptoms include sudden fever, chills, lower back pain, myalgia, perineal fullness, and arthralgia. Urination becomes increasingly frequent and urgent, and the urine may appear cloudy. Dysuria, nocturia, and some degree of urinary obstruction may also occur. The prostate may be tense, boggy, tender, and warm. Prostate massage to obtain prostatic fluid is contraindicated.

Chronic prostatitis, although commonly producing no symptoms, may produce a persistent urethral discharge that's thin, milky, or clear and sometimes sticky. The discharge appears at the meatus after a long interval between voidings, as in the morning. Associated effects include a dull aching in the prostate or rectum, sexual dysfunction such as ejaculatory pain, and urinary disturbances such as frequency, urgency, and dysuria.

Reiter's syndrome. In Reiter's syndrome (also known as *reactive arthritis*), urethral discharge and other signs of acute urethritis occur 1 to 2 weeks after sexual contact. Asymmetrical arthritis, conjunctivitis of one or both eyes, and ulcerations on the oral mucosa, glans

Collecting a urethral discharge specimen

To obtain a urethral specimen from a male patient, follow these steps:

Instruct the patient not to void for 1 hour before specimen collection to prevent flushing of secretions from the urethra.

▼

Provide privacy for the patient. Help him onto an examination table and into a supine position, and expose his penis. Have him grasp and raise his penis to allow visualization of the urethra.

▼

Wash your hands, and put on sterile gloves. Then insert a thin, sterile urogenital alginate swab no more than ³⁄₄″ (2 cm) into the urethra. Rotate the swab, and leave it in place for 10 to 30 seconds to absorb organisms.

▼

Remove the swab, allow it to dry, and then send it to the laboratory. Help the patient off of the examination table, and tell him to dress.

To obtain a urethral specimen from a female patient, follow these steps:

Instruct the patient not to void for 1 hour before specimen collection to prevent flushing of secretions from the urethra.

▼

Provide privacy for the patient. Help her onto an examination table and into the lithotomy position.

▼

Wash your hands, and put on sterile gloves. Then insert a thin, sterile urogenital alginate swab into the urethral meatus. Gently rotate the swab, and leave it in place for 10 to 30 seconds to absorb organisms. Take care not to touch the swab to the area around the urethral meatus.

▼

Remove the swab, allow it to dry, and then send it to the laboratory. Assist the patient off of the table, and tell her to dress.

penis, palms, and soles may also occur with Reiter's syndrome.

Urethritis. Urethritis commonly produces scant or profuse urethral discharge that's either thin and clear, mucoid, or thick and purulent. Other effects include urinary hesitancy, urgency, and frequency; dysuria; and itching and burning around the meatus.

Nursing considerations
■ To relieve symptoms, have the patient take hot sitz baths, increase fluid intake, void frequently, and avoid caffeine, tea, and alcohol.
■ Monitor him for urine retention.

Patient teaching
■ Advise the patient with acute prostatitis to discontinue sexual activity until acute symptoms subside.
■ Encourage the patient with chronic prostatitis to regularly engage in sexual activity because ejaculation may relieve pain.

Urinary frequency

Urinary frequency refers to increased incidence of the urge to void without an increase in the total volume of urine produced. Usually resulting from decreased bladder capacity, frequency is a cardinal sign of urinary tract infection.

However, it can also stem from another urologic disorder, neurologic dysfunction, or pressure on the bladder from a nearby tumor or from organ enlargement (as with pregnancy).

History and physical examination

Ask the patient how many times per day he voids. How does this compare with his previous pattern of voiding? Ask about the onset and duration of the abnormal frequency and about any associated urinary signs or symptoms, such as dysuria, urgency, incontinence, hematuria, discharge, or lower abdominal pain with urination.

Ask also about neurologic symptoms, such as muscle weakness, numbness, or tingling. Explore his medical history for urinary tract infection, other urologic problems or recent urologic procedures, and neurologic disorders. With a male patient, ask about a history of prostatic enlargement. If the patient is a female of childbearing age, ask whether she is or could be pregnant. Obtain a complete drug history.

Obtain a clean-catch midstream specimen for urinalysis and culture and sensitivity tests. Then palpate the patient's suprapubic area, abdomen, and flanks, noting any tenderness. Examine his urethral meatus for redness, discharge, or swelling. In a male patient, the physician may palpate the prostate gland.

If the patient's medical history reveals symptoms or a history of neurologic disorders, perform a neurologic examination.

Medical causes

Benign prostatic hyperplasia. Prostatic enlargement causes urinary frequency, along with nocturia and possibly incontinence and hematuria. Initial effects are those of prostatism: reduced caliber and force of the urine stream, urinary hesitancy and tenesmus, inability to stop the urine stream, a feeling of incomplete voiding, and occasionally urine retention. Assessment reveals bladder distention.

Bladder calculus. Bladder irritation may lead to urinary frequency and urgency, dysuria, terminal hematuria, and suprapubic pain from bladder spasms. The patient may have overflow incontinence if the calculus lodges in the bladder neck. Greatest discomfort usually occurs at the end of micturition if the calculus lodges in the bladder neck. This may also cause overflow incontinence and referred pain to the lower back or heel.

Prostate cancer. In advanced stages of prostate cancer, urinary frequency may occur, along with hesitancy, dribbling, nocturia, dysuria, bladder distention, perineal pain, constipation, and a hard, irregularly shaped prostate.

Prostatitis. Acute prostatitis commonly produces urinary frequency, along with urgency, dysuria, nocturia, and purulent urethral discharge. Other findings include fever, chills, low back pain, myalgia, arthralgia, and perineal fullness. The prostate may be tense, boggy, tender, and warm. Prostate massage to obtain prostatic fluid is contraindicated. Signs and symptoms of chronic prostatitis are usually the same as those of the acute form, but to a lesser degree. The patient may also experience pain on ejaculation.

Rectal tumor. The pressure exerted by a rectal tumor on the bladder may cause urinary frequency. Early findings include changed bowel habits, commonly starting with an urgent need to defecate on arising or obstipation alternating with diarrhea; blood or mucus in the stools; and a sense of incomplete evacuation.

Reiter's syndrome. In Reiter's syndrome, urinary frequency occurs with symptoms of acute urethritis 1 to 2 weeks after sexual contact. Other symptoms of this self-limiting syndrome include asymmetrical arthritis of knees, ankles, and metatarsophalangeal joints; unilateral or bilateral conjunctivitis; and small painless ulcers on the mouth, tongue, glans penis, palms, and soles.

Reproductive tract tumor. A tumor in the female reproductive tract may compress the bladder, causing urinary frequency. Other findings vary but may include abdominal distention, menstrual disturbances, vaginal bleeding, weight loss, pelvic pain, and fatigue.

Spinal cord lesion. Incomplete cord transection results in urinary frequency, continuous overflow, dribbling, urgency when voluntary control of sphincter function weakens, urinary hesitancy, and bladder distention. Other effects occur below the level of the lesion and include weakness, paralysis, sensory disturbances, hyperreflexia, and impotence.

Urethral stricture. Bladder decompensation produces urinary frequency, along with urgency and nocturia. Early signs include hesitancy, tenesmus, and reduced caliber and force of the urine stream. Eventually, overflow incontinence may occur. Urinoma and urosepsis may develop.

Urinary tract infection. Affecting the urethra, the bladder, or the kidneys, this common cause of urinary frequency may also produce urgency, dysuria, hematuria, cloudy urine and, in males, urethral discharge. The patient may report bladder spasms or a feeling of warmth and pain during urination and fever. Women may experience suprapubic or pelvic pain.

Other causes

Diuretics. Diuretics, which include caffeine, reduce the body's total volume of water and salt by increasing urine excretion. Excessive intake of coffee, tea, and other caffeinated beverages leads to urinary frequency.

Treatments. Radiation therapy may cause bladder inflammation, leading to urinary frequency.

Nursing considerations

■ Prepare the patient for diagnostic tests, such as urinalysis, culture and sensitivity tests, imaging tests, ultrasonography, cystoscopy, cystometry, postvoid residual tests, and a complete neurologic workup.
■ If the patient's mobility is impaired, keep a bedpan or commode near his bed.
■ Document the patient's daily intake and output amounts.

Patient teaching

■ Explain to the patient the underlying disorder and treatment plan.
■ Emphasize safer sex practices.
■ Instruct the patient in proper genital hygiene.
■ Explain the importance of increasing fluid intake and the frequency of voiding.

Urinary hesitancy

Hesitancy—difficulty starting a urine stream generally followed by a decrease in the force of the stream—can result from a urinary tract infection (UTI), a partial lower urinary tract obstruction, a neuromuscular disorder, or use of certain drugs. Occurring at all ages and in both sexes, it's most common in older men with prostatic enlargement. It also occurs in women with gravid uterus, tumors in the reproductive system, such as uterine fibroids, or ovarian, uterine, or vaginal cancer. Hesitancy usually arises gradually, commonly going unnoticed until urine retention causes bladder distention and discomfort.

History and physical examination

Ask the patient when he first noticed hesitancy and if he has ever had the problem before. Ask about other urinary problems, especially reduced force or interruption of the urine stream. Ask if he has ever been treated for a prostate problem or UTI or obstruction. Obtain a drug history.

Inspect the patient's urethral meatus for inflammation, discharge, and other abnormalities. Examine the anal sphincter and test sensation in the perineum. Obtain a clean-catch specimen for urinalysis and culture. In a male patient, the prostate gland requires palpation. A female patient requires a gynecologic examination.

Medical causes

Benign prostatic hyperplasia (BPH). Signs and symptoms of BPH depend on the extent of prostatic enlargement and the lobes affected. Characteristic early findings include urinary hesitancy, reduced caliber and force of urine stream, perineal pain, a feeling of incomplete voiding, inability to stop the urine stream and, occasionally, urine retention. As obstruction increases, urination becomes more frequent, with nocturia, urinary overflow, incontinence, bladder distention, and possibly hematuria.

Prostatic cancer. In patients with advanced prostate cancer, urinary hesitancy may occur, accompanied by frequency, dribbling, nocturia, dysuria, bladder distention, perineal pain, and constipation. Digital rectal examination commonly reveals a hard, nodular prostate.

Spinal cord lesion. A lesion below the micturition center that has destroyed the sacral nerve roots causes urinary hesitancy, tenesmus, and constant dribbling from retention and overflow incontinence. Associated findings are urinary frequency and urgency, dysuria, and nocturia.

Urethral stricture. Partial obstruction of the lower urinary tract secondary to trauma or infection produces urinary hesitancy, tenesmus, and decreased force and caliber of the urine stream. Urinary frequency and urgency, nocturia, and eventually overflow incontinence may develop. Pyuria usually indicates accompanying infection. Increased obstruction may lead to urine extravasation and formation of urinomas.

UTI. Urinary hesitancy may be associated with a UTI. Characteristic urinary changes include frequency, possible hematuria, dysuria, nocturia, and cloudy urine. Associated findings include bladder spasms; costovertebral angle tenderness; suprapubic, low back, pelvic, or flank pain; urethral discharge in males; fever; chills; malaise; nausea; and vomiting.

Other causes

Drugs. Anticholinergics and drugs with anticholinergic properties (such as tricyclic antidepressants and some nasal decongestants and cold remedies) may cause urinary hesitancy. Hesitancy may also occur in those recovering from general anesthesia.

Nursing considerations

- Monitor the patient's voiding pattern and intake and output.
- Frequently palpate for bladder distention.
- Apply local heat to the perineum or the abdomen to enhance muscle relaxation and aid urination.

- Prepare the patient for tests, such as cystometrography or cystourethrography.

Patient teaching
- Explain the underlying disorder and treatment plan.
- Teach the patient how to perform a clean, intermittent self-catheterization.
- Discuss the importance of increasing fluid intake and voiding frequently.

Urinary incontinence

Urinary incontinence, the uncontrollable passage of urine, can result from a bladder abnormality, a neurologic disorder, or an alteration in pelvic muscle strength. A common urologic sign, incontinence may be transient or permanent and may involve large volumes of urine or scant dribbling. It can be classified as stress, neurogenic, overflow, urge, or total incontinence. *Stress incontinence* refers to intermittent leakage resulting from a sudden physical strain, such as a cough, sneeze, laugh, or quick movement. *Neurogenic incontinence* occurs due to an unawareness of the need to void caused by spinal cord injury. *Overflow incontinence* is a dribble resulting from urine retention, which fills the bladder and prevents it from contracting with sufficient force to expel a urine stream. *Urge incontinence* refers to the inability to suppress a sudden urge to urinate. *Total incontinence* is continuous leakage resulting from the bladder's inability to retain urine.

History and physical examination

Ask the patient when he first noticed the incontinence and whether it began suddenly or gradually. Have him describe his typical urinary pattern: Does incontinence usually occur during the day or at night? Does he have any urinary control, or is he totally incontinent? If he can occasionally control urination, ask him the usual times and amounts voided. Determine his normal fluid intake. Ask about other urinary problems, such as hesitancy, frequency, urgency, nocturia, and decreased force or interruption of the urine stream. Also ask if he has ever sought treatment for incontinence or found a way to deal with it himself.

Obtain a medical history, especially noting urinary tract infection (UTI), prostate conditions, spinal injury or tumor, stroke, or surgery involving the bladder, prostate, or pelvic floor. Ask a woman how many pregnancies she has had and how many childbirths. A diary of voiding habits for a 24- to 48-hour period may provide useful information. Obtain a complete drug history.

After completing the history, have the patient empty his bladder. Inspect the urethral meatus for obvious inflammation or anatomic defect. Have female patients bear down; note any urine leakage. Gently palpate the abdomen for bladder distention, which signals urine retention. Perform a complete neurologic assessment, noting motor and sensory function and obvious muscle atrophy.

Medical causes
Benign prostatic hyperplasia (BPH). Overflow incontinence is common with BPH as a result of urethral obstruction and urine retention. BPH begins with a group of signs and symptoms known as *prostatism*: reduced caliber and force of urine stream, urinary hesitancy, and a feeling of incomplete voiding. As obstruction increases, urination becomes more frequent, with nocturia and, possibly, hematuria. Examination reveals bladder distention and an enlarged prostate.

Bladder cancer. With bladder cancer, the patient commonly presents with urge incontinence and hematuria; obstruction by a tumor may produce overflow incontinence. The early stages may not produce symptoms. Other urinary signs and symptoms include frequency, dysuria, nocturia, dribbling, and suprapubic pain from bladder spasms after voiding. A mass may be palpable on bimanual examination.

Diabetic neuropathy. Autonomic neuropathy may cause painless bladder distention with overflow incontinence. Related findings include episodic constipation or diarrhea (which is commonly nocturnal), impotence and retrograde ejaculation, orthostatic hypotension, syncope, and dysphagia.

Multiple sclerosis (MS). Urinary incontinence, urgency, and frequency are common urologic findings in MS. In most patients, vision problems and sensory impairment occur early. Other findings include constipation, muscle weakness, paralysis, spasticity, hyperreflexia, intention tremor, ataxic gait, dysarthria, impotence, and emotional lability.

Prostate cancer. Urinary incontinence usually appears only in the advanced stages of prostate cancer. Urinary frequency and hesitancy, nocturia, dysuria, bladder distention, perineal pain, constipation, and a hard, irregularly shaped, nodular prostate are other common late findings.

Prostatitis (chronic). Urinary incontinence may occur as a result of urethral obstruction from an enlarged prostate. Other findings include urinary frequency and urgency, dysuria, hematuria, bladder distention, persistent urethral discharge, dull perineal pain that may radiate, ejaculatory pain, and decreased libido.

Spinal cord injury. Complete cord transection above the sacral level causes flaccid paralysis of the bladder. Overflow incontinence follows rapid bladder distention. Other findings include paraplegia, sexual dysfunction, sensory loss, muscle atrophy, anhidrosis, and loss of reflexes distal to the injury.

Stroke. With a stroke, urinary incontinence may be transient or permanent. Associated findings reflect the site and extent of the lesion and may include impaired mentation, emotional lability, behavioral changes, altered level of consciousness, and seizures. Headache, vomiting, visual deficits, and decreased visual acuity are possible. Sensorimotor effects include contralateral hemiplegia, dysarthria, dysphagia, ataxia, apraxia, agnosia, aphasia, and unilateral sensory loss.

Urethral stricture. Eventually, overflow incontinence may occur with a urethral stricture. As obstruction increases, urine extravasation may lead to formation of urinomas and urosepsis.

UTI. Besides incontinence, a UTI may produce urinary urgency, dysuria, hematuria, cloudy urine and, in males, urethral discharge. Bladder spasms or a feeling of warmth during urination may occur.

Other causes

Surgery. Urinary incontinence may occur after prostatectomy as a result of urethral sphincter damage.

Nursing considerations

- Prepare the patient for diagnostic tests, such as cystoscopy, cystometry, and a complete neurologic workup. Obtain a urine specimen.
- Implement a bladder retraining program. (See *Correcting incontinence with bladder retraining.*)
- If the patient's incontinence has a neurologic basis, monitor him for urine re-

Correcting incontinence with bladder retraining

The incontinent patient typically feels frustrated, embarrassed and, sometimes, hopeless. Fortunately, though, his problem may be corrected by bladder retraining—a program that aims to establish a regular voiding pattern. Here are some guidelines for establishing such a program:

■ Before you start the program, assess the patient's intake pattern, voiding pattern, and behavior (for example, restlessness or talkativeness) before each voiding episode.

■ Encourage the patient to use the toilet 30 minutes before he's usually incontinent. If this isn't successful, readjust the schedule. Once he can stay dry for 2 hours, increase the time between voidings by 30 minutes each day until he achieves a 3- to 4-hour voiding schedule.

■ When your patient voids, make sure that the sequence of conditioning stimuli is always the same.

■ Make sure that the patient has privacy while voiding—any inhibiting stimuli should be avoided.

■ Keep a record of continence and incontinence for 5 days—this may reinforce your patient's efforts to remain continent.

Tips for success

Remember that both your positive attitude and your patient's are crucial to his successful bladder retraining. Here are some additional tips that may help your patient succeed:

■ Make sure the patient is close to a bathroom or portable toilet. Leave a light on at night, and ensure there's a clear pathway to the bathroom.

■ If your patient needs assistance getting out of his bed or chair, promptly answer his call for help.

■ Encourage the patient to wear his accustomed clothing, as an indication that you're confident he can remain continent. Acceptable alternatives to diapers include a condom catheter for the male patient and incontinence pads or panties for the female patient.

■ Encourage the patient to drink 2 to 2½ qt (2 to 2.5 L) of fluid each day. Less fluid doesn't prevent incontinence but does promote bladder infection. Limiting his intake after 5 p.m., however, will help him remain continent during the night.

■ Reassure your patient that episodes of incontinence don't signal a failure of the program. Encourage him to maintain a persistent, tolerant attitude.

■ Teach the patient how to perform Kegel exercises to strengthen his pelvic muscles.

---

tention, which may require periodic catheterizations.

Patient teaching

■ Explain the underlying disorder and treatment plan.

■ To prevent stress incontinence, teach the patient how to perform Kegel exercises to help strengthen the pelvic floor muscles.

■ Teach the patient self-catheterization techniques, as appropriate.

▌Urinary urgency

A sudden compelling urge to urinate (urinary urgency), accompanied by bladder pain, is a classic symptom of a urinary tract infection (UTI). As inflammation decreases bladder capacity, discomfort results from the accumulation of even small amounts of urine. Repeated, frequent voiding in an effort to alleviate this discomfort produces urine output of only a few milliliters at each voiding.

Urgency without bladder pain may point to an upper-motor-neuron lesion that has disrupted bladder control.

History and physical examination

Ask the patient about the onset of urinary urgency and whether he has ever experienced it before. Ask about other urologic symptoms, such as dysuria and cloudy urine. Also ask about neurologic symptoms, such as paresthesia. Examine his medical history for recurrent or chronic UTIs or for surgery or procedures involving the urinary tract. Obtain a complete drug history.

Obtain a clean-catch specimen for urinalysis and culture. Note urine character, color, and odor, and use a reagent strip to test for pH, glucose, and blood. Then palpate the suprapubic area and both flanks for distention and tenderness. If the patient's history or symptoms suggest neurologic dysfunction, perform a neurologic examination.

Medical causes

Bladder calculus. Bladder irritation can lead to urinary urgency and frequency, dysuria, terminal hematuria, and suprapubic pain from bladder spasms. Pain may be referred to the penis, vulva, lower back, or heel.

Multiple sclerosis (MS). Urinary urgency can occur with or without the frequent UTIs that can accompany MS. Like MS's other variable effects, urinary urgency may wax and wane. Commonly, vision and sensory impairments are the earliest findings. Others include urinary frequency, incontinence, constipation, muscle weakness, paralysis, spasticity,

intention tremor, hyperreflexia, ataxic gait, dysphagia, dysarthria, impotence, and emotional lability.

Reiter's syndrome. In Reiter's syndrome, urinary urgency occurs with other symptoms of acute urethritis 1 to 2 weeks after sexual contact. Arthritic and ocular symptoms and skin lesions usually develop within several weeks after sexual contact. These include asymmetrical arthritis of knees, ankles, or metatarsal phalangeal joints; conjunctivitis; and ulcers on the penis, or skin, or in the mouth.

Spinal cord lesion. Urinary urgency can result from incomplete cord transection when voluntary control of sphincter function weakens. Urinary frequency, difficulty initiating and inhibiting a urine stream, and bladder distention and discomfort may also occur. Neuromuscular effects distal to the lesion include weakness, paralysis, hyperreflexia, sensory disturbances, and impotence.

Urethral stricture. Bladder decompensation produces urinary urgency, frequency, and nocturia. Early signs and symptoms include hesitancy, tenesmus, and reduced caliber and force of the urine stream. Eventually, overflow incontinence may occur.

UTI. Urinary urgency is commonly associated with a UTI. Other characteristic urinary changes include frequency, hematuria, dysuria, nocturia, and cloudy urine. Urinary hesitancy may also occur. Associated findings include bladder spasms; costovertebral angle tenderness; suprapubic, low back, or flank pain; urethral discharge in males; fever; chills; malaise; nausea; and vomiting.

Other causes

Treatments. Radiation therapy may irritate and inflame the bladder, causing urinary urgency.

Performing the three-glass urine test

If your male patient complains of urinary frequency and urgency, dysuria, flank or lower back pain, or other signs or symptoms of urethritis, and if his urine specimen is cloudy, perform the three-glass urine test.

First, ask him to void into three conical glasses labeled with numbers 1, 2, and 3. First-voided urine goes into glass #1, midstream urine into glass #2, and the remainder into glass #3. Tell the patient to avoid interrupting the stream of urine when shifting glasses, if possible.

Next, observe each glass for pus and mucus shreds. Also, note urine color and odor. Glass #1 will contain matter from the anterior urethra; glass #2, matter from the bladder; and glass #3, sediment from the prostate and seminal vesicles.

Some common findings are shown here. However, confirming diagnosis requires microscopic examination and a bacteriology report.

	Specimen 1	Specimen 2	Specimen 3
Acute or subacute urethritis	Cloudy	Clear	Clear
Acute posterior urethritis	Cloudy	Clear or cloudy	Cloudy
Chronic anterior urethritis	Small shreds	Clear	Clear
Chronic posterior urethritis	Large shreds	Clear	Clear
Chronic urethritis (anterior and posterior)	Small and large shreds	Clear	Clear
Prostatitis	Clear or large shreds	Clear	Cloudy or large shreds
Pyelonephritis and cystitis	Cloudy	Cloudy	Cloudy

Nursing considerations

- Prepare the patient for the diagnostic workup, including a complete urinalysis, culture and sensitivity studies, and possibly neurologic tests.
- Increase the patient's fluid intake and monitor intake and output.
- Administer an antibiotic and a urinary anesthetic, such as phenazopyridine.

Patient teaching

- Explain the underlying disorder and treatment plan.
- Instruct the patient in safer sex practices.

- Discuss proper genital hygiene.
- Explain the need for adequate fluid intake and frequent voidings.
- Explain how to perform Kegel exercises.

Urine cloudiness

Cloudy, murky, or turbid urine reflects the presence of bacteria, mucus, leukocytes or erythrocytes, epithelial cells, fat, or phosphates (in alkaline urine). It's characteristic of urinary tract infection (UTI) but can also result from prolonged storage of a urine specimen at room temperature.

History and physical examination

Ask about symptoms of UTI, such as dysuria; urinary urgency or frequency; or pain in the flank, lower back, or suprapubic area. Also ask about recurrent UTIs or recent surgery or treatment involving the urinary tract. Obtain a complete drug history.

Obtain a urine specimen to check for pus or mucus. (See *Performing the three-glass urine test*, page 613.) Using a reagent strip, test for blood, glucose, and pH. Palpate the suprapubic area and flanks for tenderness.

If you note cloudy urine in a patient with an indwelling urinary catheter, especially with concurrent fever, remove the catheter immediately (or change it if the patient must have one in place).

Medical causes

UTI. Cloudy urine is common with UTI. Other urinary changes include urgency, frequency, hematuria, dysuria, nocturia and, in males, urethral discharge. Urinary hesitancy; bladder spasms; costovertebral angle tenderness; and suprapubic, lower back, or flank pain may occur. Other effects include fever, chills, malaise, nausea, and vomiting.

Nursing considerations

- Collect urine specimens for urinalysis and culture and sensitivity tests.
- Increase the patient's fluid intake, and administer an antibiotic and a urinary anesthetic (such as phenazopyridine).
- Continue checking the appearance of the patient's urine to monitor the effectiveness of therapy.

Patient teaching

- Explain the underlying disorder and treatment plan.
- Teach the patient to increase his fluid intake.
- Discuss the importance of finishing the full course of antibiotics.
- Explain proper genital hygiene.

Urticaria
[Hives]

Urticaria is a vascular skin reaction characterized by the eruption of transient pruritic wheals—smooth, slightly elevated patches with well-defined erythematous margins and pale centers of various shapes and sizes. It's produced by the local release of histamine or other vasoactive substances as part of a hypersensitivity reaction.

Acute urticaria evolves rapidly and usually has a detectable cause, commonly hypersensitivity to certain drugs, foods, insect bites, inhalants, or contactants; emotional stress; or environmental factors. Although individual lesions usually subside within 12 to 24 hours, new crops of lesions may erupt continuously, thus prolonging the attack.

Urticaria lasting longer than 6 weeks is classified as *chronic*. The lesions may recur for months or years, and the underlying cause is usually unknown. Occasionally, a diagnosis of psychogenic urticaria is made.

Angioedema, or giant urticaria, is characterized by the acute eruption of wheals involving the mucous membranes and, occasionally, the arms, legs, or genitals.

ACTION STAT!

 In an acute case of urticaria, quickly evaluate respiratory status, and take the patient's vital signs. Ensure patent I.V. access if you note any respiratory difficulty or signs of impending anaphylactic shock. Also, as appropriate, give local epinephrine or apply ice to the affected site to decrease absorption through vasoconstriction. Clear and maintain the airway, give oxygen as needed, and institute cardiac monitoring. Have resuscitation equipment at hand, and be prepared to begin cardiopulmonary resuscitation. Endotracheal intubation or a tracheostomy may be required.

History and physical examination

If the patient isn't in distress, obtain a complete history. Does he have any known allergies? Does the urticaria follow a seasonal pattern? Do certain foods or drugs seem to aggravate it? Is there a relationship to physical exertion? Is the patient routinely exposed to chemicals on the job or at home? Has the patient recently changed or used new skin products or detergents? Obtain a detailed drug history, including prescription and over-the-counter drugs. Note any history of chronic or parasitic infection, skin disease, or a GI disorder.

Next, assess respiratory status. Inspect the chest for sternal retractions and accessory muscle use. Auscultate and percuss the chest. Assess cardiac status. Obtain vital signs and pulse oximetry and begin cardiac monitoring. Assess all skin surfaces.

Medical causes

Anaphylaxis. Anaphylaxis—an acute allergic reaction—is marked by the rapid eruption of diffuse urticaria and angioedema, with wheals ranging from pinpoint to palm-size or larger. Lesions are usually pruritic and stinging; paresthesia commonly precedes their eruption. Other acute findings include profound anxiety, weakness, diaphoresis, sneezing, shortness of breath, profuse rhinorrhea, nasal congestion, dysphagia, and warm, moist skin.

Hereditary angioedema. With hereditary angioedema, cutaneous involvement is manifested by nonpitting, nonpruritic edema of an extremity or the face. Respiratory mucosal involvement can produce life-threatening acute laryngeal edema.

Lyme disease. Although not diagnostic of Lyme disease, urticaria may result from the characteristic skin lesion (erythema chronicum migrans). Later effects include constant malaise and fatigue, intermittent headache, fever, chills, lymphadenopathy, neurologic and cardiac abnormalities, and arthritis.

Other causes

Drugs. Drugs that can produce urticaria include aspirin, codeine, dextrans, immune serums, insulin, morphine, penicillin, quinine, sulfonamides, and vaccines.

Radiographic contrast medium. Radiographic contrast medium, especially when administered I.V., commonly produces urticaria.

Nursing considerations

- Apply a bland skin emollient or one containing menthol and phenol to the patient's skin.
- Administer an antihistamine, a systemic corticosteroid or, if stress is a suspected contributing factor, a tranquilizer, as ordered.
- Provide tepid baths and cool compresses to enhance vasoconstriction and decrease pruritus.
- Administer oxygen and monitor respiratory status.

Patient teaching

- Explain the underlying disorder and treatment plan.
- Teach the patient to avoid the causative stimulus, if identified.
- Emphasize the importance of wearing medical identification for allergies.
- Explain signs and symptoms that require prompt medical attention.
- Stress ways to avoid anaphylaxis.
- Teach the patient and his family how to use an anaphylaxis kit.

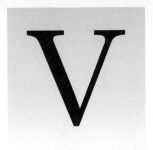

Vaginal bleeding, postmenopausal

Postmenopausal vaginal bleeding—bleeding that occurs 6 or more months after menopause—is an important, albeit not a definitive, indicator of gynecologic cancer. It can also result from infection, a local pelvic disorder, estrogenic stimulation, atrophy of the endometrium, and physiologic thinning and drying of the vaginal mucous membranes. Bleeding from the vagina may also be indicative of bleeding from another gynecologic location, such as the ovaries, fallopian tubes, uterus, cervix, or vagina. Bleeding usually occurs as slight, brown or red spotting developing either spontaneously or following coitus or douching, but it may also occur as oozing of fresh blood or as bright red hemorrhage. Many patients—especially those with a history of heavy menstrual flow—minimize the importance of this bleeding, thus delaying diagnosis.

History and physical examination

Determine the patient's age and her age at menopause. Ask when she first noticed the abnormal bleeding then obtain a thorough obstetric and gynecologic history. When did she begin menstruating? Were her menses regular? If not, ask her to describe menstrual irregulari-

ties. How old was she when she first had intercourse? How many sexual partners has she had? Has she had children? Has she had fertility problems? If possible, obtain an obstetric and gynecologic history of the patient's mother and ask about a family history of gynecologic cancer. Determine whether the patient has associated symptoms and if she's taking estrogen.

Observe the external genitalia, noting the character of vaginal discharge and the appearance of the labia, vaginal rugae, and clitoris. Carefully palpate the patient's breasts and lymph nodes for nodules or enlargement. The patient will require pelvic and rectal examinations.

Medical causes

Atrophic vaginitis. When bloody staining occurs with atrophic vaginitis, it usually follows coitus or douching. Characteristic white, watery vaginal discharge may be accompanied by pruritus, dyspareunia, and a burning sensation in the vagina and labia. Sparse pubic hair, a pale vagina with decreased rugae and small hemorrhagic spots, clitoral atrophy, and shrinking of the labia minora may also occur.

Cervical cancer. Early invasive cervical cancer causes vaginal spotting or heavier bleeding, usually after coitus or douching but occasionally spontaneously. Related findings include persistent, pink-tinged, and foul-smelling vaginal discharge and postcoital pain. As the cancer spreads, back and sciatic pain, leg swelling, anorexia, weight loss, hematuria, dysuria, rectal bleeding, and weakness may occur and the drainage may become dark and malodorous.

Cervical or endometrial polyps. Cervical or endometrial polyps are small, pedunculated growths that may cause spotting (possibly as a mucopurulent, pink discharge) after coitus, douching, or straining to defecate. Many endometrial polyps produce no symptoms.

Endometrial hyperplasia or cancer. Bleeding occurs early with endometrial hyperplasia or cancer; it can be brownish and scant or bright red and profuse, and usually follows coitus or douching. Bleeding later becomes heavier and more frequent, leading to clotting and anemia. Bleeding may be accompanied by pelvic, rectal, lower back, and leg pain. The uterus may be enlarged.

Ovarian tumors (feminizing). Ovarian tumors producing estrogen can stimulate endometrial shedding and cause heavy bleeding unassociated with coitus or douching. A palpable pelvic mass, increased cervical mucus, breast enlargement, and spider angiomas may be present.

Vaginal cancer. Characteristic spotting or bleeding with vaginal cancer may be preceded by a thin, watery vaginal discharge. Bleeding may be spontaneous but usually follows coitus or douching. A firm, ulcerated vaginal lesion may be present; dyspareunia, urinary frequency, bladder and pelvic pain, rectal bleeding, and vulvar lesions may develop later.

Other causes

Drugs. Unopposed estrogen replacement therapy is a common cause of abnormal vaginal bleeding. This can usually be reduced by adding progesterone (in women who haven't had a hysterectomy) and by adjusting the patient's estrogen dosage.

Nursing considerations

- Prepare the patient for diagnostic tests, such as ultrasonography, endometrial biopsy, colposcopy, dilatation and curettage, and vaginal and cervical cultures.
- Discontinue estrogen until a diagnosis is made.

Patient teaching

- Reassure the patient that postmenopausal vaginal bleeding may be benign, but careful assessment is needed.
- Teach the patient about the underlying cause and its treatment.

Vaginal discharge

Common in women of childbearing age, physiologic vaginal discharge is mucoid, clear or white, nonbloody, and odorless. Produced by the cervical mucosa and, to a lesser degree, by the vulvar glands, this discharge may occasionally be scant or profuse due to estrogenic stimulation and changes during the patient's menstrual cycle. However, a marked increase in discharge or a change in discharge color, odor, or consistency can signal disease. Discharge may result from infection, sexually transmitted disease, reproductive tract disease, fistulas, and certain drugs. In addition, the prolonged presence of a foreign body, such as a tampon or diaphragm, in the patient's vagina can cause irritation and an inflammatory exudate, as can frequent douching, feminine hygiene products, contraceptive products, bubble baths, and colored or perfumed toilet paper.

History and physical examination

Ask the patient to describe the onset, color, consistency, odor, and texture of her vaginal discharge. How does the dis-

Identifying causes of vaginal discharge

The color, consistency, amount, and odor of your patient's vaginal discharge provide important clues about the underlying disorder. For quick reference, use this chart to match common characteristics of vaginal discharge and their possible causes.

Characteristics	Possible causes
Thin, scant, watery white discharge	Atrophic vaginitis
Thin, green or gray-white, foul-smelling discharge	Bacterial vaginosis
White, curdlike, profuse discharge with yeasty, sweet odor	Candidiasis
Mucopurulent, foul-smelling discharge	Chancroid
Yellow, mucopurulent, odorless, or acrid discharge	Chlamydial infection
Scant, serosanguineous, or purulent discharge with foul odor	Endometritis
Copious mucoid discharge	Genital herpes
Profuse, mucopurulent discharge, possibly foul-smelling	Genital warts
Yellow or green, foul-smelling discharge from the cervix or occasionally from Bartholin's or Skene's ducts	Gonorrhea
Chronic, watery, bloody, or purulent discharge, possibly foul-smelling	Gynecologic cancer
Frothy, green-yellow, and profuse (or thin, white, and scant) foul-smelling discharge	Trichomoniasis

charge differ from her usual vaginal secretions? Is the onset related to her menstrual cycle? Ask about associated symptoms, such as dysuria and perineal pruritus and burning. Does she have spotting after coitus or douching? Ask about recent changes in her sexual habits and hygiene practices. Is she or could she be pregnant? Ask if she has had vaginal discharge before or has ever been treated for a vaginal infection or sexually transmitted disease. What treatment did she receive? Did she complete the course of medication and were all sexual contacts treated? Ask about her current use of medications, especially antibiotics, oral estrogens, and hormonal contraceptives.

Examine the external genitalia and note the character of the discharge. (See *Identifying causes of vaginal discharge.*) Observe vulvar and vaginal tissues for redness, edema, and excoriation. Palpate the inguinal lymph nodes to detect tenderness or enlargement, and palpate the abdomen for tenderness. A pelvic examination may be required. Obtain vaginal discharge specimens for testing.

Medical causes

Atrophic vaginitis. With atrophic vaginitis, a thin, scant, watery white vaginal discharge may be accompanied by pruritus, burning, tenderness, and bloody spotting after coitus or douching. Sparse pubic hair, a pale vagina with decreased rugae and small hemorrhagic spots, clitoral atrophy, and shrinking of the labia minora may also occur.

Bacterial vaginosis. Bacterial vaginosis causes a thin, foul-smelling, green or gray-white discharge, it adheres to the vaginal walls and can be easily wiped away, leaving healthy-looking tissue. Pruritus, redness, and other signs of vaginal irritation may occur but are usually minimal.

Candidiasis. Infection with *Candida albicans* causes a profuse, white, curdlike discharge with a yeasty, sweet odor. Onset is abrupt, usually just before menses or during a course of antibiotics. Exudate may be lightly attached to the labia and vaginal walls and is commonly accompanied by vulvar redness and edema. The inner thighs may be covered with a fine, red dermatitis and weeping erosions. Intense labial itching and burning may also occur. Some patients experience external dysuria.

Chancroid. Chancroid produces a mucopurulent, foul-smelling discharge and vulvar lesions that are initially erythematous and later ulcerated. Within 2 to 3 weeks, inguinal lymph nodes (usually unilateral) may become tender and enlarged, with pruritus, suppuration, and spontaneous drainage of nodes. Headache, malaise, and fever to 102.2° F (39° C) are common.

Chlamydial infection. Chlamydial infection causes a yellow, mucopurulent, odorless, or acrid vaginal discharge. Other findings include dysuria, dyspareunia, and vaginal bleeding after douching or coitus, especially following menses. Many women remain asymptomatic.

Endometritis. A scant, serosanguineous discharge with a foul odor can result from bacterial invasion of the endometrium. Associated findings include fever, lower back and abdominal pain, abdominal muscle spasm, malaise, dysmenorrhea, and an enlarged uterus.

Genital warts. Genital warts are mosaic, papular vulvar lesions that can cause a profuse, mucopurulent vaginal discharge, which may be foul-smelling if the warts are infected. Patients frequently complain of burning or paresthesia in the vaginal introitus.

Gonorrhea. Although 80% of women with gonorrhea are asymptomatic, others have a yellow or green, foul-smelling discharge that can be expressed from Bartholin's or Skene's ducts. Other findings include dysuria, urinary frequency and incontinence, bleeding, and vaginal redness and swelling. Severe pelvic and lower abdominal pain and fever may develop.

Gynecologic cancer. Endometrial or cervical cancer produces a chronic, watery, bloody or purulent vaginal discharge that may be foul-smelling. Other findings include abnormal vaginal bleeding and, later, weight loss; pelvic, back, and leg pain; fatigue; urinary frequency; and abdominal distention.

Herpes simplex (genital). A copious mucoid discharge results from genital herpes simplex, but the initial complaint is painful, indurated vesicles and ulcerations on the labia, vagina, cervix, anus, thighs, or mouth. Erythema, marked edema, and tender inguinal lymph nodes may occur with fever, malaise, and dysuria.

Trichomoniasis. Trichomoniasis can cause a foul-smelling discharge, which may be frothy, green-yellow, and profuse or thin, white, and scant. Other findings include pruritus; a red, inflamed vagina with tiny petechiae; dysuria and urinary frequency; and dyspareunia, postcoital spotting, menorrhagia, or dysmenorrhea. About 70% of patients are asymptomatic.

Other causes

Contraceptive creams and jellies. Contraceptive creams and jellies increase vaginal secretions.

Drugs. Drugs that contain estrogen, including hormonal contraceptives, can cause increased mucoid vaginal discharge. Antibiotics, such as tetracycline, may increase the risk of a candidal vaginal infection and discharge.

Radiation therapy. Irradiation of the reproductive tract can cause a watery, odorless vaginal discharge.

Nursing considerations

- Obtain cultures of the vaginal discharge.
- Give antibiotics, antivirals, or other drugs, as ordered.
- Observe standard precautions to prevent the spread of infection.

Patient teaching

- Explain to the patient the cause of vaginal discharge and its treatment.
- Teach the patient proper perineal hygiene and advise her to avoid tight-fitting clothing and nylon underwear.
- Suggest douching with vinegar and warm water to help relieve discomfort, if appropriate.
- Tell the patient to continue taking prescribed drugs even if her symptoms clear.
- Advise the patient to avoid intercourse until symptoms resolve.
- Provide information on safer sex practices.

Vertigo

Vertigo is an illusion of movement in which the patient feels that he's revolv-

ing in space (subjective vertigo) or that his surroundings are revolving around him (objective vertigo). He may complain of feeling pulled sideways, as though drawn by a magnet.

A common symptom, vertigo usually begins abruptly and may be temporary or permanent and mild or severe. It may worsen when the patient moves and subside when he lies down. It's often confused with dizziness—a sensation of imbalance and light-headedness that's nonspecific. However, unlike dizziness, vertigo is commonly accompanied by nausea and vomiting, nystagmus, and tinnitus or hearing loss. And, although the patient's limb coordination is unaffected, vertiginous gait may occur.

Vertigo may result from a neurologic or otologic disorder that affects the equilibratory apparatus (the vestibule, semicircular canals, eighth cranial nerve, vestibular nuclei in the brain stem and their temporal lobe connections, and eyes). However, this symptom may also result from alcohol intoxication, hyperventilation, and postural changes (benign postural vertigo). It may also be an adverse effect of certain drugs, tests, or procedures.

History and physical examination

Ask your patient to describe the onset and duration of his vertigo, being careful to distinguish this symptom from dizziness. Does he feel that he's moving or that his surroundings are moving around him? How often do the attacks occur? Do they follow position changes, or are they unpredictable? Find out if the patient can walk during an attack, if he leans to one side, and if he has ever fallen. Ask whether he experiences motion sickness and if he prefers one position during an attack. Obtain a recent drug history, and note evidence of alcohol abuse.

Perform a neurologic assessment, focusing particularly on eighth cranial nerve function. Observe the patient's gait and posture for abnormalities.

Medical causes

Acoustic neuroma. Acoustic neuroma causes mild, intermittent vertigo and unilateral sensorineural hearing loss. Other findings include tinnitus, postauricular or suboccipital pain, and—with cranial nerve compression—facial paralysis.

Benign positional vertigo. With benign positional vertigo, debris in a semicircular canal produces vertigo with head position change, which lasts a few minutes. It's usually temporary and can be effectively treated with positional maneuvers.

Brain stem ischemia. Brain stem ischemia produces sudden, severe vertigo that may become episodic and later persistent. Associated findings include ataxia, nausea, vomiting, increased blood pressure, tachycardia, nystagmus, and lateral deviation of the eyes toward the side of the lesion. Hemiparesis and paresthesia may also occur.

Head trauma. Persistent vertigo, occurring soon after head injury, accompanies spontaneous or positional nystagmus and, if the temporal bone is fractured, hearing loss. Associated findings include headache, nausea, vomiting, and decreased (LOC). Behavioral changes, diplopia or visual blurring, seizures, motor or sensory deficits, and signs of increased intracranial pressure may also occur.

Herpes zoster. Herpes infection of the eighth cranial nerve produces sudden onset of vertigo accompanied by facial paralysis, hearing loss in the affected ear, and herpetic vesicular lesions in the auditory canal.

Labyrinthitis. Severe vertigo begins abruptly with labyrinthitis. Vertigo may occur in a single episode or may recur over months or years. Associated findings include nausea, vomiting, progressive sensorineural hearing loss, and nystagmus.

Ménière's disease. With Ménière's disease, labyrinthine dysfunction causes abrupt onset of vertigo, lasting minutes, hours, or days. Unpredictable episodes of severe vertigo and unsteady gait may cause the patient to fall. During an attack, a sudden motion of the head or eyes can precipitate nausea and vomiting.

Multiple sclerosis (MS). With MS, episodic vertigo may occur early and become persistent. Other early findings include diplopia, visual blurring, and paresthesia. MS may also produce nystagmus, constipation, muscle weakness, paralysis, spasticity, hyperreflexia, intention tremor, and ataxia.

Seizures. Temporal lobe seizures may produce vertigo, usually associated with other symptoms of partial complex seizures.

Vestibular neuritis. With vestibular neuritis, severe vertigo usually begins abruptly and lasts several days, without tinnitus or hearing loss. Other findings include nausea, vomiting, and nystagmus.

Other causes

Diagnostic tests. Caloric testing (irrigating the ears with warm or cold water) can induce vertigo.

Drugs and alcohol. High or toxic doses of certain drugs or alcohol may produce vertigo. These drugs include salicylates, aminoglycosides, antibiotics, quinine, and hormonal contraceptives.

Surgery and other procedures. Ear surgery may cause vertigo that lasts for several days. Administration of overly warm or cold eardrops or irrigating solutions can also cause vertigo.

Nursing considerations

- Place the patient in a comfortable position.
- Monitor vital signs and LOC.
- Take measures to provide for the patient's safety.
- Darken the room and keep the patient calm.
- Administer drugs to control nausea and vomiting and decrease labyrinthine irritability.
- Prepare the patient for diagnostic tests, such as electronystagmography, EEG, and X-rays of the middle and inner ears.

Patient teaching

- Explain to the patient the underlying cause of vertigo and its treatment.
- Explain safety measures to the patient.
- Tell the patient to avoid sudden position changes and dangerous tasks.

Vesicular rash

A vesicular rash is a scattered or linear distribution of sharply circumscribed, blister-like lesions, which are filled with clear, cloudy, or bloody fluid. The lesions are usually less than 0.5 cm in diameter and may occur singly or in groups. (See *Recognizing common skin lesions,* page 459.) They may also occur with bullae—fluid-filled lesions that are larger than 0.5 cm in diameter.

A vesicular rash may be mild or severe and temporary or permanent; it may result from infection, inflammation, or allergic reactions.

History and physical examination

Ask your patient when the rash began, how it spread, and whether it has occurred before. Did other skin lesions precede eruption of the vesicles? Obtain a thorough drug history. If the patient has used a topical medication, what type did he use and when was it last applied?

Ask about associated signs and symptoms. Find out if he has a family history of skin disorders, and ask about allergies, recent infections, insect bites, and exposure to allergens.

Examine the patient's skin, noting if it's dry, oily, or moist. Observe the general distribution of the lesions and record their exact location. Note the color, shape, and size of the lesions, and check for crusts, scales, scars, macules, papules, or wheals. Palpate the vesicles or bullae to determine if they're flaccid or tense. Slide your finger across the skin to see if the outer layer of epidermis separates easily from the basal layer (Nikolsky's sign).

Medical causes

Burns (second degree). Thermal burns that affect the epidermis and part of the dermis cause vesicles and bullae, with erythema, swelling, pain, and moistness.

Dermatitis. With *contact dermatitis,* a hypersensitivity reaction produces an eruption of small vesicles surrounded by redness and marked edema. The vesicles may ooze, scale, and cause severe pruritus.

Dermatitis herpetiformis produces a chronic inflammatory eruption marked by vesicular, papular, bullous, pustular, or erythematous lesions. Usually, the rash is symmetrically distributed on the buttocks, shoulders, extensor surfaces of the elbows and knees, and sometimes on the face, scalp, and neck. Other symptoms include severe pruritus, burning, and stinging.

With *nummular dermatitis,* groups of pinpoint vesicles and papules appear on erythematous or pustular lesions that are nummular (coinlike) or annular (ringlike). Often, the pustular lesions ooze a purulent exudate, itch severely, and rapidly become crusted and scaly. Two or three lesions may develop on the hands, but the lesions typically develop on the extensor surfaces of the limbs and on the buttocks and posterior trunk.

Erythema multiforme. Erythema multiforme is heralded by a sudden eruption of erythematous macules, papules and, occasionally, vesicles and bullae. The characteristic rash appears symmetrically over the hands, arms, feet, legs, face, and neck and tends to reappear. Although vesicles and bullae may also erupt on the eyes and genitalia, vesiculobullous lesions usually appear on the mucous membranes—especially the lips and buccal mucosa—where they rupture and ulcerate, producing a thick, yellow or white exudate. Bloody, painful crusts, a foul-smelling oral discharge, and difficulty chewing may develop. Lymphadenopathy may also occur.

Herpes simplex. Herpes simplex produces groups of vesicles on an inflamed base, most commonly on the lips and lower face. In about 25% of cases, the genital region is the site of involvement. Vesicles are preceded by itching, tingling, burning, or pain; develop singly or in groups; are 2 to 3 mm in size; and don't coalesce. Eventually, they rupture, forming a painful ulcer followed by a yellowish crust.

Herpes zoster. With herpes zoster, a vesicular rash is preceded by erythema and, occasionally, by a nodular skin eruption and unilateral, sharp, pain along a dermatome. About 5 days later, the lesions erupt and the pain becomes burning. Vesicles dry and scab approximately 10 days after eruption. Associated findings include fever, malaise, pruritus, and paresthesia or hyperesthesia of the involved area. Herpes zoster involving the cranial nerves produces facial palsy, hearing loss, dizziness, loss of taste, eye pain, and impaired vision.

Insect bites. With insect bites, vesicles appear on red hivelike papules and may become hemorrhagic.

Pemphigoid (bullous). Generalized pruritus or an urticarial or eczematous eruption may precede pemphigoid—a classic bullous rash. Bullae are large, thick-walled, tense, and irregular, typically forming on an erythematous base. They usually appear on the lower abdomen, groin, inner thighs, and forearms.

Pompholyx (dyshidrosis or dyshidrosis eczema). Pompholyx is a common, recurrent disorder that produces symmetrical vesicular lesions that can become pustular. The pruritic lesions are more common on the palms than on the soles and may be accompanied by minimal erythema.

Porphyria cutanea tarda. Bullae—especially on areas exposed to sun, friction, trauma, or heat—result from abnormal porphyrin metabolism. Photosensitivity is also a common sign. Papulovesicular lesions evolving into erosions or ulcers and scars may appear. Chronic skin changes include hyperpigmentation or hypopigmentation, hypertrichosis, and sclerodermoid lesions. Urine is pink to brown.

Scabies. With scabies, small vesicles erupt on an erythematous base and may be at the end of a threadlike burrow. Burrows are a few millimeters long, with a swollen nodule or red papule that contains the mite. Pustules and excoriations may also occur. Men may develop burrows on the glans, shaft, and scrotum; women may develop burrows on the nipples. Both sexes may develop burrows on the webs of the fingers, wrists, elbows, axillae, and waistline. Associated pruritus worsens with inactivity and warmth and at night.

Smallpox (variola major). Initial signs and symptoms of smallpox include high fever, malaise, prostration, severe headache, backache, and abdominal pain. A maculopapular rash develops on the mucosa of the mouth, pharynx, face and forearms and then spreads to the trunk and legs. Within 2 days the rash becomes vesicular and later pustular. The lesions develop at the same time, appear identical, and are more prominent on the face and extremities. The pustules are round, firm, and deeply embedded in the skin. After 8 to 9 days, the pustules form a crust. Later, the scab separates from the skin, leaving a pitted scar. In fatal cases, death results from encephalitis, extensive bleeding, or secondary infection.

Tinea pedis. Tinea pedis causes vesicles and scaling between the toes and, possibly, scaling over the entire sole. Severe infection causes inflammation, pruritus, and difficulty walking.

Toxic epidermal necrolysis. Toxic epidermal necrolysis is an immune reaction to drugs or other toxins, in which vesicles and bullae are preceded by a diffuse, erythematous rash and followed by large-scale epidermal necrolysis and desquamation. Large, flaccid bullae develop after mucous membrane inflammation, a burning sensation in the conjunctivae, malaise, fever, and generalized skin tenderness. The bullae rupture easily, exposing extensive areas of denuded skin. (See *Drugs that cause toxic epidermal necrolysis.*)

Nursing considerations

■ If skin eruptions cover a large skin surface, insert an I.V. catheter to replace fluids and electrolytes.
■ Keep the environment warm and free from drafts.
■ Obtain cultures to determine the causative organism.
■ Use precautions until infection is ruled out.
■ Be alert for signs of secondary infection.

Drugs that cause toxic epidermal necrolysis

Various drugs can trigger toxic epidermal necrolysis—a rare but potentially fatal immune reaction characterized by a vesicular rash. This type of necrolysis produces large, flaccid bullae that rupture easily, exposing extensive areas of denuded skin. The resulting loss of fluid and electrolytes—along with widespread systemic involvement—can lead to such life-threatening complications as pulmonary edema, shock, renal failure, sepsis, and disseminated intravascular coagulation.

Here's a list of some drugs that can cause toxic epidermal necrolysis:
■ allopurinol
■ aspirin
■ barbiturates
■ chloramphenicol
■ chlorpropamide
■ gold salts
■ nitrofurantoin
■ penicillin
■ phenytoin
■ primidone
■ sulfonamides
■ tetracycline.

■ Give the patient an antibiotic and apply corticosteroid or antimicrobial ointment to the lesions, as ordered.

Patient teaching
■ Explain the importance of frequent handwashing.
■ Instruct the patient to avoid touching the lesions.
■ Discuss measures to relieve itching, such as tepid baths or cold compresses.

Violent behavior

Marked by sudden loss of self-control, violent behavior refers to the use of physical force to violate, injure, or abuse

Understanding family violence

Effectively managing the violent patient requires an understanding of the roots of his behavior. For example, his behavior may be spawned by a family history of corporal punishment or child or spouse abuse. His violent behavior may also be associated with drug or alcohol abuse and fixed family roles that stifle growth and individuality.

Causes of family violence

Social scientists suggest that family violence stems from cultural attitudes fostering violence and from the frustration and stress associated with overcrowded living conditions and poverty. Albert Bandura, a social learning theorist, believes that individuals learn violent behavior by observing and imitating other family members who vent their aggressive feelings through verbal abuse and physical force. (They also learn from television and the movies, especially when the violent hero gains power and recognition.) Members of families with these characteristics may have an increased potential for violent behavior, thus initiating a cycle of violence that passes from generation to generation.

---

an object or person. This behavior may also be self-directed. It may result from an organic or psychiatric disorder or from the use of certain drugs or alcohol

Someone displaying violent behavior may be wildly irrational, resulting in a situation that's difficult to diffuse. Therefore, the initial intervention should be to secure the safety of the patient and anyone in the immediate vicinity, including healthcare personnel, until the patient's violent behavior can be controlled.

History and physical examination

During your evaluation, determine whether the patient has a history of violent behavior. Is he intoxicated or suffering symptoms of alcohol or drug intoxication or withdrawal? Does he have a history of family violence, including corporal punishment and child or spouse abuse? (See *Understanding family violence*.)

Watch for clues indicating that the patient is losing control and may become violent. Has he exhibited abrupt behavioral changes? Is he unable to sit still? Increased activity may indicate an attempt to discharge aggression. Does he suddenly cease activity (suggesting the calm before the storm)? Does he make verbal threats or angry gestures? Is he jumpy, extremely tense, or laughing? Such intensifying of emotion may herald loss of control.

If your patient's violent behavior is a new development, he may have an organic disorder. Obtain a medical history and perform a physical examination. Watch for a sudden change in his level of consciousness. Disorientation, failure to recall recent events, and display of tics, jerks, tremors, and asterixis all suggest an organic disorder.

Medical causes

Organic disorders. Disorders resulting from metabolic or neurologic dysfunction can cause violent behavior. Common causes include epilepsy, brain tumor, encephalitis, head injury, endocrine disorders, metabolic disorders (such as uremia and calcium imbalance), and severe physical trauma.

Psychiatric disorders. Violent behavior occurs as a protective mechanism in response to a perceived threat in psychotic disorders such as schizophrenia. A similar response may occur in personality disorders, such as antisocial or borderline personality.

Other causes

Drugs and alcohol. Violent behavior is an adverse effect of some drugs, such as lidocaine and penicillin G. Alcohol abuse or withdrawal, hallucinogens, amphetamines, and barbiturate withdrawal may also cause violent behavior.

Nursing considerations

■ Take measures to protect yourself, such as remaining at a distance from the patient and calling for assistance.
■ Remain calm, and make sure you have enough personnel for a show of force to subdue or restrain the patient if necessary.
■ Encourage the patient to move to a quiet location—free from noise, activity, and people—to avoid frightening or stimulating him further.
■ If the patient makes violent threats, take them seriously, and inform those at whom the threats are directed.
■ If ordered, administer a psychotropic medication.

Patient teaching

■ Reassure the patient, explain what's happening, and tell him that he's safe.
■ After the patient is calm, explain the reason for his violent behavior, if known.

Vision loss

Vision loss—the inability to perceive visual stimuli—can be sudden or gradual and temporary or permanent. The deficit can range from a slight impairment of vision to total blindness. It can result from an ocular, neurologic, or systemic disorder or from trauma or the use of certain drugs. The ultimate visual outcome may depend on early, accurate diagnosis and treatment.

History and physical examination

Sudden vision loss can signal an ocular emergency. (See *Managing sudden vision loss,* page 628.) Don't touch the eye if the patient has perforating or penetrating ocular trauma.

If the patient's vision loss occurred gradually, ask him if the vision loss affects one eye or both and all or only part of the visual field. Is the visual loss transient or persistent? Did the vision loss occur abruptly or did it develop over hours, days, or weeks? What's the patient's age? Ask the patient if he has experienced photosensitivity and ask him about the location, intensity, and duration of eye pain. You should also obtain an ocular history and a family history of eye problems or systemic diseases that may lead to eye problems, such as hypertension; diabetes mellitus; thyroid, rheumatic, or vascular disease; infections; and cancer.

The first step in performing an eye examination is to assess visual acuity, with best available correction in each eye. (See *Testing visual acuity,* page 629.)

Carefully inspect both eyes, noting edema, foreign bodies, drainage, or conjunctival or scleral redness. Observe whether lid closure is complete or incomplete and check for ptosis. Using a flashlight, examine the cornea and iris for scars, irregularities, and foreign bodies. Observe the size, shape, and color of the pupils, and test the direct and consensual light reflex (See "Pupils, nonreactive," page 515.) and the effect of accommodation. Evaluate extraocular muscle function by testing the six cardinal fields of gaze. (See *Testing extraocular muscles,* page 197.)

Managing sudden vision loss

Sudden vision loss can signal central retinal artery occlusion or acute angle-closure glaucoma—ocular emergencies that require immediate intervention. If your patient reports sudden vision loss, immediately notify an ophthalmologist for an emergency examination and perform these interventions:

For a patient with suspected central retinal artery occlusion, perform light massage over his closed eyelid. Increase his carbon dioxide level by administering a set flow of oxygen and carbon dioxide through a Venturi mask, or have the pa-

tient rebreathe in a paper bag to retain exhaled carbon dioxide. These steps will dilate the artery and, possibly, restore blood flow to the retina.

For a patient with suspected acute angle-closure glaucoma, measure intraocular pressure (IOP) with a tonometer. (You can also estimate IOP without a tonometer by placing your fingers over the patient's closed eyelid. A rock-hard eyeball usually indicates increased IOP.) Expect to instill timolol drops and administer I.V. acetazolamide to help decrease IOP.

Suspected central retinal artery occlusion

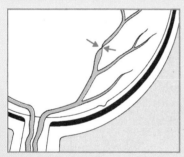

Suspected acute angle-closure glaucoma

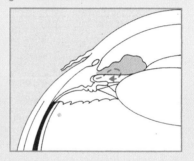

Medical causes

Amaurosis fugax. With amaurosis fugax, recurrent attacks of unilateral vision loss may last from a few seconds to a few minutes. Vision is normal at other times. Transient unilateral weakness, hypertension, and elevated intraocular pressure (IOP) in the affected eye may also occur.

Cataract. With a cataract, painless and gradual visual blurring typically precede vision loss. As the cataract progresses, the pupil turns milky white.

Concussion. Immediately or shortly after blunt head trauma, vision may be blurred, double, or lost. Generally, vision loss is temporary. Other findings

include headache, anterograde and retrograde amnesia, transient loss of consciousness, nausea, vomiting, dizziness, irritability, confusion, lethargy, and aphasia.

Diabetic retinopathy. With diabetic retinopathy, retinal edema and hemorrhage lead to visual blurring, which may progress to blindness.

Endophthalmitis. Typically, endophthalmitis follows penetrating trauma, I.V. drug use, or intraocular surgery, causing possibly permanent unilateral vision loss; a sympathetic inflammation may affect the other eye.

Glaucoma. Glaucoma produces gradual visual blurring that may pro-

ASSESSMENT TIP

Testing visual acuity

Use a Snellen letter chart (as shown below) to test visual acuity in the literate patient older than age 6. Have the patient sit or stand 20′ (6 m) from the chart. Tell him to cover his left eye and read aloud the smallest line of letters that he can see. Record the fraction assigned to that line on the chart (the numerator indicates distance from the chart; the denominator indicates the distance at which a normal eye can read the chart). Normal vision is 20/20. Repeat the test with the patient's right eye covered.

If your patient can't read the largest letter from a distance of 20′ (6 m), have him approach the chart until he can read it. Record the distance between him and the chart as the numerator of the fraction. For example, if he can see the top line of the chart at a distance of 3′ (1 m), record the test result as 3/200.

Use a Snellen symbol chart (as shown below) to test children ages 3 to 6 and patients who are illiterate. Follow the same procedure as for the Snellen letter chart, but ask the patient to indicate the direction of the E's "fingers" as you point to each symbol (for example, right or left, up or down).

Snellen letter chart

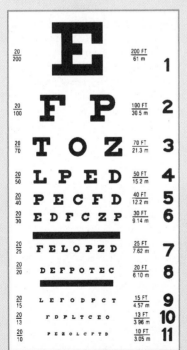

Snellen symbol chart

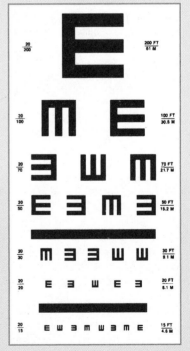

gress to total blindness. *Acute angle-closure glaucoma* is an ocular emergency that may produce blindness within 3 to 5 days. Findings are rapid onset of unilateral inflammation and pain, pressure over the eye, moderate pupil dilation, nonreactive pupillary response, a cloudy cornea, reduced visual acuity, photophobia, and perception of blue or red halos around lights. Nausea and vomiting may also occur.

Chronic angle-closure glaucoma has a gradual onset and usually produces no symptoms, although blurred or halo vision may occur. If untreated, it progresses to blindness and extreme pain.

Chronic open-angle glaucoma is usually bilateral, with an insidious onset and a slowly progressive course. It causes peripheral vision loss, aching eyes, halo vision, and reduced visual acuity (especially at night).

Ocular trauma. Following eye injury, sudden unilateral or bilateral vision loss may occur. Vision loss may be total or partial and permanent or temporary. The eyelids may be reddened, edematous, and lacerated; intraocular contents may be extruded.

Optic atrophy. Optic atrophy can develop spontaneously or follow inflammation or edema of the nerve head, causing irreversible loss of the visual field with changes in color vision. Pupillary reactions are sluggish and optic disk pallor is evident.

Optic neuritis. An umbrella term for inflammation, degeneration, or demyelinization of the optic nerve, optic neuritis usually produces temporary but severe unilateral vision loss. Pain around the eye occurs, especially with movement of the globe. This may occur with visual field defects and a sluggish pupillary response to light. Ophthalmoscopic examination commonly reveals hyperemia of the optic disk, blurred disk margins, and filling of the physiologic cup.

Paget's disease. With Paget's disease, bilateral vision loss may develop as a result of bony impingements on the cranial nerves. This occurs with hearing loss, tinnitus, vertigo, and severe, persistent bone pain. Cranial enlargement may be noticeable frontally and occipitally, and headaches may occur. Sites of bone involvement are warm and tender and impaired mobility and pathologic fractures are common.

Pituitary tumor. As a pituitary adenoma grows, blurred vision progresses to hemianopsia and, possibly, unilateral blindness. Double vision, nystagmus, ptosis, limited eye movement, and headaches may also occur.

Retinal artery occlusion (central). Retinal artery occlusion is a painless ocular emergency that causes sudden unilateral vision loss, which may be partial or complete. Pupil examination reveals a sluggish direct pupillary response and a normal consensual response. Permanent blindness may occur within hours.

Retinal detachment. Depending on the degree and location of retinal detachment, painless vision loss may be gradual or sudden and total or partial. Macular involvement causes total blindness.

With partial vision loss, the patient may describe visual field defects or a shadow or curtain over the visual field as well as visual floaters.

Retinal vein occlusion (central). Retinal vein occlusion causes a unilateral decrease in visual acuity with variable vision loss. IOP may be elevated in both eyes.

Rift Valley fever. Rift Valley fever causes inflammation of the retina and may result in some permanent vision loss. Typical signs and symptoms include fever, myalgia, weakness, dizziness, and back pain. A small percentage of patients may develop encephalitis or may progress to hemorrhagic fever that can lead to shock and hemorrhage.

Senile macular degeneration. Senile macular degeneration causes painless blurring or loss of central vision. Vision loss may proceed slowly or rapidly, eventually affecting both eyes. Visual acuity may be worse at night.

Stevens-Johnson syndrome. With Stevens-Johnson syndrome, corneal scarring from associated conjunctival lesions produces marked vision loss. Purulent conjunctivitis, eye pain, and difficulty opening the eyes occur. Additional findings include widespread bullae, fever, malaise, cough, drooling, inability to eat, sore throat, chest pain, vomiting, diarrhea, myalgias, arthralgias, hematuria, and signs of renal failure.

Temporal arteritis. Vision loss and visual blurring with a throbbing, unilateral headache characterize temporal arteritis. Other findings include malaise, anorexia, weight loss, weakness, low-grade fever, generalized muscle aches, and confusion.

Vitreous hemorrhage. With vitreous hemorrhage, sudden unilateral vision loss may result from intraocular trauma, ocular tumors, or systemic disease (especially diabetes, hypertension, sickle cell anemia, or leukemia). Visual floaters and partial vision with a reddish haze may occur. The patient's vision loss may be permanent.

Other causes

Drugs. Chloroquine therapy may cause patchy retinal pigmentation that typically leads to blindness. Phenylbutazone may cause vision loss and increased susceptibility to retinal detachment. Digoxin, indomethacin, ethambutol, quinine sulfate, and methanol toxicity may also cause vision loss.

Nursing considerations
- Take measures to ensure the patient's safety.
- If the patient reports photophobia, darken the room and suggest that he wear sunglasses during the day.
- Obtain cultures of eye drainage.
- Announce your presence each time you approach the patient.
- If necessary, prepare the patient for surgery.

Patient teaching
- Orient the patient to his environment and explain safety measures.
- Instruct the patient to wash his hands often and to avoid rubbing his eyes.
- Explain to the patient the cause of vision loss and its treatment.
- If vision loss is progressive or permanent, refer the patient to appropriate social service agencies for assistance with adaptation and equipment.

Visual blurring

Visual blurring is a common symptom that refers to the loss of visual acuity with indistinct visual details. It may result from eye injury, a neurologic or eye disorder, or a disorder with vascular complications, such as diabetes mellitus. Visual blurring may also result from mucus passing over the cornea, a refractive error, improperly fitted contact lenses, or certain drugs.

History and physical examination

If your patient has visual blurring accompanied by sudden, severe eye pain, a history of trauma, or sudden vision loss, order an ophthalmologic examination. (See *Managing sudden vision loss*, page 628.) If the patient has a penetrating or perforating eye injury, don't touch the eye.

If the patient isn't in distress, ask him how long he has had the visual blurring. Does it occur only at certain times? Ask about associated signs and symptoms, such as pain or discharge. If visual blurring followed injury, obtain details of the accident and ask if vision was impaired immediately after the injury. Obtain a medical and drug history.

Inspect the patient's eye, noting lid edema, drainage, or conjunctival or scleral redness. Also note an irregularly shaped iris, which may indicate previous trauma, and excessive blinking, which may indicate corneal damage. Assess the patient for pupillary changes, and test visual acuity in both eyes. (See *Testing visual acuity,* page 629.)

Medical causes

Brain tumor. Visual blurring may occur with a brain tumor. Associated findings include decreased level of consciousness (LOC), headache, apathy, behavioral changes, memory loss, decreased attention span, dizziness, and confusion. A tumor can also cause aphasia, seizures, ataxia, and signs of hormonal imbalance. Its later effects are papilledema, vomiting, increased systolic blood pressure, widened pulse pressure, and decorticate posture.

Cataract. A cataract causes gradual visual blurring. Other effects include halo vision (an early sign), visual glare in bright light, progressive vision loss, and a gray pupil that later turns milky white.

Concussion. Immediately or shortly after blunt head trauma, vision may be blurred, double, or temporarily lost. Other findings include changes in LOC and behavior.

Corneal abrasions. With corneal abrasions, visual blurring may occur with severe eye pain, photophobia, redness, and excessive tearing.

Corneal foreign bodies. With a corneal foreign body, visual blurring may accompany a foreign-body sensation, excessive tearing, photophobia, intense eye pain, miosis, conjunctival injection, and a dark corneal speck.

Diabetic retinopathy. With diabetic retinopathy, retinal edema and hemorrhage produce gradual blurring, which may progress to blindness.

Dislocated lens. Dislocation of the lens, especially beyond the line of vision, causes visual blurring and (with trauma) redness.

Eye tumor. If an eye tumor involves the macula, visual blurring may be the presenting symptom. Related findings include varying visual field losses.

Glaucoma. With *acute angle-closure glaucoma,* an ocular emergency, unilateral visual blurring and severe pain begin suddenly. Other findings include halo vision; a moderately dilated, nonreactive pupil; conjunctival injection; a cloudy cornea; and decreased visual acuity. Severely elevated intraocular pressure may cause nausea and vomiting.

With *chronic angle-closure glaucoma,* transient visual blurring and halo vision may precede pain and blindness.

Hereditary corneal dystrophies. With hereditary corneal dystrophy, visual blurring may remain stable or may progressively worsen throughout life. Some dystrophies cause associated pain, vision loss, photophobia, tearing, and corneal opacities.

Hypertension. Hypertension may cause visual blurring and a constant morning headache that decreases in severity during the day. If diastolic blood pressure exceeds 120 mm Hg, the patient may report a severe, throbbing headache. Associated findings include restlessness, confusion, nausea, vomiting, seizures, and decreased LOC.

Hyphema. With hyphema, blunt eye trauma with hemorrhage into the anterior chamber causes visual blurring. Other effects include moderate pain, diffuse conjunctival injection, visible blood in the anterior chamber, ecchymoses, eyelid edema, and a hard eye.

Iritis. Acute iritis causes sudden visual blurring, moderate to severe eye pain, photophobia, conjunctival injection, and a constricted pupil.

Optic neuritis. Inflammation, degeneration, or demyelinization of the optic nerve usually causes an acute attack of visual blurring and vision loss. Related findings include scotomas and eye pain. Ophthalmoscopic examination reveals hyperemia of the optic disk, large vein distention, blurred disk margins, and filling of the physiologic cup.

Retinal detachment. Sudden visual blurring may be the initial symptom of retinal detachment. Blurring worsens, accompanied by visual floaters and recurring flashes of light. Progressive detachment increases vision loss.

Retinal vein occlusion (central). Retinal vein occlusion causes gradual unilateral visual blurring and varying degrees of vision loss.

Senile macular degeneration. Senile macular degeneration may cause visual blurring (initially worse at night) and slowly or rapidly progressive vision loss.

Stroke. Brief attacks of bilateral visual blurring may precede or accompany a stroke. Associated findings include decreased LOC, contralateral hemiplegia, dysarthria, dysphagia, ataxia, unilateral sensory loss, and apraxia. Stroke may also cause agnosia, aphasia, homonymous hemianopsia, diplopia, disorientation, memory loss, and poor judgment. Other features include urine retention or urinary incontinence, constipation, personality changes, emotional lability, headache, vomiting, and seizures.

Temporal arteritis. Temporal arteritis causes sudden blurred vision accompanied by vision loss and a throbbing unilateral headache in the temporal or frontotemporal region. Prodromal signs and symptoms include malaise, anorexia, weight loss, weakness, low-grade fever, and generalized muscle aches. Other findings include confusion; disorientation; swollen, nodular, tender temporal arteries; and erythema of overlying skin.

Vitreous hemorrhage. Sudden unilateral visual blurring and varying vision loss occur with this condition. Visual floaters or dark streaks may also occur.

Other causes

Drugs. Visual blurring may stem from the effects of cycloplegics, guanethidine, reserpine, clomiphene, phenylbutazone, thiazide diuretics, antihistamines, anticholinergics, or phenothiazines.

Nursing considerations

- Prepare the patient for diagnostic tests, such as tonometry, slit-lamp examination, X-rays of the skull and orbit and, if a neurologic lesion is suspected, a computed tomography scan.
- Initiate safety measures to prevent injury.
- If visual blurring leads to permanent vision loss, provide emotional support.
- If necessary, prepare the patient for surgery.

Patient teaching

- Explain to the patient the cause of visual blurring and its treatment.
- Teach the patient how to instill eyedrops properly.
- Discuss safety measures.

Visual floaters

Visual floaters are particles of blood or cellular debris that move about in the vitreous. As these floaters enter the visual field, they appear as spots or dots. *Chronic* floaters may occur normally in elderly or myopic patients; however, the *sudden* onset of visual floaters commonly signals retinal detachment, an ocular emergency.

 Sudden onset of visual floaters may signal retinal detachment. Does the patient also see flashing lights or spots in the affected eye? Is he experiencing a curtainlike loss of vision? If so, notify an ophthalmologist immediately and restrict the patient's eye movements until the diagnosis is made.

History and physical examination

If the patient's condition permits, obtain a drug and allergy history. Ask about nearsightedness (a predisposing factor), use of corrective lenses, eye trauma, or other eye disorders. Ask about a history of granulomatous disease, diabetes mellitus, or hypertension, which may have predisposed him to retinal detachment, vitreous hemorrhage, or uveitis. If appropriate, inspect the patient's eyes for signs of injury, such as bruising or edema, and determine his visual acuity. (See *Testing visual acuity,* page 629.)

Medical causes

Retinal detachment. With retinal detachment, floaters and light flashes appear suddenly in the portion of the visual field where the retina is detached from the choroid. As the retina detaches further (a painless process), gradual vision loss occurs, likened to a cloud or curtain falling in front of the eyes. Ophthalmoscopic examination reveals a gray, opaque, detached retina with an indefinite margin. Retinal vessels appear almost black.

Uveitis (posterior). Uveitis may cause visual floaters accompanied by gradual eye pain, photophobia, blurred vision, and conjunctival injection.

Vitreous hemorrhage. Rupture of retinal vessels produces a shower of red or black dots or a red haze across the visual field. Vision is suddenly blurred in the affected eye and visual acuity may be greatly reduced.

Nursing considerations

- Place the patient on bed rest and provide a calm environment.
- Place a patch over one or both of the patient's eyes, as ordered.
- If bilateral eye patches are necessary, take measures to ensure the patient's safety.
- Prepare the patient for surgery, as necessary.
- Administer medications, as ordered.
- Provide sensory stimulation, such as music, if the patient desires.
- Place pillows or towels behind the patient's head to maintain appropriate patient position.
- Identify yourself when you approach the patient.
- Orient the patient to time frequently.

Patient teaching

- Tell the patient not to touch or rub his eyes and to avoid straining or sudden movements.

Vomiting

Vomiting is the forceful expulsion of gastric contents through the mouth. Characteristically preceded by nausea, vomiting results from a coordinated sequence of abdominal muscle contractions and reverse esophageal peristalsis.

A common sign of GI disorders, vomiting also occurs with fluid and electrolyte imbalances; infections; and metabolic, endocrine, labyrinthine, central nervous system (CNS), and cardiac disorders. It can also result from drug therapy, surgery, or radiation.

Vomiting occurs normally during the first trimester of pregnancy, but its subsequent development may also signal complications. It can also result from stress, anxiety, pain, alcohol intoxication, overeating, or ingestion of distasteful foods or liquids.

History and physical examination

Ask your patient to describe the onset, duration, and intensity of his vomiting. What started the vomiting? What makes it subside? If possible, collect, measure, and inspect the character of the vomitus. (See *Vomitus: Characteristics and causes.*) Explore associated complaints, particularly nausea, abdominal pain, anorexia and weight loss, changes in bowel habits or stools, excessive belching or flatus, and bloating or fullness.

Obtain a medical history, noting GI, endocrine, and metabolic disorders; recent infections; and cancer, including chemotherapy or radiation therapy. Ask the patient about current medication use and alcohol consumption. If the patient is a female of childbearing age, ask if she is or could be pregnant or which contraceptive method she's using.

Inspect the patient's abdomen for distention and localized bulging, and auscultate for bowel sounds and bruits. Palpate for rigidity and tenderness and test for rebound tenderness. Palpate and percuss the liver for enlargement. Assess the patient's other body systems as appropriate.

During the examination, keep in mind that projectile vomiting unaccompanied by nausea may be an indication of increased intracranial pressure, a life-threatening emergency. If this occurs in a patient with CNS injury, you should

Vomitus: Characteristics and causes

When you collect a sample of the patient's vomitus, observe it carefully for clues to the underlying disorder. Here's what vomitus may indicate.

Bile-stained (greenish) vomitus
Obstruction below the pylorus, as from a duodenal lesion

Bloody vomitus
Upper GI bleeding (if bright red, may result from gastritis or a peptic ulcer; if dark red, from esophageal or gastric varices)

Brown vomitus with a fecal odor
Intestinal obstruction or infarction

Burning, bitter-tasting vomitus
Excessive hydrochloric acid in gastric contents

Coffee-ground vomitus
Digested blood from slowly bleeding gastric or duodenal lesion

Undigested food
Gastric outlet obstruction, as from gastric tumor or ulcer

quickly check his vital signs. Be alert for widened pulse pressure or bradycardia.

Medical causes
Adrenal insufficiency. Common GI findings with adrenal insufficiency include vomiting, nausea, anorexia, and diarrhea. Other findings include weakness; fatigue; weight loss; bronze skin; orthostatic hypotension; and weak, irregular pulse.

Anthrax (GI). Initial signs and symptoms after eating contaminated meat from an animal infected with anthrax include vomiting, loss of appetite, nausea, and fever. Signs and symptoms may progress to abdominal pain, severe bloody diarrhea, and hematemesis.

Appendicitis. Vomiting and nausea may follow or accompany abdominal pain from appendicitis. Pain typically begins as vague epigastric or periumbilical discomfort and rapidly progresses to severe, stabbing pain in the right lower quadrant. The patient generally has a positive McBurney's sign—severe pain and tenderness on palpation about 2″ (5 cm) from the right anterior superior spine of the ilium, on a line between that spine and the umbilicus. Associated findings usually include abdominal rigidity and tenderness, anorexia, constipation or diarrhea, cutaneous hyperalgesia, fever, tachycardia, and malaise.

Cholecystitis (acute). With cholecystitis, nausea and mild vomiting commonly follow severe right-upper-quadrant pain that may radiate to the back or shoulders. Associated findings include abdominal tenderness and, possibly, rigidity and distention, fever, and diaphoresis.

Cholelithiasis. With cholelithiasis, nausea and vomiting accompany severe, unlocalized right-upper-quadrant or epigastric pain after ingestion of fatty foods. Other findings include abdominal tenderness and guarding, flatulence, belching, epigastric burning, pyrosis, tachycardia, and restlessness.

Cholera. Signs and symptoms of cholera include vomiting and abrupt watery diarrhea. Severe water and electrolyte loss leads to thirst, weakness, muscle cramps, decreased skin turgor, oliguria, tachycardia, and hypotension. Without treatment, death can occur within hours.

Cirrhosis. Insidious early signs and symptoms of cirrhosis typically include nausea and vomiting, anorexia, aching abdominal pain, and constipation or diarrhea. Later findings include jaundice, hepatomegaly, and abdominal distention.

Electrolyte imbalances. Such electrolyte disturbances as hyponatremia, hypernatremia, hypokalemia, and hypercalcemia frequently cause nausea and vomiting. Other effects include arrhythmias, tremors, seizures, anorexia, malaise, and weakness.

Escherichia coli O157:H7. The signs and symptoms of *E.coli* include vomiting, watery or bloody diarrhea, nausea, fever, and abdominal cramps. In children younger than age 5 and the elderly, hemolytic uremic syndrome may develop in which the red blood cells are destroyed, which may ultimately lead to acute renal failure.

Food poisoning. Vomiting is a common finding of food poisoning, caused by preformed toxins produced by bacteria typically found in foods, such as *Bacillus cereus*, *Clostridium*, and *Staphylococcus*. Diarrhea and fever also usually occur.

Gastric cancer. This rare cancer may produce mild nausea, vomiting (possibly of mucus or blood), anorexia, upper abdominal discomfort, and chronic dyspepsia. Fatigue, weight loss, melena, and altered bowel habits are also common.

Gastritis. Nausea and vomiting of mucus or blood are common with gastritis, especially after ingestion of alcohol, aspirin, spicy foods, or caffeine. Epigastric pain, belching, and fever may occur.

Gastroenteritis. Gastroenteritis causes nausea, vomiting (commonly of undigested food), diarrhea, and abdominal cramping. Fever, malaise, hyperactive bowel sounds, and abdominal pain and tenderness may also occur.

Heart failure. Nausea and vomiting may occur heart failure, especially with right-sided heart failure. Associated findings include tachycardia, ventricular gallop, fatigue, dyspnea, crackles, peripheral edema, and jugular vein distention.

Hepatitis. Vomiting commonly follows nausea as an early sign of viral hepatitis. Other early findings include fatigue, myalgia, arthralgia, headache, photophobia, anorexia, pharyngitis, cough, and fever.

Hyperemesis gravidarum. Unremitting nausea and vomiting that last beyond the first trimester characterize this disorder of pregnancy. Vomitus contains undigested food, mucus, and small amounts of bile early in the disorder; later, it has a coffee-ground appearance. Associated findings include weight loss, headache, delirium, and electrolyte imbalance. Thyroid dysfunction may be associated with this condition.

Increased intracranial pressure. Projectile vomiting that isn't preceded by nausea is a sign of increased intracranial pressure. The patient may exhibit a decreased level of consciousness (LOC) and Cushing's triad (bradycardia, hypertension, and respiratory pattern changes). He may also have headache, widened pulse pressure, impaired motor movement, vision disturbances, pupillary changes, and papilledema.

Intestinal obstruction. Nausea and vomiting (bilious or fecal) are common with intestinal obstruction, especially of the upper small intestine. Abdominal pain is usually episodic and colicky but can become severe and steady. Constipation occurs early in large intestinal obstruction and late in small intestinal obstruction. Obstipation, however, may signal complete obstruction. In partial obstruction, bowel sounds are typically high pitched and hyperactive; in complete obstruction, bowel sounds are typically hypoactive or absent. Abdominal distention and tenderness also occur, possibly with visible peristaltic waves and a palpable abdominal mass.

Labyrinthitis. Nausea and vomiting commonly occur with labyrinthitis. Other findings include severe vertigo, progressive hearing loss, nystagmus, and possibly otorrhea.

Listeriosis. After the ingestion of food contaminated with the bacterium *Listeria monocytogenes*, vomiting, fever, myalgias, abdominal pain, nausea, and diarrhea occur. If the infection spreads to the nervous system, meningitis may develop. Signs and symptoms may include fever, headache, nuchal rigidity, and change in LOC. The food-borne illness primarily affects pregnant women, neonates, and those with weakened immune systems.

Mesenteric venous thrombosis. Insidious or acute onset of nausea, vomiting, and abdominal pain occurs with mesenteric venous thrombosis. Other findings include diarrhea or constipation, abdominal distention, hematemesis, and melena.

Migraine headache. Nausea and vomiting are prodromal signs of a migraine headache, along with such accompanying symptoms as fatigue, photophobia, light flashes, increased noise sensitivity, and possibly partial vision loss and paresthesia.

Motion sickness. With motion sickness, nausea and vomiting may be accompanied by headache, vertigo, dizziness, fatigue, diaphoresis, and dyspnea.

Norovirus infection. Violent vomiting may occur frequently and without warning with norovirus infection. Additional symptoms include nausea, diarrhea, and abdominal pain or cramping.

Pancreatitis (acute). Vomiting, usually preceded by nausea, is an early sign of pancreatitis. Associated findings include steady, severe epigastric or left-upper-quadrant pain that may radiate to the back, abdominal tenderness and rigidity, anorexia, hypoactive bowel sounds, vomiting, and fever. Tachycardia, restlessness, hypotension, skin mottling, and cold, sweaty extremities may occur in severe cases.

Peritonitis. With peritonitis, nausea and vomiting usually accompany acute abdominal pain in the area of inflammation. Other findings include high fever with chills; tachycardia; hypoactive or absent bowel sounds; abdominal distention, rigidity, and tenderness; weakness; pale, cold skin; diaphoresis; hypotension; signs of dehydration; and shallow respirations.

Preeclampsia. Nausea and vomiting are common with preeclampsia. Rapid weight gain, epigastric pain, generalized edema, elevated blood pressure, oliguria, proteinuria, severe frontal headache, and blurred or double vision also occur.

Q fever. Signs and symptoms of Q fever include vomiting, fever, chills, severe headache, malaise, chest pain, nausea, and diarrhea. Fever may last up to 2 weeks. In severe cases, the patient may develop hepatitis or pneumonia.

Renal and urologic disorders. Cystitis, pyelonephritis, calculi, and other disorders of this system can cause vomiting. Accompanying findings reflect the specific disorder. Persistent nausea and vomiting are typical findings in patients with acute or worsening chronic renal failure.

Rhabdomyolysis. Signs and symptoms of rhabdomyolisis include vomiting, muscle weakness or pain, fever, nausea, malaise, and dark urine. Acute renal failure is the most commonly reported complication of the disorder. It results from renal structure obstruction and injury during the kidney's attempt to filter the myoglobin from the bloodstream.

Typhus. Initial symptoms of typhus include headache, myalgia, arthralgia, and malaise, followed by an abrupt onset of vomiting, nausea, chills, and fever.

A maculopapular rash may be present in some cases.

Other causes

Drugs. Drugs that commonly cause vomiting include antineoplastics, opiates, ferrous sulfate, levodopa, oral potassium, chloride replacements, estrogens, sulfasalazine, antibiotics, quinidine, anesthetics, and overdoses of cardiac glycosides and theophylline. Syrup of ipecac is used to treat overdoses by inducing vomiting.

Radiation and surgery. Radiation therapy may cause nausea and vomiting if it disrupts the gastric mucosa. Postoperative nausea and vomiting are common, especially after abdominal surgery.

Nursing considerations
- Draw blood to determine fluid, electrolyte, and acid-base balance.
- Keep the patient's room clean smelling by removing bedpans and emesis basins promptly after use.
- Elevate the patient's head or position him on his side to prevent aspiration of vomitus.
- Monitor vital signs and intake and output (including vomitus and liquid stools).
- If necessary, administer I.V. fluids, or have the patient sip clear liquids to maintain hydration.
- Because pain can precipitate or intensify nausea and vomiting, administer pain medications promptly.
- Insert a nasogastric tube, as ordered.

Patient teaching
- Teach the patient deep-breathing exercises to ease nausea.
- Explain the importance of replacing fluid losses.
- Teach the patient about dietary restrictions and how to advance the diet.

Vulvar lesions

Vulvar lesions are cutaneous lumps, nodules, papules, vesicles, or ulcers that result from benign or malignant tumors, dystrophies, dermatoses, or infection. They can appear anywhere on the vulva and may go undetected until a gynecologic examination. Usually, however, the patient notices lesions because of associated symptoms, such as pruritus, dysuria, or dyspareunia.

History and physical examination

Ask the patient when she first noticed a vulvar lesion and find out about associated features, such as swelling, pain, tenderness, itching, or discharge. Does she have lesions elsewhere on her body? Ask about signs and symptoms of systemic illness, such as malaise, fever, or rash on other body areas. Is the patient sexually active? Ask whether she could have been exposed to sexually transmitted disease.

Examine the lesion, do a pelvic examination, and obtain cultures. (See *Recognizing common vulvar lesions,* page 640.)

Medical causes

Basal cell carcinoma. This nodular tumor has a central ulcer and a raised, poorly rolled border. Typically producing no symptoms, the tumor may occasionally cause pruritus, bleeding, discharge, and a burning sensation.

Benign cysts. Epidermal inclusion cysts, the most common vulvar cysts, appear primarily on the labia majora and are usually round and produces no symptoms. Occasionally, they become erythematous and tender.

Bartholin's duct cysts are usually unilateral, tense, nontender, and palpable; they appear on the posterior labia minora and may cause minor discomfort during intercourse or, when large, difficulty with intercourse or even walking. *Bartholin's abscess,* infection of a Bartholin's duct cyst, causes gradual pain and tenderness and possibly vulvar swelling, redness, and deformity.

Benign vulvar tumors. Cystic or solid, benign vulvar tumors usually produce no symptoms.

Chancroid. Chancroid causes painful vulvar lesions. Headache, malaise, and fever to 102.2° F (39° C) may occur, with enlarged, tender inguinal lymph nodes.

Genital warts. Genital warts are painless warts on the vulva, vagina, and cervix. They start as tiny red or pink swellings that grow and become pedunculated. Multiple swellings with a cauliflower appearance are common. Other findings include pruritus, erythema, and a profuse, mucopurulent vaginal discharge. Patients frequently complain of burning or paresthesia in the vaginal introitus.

Gonorrhea. Vulvar lesions, which usually are confined to Bartholin's glands, may develop along with pruritus, a burning sensation, pain, and a green-yellow vaginal discharge, but most patients are asymptomatic. Other findings include dysuria and urinary incontinence; vaginal redness, swelling, bleeding, and engorgement; and severe pelvic and lower abdominal pain.

Granuloma inguinale. With granuloma inguinale, a single painless macule or papule initially appears on the vulva, ulcerating into a raised, beefy-red lesion with a granulated, friable border. Other painless and possibly foul-smelling lesions may occur on the labia, vagina, or cervix. These become infected and painful, and regional lymph nodes enlarge and may become tender. Systemic effects include fever, weight loss, and malaise.

Recognizing common vulvar lesions

Various disorders can cause vulvar lesions. For example, sexually transmitted diseases account for most vulvar lesions in premenopausal women, whereas vulvar tumors and cysts account for most lesions in women ages 50 to 70. These illustrations will help you recognize some of the most common lesions.

Primary genital herpes produces multiple ulcerated lesions surrounded by red halos.

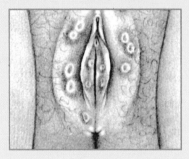

Basal cell carcinoma can produce an ulcerated lesion with raised, poorly rolled edges.

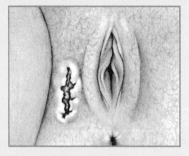

Primary syphilis produces chancres that appear as ulcerated lesions with raised borders.

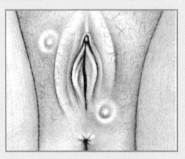

Epidermal inclusion cysts produce a round lump that usually appears on the labia majora.

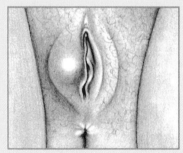

Squamous cell carcinoma can produce a large, granulomatous-appearing ulcer.

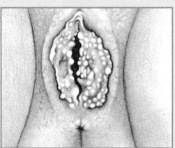

Bartholin's duct cysts produce a tense, nontender, palpable lump that usually appears on the labia minora.

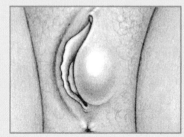

Herpes simplex (genital). With herpes simplex, fluid-filled vesicles appear on the cervix, the vulva, labia, perianal skin, vagina, or mouth. The vesicles, which may initially be painless, may rupture and develop into extensive, shallow, painful ulcers, with redness, marked edema, and tender swollen inguinal lymph nodes. Other findings include fever, malaise, and dysuria. Secondary infections may also occur.

Lymphogranuloma venereum. Lymphogranuloma venereum is a bacterial infection commonly present with a single, painless papule or ulcer on the posterior vulva that heals in a few days. Painful, swollen lymph nodes, usually unilateral, develop 2 to 6 weeks later. Other findings include fever, chills, headache, anorexia, myalgias, arthralgias, weight loss, and perineal edema.

Squamous cell carcinoma. Invasive carcinoma occurs primarily in postmenopausal women and may produce vulvar pruritus, pain, and a vulvar lump. As the tumor enlarges, it may encroach on the vagina, anus, and urethra, causing bleeding, discharge, or dysuria. Carcinoma in situ is most common in premenopausal women, producing a vulvar lesion that may be white or red, raised, well defined, moist, crusted, and isolated.

Squamous cell hyperplasia. Formerly known as *hyperplastic dystrophy,* these vulvar lesions may be well delineated or poorly defined; localized or extensive; and red, brown, white, or both red and white. However, intense pruritus, possibly with vulvar pain, intense burning, and dyspareunia, is the cardinal symptom. With lichen sclerosis, a type of vulvar dystrophy, vulvar skin has a parchmentlike appearance. Fissures may develop between the clitoris and urethra or other vulvar areas.

Syphilis. Chancres, the primary vulvar lesions of syphilis, may appear on the vulva, vagina, or cervix 10 to 90 days after initial contact. Usually painless, they start as papules that then erode, with indurated, raised edges and clear bases. Condylomata lata, highly contagious secondary vulvar lesions, are raised, gray, flat topped, and commonly ulcerated. Other findings include a maculopapular, pustular, or nodular rash; headache; malaise; anorexia; weight loss; fever; nausea; vomiting; generalized lymphadenopathy; and a sore throat.

Viral disease (systemic). Varicella, measles, and other systemic viral diseases may produce vulvar lesions.

Nursing considerations

- Give a systemic antibiotic, antiviral, topical corticosteroid, topical testosterone, or an antipruritic, as ordered.
- Follow standard precautions.

Patient teaching

- Teach the patient comfort measures, such as a sitz bath.
- Discuss safer sex practices with the patient.
- Tell the patient with a sexually transmitted disease that her sexual contacts will also need testing and treatment.
- Explain to the patient the cause of vulvar lesions and its treatment.

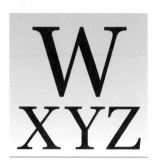

Weight gain, excessive

Weight gain occurs when ingested calories exceed body requirements for energy, causing increased adipose tissue storage. It can also occur when fluid retention causes edema. When weight gain results from overeating, emotional factors—most commonly anxiety, guilt, and depression—and social factors may be the primary causes.

Among elderly people, weight gain commonly reflects a sustained food intake in the presence of a normal, progressive fall in basal metabolic rate. Among women, a progressive weight gain occurs with pregnancy, whereas a periodic weight gain usually occurs with menstruation.

Also a primary sign of many endocrine disorders, weight gain may occur with conditions that limit activity, especially cardiovascular and pulmonary disorders. It can also result from drug therapy that increases appetite or causes fluid retention or from cardiovascular, hepatic, and renal disorders that cause edema.

History and physical examination

Determine your patient's previous patterns of weight gain and loss. Does he have a family history of obesity, thyroid disease, or diabetes mellitus? Assess his eating and activity patterns. Has his appetite increased? Does he exercise regularly or at all? Ask about associated symptoms. Has the patient experienced vision disturbances, hoarseness, paresthesia, or increased urination and thirst? Has he become impotent? If the patient is female, has she had menstrual irregularities or experienced weight gain during menstruation? Is she menopausal or postmenopausal?

Form an impression of the patient's mental status. Is he anxious or depressed? Does he respond slowly? Is his memory poor? What medications is he taking?

During your physical examination, measure skin-fold thickness to estimate fat reserves. (See *Evaluating nutritional status,* pages 644 and 645.) Note fat distribution and the presence of localized or generalized edema and overall nutritional status. Inspect for other abnormalities, such as abnormal body hair distribution or hair loss and dry skin. Take and record the patient's vital signs.

Medical causes

Acromegaly. Acromegaly causes moderate weight gain. Other findings include coarsened facial features, prognathism, enlarged hands and feet, increased sweating, oily skin, deep voice, back and joint pain, lethargy, sleepiness, and heat intolerance. Occasionally, hirsutism may occur.

Diabetes mellitus. The increased appetite associated with diabetes mellitus may lead to weight gain, although weight loss sometimes occurs initially. Other findings include fatigue, polydipsia, polyuria, nocturia, weakness, polyphagia, and somnolence.

Hypercortisolism. Excessive weight gain, usually over the trunk and the back of the neck (buffalo hump), characteristically occurs in hypercortisolism. Other cushingoid features include slender extremities, moon face, weakness, purple striae, emotional lability, and increased susceptibility to infection. Gynecomastia may occur in men; hirsutism, acne, and menstrual irregularities may occur in women.

Hyperinsulinism. Hyperinsulinism increases appetite, leading to weight gain. Emotional lability, indigestion, weakness, diaphoresis, tachycardia, vision disturbances, and syncope also occur.

Hypogonadism. Weight gain is common in hypogonadism. Prepubertal hypogonadism causes eunuchoid body proportions with relatively sparse facial and body hair and a high-pitched voice. Postpubertal hypogonadism causes loss of libido, impotence, and infertility.

Hypothalamic dysfunction. Conditions such as Laurence-Moon-Biedl syndrome cause a voracious appetite with subsequent weight gain, along with altered body temperature and sleep rhythms.

Hypothyroidism. With hypothyroidism, weight gain occurs despite anorexia. Related signs and symptoms include fatigue; cold intolerance; constipation; menorrhagia; slowed intellectual and motor activity; dry, pale, cool skin; dry, sparse hair; and thick, brittle nails. Myalgia, hoarseness, hypoactive deep tendon reflexes, bradycardia, and abdominal distention may occur. Eventually, the face assumes a dull expression with periorbital edema.

Metabolic syndrome. Metabolic syndrome, previously called *syndrome X*, consists of a group of disorders that affect metabolism, including excessive weight gain (usually in the central abdomen), hypertension (blood pressure greater than 135/85 mm Hg), abnormal cholesterol levels (high low-density lipoprotein and triglyceride levels, low high-density lipoprotein level), and high insulin levels.

Nephrotic syndrome. With nephrotic syndrome, weight gain results from edema. In severe cases, anasarca develops—increasing body weight up to 50%. Related effects include abdominal distention, orthostatic hypotension, and lethargy.

Pancreatic islet cell tumor. Pancreatic islet cell tumor causes excessive hunger, which leads to weight gain. Other findings include emotional lability, weakness, malaise, fatigue, restlessness, diaphoresis, palpitations, tachycardia, vision disturbances, and syncope.

Preeclampsia. With preeclampsia, rapid weight gain (exceeding the normal weight gain of pregnancy) may accompany nausea and vomiting, epigastric pain, elevated blood pressure, and blurred or double vision.

Sheehan's syndrome. Most common in women who experience severe obstetric hemorrhage, Sheehan's syndrome may cause weight gain.

Other causes

Drugs. Corticosteroids, phenothiazines, and tricyclic antidepressants cause weight gain from fluid retention and increased appetite. Other drugs that can lead to weight gain include hormonal contraceptives, which cause fluid retention; cyproheptadine, which increases appetite; and lithium, which can induce hypothyroidism.

Nursing considerations

- Refer the patient for psychological counseling, as necessary.
- If the patient is obese or has a cardiopulmonary disorder, monitor exercise closely.
- Perform studies to rule out possible secondary causes should include serum thyroid-stimulating hormone determination and dexamethasone suppression testing.
- Perform laboratory tests for thyroid function and serum cholesterol, triglyceride, and glucose levels.

Patient teaching

- Explain to the patient the cause of weight gain, if known.
- Teach the patient about appropriate dietary choices and discuss an individualized exercise plan.

Weight loss, excessive

Weight loss can reflect decreased food intake, decreased food absorption, increased metabolic requirements, or a combination of the three. Its causes include endocrine, neoplastic, GI, and psychiatric disorders; nutritional deficiencies; infections; and neurologic lesions that cause paralysis and dysphagia. Weight loss may accompany conditions that prevent sufficient food intake, such as painful oral lesions, ill-fitting dentures, and loss of teeth. It may be the metabolic effect of poverty, fad diets, excessive exercise, or certain drugs.

Weight loss may occur as a late sign in such chronic diseases as heart failure and renal disease. In these diseases, however, it's the result of anorexia. (See "Anorexia," page 35.)

Evaluating nutritional status

If your patient exhibits excessive weight loss or gain, you can help assess his nutritional status by measuring his skin-fold thickness and midarm circumference and by calculating his midarm muscle circumference. Skin-fold measurements reflect adipose tissue mass (subcutaneous fat accounts for about 50% of the body's adipose tissue). Midarm measurements reflect both skeletal muscle and adipose tissue mass.

Use the steps described here to gather these measurements and express them as a percentage of standard by using this formula:

$$\frac{\text{Actual measurement}}{\text{Standard measurement}} \times 100 = \underline{\hspace{1cm}} \%$$

Standard anthropometric measurements vary according to the patient's age and gender and can be found in a chart of normal anthropometric values. The abridged chart below lists standard arm measurements for adult men and women.

Test	Standard	
Triceps skin fold	Men	12.5 mm
	Women	16.5 mm
Midarm circumference	Men	29.3 mm
	Women	28.5 mm
Midarm muscle circumference	Men	25.3 mm
	Women	23.2 mm

A triceps or subscapular skin-fold measurement below 60% of the standard value indicates severe depletion of fat reserves; measurement between 60% and 90% indicates moderate to mild depletion; and above 90% indicates significant fat reserves. A midarm circumference of less than 90% of the standard value indicates caloric deprivation; greater than 90% indicates adequate or ample muscle and fat. A midarm muscle circumference of less than 90% indicates protein depletion; greater than 90% indicates adequate or ample protein reserves.

To measure the triceps skin fold, locate the midpoint of the patient's upper arm, using a nonstretch tape measure. Mark the midpoint with a felt-tip pen. Grasp the skin with your thumb and forefinger about 1 cm above the midpoint. Place the calipers at the midpoint and squeeze them for about 3 seconds. Record the measurement registered on the handle gauge to the nearest 0.5 mm. Take two more readings and average all three to compensate for measurement error.

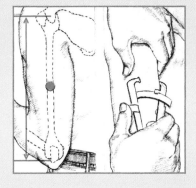

To measure the subscapular skin fold, use your thumb and forefinger to grasp the skin just below the angle of the scapula, in line with the natural cleavage of the skin. Apply the calipers and proceed as you would when measuring the triceps skin fold. Both subscapular and triceps skin-fold measurements are reliable measurements of fat loss or gain during hospitalization.

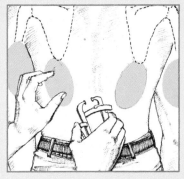

To measure midarm circumference, return to the midpoint you marked on the patient's upper arm and use a tape measure to determine the arm circumference at this point. This measurement reflects both skeletal muscle and adipose tissue mass and helps evaluate protein and calorie reserves. To calculate midarm muscle circumference, multiply the triceps skin-fold thickness (in centimeters) by 3.143 and subtract this figure from the midarm circumference. Midarm muscle circumference reflects muscle mass alone, providing a more sensitive index of protein reserves.

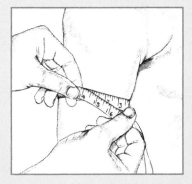

History and physical examination

Begin with a thorough diet history because weight loss is almost always caused by inadequate caloric intake. If the patient hasn't been eating properly, try to determine why. Ask him about previous weight and whether the recent loss was intentional. Determine how long the weight loss has been taking place. Be alert to lifestyle or occupational changes that may be a source of anxiety or depression. Has the patient recently experienced a loss?

Inquire about recent changes in bowel habits, such as diarrhea or bulky, floating stools. Has the patient had nausea, vomiting, or abdominal pain, which may indicate a GI disorder? Has he had excessive thirst, excessive urination, or heat intolerance, which may signal an endocrine disorder? Has he been experiencing other pain? If so, ask about the location of the pain and how long he has had it. Take a careful drug history, noting especially use of diet pills and laxatives.

Carefully check the patient's height and weight and ask about his previous weight. Take his vital signs and note his general appearance: Is he well nourished? Do his clothes fit? Is muscle wasting evident? Ask about exact weight changes (with approximate dates).

Examine the patient's skin for turgor and abnormal pigmentation, especially around the joints. Does he have pallor or jaundice? Examine his mouth, including the condition of his teeth or dentures. Look for signs of infection or irritation on the roof of the mouth and note hyperpigmentation of the buccal mucosa. Check the patient's eyes for exophthalmos and his neck for swelling; evaluate his lungs for adventitious sounds. Inspect his abdomen for signs of wasting, and palpate for masses, tenderness, and an enlarged liver.

Conventional laboratory and radiologic investigations such as complete blood count, serum albumin levels, urinalysis, chest X-ray, and upper GI series usually reveal the cause. Almost all physical causes are clinically evident during the initial evaluation. Cancer, GI disorders, and depression are the most common pathologic causes.

Medical causes

Adrenal insufficiency. Weight loss occurs with adrenal insufficiency, along with anorexia, weakness, fatigue, irritability, syncope, nausea, vomiting, abdominal pain, and diarrhea or constipation. Hyperpigmentation may occur at the joints, belt line, palmar creases, lips, gums, tongue, and buccal mucosa.

Anorexia nervosa. Anorexia nervosa is characterized by a severe, self-imposed weight loss ranging from 10% to 50% of premorbid weight, which typically was normal or not more than 5 lb (2.3 kg) over ideal weight. Related findings include skeletal muscle atrophy, loss of fatty tissue, hypotension, constipation, dental caries, susceptibility to infection, blotchy or sallow skin, cold intolerance, hairiness on the face and body, dryness or loss of scalp hair, and amenorrhea. The patient usually demonstrates restless activity and vigor and may also have a morbid fear of becoming fat. Self-induced vomiting or use of laxatives or diuretics may lead to dehydration or to metabolic alkalosis or acidosis.

Cancer. Weight loss is often a sign of cancer. Other findings reflect the type, location, and stage of the tumor and can include fatigue, pain, nausea, vomiting, anorexia, abnormal bleeding, and a palpable mass.

Crohn's disease. With Crohn's disease, weight loss occurs with chronic cramping, abdominal pain, and anorexia. Other signs and symptoms include diarrhea, nausea, fever, tachycardia, abdominal tenderness and guarding, hyperactive bowel sounds, abdominal distention, and pain. Perianal lesions and a palpable mass in the right or left lower quadrant may also be present.

Cryptosporidiosis. Weight loss may occur with cryptosporidiosis. Other findings include profuse watery diarrhea, abdominal cramping, flatulence, anorexia, malaise, fever, nausea, vomiting, and myalgia.

Depression. Weight loss or weight gain may occur with severe depression, along with insomnia or hypersomnia, anorexia, apathy, fatigue, and feelings of worthlessness. Indecisiveness, incoherence, and suicidal thoughts or behavior may also occur.

Diabetes mellitus. Weight loss may occur with diabetes mellitus, despite increased appetite. Other findings include polydipsia, weakness, fatigue, and polyuria with nocturia.

Esophagitis. Painful inflammation of the esophagus leads to temporary avoidance of eating and subsequent weight loss. Intense pain in the mouth and anterior chest occurs, along with hypersalivation, dysphagia, tachypnea, and hematemesis. If a stricture develops, dysphagia and weight loss will recur.

Gastroenteritis. Malabsorption and dehydration cause weight loss in gastroenteritis. The loss may be sudden in acute viral infections or reactions or gradual in parasitic infection. Other findings include poor skin turgor, dry mucous membranes, tachycardia, hypotension, diarrhea, abdominal pain and tenderness, hyperactive bowel sounds, nausea, vomiting, fever, and malaise.

Leukemia. *Acute leukemia* causes progressive weight loss accompanied by severe prostration; high fever; swollen, bleeding gums; and bleeding tendencies. Dyspnea, tachycardia, palpitations, and abdominal or bone pain may occur. As

the disease progresses, neurologic symptoms may eventually develop.

Chronic leukemia causes progressive weight loss with malaise, fatigue, pallor, enlarged spleen, bleeding tendencies, anemia, skin eruptions, anorexia, and fever.

Lymphoma. Hodgkin's disease and non-Hodgkin's lymphoma cause gradual weight loss. Associated findings include fever, fatigue, night sweats, malaise, hepatosplenomegaly, and lymphadenopathy. Scaly rashes and pruritus may develop.

Pulmonary tuberculosis. Pulmonary tuberculosis causes gradual weight loss, along with fatigue, weakness, anorexia, night sweats, and low-grade fever. Other clinical effects include a cough with bloody or mucopurulent sputum, dyspnea, and pleuritic chest pain. Examination may reveal dullness on percussion, crackles after coughing, increased tactile fremitus, and amphoric breath sounds.

Stomatitis. Inflammation of the oral mucosa (usually red, swollen, and ulcerated) in stomatitis causes weight loss due to decreased eating. Associated findings include fever, increased salivation, malaise, mouth pain, anorexia, and swollen, bleeding gums.

Thyrotoxicosis. With thyrotoxicosis, increased metabolism causes weight loss. Other characteristic signs and symptoms include nervousness, heat intolerance, diarrhea, increased appetite, palpitations, tachycardia, diaphoresis, fine tremor and, possibly, an enlarged thyroid and exophthalmos. A ventricular or atrial gallop may be heard.

Other causes

Drugs. Amphetamines and inappropriate dosage of thyroid preparations commonly lead to weight loss. Laxative abuse may cause a malabsorptive state that leads to weight loss. Chemotherapeutic agents cause stomatitis or nausea and vomiting, which, when severe, causes weight loss.

Nursing considerations

- Take daily calorie counts and weigh the patient weekly.
- Consult a nutritionist to determine an appropriate diet and nutritional supplements with adequate calories.
- Administer hyperalimentation or tube feedings to maintain nutrition, as needed.

Patient teaching

- Provide instruction in proper nutrition and keeping a food diary.
- Instruct the patient in proper oral hygiene.

Wheezing
[Sibilant rhonchi]

Wheezes are adventitious breath sounds with a high-pitched, musical, squealing, creaking, or groaning quality. They're caused by air flowing at a high velocity through a narrowed airway. When they originate in the large airways, they can be heard by placing an unaided ear over the chest wall or at the mouth. When they originate in smaller airways, they can be heard by placing a stethoscope over the anterior or posterior chest. Unlike crackles and rhonchi, wheezes can't be cleared by coughing.

Usually, prolonged wheezing occurs during expiration when bronchi are shortened and narrowed. Causes of airway narrowing include bronchospasm; mucosal thickening or edema; partial obstruction from a tumor, a foreign body, or secretions; and extrinsic pressure, as in tension pneumothorax or goiter. With airway obstruction, wheezing occurs during inspiration.

 Examine the degree of the patient's respiratory distress. Is he responsive? Is he restless, confused, anxious, or afraid? Are his respirations abnormally fast, slow, shallow, or deep? Are they irregular? Can you hear wheezing through his mouth? Does he exhibit increased use of accessory muscles; increased chest wall motion; intercostal, suprasternal, or supraclavicular retractions; stridor; or nasal flaring? Take his other vital signs, noting hypotension or hypertension and decreased oxygen saturation or an irregular, weak, rapid, or slow pulse.

Help the patient relax, administer humidified oxygen by face mask, and encourage him to take slow, deep breaths. Have endotracheal intubation and emergency resuscitation equipment readily available. Provide intermittent positive-pressure breathing and nebulization treatments with bronchodilators, if ordered. Insert an I.V. catheter for administration of drugs, such as diuretics, steroids, bronchodilators, and sedatives. Perform the abdominal thrust maneuver, as indicated, for airway obstruction.

History and physical examination

If the patient isn't in respiratory distress, obtain a history. What provokes his wheezing? Does he have asthma or allergies? Does he smoke or have a history of a pulmonary, cardiac, or circulatory disorder? Does he have cancer? Ask about recent surgery, illness, or trauma or changes in appetite, weight, exercise tolerance, or sleep patterns. Obtain a drug history. Ask about exposure to toxic fumes or respiratory irritants. If he has a cough, ask how it sounds, when it starts, and how often it occurs. Does he have paroxysms of coughing? Is his cough dry, sputum producing, or bloody?

Ask the patient about chest pain. If he reports pain, determine its quality, onset, duration, intensity, and radiation. Does it increase with breathing, coughing, or certain positions?

Examine the patient's nose and mouth for congestion, drainage, or signs of infection, such as halitosis. If he produces sputum, obtain a sample for examination. Check for cyanosis, pallor, clamminess, masses, tenderness, swelling, distended jugular veins, and enlarged lymph nodes. Inspect the patient's chest for abnormal configuration and asymmetrical motion, and determine if the trachea is midline. (See *Detecting slight tracheal deviation,* page 597.) Percuss for dullness or hyperresonance, and auscultate for crackles, rhonchi, or pleural friction rubs. Note absent or hypoactive breath sounds, abnormal heart sounds, gallops, or murmurs. Also note arrhythmias, bradycardia, or tachycardia. (See *Evaluating breath sounds,* pages 650 and 651.)

Medical causes

Anaphylaxis. Anaphylaxis can cause tracheal edema or bronchospasm, resulting in severe wheezing and stridor. Initial signs and symptoms include fright, weakness, sneezing, dyspnea, nasal pruritus, urticaria, erythema, and angioedema. Respiratory distress occurs with nasal flaring, accessory muscle use, and intercostal retractions. Other findings include nasal edema and congestion; profuse, watery rhinorrhea; chest or throat tightness; and dysphagia. Cardiac effects include arrhythmias and hypotension.

Aspiration pneumonitis. With aspiration pneumonitis, wheezing may accompany tachypnea, marked dyspnea, cyanosis, tachycardia, fever, productive (eventually purulent) cough, and pink, frothy sputum.

Asthma. Wheezing is an initial and cardinal sign of asthma. It's heard at the mouth during expiration. An initially dry cough later becomes productive with thick mucus. Other findings include apprehension, prolonged expiration, intercostal and supraclavicular retractions, rhonchi, accessory muscle use, nasal flaring, and tachypnea. Asthma also produces tachycardia, diaphoresis, and flushing or cyanosis.

Blast lung injury. Wheezing is a common symptom of blast lung injury, which is characterized by hypoxia and respiratory difficulty. The forceful blast wave that follows an explosive detonation can cause serious lung injury, including hemorrhage, contusion, edema, and tearing. In addition to wheezing, patients may exhibit chest pain, dyspnea, cyanosis, and hemoptysis. The diagnosis is confirmed by chest X-rays that show a classic "butterfly" pattern.

Bronchial adenoma. Bronchial adenoma produces unilateral, possibly severe wheezing. Common features are chronic cough and recurring hemoptysis. Symptoms of airway obstruction may occur later.

Bronchiectasis. With bronchiectasis, excessive mucus commonly causes intermittent and localized or diffuse wheezing. A copious, foul-smelling, mucopurulent cough is classic. It's accompanied by hemoptysis, rhonchi, and coarse crackles. Weight loss, fatigue, weakness, exertional dyspnea, fever, malaise, halitosis, and late-stage clubbing may also occur.

Bronchitis (chronic). Bronchitis causes wheezing that varies in severity, location, and intensity. Associated findings include prolonged expiration, coarse crackles, scattered rhonchi, and a hacking cough that later becomes productive. Other effects include dyspnea, accessory muscle use, barrel chest, tachy-

Evaluating breath sounds

Diminished or absent breath sounds indicate some interference with airflow. If pus, fluid, or air fills the pleural space, breath sounds will be quieter than normal. If a foreign body or secretions obstruct a bronchus, breath sounds will be diminished or absent over distal lung tissue. Increased thickness of the chest wall, such as with a patient who's obese or extremely muscular, may cause breath sounds to be decreased, distant, or inaudible. Absent breath sounds typically indicate loss of ventilation power.

When air passes through narrowed airways or through moisture, or when the membranes lining the chest cavity become inflamed, adventitious breath sounds will be heard. These include crackles, rhonchi, wheezes, and pleural friction rubs. Usually these sounds indicate pulmonary disease.

Follow the auscultation sequences shown in the illustrations here to assess the patient's breath sounds. Have the patient take full, deep breaths, and compare sound variations from one side to the other. Note the location, timing, and character of any abnormal breath sounds.

Posterior

pnea, clubbing, edema, weight gain, and cyanosis.

Bronchogenic carcinoma. Obstruction from bronchogenic carcinoma may cause localized wheezing. Typical findings include a productive cough, dyspnea, hemoptysis (initially blood-tinged sputum, possibly leading to massive hemorrhage), anorexia, and weight loss. Upper extremity edema and chest pain may also occur.

Emphysema. Mild to moderate wheezing may occur with emphysema. Related findings include dyspnea, tachypnea, diminished breath sounds, pe-

ripheral cyanosis, pursed-lip breathing, anorexia, and malaise. Accessory muscle use, barrel chest, a chronic productive cough, and clubbing may also occur.

Pulmonary coccidioidomycosis. Pulmonary coccidioidomycosis may cause wheezing and rhonchi along with cough, fever, chills, pleuritic chest pain, headache, weakness, malaise, anorexia, and macular rash.

Pulmonary edema. Wheezing may occur with pulmonary edema, a life-threatening disorder. Other signs and symptoms include coughing, exertional and paroxysmal nocturnal dyspnea and,

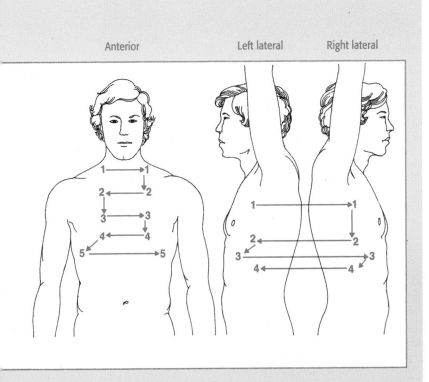

Anterior　　　Left lateral　　　Right lateral

later, orthopnea. Examination reveals tachycardia, tachypnea, dependent crackles, and a diastolic gallop. Severe pulmonary edema produces rapid, labored respirations; diffuse crackles; a productive cough with frothy, bloody sputum; arrhythmias; cold, clammy, cyanotic skin; hypotension; and thready pulse.

Respiratory syncytial virus (RSV). Individuals infected with RSV commonly develop wheezing and other symptoms within 4 to 6 days of exposure to this virus. Healthy adults and children older than age 3 usually have mild cases of RSV and experience wheezing along with other common cold-like symptoms of runny nose, cough, and low-grade fever. In children ages 3 and younger, high-pitched expiratory wheezing can accompany a severe cough, rapid breathing, and high-grade fever.

Tracheobronchitis. With tracheobronchitis, auscultation may detect wheezing, rhonchi, and crackles. The patient also has a cough, slight fever, sudden chills, muscle and back pain, and substernal tightness.

Wegener's granulomatosis. Wegener's granulomatosis may cause mild to moderate wheezing if it compresses major airways. Other findings include a cough (possibly bloody), dyspnea, pleuritic chest pain, hemorrhagic skin lesions, and progressive renal failure. Epistaxis and severe sinusitis are common.

Other causes

Foreign body aspiration. Partial obstruction by a foreign body produces sudden onset of wheezing and possibly stridor; a dry, paroxysmal cough; gagging; and hoarseness. Other findings include tachycardia, dyspnea, decreased breath sounds and, possibly, cyanosis. A retained foreign body may cause inflammation leading to fever, pain, and swelling.

Nursing considerations

- Prepare the patient for diagnostic tests, such as chest X-rays, arterial blood gas analysis, pulmonary function tests, and sputum culture.
- Ease the patient's breathing by placing him in a semi-Fowler's position.
- Perform pulmonary physiotherapy as necessary.
- Administer an antibiotic, bronchodilator, steroid, and mucolytic or expectorant, as ordered.
- Provide humidification to thin secretions.

Patient teaching

- Explain to the patient the underlying cause of wheezing and its treatment.
- Teach the patient how to promote drainage and prevent pooling of secretions.
- Explain deep-breathing and coughing techniques.
- Explain the importance of increasing fluid intake, if appropriate.
- Teach the patient how to take prescribed drugs correctly.

Web resources

Al-Anon (for friends and family
members of alcoholics)
www.al-anon.alateen.org

Alcoholics Anonymous World Services
www.alcoholics-anonymous.org

Alzheimer's Association
www.alz.org

American Academy of Allergy, Asthma
and Immunology
www.aaaai.org

American Academy of Ophthalmology
www.eyenet.org

American Cancer Society
www.cancer.org

American Chronic Pain Association
www.theacpa.org

American Diabetes Association
www.diabetes.org

American Foundation for AIDS Research
www.amfar.org

American Foundation for Urologic
Disease
www.afud.org

American Heart Association
www.americanheart.org

American Kidney Fund
www.kidneyfund.org

American Liver Foundation
www.liverfoundation.org

American Pain Society
www.ampainsoc.org

American Parkinson Disease Association
www.apdaparkinson.com

Amyotrophic Lateral Sclerosis
Association
www.alsa.org

Arthritis Foundation
www.arthritis.org

Arthritis National Research Foundation
www.curearthritis.org

Asthma and Allergy Foundation of
America
www.aafa.org

Carpal Tunnel Syndrome
www.ctsplace.com

Centers for Disease Control and
Prevention
www.cdc.gov

Crohn's and Colitis Foundation of
America
www.ccfa.org

Cystic Fibrosis Foundation
www.cff.org

Epilepsy Foundation of America
www.efa.org

Glaucoma Research Foundation
www.glaucoma.org

Heartlife
www.heartlife.com

Leukemia & Lymphoma Society
www.leukemia.org

Lupus Foundation of America
www.lupus.org

Muscular Dystrophy Association
www.mdausa.org

Myasthenia Gravis Foundation
www.myasthenia.org

National Cancer Institute
www.cancer.gov

National Coalition for Cancer
Survivorship
www.canceradvocacy.org

National Headache Foundation
www.headaches.org

National Hemophilia Foundation (NHF)
www.hemophilia.org

National Hospice and Palliative Care
Organization
www.nhpco.org

National Institute of Neurological
Disorders and Stroke
www.ninds.nih.gov

National Kidney Foundation
www.kidney.org

National Multiple Sclerosis Society
www.nationalmssociety.org

National Osteoporosis Foundation
www.nof.org

National Parkinson Foundation
www.parkinson.org

National Psoriasis Foundation
www.psoriasis.org

National Stroke Association
www.stroke.org

Scleroderma Foundation
www.scleroderma.org

Skin Cancer Foundation
www.skincancer.org

Selected references

Anatomy & Physiology Made Incredibly Easy. Philadelphia: Lippincott Williams & Wilkins, 2005.

Baranoski, S., and Ayello, E.A. *Wound Care Essentials: Practice Principles.* Philadelphia: Lippincott Williams & Wilkins, 2004.

Beers, M., et al. *The Merck Manual of Diagnosis and Therapy,* 18th ed. Hoboken, N.J.: John Wiley & Sons, 2006.

Bender, K., and Thompson, F. E., Jr. "West Nile Virus: A Growing Challenge," *AJN* 103(6):32-40, June 2003.

Bickley, L., and Szilagyi, P. *Bates' Guide to Physical Examination and History Taking.* 9th ed. Philadelphia: Lippincott Williams & Wilkins, 2007.

Craven, R., and Hirnle, C. *Fundamentals of Nursing Human Health and Function,* 5th ed. Philadelphia: Lippincott Williams & Wilkins, 2007.

D'Amico, D., and Barbito, C. *Health & Physical Assessment in Nursing.* Upper Saddle River, N.J.: Prentice Hall Health, 2006.

ECG Interpretation Made Incredibly Easy, 3rd ed. Philadelphia: Lippincott Williams & Wilkins, 2005.

Ferri, F. *Ferri's Clinical Advisor: Instant Diagnosis and Treatment.* St. Louis: Mosby–Year Book, Inc., 2004.

Handbook of Signs & Symptoms. Philadelphia: Lippincott Williams & Wilkins, 2005.

Hickey, J. *The Clinical Practice of Neurological and Neurosurgical Nursing,* 5th ed. Philadelphia: Lippincott Williams & Wilkins, 2003.

Kasper, D.L., et al., eds. *Harrison's Principles of Internal Medicine,* 16th ed. New York: McGraw-Hill Book Co., 2005.

Kozier, B., et al. *Fundamentals of Nursing Concepts, Process, and Practice,* 7th ed. Upper Saddle River, N.J.: Prentice Hall Health, 2004.

Legg, V. "Complications of Chronic Kidney Disease," *AJN* 105(6):40-49, June 2005.

Nurse's Quick Check, Diseases. Philadelphia: Lippincott Williams & Wilkins, 2005.

Nurse's Quick Check, Signs & Symptoms. Philadelphia: Lippincott Williams & Wilkins, 2006.

Nursing2007 Drug Handbook, 27th ed. Philadelphia: Lippincott Williams & Wilkins, 2007.

Nutrition Made Incredibly Easy, 2nd ed. Philadelphia: Lippincott Williams & Wilkins, 2007.

Porth, C.M. *Pathophysiology Concepts of Altered Health States,* 7th ed. Philadelphia: Lippincott Williams & Wilkins, 2005.

Rubin, E. *Rubin's Pathophysiology: Clinicopathologic Foundations of Medicine,* 4th ed. Philadelphia: Lippincott Williams & Wilkins, 2005.

Shives, L. *Basic Concepts of Psychiatric-Mental Health Nursing,* 6th ed. Philadelphia: Lippincott Williams & Wilkins, 2005.

Smeltzer, S.C., and Bare, B.G. *Brunner and Suddarth's Textbook of Medical-Surgical Nursing,* 10th ed. Philadelphia: Lippincott Williams & Wilkins, 2004.

Tierney, L., et al. *Current Medical Diagnosis and Treatment*, 45th ed. New York: McGraw-Hill Book Co., 2006.

Waldman, S. *Physical Diagnosis of Pain: An Atlas of Signs and Symptoms.* Philadelphia: Elsevier, 2006.

Woods, S.L., et al. *Cardiac Nursing,* 5th ed. Philadelphia: Lippincott Williams & Wilkins, 2005.

Index

---

i refers to an illustration; t refers to a table.

---

i refers to an illustration; t refers to a table.

i refers to an illustration; t refers to a table.

i refers to an illustration; t refers to a table.

i refers to an illustration; t refers to a table.

i refers to an illustration; t refers to a table.